EDITOR

Judith A. Barberio, PhD, APN,C, ANP, FNP, GNP
Assistant Professor
Rutgers, The State University of New Jersey
College of Nursing
Newark, New Jersey

CONSULTING EDITOR

Leonard G. Gomella, MD, FACS
The Bernard W. Godwin, Jr., Professor
Chairman, Department of Urology
Jefferson Medical College
Thomas Jefferson University
Philadelphia, Pennsylvania

ASSOCIATE EDITORS

Steven A. Haist, MD, MS, FACP
Professor of Medicine
Division of General Medicine
Department of Internal Medicine
University of Kentucky Medical Center
Lexington, Kentucky

Aimee Gelhot Adams, PharmD
Director, Primary Care Pharmacy Practice Residency
University of Kentucky Medical Center
Assistant Professor
College of Pharmacy and Department of Medicine
University of Kentucky
Lexington, Kentucky

Kelly M. Smith, PharmD
Associate Professor
Division of Pharmacy Practice and Science
University of Kentucky College of Pharmacy
Director, Drug Information Center
University of Kentucky Medical Center
Lexington, Kentucky

PREFACE

WE ARE PLEASED to present the fourth edition of the *Nurse's Pocket Drug Guide*. Our goal is to identify the most frequently used and clinically important medications based on input from our readers and editorial board. The book includes over 1000 generic medications and is designed to represent a cross section of those used in health care practices across the country.

The style of drug presentation includes key "must know" facts of commonly used medications and herbs, essential information for the student, practicing nurse, and health care provider. A unique feature is the inclusion of common uses of medications and herbs rather than just the official labeled indications. These recommendations are based on the actual uses of the medication and herbs supported by publications and community standards of care. All uses have been reviewed by our editorial board.

It is essential that students, registered nurses, and advanced-practice nurses learn more than the name and dose of the medications they prescribe. Certain common side effects and significant contraindications are associated with most prescription medications. Although nurses and other health care practitioners should ideally be completely familiar with the entire package insert of any medication prescribed, such a requirement is unreasonable. References such as the *Physician's Desk Reference* and the drug manufacturer's Web site make package inserts readily available for many medications, but may not highlight clinically significant facts or provide key data for generic drugs and those available over the counter.

The limitations of difficult-to-read package inserts were acknowledged by the Food and Drug Administration in early 2001, when it noted that health care providers do not have time to read the many pages of small print in the typical package insert. In the future, package inserts will likely be redesigned to ensure that important drug interactions, contraindications, and common side effects are highlighted for easier practitioner reference. The editorial board has analyzed the information on both brand and generic medications and has made this key prescribing information available in this pocket-sized book. Information in this book is meant for use by health care professionals who are familiar with these commonly prescribed medications.

This 2008 edition has been completely reviewed and updated by our editorial board. Over 50 new drugs and herbs have been added, and changes in other medications based on FDA actions have been incorporated. New to this edition are the therapeutic and pharmacologic classifications for each drug and a section on commonly used vitamin combinations.

We express special thanks to our families for their long-term support of this book. The contributions of the members of the editorial board are deeply appreciated. The assistance of Quincy McDonald, and the team at McGraw-Hill are also to be thanked for their support in our goal of creating a pocket drug guide for nursing professionals.

Your comments and suggestions are always welcome and encouraged because improvements to this book would be impossible without the interest and feedback of our readers. We hope this book will help you learn some of the key elements in prescribing medications and allow you to care for your patients in the best way possible.

Judith A. Barberio, PhD, APN,C, ANP, FNP, GNP
Newark, New Jersey
JABPHD83@aol.com

Leonard G. Gomella, MD, FACS
Philadelphia, PA
Leonard.Gomella@jefferson.edu

MEDICATION KEY

Medications are listed by prescribing class, and the individual medications are then listed in alphabetical order by generic name. Some of the more commonly recognized trade names are listed for each medication (in parentheses after the generic name).

Generic Drug Name (Selected Common Brand Names [Controlled Substance]) WARNING: Summarized version of the "Black Box" precautions deemed necessary by the FDA. These are significant precautions and contraindications concerning the individual medication. **Therapeutic and/or Pharmacologic Class:** Class is presented in brackets immediately following the brand name drug. The therapeutic drug class appears first and describes the disease state that the drug treats. The pharmacologic drug class follows and is based on the drug's mechanism of action. **Uses:** This includes both FDA labeled indications bracketed by * and other "off label" uses of the medication. Because many medications are used to treat various conditions based on the medical literature and not listed in their package insert, we list common uses of the medication rather than the official "labeled indications" (FDA approved) based on input from our editorial board **Action:** How the drug works. This information is helpful in comparing classes of drugs and understanding side effects and contraindications. *Spectrum:* Specifies activity against selected microbes **Dose:** *Adults.* Where no specific pediatric dose is given, the implication is that this drug is not commonly used or indicated in that age group. At the end of the dosing line, important dosing modifications may be noted (ie, take with food, avoid antacids, etc) **Caution:** [pregnancy/fetal risk categories, breast-feeding (as noted above)] cautions concerning the use of the drug in specific settings **Contra:** Contraindications **Disp:** Common dosing forms **SE:** Common or significant side effects **Notes:** Other key information about the drug **Interactions:** Common drug—drug, drug—herb, and drug—food interactions that may change the drug response **Labs:** Common laboratory test results that are changed by the drug or significant lab monitoring requirements **NIPE:** Nursing Indications and/or Patient Education) Significant information that the nurse must be aware of with administration of the drug or information that should be given to any patient taking the drug.

CONTROLLED SUBSTANCE CLASSIFICATION

Medications under the control of the US Drug Enforcement Agency (Schedule I–V controlled substances) are indicated by the symbol [C]. Most medications are "uncontrolled" and do not require a DEA prescriber number on the prescription. The following is a general description for the schedules of DEA controlled substances:

Schedule (C-I) I: All nonresearch use forbidden (eg, heroin, LSD, mescaline, etc).

Schedule (C-II) II: High addictive potential; medical use accepted. No telephone call-in prescriptions; no refills. Some states require special prescription form (eg, cocaine, morphine, methadone).

Schedule (C-III) III: Low to moderate risk of physical dependence, high risk of psychologic dependence; prescription must be rewritten after 6 months or five refills (eg, acetaminophen plus codeine).

Schedule (C-IV) IV: Limited potential for dependence; prescription rules same as for schedule III (eg, benzodiazepines, propoxyphene).

Schedule (C-V) V: Very limited abuse potential; prescribing regulations often same as for uncontrolled medications; some states have additional restrictions.

FDA FETAL RISK CATEGORIES

Category A: Adequate studies in pregnant women have not demonstrated a risk to the fetus in the first trimester of pregnancy; there is no evidence of risk in the last two trimesters.

Category B: Animal studies have not demonstrated a risk to the fetus, but no adequate studies have been done in pregnant women.

or

Animal studies have shown an adverse effect, but adequate studies in pregnant women have not demonstrated a risk to the fetus during the first trimester of pregnancy and there is no evidence of risk in the last two trimesters.

Category C: Animal studies have shown an adverse effect on the fetus, but no adequate studies have been done in humans. The benefits from the use of the drug in pregnant women may be acceptable despite its potential risks.

or

No animal reproduction studies and no adequate studies in humans have been done.

Category D: There is evidence of human fetal risk, but the potential benefits from the use of the drug in pregnant women may be acceptable despite its potential risks.

Category X: Studies in animals or humans or adverse reaction reports, or both, have demonstrated fetal abnormalities. The risk of use in pregnant women clearly outweighs any possible benefit.

Category ?: No data available (not a formal FDA classification; included to provide complete data set).

BREAST-FEEDING

No formally recognized classification exists for drugs and breast-feeding. This shorthand was developed for the Nurse's *Pocket Drug Guide*.

+   Compatible with breast-feeding
M   Monitor patient or use with caution
±   Excreted, or likely excreted, with unknown effects or at unknown concentrations
?/–   Unknown excretion, but effects likely to be of concern
–   Contraindicated in breast-feeding
?   No data available

ABBREVIATIONS

Ab: Antibody
ABMT: autologous bone marrow transplantation
Ac: before meals
ACE: angiotensin-converting enzyme
ACEI: angiotensin-converting enzyme inhibitor
ACLS: advanced cardiac life support
ACS: acute coronary syndrome, American Cancer Society, American College of Surgeons
ADH: antidiuretic hormone
ADHD: attention-deficit hyperactivity disorder
ADR: adverse drug reaction
AF: atrial fibrillation
Al: aluminum
ALL: acute lymphocytic leukemia
ALT: alanine aminotransferase
AMI: acute myocardial infarction
AML: acute myelogenous leukemia
amp: ampule
ANC: absolute neutrophil count
APAP: acetaminophen [N-acetyl-p-aminophenol]
aPTT: activated partial thromboplastin time
ARB: angiotensin II receptor blocker
ARDS: adult respiratory distress syndrome
ASA: aspirin (acetylsalicylic acid)
AUC: area under the curve

AV: atrioventricular
AVM: arteriovenous malformation
BCL: B-cell lymphoma
BM: bone marrow; bowel movement
BMT: bone marrow transplantation
BOO: bladder outlet obstruction
BP: blood pressure
BSA: body surface area
BUN: blood urea nitrogen
Ca: calcium
CA: cancer
CAD: coronary artery disease
CAP: cancer of the prostate
CBC: complete blood count
CCB: calcium channel blocker
CF: cystic fibrosis
CHF: congestive heart failure
CLA: Cis-linoleic acid
CLL: chronic lymphocytic leukemia
CML: chronic myelogenous leukemia
CMV: cytomegalovirus
CNS: central nervous system
COMT: catechol-O-methyltransferase
Contra: contraindicated
COPD: chronic obstructive pulmonary disease
CP: chest pain
CPK: creatine phosphokinase
CPP: central precocious puberty
CR: controlled release
CrCl: creatinine clearance
CRF: chronic renal failure

CV: cardiovascular

CVA: cerebrovascular accident, costovertebral angle

CVH: common variable hypergammaglobulinemia

D: diarrhea

D/C: discontinue

D_5LR: 5% dextrose in lactated Ringer's solution

D_5NS: 5% dextrose in normal saline

D_5W: 5% dextrose in water

DI: diabetes insipidus

Disp: dispensed as, how the drug is supplied

DKA: diabetic ketoacidosis

dL: deciliter

DM: diabetes mellitus

DMARD (Disease-modifying antirheumatic drug)drugs defined in randomized trials to decrease erosions and joint space narrowing in rheumatoid arthritis (eg, D-penicillamine, methotrexate, azathioprine0

DN: diabetic nephropathy

DOT: directly observed therapy

dppr: dropper

d/t: due to

DVT: deep venous thrombosis

Dz: disease

EC: enteric-coated

ECC: emergency cardiac care

ECG: electrocardiogram

ED: erectile dysfunction

EGFR: epidermal growth factor receptor

ELISA: enzyme-linked immunosorbent assay

EMIT: enzyme-multiplied immunoassay text

EPS: extrapyramidal symptoms (tardive dyskinesia, tremors and rigidity, restlessness [akathisia], muscle contractions [dystonia], changes in breathing and heart rate)

ER: extended release

ESRD: end-stage renal disease

ET: endotracheal

EtOH: ethanol

FSH: follicle-stimulating hormone

5-FU: fluorouracil

Fxn: function

g: gram

GABA: gamma-aminobutyric acid

G-CSF: granulocyte colony-stimulating factor

gen: generation

GERD: gastroesophageal reflux disease

GF: growth factor

GFR: glomerular filtration rate

GH: growth hormone

GI: gastrointestinal

GIST: Gastrointestinal stromal tumor

GLA: Gamma-linoleic Acid

GM-CSF: granulocyte-macrophage colony-stimulating factor

GnRH: gonadotropin-releasing hormone

gt, gtt: drop, drops (*gutta*)

GTT: Glucose Tolerance Test

HA: headache

HCG human chorionic gonadotropin

HCL: hairy cell leukemia

Hct: hematocrit

HCTZ: hydrochlorothiazide

HD: hemodialysis

HF: heart failure

Hgb: hemoglobin

HIT: heparin-induced thrombocytopenia

HIV: human immunodeficiency virus

HMG-CoA: hydroxymethylglutaryl coenzyme A

h/o: history of

hs: at bedtime (*hora somni*)

HSV: herpes simplex virus

5-HT: 5-hydroxytryptamine

HTN: hypertension

Hx: history of

I: iodine

IBD: irritable bowel disease

IBS: irritable bowel syndrome

ICP: intracranial pressure

IFIS: Intraoperative Floppy Iris Syndrome

Ig: immunoglobulin

IM: intramuscular

Inf: infusion

Infxn: infection

Inh: inhalation

INH: isoniazid

INR: international normalized ratio

Insuff: insufficiency

intravag: intravaginal

I&O: intake & output

IOP: intraocular pressure

ISA: intrinsic sympathomimetic activity

IT: intrathecal

ITP: idiopathic thrombocytopenic purpura

IV: intravenous

K: potassium

L/d: liters per day

LDL: low-density lipoprotein

LFT: liver function test

LH: luteinizing hormone

LHRH: luteinizing hormone-releasing hormone

Li: lithium

Liq: liquid

LMW: low molecular weight

LVD: left ventricular dysfunction

LVEF: left ventricular ejection fraction

LVSD: left ventricular systolic dysfunction

MAC: *Mycobacterium avium* complex

MAO/MAOI: monoamine oxidase/inhibitor

mEq: milliequivalent

Mg: magnesium

MI: myocardial infarction, mitral insufficiency

mL: milliliter

MoAb: monoclonal antibody

MRSA: methicillin-resistant *Staphylococcus aureus*

MS: multiple sclerosis

MSSA: methicillin-sensitive *Staphylococcus aureus*

MTT: monotetrazolium

MTX: methotrexate

MyG: myasthenia gravis

N: nausea

na: sodium

NA: narrow angle

NAG: narrow angle glaucoma

ng: nanogram

NG: nasogastric

NHL: non-Hodgkin's lymphoma

NIDDM: non-insulin-dependent diabetes mellitus

nl: normal

NMDA: N-Methyl-D-Aspartate

NNRTI: nonnucleoside reverse transcriptase inhibitor

NO: nitric oxide

NPO: nothing by mouth (*nil per os*)

NRTI: nucleoside reverse transcriptase inhibitor

NS: normal saline

NSAID: nonsteroidal antiinflammatory drug

NSCLC: non-small-cell lung cancer

N/V: nausea and vomiting

N/V/D: nausea, vomiting, diarrhea

OAB: overactive bladder

OCP: oral contraceptive pill

OD: overdose

ODT: orally disintegrating tablets

OK: recommended

OTC: over the counter

P: phosphorus

PABA: para-amino benzoic acid

PAT: paroxysmal atrial tachycardia

pc: after eating (*post cibum*)

PCN: penicillin

PCP: *Pneumocystis jiroveci* (formerly *carinii*) pneumonia

PCWP: pulmonary capillary wedge pressure

PDE5: phosphodiesterase type 5

PDGF: platelet-derived growth factor

PE: pulmonary embolus, physical examination, pleural effusion

PFT: pulmonary function test

pg: picogram

PID: pelvic inflammatory disease

plt: platelet

PMDD: premenstrual dysphoric disorder

PO: by mouth (*per os*)

PPD: purified protein derivative

PR: by rectum

Prep: preparation

PRG: pregnancy

PRN: as often as needed (*pro re nata*)

PSVT: paroxysmal supraventricular tachycardia

pt: patient

PT: prothrombin time

PTCA: percutaneous transluminal coronary angioplasty

PTH: parathyroid hormone

PTT: partial thromboplastin time

PUD: peptic ulcer disease

PVC: premature ventricular contraction

PVD: peripheral vascular disease

PWP: pulmonary wedge pressure

Px: prevention

q: every (*quaque*)

q_h: every _ hours

qd: every day

qh: every hour

qhs: every hour of sleep (before bedtime)

qid: four times a day (*quater in die*)

qod: every other day

RA: rheumatoid arthritis

RCC: renal cell carcinoma

RDA: recommended dietary allowance

RDS: respiratory distress syndrome

resp: respiratory

RSV: respiratory syncytial virus

RT: reverse transcriptase

RTA: renal tubular acidosis

Rx: prescription or therapy

Rxn: reaction

SCr: serum creatinine

SDV: Single Dose Vial

SIADH: syndrome of inappropriate antidiuretic hormone

SL: sublingual

SLE: systemic lupus erythematosus

soln: solution

SPAG: small particle aerosol generator

Sp: species

SQ: subcutaneous

SR: sustained release

SSRI: selective serotonin reuptake inhibitor

SSS: sick sinus syndrome

S/Sys: signs & symptoms

stat: immediately (*statim*)

supl: supplement
supp: suppository
SVT: supraventricular tachycardia
Sx: symptom
Sz: seizure
tab/tabs: tablet/tablets
TB: tuberculosis
TCA: tricyclic antidepressant
TFT: thyroid function test
TIA: transient ischemic attack
tid: three times a day (*ter in die*)
tinc: tincture
TMP: trimethoprim
TMP–SMX:
  trimethoprim–sulfamethoxazole
TNF: tumor necrosis factor
tox: toxicity
TPA: tissue plasminogen activator
tri: trimester
TSH thyroid stimulating hormone
Tsp: teaspoon
TTP: thrombotic thrombocytopenic
  purpura
TTS: transdermal therapeutic
  system
Tx: treatment

uln: upper limits of normal
UPA pyrrolizidine alkaloids
URI: upper respiratory infection
UTI: urinary tract infection
Vag: vaginal
VF: ventricular fibrillation
VRE: vancomycin-resistant
  Enterococcus
VT: ventricular tachycardia
W/: with
WHI: Women's Health Initiative
W/in: within
Wk: week
WNL: within normal limits
w/o: without
WPW: Wolff–Parkinson–White
  syndrome
Wt: weight
XR: extended release
ZE: Zollinger—Ellison (syndrome)
>: greater than; older than
↑: increase
↓: decrease
∅: not recommended; do not take
÷/%: divided dose

CLASSIFICATION (Generic and common brand names)

ALLERGY

Antihistamines

Azelastine (Astelin, Optivar)
Cetirizine (Zyrtec, Zyrtec D)
Chlorpheniramine (Chlor-Trimeton)
Clemastine Fumarate (Tavist)
Cyproheptadine (Periactin)
Desloratadine (Clarinex)
Diphenhydramine (Benadryl)
Fexofenadine (Allegra)
Hydroxyzine (Atarax, Vistaril)
Loratadine (Claritin, Alavert)

Miscellaneous Antiallergy Agents

Budesonide (Rhinocort, Pulmicort)
Cromolyn Sodium (Intal, NasalCrom, Opticrom)
Montelukast (Singulair)

ANTIDOTES

Acetylcysteine (Aceta-dote, Mucomyst)
Amifostine (Ethyol)
Charcoal (Superchar, Actidose, Liqui-Char Activated)
Deferasirox (Exjade)
Dexrazoxane (Zinecard)
Digoxin Immune Fab (Digibind)
Flumazenil (Romazicon)
Ipecac Syrup (OTC Syrup)
Mesna (Mesnex)
Naloxone (Narcan)
Physostigmine (Antilirium)
Succimer (Chemet)

ANTIMICROBIAL AGENTS

Antibiotics

AMINOGLYCOSIDES
Amikacin (Amikin)
Gentamicin (Garamycin, G-Mycitin)
Neomycin
Streptomycin
Tobramycin (Nebcin)

CARBAPENEMS
Ertapenem (Invanz)
Imipenem–Cilastatin (Primaxin)
Meropenem (Merrem)

1

CEPHALOSPORINS, FIRST GENERATION

Cefadroxil (Duricef, Ultracef)

Cefazolin (Ancef, Kefzol)

Cephalexin (Keflex, Keftab)

Cephradine (Velosef)

CEPHALOSPORINS, SECOND GENERATION

Cefaclor (Ceclor)

Cefmetazole (Zefazone)

Cefonicid (Monocid)

Cefotetan (Cefotan)

Cefoxitin (Mefoxin)

Cefprozil (Cefzil)

Cefuroxime (Ceftin [oral], Zinacef [parenteral])

Loracarbef (Lorabid)

CEPHALOSPORINS, THIRD GENERATION

Cefdinir (Omnicef)

Cefditoren (Spectracef)

Cefixime (Suprax)

Cefoperazone (Cefobid)

Cefotaxime (Claforan)

Cefpodoxime (Vantin)

Ceftazidime (Fortaz, Ceptaz, Tazidime, Tazicef)

Ceftibuten (Cedax)

Ceftizoxime (Cefizox)

Ceftriaxone (Rocephin)

CEPHALOSPORINS, FOURTH GENERATION

Cefepime (Maxipime)

FLUOROQUINOLONES

Ciprofloxacin (Cipro)

Gatifloxacin (Tequin)

Gemifloxacin (Factive)

Levofloxacin (Levaquin, Quixin Ophthalmic)

Lomefloxacin (Maxaquin)

Moxifloxacin (Avelox)

Norfloxacin (Noroxin, Chibroxin Ophthalmic)

Ofloxacin (Floxin, Ocuflox Ophthalmic)

Sparfloxacin (Zagam)

Trovafloxacin (Trovan)

MACROLIDES

Azithromycin (Zithromax)

Clarithromycin (Biaxin)

Dirithromycin (Dynabac)

Erythromycin (E-Mycin, E.E.S., Ery-Tab)

Erythromycin & Sulfisoxazole (Eryzole, Pediazole)

KETOLIDE

Telithromycin (Ketek)

PENICILLINS

Amoxicillin (Amoxil, Polymox)

Amoxicillin & Clavulanic Acid (Augmentin)

Ampicillin (Amcill, Omnipen)

Ampicillin–Sulbactam (Unasyn)

Dicloxacillin (Dynapen, Dycill)

Mezlocillin (Mezlin)

Nafcillin (Nallpen)

Oxacillin (Bactocill, Prostaphlin)

Penicillin G, Aqueous (Potassium or Sodium) (Pfizerpen, Pentids)

Penicillin G Benzathine (Bicillin)
Penicillin G Procaine (Wycillin)

Penicillin V (Pen-Vee K, Veetids)
Piperacillin (Pipracil)
Piperacillin–Tazobactam (Zosyn)

Ticarcillin (Ticar)
Ticarcillin/Potassium Clavulanate (Timentin)

TETRACYCLINES

Doxycycline (Vibramycin)

Tetracycline (Achromycin V, Sumycin)

Tigecycline (Tygacil)

Miscellaneous Antibiotic Agents

Aztreonam (Azactam)
Clindamycin (Cleocin, Cleocin-T)
Fosfomycin (Monurol)
Linezolid (Zyvox)
Metronidazole (Flagyl, MetroGel)

Quinupristin–Dalfopristin (Synercid)
Rifaximin (Xifaxan)
Trimethoprim–Sulfamethoxazole [Co-Trimoxazole] (Bactrim, Septra)

Vancomycin (Vancocin, Vancoled)

Antifungals

Amphotericin B (Fungizone)
Amphotericin B Cholesteryl (Amphotec)
Amphotericin B Lipid Complex (Abelcet)
Amphotericin B Liposomal (AmBisome)
Anidulafungin (Eraxis)

Caspofungin (Cancidas)
Clotrimazole (Lotrimin, Mycelex)
Clotrimazole & Betamethasone (Lotrisone)
Econazole (Spectazole)
Fluconazole (Diflucan)
Itraconazole (Sporanox)
Ketoconazole (Nizoral)

Miconazole (Monistat)
Nystatin (Mycostatin)
Oxiconazole (Oxistat)
Posaconazole (Noxafil)
Sertaconazole (Ertaczo)
Terbinafine (Lamisil)
Triamcinolone & Nystatin (Mycolog-II)
Voriconazole (VFEND)

Antimycobacterials

Clofazimine (Lamprene)
Dapsone (Avlosulfon)
Ethambutol (Myambutol)

Isoniazid (INH)
Pyrazinamide
Rifabutin (Mycobutin)

Rifampin (Rifadin)
Rifapentine (Priftin)
Streptomycin

Antiprotozoals

Nitazoxanide (Alinia)

Tinidazole (Tindamax)

Antiretrovirals

Abacavir (Ziagen)
Amprenavir (Agenerase)

Delavirdine (Rescriptor)
Didanosine [ddI] (Videx)

Efavirenz (Sustiva)

Efavirenz, 600 mg, Emtricitabine, 200 mg, Tenofovir Disoproxil Fumarate, 300 mg (Atripla)
Fosamprenavir (Lexiva)
Indinavir (Crixivan)
Lamivudine (Epivir, Epivir-HBV)

Lopinavir/Ritonavir (Kaletra)
Nelfinavir (Viracept)
Nevirapine (Viramune)
Ritonavir (Norvir)
Saquinavir (Fortovase)
Stavudine (Zerit)
Telbivudine (Tyzeka)
Tenofovir (Viread)

Tenofovir/Emtricitabine (Truvada)
Tipranavir (Aptivus)
Zalcitabine (Hivid)
Zidovudine (Retrovir)
Zidovudine & Lamivudine (Combivir)

Antivirals

Acyclovir (Zovirax)
Adefovir (Hepsera)
Amantadine (Symmetrel)
Atazanavir (Reyataz)
Cidofovir (Vistide)
Emtricitabine (Emtriva)
Enfuvirtide (Fuzeon)
Famciclovir (Famvir)

Foscarnet (Foscavir)
Ganciclovir (Cytovene, Vitrasert)
Interferon Alfa-2b & Ribavirin Combo (Rebetron)
Oseltamivir (Tamiflu)
Palivizumab (Synagis)

Peg Interferon Alfa 2a (Peg Intron)
Penciclovir (Denavir)
Ribavirin (Virazole)
Rimantadine (Flumadine)
Valacyclovir (Valtrex)
Valganciclovir (Valcyte)
Zanamivir (Relenza)

Miscellaneous Antimicrobial Agents

Atovaquone (Mepron)
Atovaquone/Proguanil (Malarone)

Daptomycin (Cubicin)
Pentamidine (Pentam 300, NebuPent)

Trimetrexate (Neutrexin)

ANTINEOPLASTIC AGENTS

Alkylating Agents

Altretamine (Hexalen)
Busulfan (Myleran, Busulfex)
Carboplatin (Paraplatin)

Cisplatin (Platinol)
Oxaliplatin (Eloxatin)
Procarbazine (Matulane)

Triethylenetriphosphamide (Thio-Tepa)

NITROGEN MUSTARDS

Chlorambucil (Leukeran)
Cyclophosphamide (Cytoxan, Neosar)

Ifosfamide (Ifex, Holoxan)
Mechlorethamine (Mustargen)

Melphalan [L-PAM] (Alkeran)

NITROSOUREAS

Carmustine [BCNU] (BiCNU, Gliadel)

Streptozocin (Zanosar)

Antibiotics

Bleomycin Sulfate
(Blenoxane)
Dactinomycin
(Cosmegen)

Daunorubicin (Dauno-
mycin, Cerubidine)
Doxorubicin
(Adriamycin, Rubex)

Epirubicin (Ellence)
Idarubicin (Idamycin)
Mitomycin (Mutamycin)

Antimetabolites

Clofarabine (Clolar)
Cytarabine [ARA-C]
(Cytosar-U)
Cytarabine Liposome
(DepoCyt)
Floxuridine (FUDR)

Fludarabine Phosphate
(Flamp, Fludara)
Fluorouracil [5-FU]
(Adrucil)
Gemcitabine (Gemzar)
Mercaptopurine [6-MP]
(Purinethol)

Methotrexate (Folex,
Rheumatrex)
Nelarabine (Arranon)
Pemetrexed (Alimta)
6-Thioguanine [6-TG]

Hormones

Anastrozole (Arimidex)
Bicalutamide (Casodex)
Estramustine Phosphate
(Estracyt, Emcyt)
Exemestane (Aromasin)
Fluoxymesterone
(Halotestin)

Flutamide (Eulexin)
Fulvestrant (Faslodex)
Goserelin (Zoladex)
Leuprolide (Lupron,
Viadur, Eligard)
Levamisole (Ergamisol)

Megestrol Acetate
(Megace)
Nilutamide (Nilandron)
Tamoxifen (Nolvadex)
Triptorelin (Trelstar
Depot, Trelstar LA)

Mitotic Inhibitors

Etoposide [VP-16]
(VePesid)
Vinblastine (Velban,
Velbe)

Vincristine (Oncovin,
Vincasar PFS)

Vinorelbine (Navelbine)

Monoclonal Antibodies

Cetuximab (Erbitux)

Erlotinib (Tarceva)

Trastuzumab (Herceptin)

Miscellaneous Antineoplastic Agents

Aldesleukin [Interleukin-2,
IL-2] (Proleukin)
Aminoglutethimide
(Cytadren)

L-Asparaginase (Elspar,
Oncaspar)
BCG [Bacillus Calmette-
Guérin] (TheraCys,
Tice BCG)

Bevacizumab (Avastin)
Bortezomib (Velcade)
Cladribine (Leustatin)
Dacarbazine (DTIC)
Docetaxel (Taxotere)

Gefitinib (Iressa)
Gemtuzumab Ozogam-
    icin (Mylotarg)
Hydroxyurea (Hydrea,
    Droxia)
Imatinib (Gleevec)
Irinotecan (Camptosar)
Letrozole (Femara)

Leucovorin (Wellcovorin)
Mitoxantrone
    (Novantrone)
Paclitaxel (Taxol,
    Abraxane)
Pemetrexed (Alimta)
Rasburicase (Elitek)
Sorafenib (Nexavar)

Sunitinib (Sutent)
Thalidomide (Thalomid)
Topotecan (Hycamtin)
Tretinoin, Topical
    [Retinoic Acid]
    (Retin-A, Avita,
    Renova)

CARDIOVASCULAR (CV) AGENTS

Aldosterone Antagonist

Eplerenone (Inspra)

Alpha$_1$-Adrenergic Blockers

Doxazosin (Cardura)   Prazosin (Minipress)   Terazosin (Hytrin)

Angiotensin-Converting Enzyme (ACE) Inhibitors

Benazepril (Lotensin)
Captopril (Capoten)
Enalapril (Vasotec)
Fosinopril (Monopril)

Lisinopril (Prinivil,
    Zestril)
Moexipril (Univasc)
Perindopril Erbumine
    (Aceon)

Quinapril (Accupril)
Ramipril (Altace)
Trandolapril (Mavik)

Angiotensin II Receptor Antagonists

Candesartan (Atacand)
Eprosartan (Teveten)

Irbesartan (Avapro)
Losartan (Cozaar)

Telmisartan (Micardis)
Valsartan (Diovan)

Antiarrhythmic Agents

Adenosine (Adenocard)
Amiodarone (Cordarone,
    Pacerone)
Atropine
Digoxin (Lanoxin,
    Lanoxicaps)
Disopyramide (Norpace,
    NAPamide)

Dofetilide (Tikosyn)
Esmolol (Brevibloc)
Flecainide (Tambocor)
Ibutilide (Corvert)
Lidocaine (Anestacon
    Topical, Xylocaine)
Mexiletine (Mexitil)

Procainamide (Pronestyl,
    Procan)
Propafenone (Rythmol)
Quinidine (Quinidex,
    Quinaglute)
Sotalol (Betapace,
    Betapace AF)

Beta-Adrenergic Blockers

Acebutolol (Sectral)
Atenolol (Tenormin)
Atenolol & Chlorthalidone (Tenoretic)
Betaxolol (Kerlone)
Bisoprolol (Zebeta)

Carteolol (Cartrol, Ocupress Ophthalmic)
Carvedilol (Coreg)
Labetalol (Trandate, Normodyne)
Metoprolol (Lopressor, Toprol XL)

Nadolol (Corgard)
Penbutolol (Levatol)
Pindolol (Visken)
Propranolol (Inderal)
Timolol (Blocadren)

Calcium Channel Antagonists

Amlodipine (Norvasc)
Diltiazem (Cardizem, Cartia XT, Dilacor, Diltia XT, Tiamate, Tiazac)
Felodipine (Plendil)

Isradipine (DynaCirc)
Nicardipine (Cardene)
Nifedipine (Procardia, Procardia XL, Adalat, Adalat CC)
Nimodipine (Nimotop)

Nisoldipine (Sular)
Verapamil (Calan, Isoptin)

Centrally Acting Antihypertensive Agents

Clonidine (Catapres)

Methyldopa (Aldomet)

Diuretics

Acetazolamide (Diamox)
Amiloride (Midamor)
Bumetanide (Bumex)
Chlorothiazide (Diuril)
Chlorthalidone (Hygroton)
Furosemide (Lasix)
Hydrochlorothiazide (HydroDIURIL, Esidrix)

Hydrochlorothiazide & Amiloride (Moduretic)
Hydrochlorothiazide & Spironolactone (Aldactazide)
Hydrochlorothiazide & Triamterene (Dyazide, Maxzide)
Indapamide (Lozol)

Mannitol
Metolazone (Mykrox, Zaroxolyn)
Spironolactone (Aldactone)
Torsemide (Demadex)
Triamterene (Dyrenium)

Inotropic/Pressor Agents

Digoxin (Lanoxin, Lanoxicaps)
Dobutamine (Dobutrex)
Dopamine (Intropin)

Epinephrine (Adrenalin, Sus-Phrine, EpiPen)
Inamrinone (Inocor)
Isoproterenol (Isuprel)
Milrinone (Primacor)

Nesiritide (Natrecor)
Norepinephrine (Levophed)
Phenylephrine (Neo-Synephrine)

Antihypertensive Combination Agents

Amlodipine Besylate & Benazepril Hydrochloride (Lotrel)

Isosorbide Dinitrate & Hydralazine HCL (BiDil)

Lipid-Lowering Agents

Atorvastatin (Lipitor)
Cholestyramine (Questran, LoCHOLEST)
Colesevelam (WelChol)
Colestipol (Colestid)

Ezetimibe (Zetia)
Fenofibrate (TriCor)
Fluvastatin (Lescol)
Gemfibrozil (Lopid)
Lovastatin (Mevacor, Altocor)

Niacin (Niaspan)
Pravastatin (Pravachol)
Rosuvastatin (Crestor)
Simvastatin (Zocor)

Lipid-Lowering/Antihypertensive Combos

Amlodipine/Atorvastatin (Caduet)

Vasodilators

Alprostadil [Prostaglandin E_1] (Prostin VR)
Epoprostenol (Flolan)
Fenoldopam (Corlopam)
Hydralazine (Apresoline)
Iloprost (Ventavis)
Isosorbide Dinitrate (Isordil, Sorbitrate, Dilatrate-SR)

Isosorbide Mononitrate (Ismo, Imdur)
Minoxidil (Loniten, Rogaine)
Nitroglycerin (Nitrostat, Nitrolingual, Nitro-Bid Ointment, Nitro-Bid IV, Nitrodisc, Transderm-Nitro)

Nitroprusside (Nipride, Nitropress)
Tolazoline (Priscoline)
Treprostinil Sodium (Remodulin)

Miscellaneous Cardiovascular Agents

Conivaptan (Vaprisol)

Ranolazine (Ranexa)

CENTRAL NERVOUS SYSTEM AGENTS

Antianxiety Agents

Alprazolam (Xanax)
Buspirone (BuSpar)
Chlordiazepoxide (Librium, Mitran, Libritabs)
Clorazepate (Tranxene)

Diazepam (Valium)
Doxepin (Sinequan, Adapin)
Hydroxyzine (Atarax, Vistaril)

Lorazepam (Ativan)
Meprobamate (Equanil, Miltown)
Oxazepam (Serax)

Anticonvulsants

Carbamazepine (Tegretol)
Clonazepam (Klonopin)
Diazepam (Valium)
Ethosuximide (Zarontin)
Fosphenytoin (Cerebyx)
Gabapentin (Neurontin)

Lamotrigine (Lamictal)
Levetiracetam (Keppra)
Lorazepam (Ativan)
Oxcarbazepine (Trileptal)
Pentobarbital (Nembutal)
Phenobarbital

Phenytoin (Dilantin)
Tiagabine (Gabitril)
Topiramate (Topamax)
Valproic Acid (Depakene, Depakote)
Zonisamide (Zonegran)

Antidepressants

Amitriptyline (Elavil)
Bupropion (Wellbutrin, Zyban)
Citalopram (Celexa)
Desipramine (Norpramin)
Doxepin (Sinequan, Adapin)
Duloxetine (Cymbalta)

Escitalopram (Lexapro)
Fluoxetine (Prozac, Sarafem)
Fluvoxamine (Luvox)
Imipramine (Tofranil)
Mirtazapine (Remeron)
Nefazodone (Serzone)
Nortriptyline (Aventyl, Pamelor)

Paroxetine (Paxil)
Phenelzine (Nardil)
Selegiline transdermal (Emsam)
Sertraline (Zoloft)
Trazodone (Desyrel)
Venlafaxine (Effexor, Effexor XR)

Antiparkinson Agents

Amantadine (Symmetrel)
Apomorphine (Apokyn)
Benztropine (Cogentin)
Bromocriptine (Parlodel)
Carbidopa/Levodopa (Sinemet)

Entacapone (Comtan)
Pergolide (Permax)
Pramipexole (Mirapex)
Rasagiline mesylate (Azilect)
Ropinirole (Requip)

Selegiline (Eldepryl)
Selegiline HCL (Zelapar)
Tolcapone (Tasmar)
Trihexyphenidyl (Artane)

Antipsychotics

Aripiprazole (Abilify)
Chlorpromazine (Thorazine)
Clozapine (Clozaril)
Fluphenazine (Prolixin, Permitil)
Haloperidol (Haldol)

Lithium Carbonate (Eskalith, Lithobid)
Mesoridazine (Serentil)
Molindone (Moban)
Olanzapine (Zyprexa)
Perphenazine (Trilafon)
Prochlorperazine (Compazine)

Quetiapine (Seroquel)
Risperidone (Risperdal)
Thioridazine (Mellaril)
Thiothixene (Navane)
Trifluoperazine (Stelazine)
Ziprasidone (Geodon)

Sedative Hypnotics

Chloral Hydrate (Aquachloval, Supprettes)

Diphenhydramine (Benadryl)

Estazolam (ProSom)
Eszopiclone (Lunesta)

Flurazepam (Dalmane)
Hydroxyzine (Atarax,
    Vistaril)
Midazolam (Versed)
Pentobarbital (Nembutal)

Phenobarbital
Propofol (Diprivan)
Ramelteon (Rozerem)
Quazepam (Doral)
Secobarbital (Seconal)

Temazepam (Restoril)
Triazolam (Halcion)
Zaleplon (Sonata)
Zolpidem (Ambien)

Miscellaneous CNS Agents

Atomoxetine (Strattera)
Galantamine (Reminyl)
Interferon beta 1a
    (Rebif)
Memantine (Namenda)

Methylphenidate, Oral
    (Concerta, Ritalin,
    Ritalin-SR, others)
Methylphenidate, Trans-
    dermal (Daytrana)
Natalizumab (Tysabri)

Nimodipine (Nimotop)
Rivastigmine (Exelon)
Sodium Oxybate
    (Xyrem)
Tacrine (Cognex)

DERMATOLOGIC AGENTS

Acitretin (Soriatane)
Acyclovir (Zovirax)
Alefacept (Amevive)
Anthralin (Anthra-Derm)
Amphotericin B
    (Fungizone)
Bacitracin, Topical
    (Baciguent)
Bacitracin & Poly-
    myxin B, Topical
    (Polysporin)
Bacitracin, Neomycin, &
    Polymyxin B, Topical
    (Neosporin Ointment)
Bacitracin, Neomycin,
    Polymyxin B, &
    Hydrocortisone,
    Topical (Cortisporin)
Bacitracin, Neomycin,
    Polymyxin B, &
    Lidocaine, Topical
    (Clomycin)
Calcipotriene (Dovonex)
Capsaicin (Capsin,
    Zostrix)

Ciclopirox (Loprox)
Ciprofloxacin (Cipro)
Clindamycin (Cleocin)
Clotrimazole & Beta-
    methasone (Lotrisone)
Dibucaine (Nupercainal)
Doxepin, Topical
    (Zonalon)
Econazole (Spectazole)
Efalizumab (Raptiva)
Erythromycin, Topical
    (A/T/S, Eryderm,
    Erycette, T-Stat)
Finasteride (Proscar,
    Propecia)
Gentamicin, Topical
    (Garamycin,
    G-Mycitin)
Haloprogin (Halotex)
Imiquimod Cream, 5%
    (Aldara)
Isotretinoin [13-*cis*
    Retinoic acid]
    (Accutane, Amnes-
    teem, Claravis, Sotret)

Ketoconazole (Nizoral)
Lactic Acid & Ammo-
    nium Hydroxide
    [Ammonium Lactate]
    (Lac-Hydrin)
Lindane (Kwell)
Metronidazole (Flagyl,
    MetroGel)
Miconazole (Monistat)
Minoxidil (Loniten,
    Rogaine)
Mupirocin (Bactroban)
Naftifine (Naftin)
Neomycin Sulfate
    (Myciguent)
Nystatin (Mycostatin)
Oxiconazole (Oxistat)
Penciclovir (Denavir)
Permethrin (Nix, Elimite)
Pimecrolimus (Elidel)
Podophyllin (Podocon-
    25, Condylox Gel
    0.5%, Condylox)

Pramoxine (Anusol
Ointment,
Proctofoam-NS)
Pramoxine & Hydro-
cortisone (Enzone,
Proctofoam-HC)
Selenium Sulfide (Exsel
Shampoo, Selsun Blue

Shampoo, Selsun
Shampoo)
Silver Sulfadiazine
(Silvadene)
Steroids, Topical (Table 5)
Tacrolimus (Prograf,
Protopic)
Tazarotene (Tazorac)

Terbinafine (Lamisil)
Tolnaftate (Tinactin)
Tretinoin, Topical
[Retinoic Acid]
(Retin-A, Avita,
Renova)

DIETARY SUPPLEMENTS

Calcium Acetate
(Calphron, Phos-Ex,
PhosLo)
Calcium Glubionate
(Neo-Calglucon)
Calcium Salts [Chloride,
Gluconate, Gluceptate]
Cholecalciferol [Vitamin
D_3] (Delta D)
Cyanocobalamin
[Vitamin B_{12}]

Ferric Gluconate
Complex (Ferrlecit)
Ferrous Gluconate
(Fergon)
Ferrous Sulfate
Folic Acid
Iron Dextran
(DexFerrum, InFeD)
Iron Sucrose (Venofer)
Magnesium Oxide
(Mag-Ox 400)
Magnesium Sulfate

Multivitamins (Table 15)
Phytonadione [Vitamin K]
(Aqua-MEPHYTON)
Potassium Supplements
(Kaon, Kaochlor,
K-Lor, Slow-K,
Micro-K, Klorvess)
Pyridoxine [Vitamin B_6]
Sodium Bicarbonate
[$NaHCO_3$]
Thiamine [Vitamin B_1]

EAR (OTIC) AGENTS

Acetic Acid &
Aluminum Acetate
(Otic Domeboro)
Benzocaine &
Antipyrine (Auralgan)
Ciprofloxacin, Otic
(Cipro HC Otic)

Neomycin, Colistin, &
Hydrocortisone
(Cortisporin-TC Otic
Drops)
Neomycin, Colistin, Hy-
drocortisone, & Thon-
zonium (Cortisporin-TC
Otic Suspension)

Polymyxin B & Hydro-
cortisone (Otobiotic
Otic)
Sulfacetamide & Pred-
nisolone (Blephamide)
Triethanolamine
(Cerumenex)

ENDOCRINE SYSTEM AGENTS

Antidiabetic Agents

Acarbose (Precose)
Chlorpropamide
(Diabinese)
Glimepiride (Amaryl)
Glipizide (Glucotrol)

Glyburide (DiaBeta,
Micronase, Glynase)
Glyburide/Metformin
(Glucovance)
Insulins (Table 6)

Insulin Human Inhala-
tion Powder (Exubera)
Metformin (Glucophage,
Glucophage XR,
Glumetza)

Miglitol (Glyset)
Nateglinide (Starlix)
Pioglitazone (Actos)
Pioglitazone HCL/
  Glimepiride (Duetact)

Pioglitazone/Metformin
  (ActoPlus Met)
Repaglinide (Prandin)
Rosiglitazone (Avandia)
Rosiglitazone/Metformin
  (Arandamet)

Sitagliptin Phosphate
  (Januvia)
Tolazamide (Tolinase)
Tolbutamide (Orinase)

Hormone & Synthetic Substitutes

Calcitonin (Cibacalcin,
  Miacalcin)
Calcitriol (Rocaltrol)
Cortisone Systemic,
  Topical
Desmopressin (DDAVP,
  Stimate)
Dexamethasone
  (Decadron)

Fludrocortisone Acetate
  (Florinef)
Glucagon
Hydrocortisone Topical
  & Systemic (Cortef,
  Solu-Cortef)
Methylprednisolone
  (Solu-Medrol)

Prednisolone
Prednisone
Testosterone (AndroGel,
  Androderm, Striant,
  Testim, Testoderm)
Vasopressin [Antidi-
  uretic Hormone,
  ADH] (Pitressin)

Hypercalcemia/Osteoporosis Agents

Etidronate Disodium
  (Didronel)
Gallium Nitrate (Ganite)

Ibandronate (Boniva)
Pamidronate (Aredia)

Zoledronic acid
  (Zometa)

Obesity

Sibutramine (Meridia)

Osteoporosis Agents

Alendronate (Fosamax)
Raloxifene (Evista)

Risedronate (Actonel)
Teriparatide (Forteo)

Zoledronic Acid
  (Zometa)

Thyroid/Antithyroid

Levothyroxine (Syn-
  throid, Levoxyl)
Liothyronine (Cytomel)
Methimazole (Tapazole)

Potassium iodide [Lugol
  Solution] (SSKI,
  Thyro-Block)

Propylthiouracil [PTU]

Miscellaneous Endocrine Agents

Cinacalcet (Sensipar)

Demeclocycline
  (Declomycin)

Diazoxide (Hyperstat,
  Proglycem)

EYE (OPHTHALMIC) AGENTS

Glaucoma Agents

Acetazolamide (Diamox)
Apraclonidine (Iopidine)
Betaxolol, Ophthalmic (Betopic)
Brimonidine (Alphagan)
Brinzolamide (Azopt)
Carteolol (Cartrol, Ocupress Ophthalmic)
Ciprofloxacin, Ophthalmic (Ciloxan)
Cyclosporine, Ophthalmic (Restasis)
Dipivefrin (Propine)
Dorzolamide (Trusopt)

Dorzolamide & Timolol (Cosopt)
Echothiophate Iodine (Phospholine Ophthalmic)
Epinastine (Elestat)
Gatifloxacin Ophthalmic (Zymar Ophthalmic)
Latanoprost (Xalatan)
Levobunolol (A-K Beta, Betagan)
Levocabastine (Livostin)
Levofloxacin (Levaquin, Quixin & Iquix Ophthalmic)

Lodoxamide (Alomide)
Moxifloxacin (Vigamox)
Neomycin, Polymyxin, & Hydrocortisone (Cortisporin Ophthalmic & Otic)
Norfloxin (Chibroxin)
Ofloxacin (Ocuflox Ophthalmic)
Rimexolone (Vexol Ophthalmic)
Timolol, Ophthalmic (Timoptic)
Trifluridine, Ophthalmic (Viroptic)

Ophthalmic Antibiotics

Bacitracin, Ophthalmic (AK-Tracin Ophthalmic)
Bacitracin & Polymyxin B, Ophthalmic (AK Poly Bac Ophthalmic, Polysporin Ophthalmic)
Bacitracin, Neomycin, & Polymyxin B (AK Spore Ophthalmic, Neosporin Ophthalmic)
Bacitracin, Neomycin, Polymyxin B, & Hydrocortisone, Ophthalmic (AK Spore HC Ophthalmic, Cortisporin Ophthalmic)

Ciprofloxacin, Ophthalmic (Ciloxan)
Erythromycin, Ophthalmic (Ilotycin Ophthalmic)
Gentamicin, Ophthalmic (Garamycin, Genoptic, Gentacidin, Gentak)
Neomycin & Dexamethasone (AK-Neo-Dex Ophthalmic, NeoDecadron Ophthalmic)
Neomycin, Polymyxin B, & Dexamethasone (Maxitrol)

Neomycin, Polymyxin B, & Prednisolone (Poly-Pred Ophthalmic)
Ofloxacin (Floxin, Ocuflox Ophthalmic)
Silver Nitrate (Dey-Drop)
Sulfacetamide (Bleph-10, Cetamide, Sodium Sulamyd)
Sulfacetamide & Prednisolone (Blephamide)
Tobramycin, Ophthalmic (AKTob, Tobrex)
Tobramycin & Dexamethasone (TobraDex)
Trifluridine (Viroptic)

Miscellaneous Ophthalmic Agents

Artificial Tears (Tears Naturale)

Cromolyn Sodium (Opticrom)

Cyclopentolate (Cyclogyl)

Cyclopentolate with phenylephrine (Cyclomydril)
Cyclosporine Ophthalmic (Restasis)
Dexamethasone, Ophthalmic (AK-Dex Ophthalmic, Decadron Ophthalmic)

Emedastine (Emadine)
Ketorolac, Ophthalmic (Acular)
Ketotifen (Zaditor)
Lodoxamide (Alomide)
Naphazoline & Antazoline (Albalon-A Ophthalmic)

Naphazoline & Pheniramine Acetate (Naphcon A)
Nepafenac (Nevanac)
Olopatadine (Patanol)
Pemirolast (Alamast)
Rimexolone (Vexol Ophthalmic)

GASTROINTESTINAL AGENTS

Antacids

Alginic Acid (Gaviscon)
Aluminum Hydroxide (Amphojel, AlternaGEL)
Aluminum Hydroxide with Magnesium Carbonate (Gaviscon)
Aluminum Hydroxide with Magnesium Hydroxide (Maalox)

Aluminum Hydroxide with Magnesium Hydroxide & Simethicone (Mylanta, Mylanta II, Maalox Plus)
Aluminum Hydroxide with Magnesium Trisilicate (Gaviscon, Gaviscon-2)

Calcium Carbonate (Tums, Alka-Mints)
Magaldrate (Riopan, Lowsium)
Simethicone (Mylicon)

Antidiarrheals

Bismuth Subsalicylate (Pepto-Bismol)
Diphenoxylate with Atropine (Lomotil)

Kaolin-Pectin (Kaodene, Kao-Spen, Kapectolin, Parepectolin)
Lactobacillus (Lactinex Granules)

Loperamide (Imodium)
Octreotide (Sandostatin, Sandostatin LAR)
Paregoric [Camphorated Tincture of Opium]

Antiemetics

Aprepitant (Emend)
Chlorpromazine (Thorazine)
Dimenhydrinate (Dramamine)
Dolasetron (Anzemet)
Dronabinol (Marinol)
Droperidol (Inapsine)

Granisetron (Kytril)
Meclizine (Antivert)
Metoclopramide (Reglan, Clopra, Octamide)
Nabilone (Cesamet)
Ondansetron (Zofran)
Palonosetron (Aloxi)

Prochlorperazine (Compazine)
Promethazine (Phenergan)
Scopolamine (Scopace)
Thiethylperazine (Torecan)
Trimethobenzamide (Tigan)

Antiulcer Agents

Cimetidine (Tagamet)
Esomeprazole (Nexium)
Famotidine (Pepcid)
Lansoprazole (Prevacid)

Nizatidine (Axid)
Omeprazole (Prilosec, Zegerid)
Pantoprazole (Protonix)

Rabeprazole (Aciphex)
Ranitidine Hydrochloride (Zantac)
Sucralfate (Carafate)

Cathartics/Laxatives

Bisacodyl (Dulcolax)
Docusate Calcium (Surfak)
Docusate Potassium (Dialose)
Docusate Sodium (Doss, Colace)
Glycerin Suppository

Lactulose (Constulose, Generlac, Chronulac, Cephulac, Enulose)
Magnesium Citrate
Magnesium Hydroxide (Milk of Magnesia)
Mineral Oil

Polyethylene Glycol-Electrolyte Solution (GoLYTELY, CoLyte)
Psyllium (Metamucil, Serutan, Effer-Syllium)
Sodium Phosphate (Visicol)
Sorbitol

Enzymes

Pancreatin (Pancrease, Cotazym, Creon, Ultrase)

Miscellaneous GI Agents

Alosetron (Lotronex)
Balsalazide (Colazal)
Dexpanthenol (Ilopan-Choline Oral, Ilopan)
Dibucaine (Nupercainal)
Dicyclomine (Bentyl)
Hydrocortisone, Rectal (Anusol-HC Suppository, Cortifoam Rectal, Proctocort)
Hyoscyamine (Anaspaz, Cystospaz, Levsin)

Hyoscyamine, Atropine, Scopolamine, & Phenobarbital (Donnatal)
Infliximab (Remicade)
Lubiprostone (Amitiza)
Mesalamine (Rowasa, Asacol, Pentasa)
Metoclopramide (Reglan, Clopra, Octamide)
Misoprostol (Cytotec)
Olsalazine (Dipentum)

Pramoxine (Anusol Ointment, Proctofoam-NS)
Pramoxine with Hydrocortisone (Enzone, Proctofoam-HC)
Propantheline (Pro-Banthine)
Sulfasalazine (Azulfidine)
Tegaserod Maleate (Zelnorm)
Vasopressin (Pitressin)

HEMATOLOGIC AGENTS

Anticoagulants

Ardeparin (Normiflo)
Argatroban (Acova)
Bivalirudin (Angiomax)
Dalteparin (Fragmin)

Enoxaparin (Lovenox)
Fondaparinux (Arixtra)
Heparin
Lepirudin (Refludan)

Protamine
Tinzaparin (Innohep)
Warfarin (Coumadin)

Antiplatelet Agents

Abciximab (ReoPro)
Aspirin (Bayer, Ecotrin, St. Joseph's)
Clopidogrel (Plavix)
Dipyridamole (Persantine)
Dipyridamole & Aspirin (Aggrenox)
Eptifibatide (Integrilin)
Reteplase (Retavase)
Ticlopidine (Ticlid)
Tirofiban (Aggrastat)

Antithrombotic Agents

Alteplase, Recombinant [tPA] (Activase)
Aminocaproic Acid (Amicar)
Anistreplase (Eminase)
Aprotinin (Trasylol)
Danaparoid (Orgaron)
Dextran 40 (Rheomacrodex)
Reteplase (Retavase)
Streptokinase (Streptase, Kabikinase)
Tenecteplase (TNKase)
Urokinase (Abbokinase)

Hematopoietic Stimulants

Darbepoetin Alfa (Aranesp)
Epoetin Alfa [Erythropoietin, EPO] (Epogen, Procrit)
Filgrastim [G-CSF] (Neupogen)
Oprelvekin (Neumega)
Pegfilgrastim (Neulasta)
Sargramostim [GM-CSF] (Prokine, Leukine)

Volume Expanders

Albumin (Albuminar, Buminate, Albutein)
Dextran 40 (Rheomacrodex)
Hetastarch (Hespan)
Plasma Protein Fraction (Plasmanate)

Miscellaneous Hematologic Agents

Antihemophilic Factor VIII (Monoclate)
Decitabine (Dacogen)
Desmopressin (DDAVP, Stimate)
Lenalidomide (Revlimid)
Pentoxifylline (Trental)

IMMUNE SYSTEM AGENTS

Immunomodulators

Abatacept (Orencia)
Adalimumab (Humira)
Anakinra (Kineret)
Etanercept (Enbrel)
Interferon Alfa (Roferon-A, Intron A)
Interferon Alfacon-1 (Infergen)
Interferon Beta-1b (Betaseron)
Interferon Gamma-1b (Actimmune)
Mycophenolic Acid (Myfortic)
Natalizumab (Tysabri)
Peg Interferon Alfa-2b (PEG-Intron)

Immunosuppressive Agents

Azathioprine (Imuran)
Basiliximab (Simulect)
Cyclosporine (Sandimmune, NePO)
Daclizumab (Zenapax)
Lymphocyte Immune Globulin [Antithymocyte Globulin, ATG] (Atgam)
Muromonab-CD3 (Orthoclone OKT3)
Mycophenolate Mofetil (CellCept)
Sirolimus (Rapamune)
Steroids, Systemic (Table 4)
Tacrolimus (Prograf, Protopic)

Vaccines/Serums/Toxoids

Cytomegalovirus Immune Globulin [CMV-IG IV] (CytoGam)
Diphtheria, Tetanus Toxoids, & Acellular Pertussis Adsorbed, Hepatitis B (recombinant), & Inactivated Poliovirus Vaccine (IPV) Combined (Pediarix)
Haemophilus B Conjugate Vaccine (ActHIB, HibTITER, Pedvax-HIB, Prohibit)
Hepatitis A Vaccine (Havrix, Vaqta)
Hepatitis A (Inactivated) & Hepatitis B Recombinant Vaccine (Twinrix)
Hepatitis B Immune Globulin (HyperHep, H-BIG)
Hepatitis B Vaccine (Engerix-B, Recombivax HB)
Human Papillomavirus (Types 6, 11, 16, 18) Recombinant Vaccine (Gardasil)
Immune Globulin, IV (Gamimune N, Sandoglobulin, Gammar IV)
Influenza Vaccine (Fluzone, FluShield, Fluvirin)
Influenza Virus Vaccine Live, Intranasal (FluMist)
Measles, Mumps, Rubella and Varicella
Virus Vaccine Live (Proquad)
Meningococcal Polysaccharide Vaccine (Menomune)
Pneumococcal 7-Valent Conjugate Vaccine (Prevnar)
Pneumococcal Vaccine, Polyvalent (Pneumovax-23)
Rotavirus vaccine, live, oral, pentavalent (RotaTeq)
Tetanus Immune Globulin
Tetanus Toxoid
Varicella Virus Vaccine (Varivax)
Zoster vaccine, live (Zostavax)

MUSCULOSKELETAL AGENTS

Antigout Agents

Allopurinol (Zyloprim, Lopurin, Alloprim)
Colchicine
Probenecid (Benemid)
Sulfinpyrazone (Anturane)

Muscle Relaxants

Baclofen (Lioresal)
Carisoprodol (Soma)
Chlorzoxazone (Paraflex, Parafon Forte DSC)
Cyclobenzaprine (Flexeril)

Dantrolene (Dantrium)
Diazepam (Valium)

Metaxalone (Skelaxin)
Methocarbamol (Robaxin)

Orphenadrine (Norflex)

Neuromuscular Blockers

Atracurium (Tracrium)
Pancuronium (Pavulon)
Rocuronium (Zemuron)

Succinylcholine
(Anectine, Quelicin,
Sucostrin)

Vecuronium (Norcuron)

Miscellaneous Musculoskeletal Agents

Edrophonium (Tensilon)

Leflunomide (Arava)

Methotrexate (Folex,
Rheumatrex)

OB/GYN AGENTS

Contraceptives

Drospirenone/Ethinyl
Estradiol (YAZ)
Estradiol Cypionate &
Medroxyprogesterone
Acetate (Lunelle)
Etonogestrel/Ethinyl
Estradiol (NuvaRing)
Levonorgestrel Implant
(Norplant)

Levonorgestrel/Ethinyl
Estradiol (Seasonale)
Medroxyprogesterone
(Provera, Depo-
Provera)
Norgestrel (Ovrette)
Oral Contraceptives,
Monophasic (Table 7)

Oral Contraceptives,
Multiphasic (Table 7)
Oral Contraceptives,
Progestin Only
(Table 7)

Emergency Contraceptives

Ethinyl Estradiol, &
Levonorgestrel (Preven)

Levonorgestrel (Plan B)

Estrogen Supplementation Agents

Drospirenone/Estradiol
(Angelia)
Esterified Estrogens
(Estratab, Menest)
Esterified Estrogens with
Methyltestosterone
(Estratest)
Estradiol (Estrace)
Estradiol, Transdermal
(Estraderm, Climara,
Vivelle)

Estrogen, Conjugated
(Premarin)
Estrogen, Conjugated-
Synthetic (Cenestin)
Estrogen, Conjugated
with Medroxyproges-
terone (Prempro,
Premphase)
Estrogen, Conjugated
with Methylproges-

terone (Premarin with
Methylprogesterone)
Estrogen, Conjugated
with Methyltestos-
terone (Premarin with
Methyltestosterone)
Ethinyl Estradiol
(Estinyl, Feminone)
Norethindrone
Acetate/Ethinyl Estra-
diol (FemHRT)

Vaginal Preparations

Amino-Cerv pH 5.5
Cream

Miconazole (Monistat)
Nystatin (Mycostatin)

Terconazole (Terazol 7)
Tioconazole (Vagistat)

Miscellaneous Ob/Gyn Agents

Dinoprostone (Cervidil
Vaginal Insert, Pre-
pidil Vaginal Gel)
Gonadorelin (Lutrepulse)
Leuprolide (Lupron)
Lutropin Alfa (Luveris)

Magnesium Sulfate
Medroxyprogesterone
(Provera, Depo-
Provera)
Methylergonovine
(Methergine)

Mifepristone [RU 486]
(Mifeprex)
Oxytocin (Pitocin)
Terbutaline (Brethine,
Bricanyl)

PAIN MEDICATIONS

Local Anesthetics (See Table 3)

Benzocaine &
Antipyrine (Auralgan)
Bupivacaine (Marcaine)
Capsaicin (Capsin,
Zostrix)
Cocaine

Dibucaine (Nupercainal)
Lidocaine (Anestacon
Topical, Xylocaine)
Lidocaine & Prilocaine
(EMLA, LMX)

Lidocaine/Tetracaine
(Synera)
Pramoxine (Anusol
Ointment, Procto-
foam-NS)

Migraine Headache Medications

Acetaminophen with Bu-
talbital w/wo Caffeine
(Fioricet, Medigesic,
Repan, Sedapap-10
Two-Dyne, Triapin, Ax-
ocet, Phrenilin Forte)
Almotriptan (Axert)

Aspirin & Butalbital
Compound (Fiorinal)
Aspirin with Butalbital,
Caffeine, & Codeine
(Fiorinal with
Codeine)
Eletriptan (Relpax)

Frovatriptan (Frova)
Naratriptan (Amerge)
Serotonin 5-HT$_1$ Recep-
tor Agonists (See
Table 11)
Sumatriptan (Imitrex)
Zolmitriptan (Zomig)

Narcotic Analgesics

Acetaminophen with
Codeine (Tylenol No.
1, 2, 3, 4)
Alfentanil (Alfenta)
Aspirin with Codeine
(Empirin No. 2, 3, 4)
Buprenorphine
(Buprenex)
Butorphanol (Stadol)
Codeine

Dezocine (Dalgan)
Fentanyl (Sublimaze)
Fentanyl, Transdermal
(Duragesic)
Fentanyl, Transmucosal
(Actiq System)
Hydrocodone & Aceta-
minophen (Lorcet,
Vicodin)

Hydrocodone & Aspirin
(Lortab ASA)
Hydrocodone & Ibupro-
fen (Vicoprofen)
Hydromorphone
(Dilaudid)
Levorphanol (Levo-
Dromoran)
Meperidine (Demerol)
Methadone (Dolophine)

Morphine (Avinza XR, Duramorph, Infumorph, MS Contin, Kadian SR, Oramorph SR, Palladone, Roxanol)

Morphine, Liposomal (DepoDur)

Nalbuphine (Nubain)

Oxycodone (OxyContin, OxyIR, Roxicodone)

Oxycodone & Acetaminophen (Percocet, Tylox)

Oxycodone & Aspirin (Percodan, Percodan-Demi)

Oxymorphone (Numorphan)

Pentazocine (Talwin)

Propoxyphene (Darvon)

Propoxyphene & Acetaminophen (Darvocet)

Propoxyphene & Aspirin (Darvon Compound-65, Darvon-N with Aspirin)

Nonnarcotic Analgesics

Acetaminophen [APAP] (Tylenol)

Aspirin (Bayer, Ecotrin, St. Joseph's)

Tramadol (Ultram)

Tramadol/Acetaminophen (Ultracet)

Nonsteroidal Antiinflammatory Agents

Celecoxib (Celebrex)

Diclofenac (Cataflam, Voltaren)

Diflunisal (Dolobid)

Etodolac (Lodine)

Fenoprofen (Nalfon)

Flurbiprofen (Ansaid)

Ibuprofen (Motrin, Rufen, Advil)

Indomethacin (Indocin)

Ketoprofen (Orudis, Oruvail)

Ketorolac (Toradol)

Meloxicam (Mobic)

Nabumetone (Relafen)

Naproxen (Aleve, Naprosyn, Anaprox)

Oxaprozin (Daypro)

Piroxicam (Feldene)

Sulindac (Clinoril)

Tolmetin (Tolectin)

Miscellaneous Pain Medications

Amitriptyline (Elavil)

Imipramine (Tofranil)

Pregabalin (Lyrica)

Tramadol (Ultram)

Ziconotide (Prialt)

RESPIRATORY AGENTS

Antitussives, Decongestants, & Expectorants

Acetylcysteine (Acetadote, Mucomyst)

Benzonatate (Tessalon Perles)

Codeine

Dextromethorphan (Mediquell, Benylin DM, PediaCare 1)

Guaifenesin (Robitussin)

Guaifenesin & Codeine (Robitussin AC, Brontex)

Guaifenesin & Dextromethorphan

Hydrocodone & Guaifenesin (Hycotuss Expectorant)

Hydrocodone & Homatropine (Hycodan, Hydromet)

Hydrocodone & Pseudoephedrine (Detussin, Histussin-D)

Hydrocodone, Chlorpheniramine, Phenylephrine, Acetaminophen, & Caffeine (Hycomine)

Potassium Iodide (SSKI, Thyro-Block)

Pseudoephedrine (Sudafed, Novafed, Afrinol)

Bronchodilators

Albuterol (Proventil, Ventolin, Volmax)
Albuterol & Ipratropium (Combivent)
Aminophylline
Bitolterol (Tornalate)
Ephedrine

Epinephrine (Adrenalin, Sus-Phrine, EpiPen)
Formoterol (Foradil Aerolizer)
Isoproterenol (Isuprel)
Levalbuterol (Xopenex)
Metaproterenol (Alupent, Metaprel)

Pirbuterol (Maxair)
Salmeterol (Serevent)
Terbutaline (Brethine, Bricanyl)
Theophylline (Theo24, TheoChron)

Respiratory Inhalants

Acetylcysteine (Aceta-dote, Mucomyst)
Beclomethasone (Beconase, Vancenase Nasal Inhaler)
Beclomethasone (QVAR)
Beractant (Survanta)
Budesonide (Rhinocort, Pulmicort)

Calfactant (Infasurf)
Cromolyn Sodium (Intal, Nasalcrom, Opticrom)
Dexamethasone, Nasal (Dexacort Phosphate Turbinaire)
Flunisolide (AeroBid, Nasalide)
Fluticasone, Oral, Nasal (Flonase, Flovent)

Fluticasone Propionate & Salmeterol Xinafoate (Advair Diskus)
Ipratropium (Atrovent)
Nedocromil (Tilade)
Tiotropium (Spiriva)
Triamcinolone (Azmacort)

Miscellaneous Respiratory Agents

Alpha$_1$-Protease Inhibitor (Prolastin)

Dornase Alfa (Pulmozyme)
Montelukast (Singulair)

Omalizumab (Xolair)
Zafirlukast (Accolate)
Zileuton (Zyflo)

URINARY/GENITOURINARY AGENTS

Alprostadil, Intracaver-nosal (Caverject, Edex)
Alprostadil, Urethral Suppository (Muse)
Ammonium Aluminum Sulfate [Alum]
Belladonna & Opium Suppositories (B & O Supprettes)
Bethanechol (Ure-choline, Duvoid)
Darifenacin (Enablex)
Dimethyl Sulfoxide [DMSO] (Rimso 50)

Flavoxate (Urispas)
Hyoscyamine (Anaspaz, Cystospaz, Levsin)
Methenamine (Hiprex, Urex)
Neomycin-Polymyxin Bladder Irrigant [Neosporin GU Irrigant]
Nitrofurantoin (Macro-dantin, Furadantin, Macrobid)
Oxybutynin (Ditropan, Ditropan XL)

Oxybutynin Transdermal System (Oxytrol)
Pentosan Polysulfate (Elmiron)
Phenazopyridine (Pyridium)
Potassium Citrate (Urocit-K)
Potassium Citrate & Citric Acid (Polycitra-K)
Sildenafil (Viagra)
Solifenacin (VESIcare)
Sodium Citrate (Bicitra)
Tadalafil (Cialis)

Tolterodine (Detrol, Detrol LA)

Trimethoprim (Trimpex, Proloprim)

Trospium Chloride (Sanctura)
Vardenafil (Levitra)

Benign Prostatic Hyperplasia Medications

Alfuzosin (Uroxatral)
Doxazosin (Cardura)
Dutasteride (Avodart)

Finasteride (Proscar, Propecia)

Tamsulosin (Flomax)
Terazosin (Hytrin)

WOUND CARE

Becaplermin (Regranex Gel)

Silver Nitrate (Dey-Drop)

MISCELLANEOUS THERAPEUTIC AGENTS

Acamprosate (Campral)
Alglucosidase alfa (Myozyme)
Cilostazol (Pletal)
Drotrecogin Alfa (Xigris)
Lanthanum Carbonate (Fosrenol)
Megestrol Acetate (Megace)
Mecasermin (Increlex)

Naltrexone (ReVia)
Nicotine Gum (Nicorette)
Nicotine Nasal Spray (Nicotrol NS)
Nicotine Transdermal (Habitrol, Nicoderm, Nicotrol)
Orlistat (Xenical)

Palifermin (Kepivance)
Potassium Iodide [Lugol Solution] (SSKI, Thyro-Block)
Sevelamer (Renagel)
Sodium Polystyrene Sulfonate (Kayexalate)
Talc (Sterile Talc Powder)
Varenicline (Chantix)

NATURAL AND HERBAL AGENTS (see page 286)

Aloe Vera (*Aloe barbadensis*)
Arnica (*Arnica montana*)
Butcher's Broom (*Ruscus aculeatus*)
Black Cohosh (*Cimicifuga racemosa*)
Bilberry (*Vaccinium myrtillus*)
Bogbean (*Menyanthes trifoliate*)
Borage (*Borago officinalis*)

Bugleweed (*Lycopus virginicus*)
Capsicum (*Capsicum frutescens*)
Cascara Sagrada (*Rhamnus purshiana*)
Chamomile (*Matricaria recutita*)
Chondroitin Sulfate
Comfrey (*Symphytum officinale*)
Coriander (*Coriandrum sativum*)

Cranberry (*Vaccinium macrocarpon*)
Dong Quai (*Angelica polymorpha, sinensis*)
Echinacea (*Echinacea purpurea*)
Ephedra/Ma Huang
Evening Primrose Oil (*Oenothera biennis*)
Feverfew (*Tanacetum parthenium*)
Garlic (*Allium sativum*)
Gentian (*Gentiana lutea*)

Ginger (*Zingiber officinale*)

Ginkgo biloba

Ginseng (*Panax quinquefolius*)

Glucosamine Sulfate (Chitosamine)

Green Tea (*Camellia sinensis*)

Guarana (*Paullinia cupana*)

Hawthorn (*Crataegus laevigata*)

Horsetail (*Equisetum arvense*)

Kava Kava (*Piper methysticum*)

Licorice (*Glycyrrhiza glabra*)

Melatonin (MEL)

Milk thistle (*Silybum marianum*)

Nettle (*Urtica dioica*)

Rue (*Ruta graveolens*)

Saw Palmetto (*Serenoa repens*)

Spirulina (*Spirulina* spp)

Stevia (*Stevia rebaudiana*)

St. John's Wort (*Hypericum perforatum*)

Tea Tree (*Melaleuca alternifolia*)

Valerian (*Valeriana officinalis*)

Yohimbine (*Pausinystalia yohimbe*)

GENERIC DRUG DATA

Abacavir (Ziagen) [Antiretroviral/NRTI] WARNING: Allergy (fever, rash, fatigue, GI, resp) reported; stop drug immediately & do not rechallenge; lactic acidosis & hepatomegaly/steatosis reported **Uses:** *HIV Infxn* **Action:** Nucleoside RT inhibitor **Dose:** *Adults.* 300 mg PO bid or 600 mg PO daily *Peds.* 8 mg/kg bid **Caution:** [C, -] CDC recommends HIV-infected mothers not breast-feed (risk of infant transmission) **Disp:** Tabs 300 mg; soln 20 mg/mL **SE:** See Warning, ↑ LFTs, fat redistribution **Notes:** Numerous drug interactions **Interactions:** EtOH ↓ drug elimination and ↑ drug exposure **Labs:** Monitor LFTs, FBS, CBC, & differential, BUN & creatinine, triglycerides **NIPE:** ⊘ EtOH; monitor & teach pt about hypersensitivity Rxns; DC drug immediately if hypersensitivity Rxn occurs and ⊘ rechallenge; take w/ or w/o food

Abatacept (Orencia) [Immunomodulator] **Uses:** *Mod/severe RA w/inadequate response to one or more DMARDs* **Action:** Selective costimulation modulator, ↓ T-cell activation **Dose:** Initial 500 mg (<60 kg), 750 mg (60–100 kg); 1 gm (>100kg) IV over 30 min; repeat at 2 and 4 wk, then every 4 wk **Caution:** [C; ?/-] COPD h/o recurrent, localized, chronic, or predisposition to Infxn **Contra:** w/TNF antagonists (↑ Infxn) **Disp:** Powder for IV: 250 mg/15 mL **SE:** HA, URI, N, nasopharyngitis, Infxn, malignancy, infusion Rxns (dizziness, HA, HTN), hypersensitivity, COPD exacerbations, cough, rhonchi, dyspnea **Interactions:** Do not give w/ live vaccines w/ or w/in 3 mo discontinuing abatacept **NIPE:** Screen for TB prior to use; d/c if serious infection occurs

Abciximab (ReoPro) [Platelet-aggregation inhibitor/Antiplatelet] **Uses:** *Prevent acute ischemic complications in PTCA,* *MI* **Action:** ↓ plt aggregation (glycoprotein IIb/IIIa inhibitor) **Dose:** Unstable angina w/ PCI: 0.25 mg/kg bolus followed by 10 mcg/min cont inf ¥ 18–24 h, stopping 1 h after PCI; PCI: 0.25 mg/kg bolus 10–60 min pre PTCA, then 0.125 mcg/kg/min (max = 10 mcg/min) cont inf for 12 h **Caution:** [C, ?/-] **Contra:** Active or recent (w/in 6 wk) internal hemorrhage, CVA w/in 2 y or CVA w/ significant neurologic deficit, bleeding diathesis or PO anticoagulants use w/in 7 d (unless PT <1.2× control), thrombocytopenia (<100,000 cells/mcL), recent trauma or major surgery (w/in 6 wk), CNS tumor, AVM, aneurysm, severe uncontrolled HTN, vasculitis, use of dextran prior to or during PTCA, allergy to murine proteins **Disp:** Inj 2 mg/mL **SE:** Allergic Rxns, bleeding, thrombocytopenia possible **Notes:** Use w/ heparin **Interactions:** May ↑ bleeding w/ anticoagulants, antiplts, NSAIDs, thrombolytics **Labs:** Monitor CBC, PT, PTT, INR, guaiac stools, urine for blood **NIPE:** Monitor for ↑ bleeding & bruising; ⊘ shake vial or mix w/ another drug, contact sports ⊘

24

Acamprosate (Campral) [Hypoglycemic/Alpha-glucosidase Inhibitor]

Uses: *Maint abstinence from EtOH* Action: ↓ Glutamatergic transmission; modulates neuronal hyperexcitability; related to GABA Dose: 666 mg PO tid; CrCl 30-50 mL/min: 333 mg PO tid Caution: [C; ?/-] Contra: CrCl ≤ 30 mL/min Disp: Tabs 333 mg EC (enteric coated) SE: N/D, depression, anxiety, insomnia Notes: Does not eliminate EtOH withdrawal Sx; continue even if relapse occurs Interactions: None Labs: BS, LFTs, Uric Acid; ↑ hgb, hct, platelets; NIPE: Caution w/ elderly & pts w/ h/o suicide ideations or depression; take without regard to food & swallow whole; ⊘ make up missed dose or take >3 doses in 24 h.

Acarbose (Precose) [Hypoglycemic/Alpha-glucosidase Inhibitor]

Uses: *Type 2 DM* Action: α-Glucosidase inhibitor; delays digestion of carbohydrates Dose: 25-100 mg PO tid (w/ 1st bite each meal) Caution: [B, ?] Avoid if CrCl <25 mL/min can affect digoxin levels Contra: IBD, cirrhosis Disp: Tabs 25, 50, 100 mg SE: Abdominal pain, D, flatulence, ↑ LFTs Notes: OK w/ sulfonylureas; LFTs q3mo for 1st y Interactions: ↑ Hypoglycemic effect w/ sulfonylureas, juniper berries, ginseng, garlic, coriander, celery; ↓ effects w/ intestinal absorbents, digestive enzyme preps, diuretics, corticosteroids, phenothiazines, estrogens, phenytoin, INH, sympathomimetics, CCBs, thyroid hormones; ↓ conc OF digoxin Labs: LFTs, FBS, HbA1c, LFTs, Hgb & Hct, monitor digoxin levels NIPE: Take drug tid w/ first bite of food, ↓ GI side effects by ↓ dietary starch, treat hypoglycemia w/ dextrose instead of sucrose, continue diet & exercise program

Acebutolol (Sectral) [Antihypertensive, Antiarrhythmic/ Beta Blocker]

Uses: *HTN, arrhythmias* angina Action: Competitively blocks β-adrenergic receptors, β₁, w/ ISA Dose: HTN: 200-800 mg/d; arrhythmia: 400–1200 mg/day in divided doses; ↓ if CrCl >50 mL/min Caution: [B, D in 2nd & 3rd tri, +] Can exacerbate ischemic heart Dz, do not D/C abruptly Contra: 2nd-, 3rd-degree heart block Disp: Caps 200, 400 mg SE: Fatigue, HA, dizziness, bradycardia Interactions: ↓ Antihypertensive effect w/ NSAIDs, salicylates, thyroid preps, anesthetics, antacids, α-adrenergic stimulants, ma-huang, ephedra, licorice; ↓ hypoglycemic effect OF glyburide; ↑ hypotensive response w/ other antihypertensives, nitrates, EtOH, diuretics, black cohosh, hawthorn, goldenseal, parsley; ↑ bradycardia w/ digoxin, amiodarone; ↑ hypoglycemic effect OF insulin Labs: Monitor lipids, uric acid, K⁺, FBS, LFTs, thyroxin, ECG NIPE: Teach pt to monitor BP, pulse, S/Sxs CHF

Acetaminophen [APAP, N-acetyl-p-aminophenol] (Tylenol, other generic) [OTC] [Analgesic, Antipyretic]

Uses: *Mild–moderate pain, HA, fever* Action: Nonnarcotic analgesic; ↓ CNS synthesis of prostaglandins & hypothalamic heat-regulating center Dose: *Adults.* 650 mg PO or PR q4–6h or 1000 mg PO q6h; max 4 g/24 h. *Peds.* <12 y. 10–15 mg/kg/dose PO or PR q4–6h; max 2.6 g/24 h. Quick dosing Table 1. Administer q6h if CrCl 10–50 mL/min & q8h if CrCl <10 mL/min Caution: [B, +] Hepatotoxic in elderly & w/

EtOH use w/ >4 g/day; alcoholic liver Dz **Contra:** G6PD deficiency **Disp:** Tabs meltaway/dissolving 160; Tabs: 325, 500, 650 mg; chew tabs 80, 160 mg; liq 100 mg/mL, 120 mg/2.5 mL, 120 mg/5 mL, 160 mg/5 mL, 167 mg/5 mL, 325 mg/5 mL, 500 mg/15 mL; 80 mg/0.8 mL supp 80, 120, 125, 325, 650 mg **SE:** OD causes hepatotox at 10 g dose; 15 g is potentially lethal Rx w/ *N*-acetylcysteine **Notes:** No antiinflammatory or plt-inhibiting action; **Interactions:** ↑ Hepatotoxicity w/ ETOH, barbiturates, carbamazepine, INH, rifampin, phenytoin; ↑ risk of bleeding w/ NSAIDs, salicylates, warfarin, feverfew, ginkgo biloba, red clover; ↓ absorption w/ antacids, cholestyramine, colestipol **Labs:** Monitor LFTs, CBC, BUN, creatinine, PT, INR; false ↑ urine 5-HIAA, urine glucose, serum uric acid; false ↓ serum glucose, amylase **NIPE:** Delayed absorption if given w/ food, ⊘ EtOH, teach S/Sxs hepatotoxicity, consult health provider if temp ↑103° F/>3 d

Acetaminophen + Butalbital ± Caffeine (Fioricet, Medigesic, Repan, Sedapap-10, Two-Dyne, Triapin, Axocet, Phrenilin Forte) [C-III] [Analgesic, Antipyretic/Barbiturate]

Uses: *Tension HA,* mild pain **Action:** Nonnarcotic analgesic w/ barbiturate **Dose:** 1-2 tabs or caps PO q4/6h PRN; ↓ in renal/hepatic impair; 4 g/24 h APAP max **Caution:** [C, D, +] Alcoholic liver Dz **Contra:** G6PD deficiency **Disp:** Caps Dolgic Plus butalbital 50 mg, caffeine 40 mg, APAP 750 mg; Caps Medigesic, Repan, Two-Dyne: butalbital 50 mg, caffeine 40 mg, + APAP 325 mg; Caps Axocet, Phrenilin Forte: butalbital 50 mg + APAP 650 mg; Caps: Esgic-Plus, Zebutral: butalbital 50 mg, caffeine 40 mg, APAP 500 mg; Liq. Dolgic LQ: butalbital 50 mg, caffeine 40 mg, APAP 325 mg/15 mL; Tabs Medigesic, Fioricet, Repan: butalbital 50 mg, caffeine 40 mg, APAP 325 mg; Phrenilin: butalbital 50 mg + APAP 325 mg; Sedapap-10: butalbital 50 mg + APAP 650 mg **SE:** Drowsiness, dizziness, "hangover" effect **Notes:** Butalbital habit-forming; avoid EtOH **Interactions:** ↑ Effects OF benzodiazepines, opioid analgesics, sedatives/hypnotics, ETOH, methylphenidate hydrochloride; ↓ effects OF MAOIs, TCAs, corticosteroids, theophylline, oral contraceptives, BBs, doxycycline **NIPE:** ⊘ EtOH & CNS depressants, may impair coordination, monitor for depression, use barrier-protection contraception

Acetaminophen + Codeine (Tylenol No. 3, No. 4) [Analgesic, Antipyretic/Opioid] [C-III, C-V]

Uses: *Mild-moderate pain (No. 3); moderate-severe pain (No. 4)* **Action:** Combined APAP & narcotic analgesic **Dose:** *Adults.* 1-2 tabs q3-4h PRN (max dose APAP = 4 g/d). *Peds.* APAP 10-15 mg/kg/dose; codeine 0.5-1 mg/kg dose q4-6h (dosing guide: 3-6 y, 5 mL/dose; 7-12 y, 10 mL/dose); ↓ in renal/hepatic impair **Caution:** [C, +] Alcoholic liver Dz **Contra:** G6PD deficiency **Disp:** Tabs 300 mg APAP + codeine; caps 325 mg APAP + codeine; susp (C-V) APAP 120 mg + codeine 12 mg/5 mL **SE:** Drowsiness, dizziness, N/V **Notes:** Codeine in No. 3 = 30 mg, No. 4 = 60 mg **Interactions:** ↑ Effects OF benzodiazepines, opioid analgesics, sedatives/hypnotics, EtOH, methylphenidate hydrochloride; ↓ effects OF MAOIs, TCAs, corticosteroids, theophylline, oral contraceptives, BBs, doxycycline **NIPE:** ⊘ EtOH &

CNS depressants, may impair coordination, monitor for depression, use barrier-protection contraception

Acetazolamide (Diamox) [Anticonvulsant, Diuretic/Carbonic Anhydrase Inhibitor]

Uses: *Diuresis, glaucoma, prevent high-altitude sickness, refractory epilepsy* **Action:** Carbonic anhydrase inhibitor; ↓ renal excretion of hydrogen & ↑ renal excretion of Na^+, K^+, HCO_3^-, & H_2O **Dose:** *Adults. Diuretic:* 250-375 mg IV or PO q24h. *Glaucoma:* 250–1000 mg PO q24h in ÷ doses. *Epilepsy:* 8–30 mg/kg/d PO in ÷ doses. *Altitude sickness:* 250 mg PO q8–12h or SR 500 mg PO q12–24h start 24–48 h before & 48 h after highest ascent. *Peds.* Epilepsy: 8–30 mg/kg/24 h PO in ÷ doses; max 1 g/d. *Diuretic:* 5 mg/kg/24 h PO or IV. *Alkalinization of urine:* 5 mg/kg/dose PO bid–tid. *Glaucoma:* 5–15 mg/kg/24 h PO in ÷ doses; max 1 g/d; adjust in renal impair; avoid if CrCl <10 mL/min **Caution:** [C, +] **Contra:** Renal/hepatic failure, sulfa allergy **Disp:** Tabs 125, 250 mg; SR caps 500 mg; inj 500 mg/vial, powder for reconstitution **SE:** Malaise, metallic taste, drowsiness, photosensitivity, hyperglycemia **Notes:** Follow Na^+ & K^+; watch for metabolic acidosis; SR forms not for epilepsy **Interactions:** Causes ↑ effects OF amphetamines, quinidine, procainamide, TCAs, ephedrine; ↓ effects OF Li, phenobarbital, salicylates, barbiturates; ↑ K^+ loss w/ corticosteroids and amphotericin B **Labs:** Monitor serum electrolytes, FBS, CBC, creatinine, intraocular pressure; false + for urinary protein, urinary urobilinogen; ↓ I uptake; ↑ serum and urine glucose, uric acid, Ca^{2+}, serum ammonia **NIPE:** ↓ GI distress w/ food, monitor for S/Sxs metabolic acidosis, ↑ fluid to ↓ risk of kidney stones

Acetic Acid & Aluminum Acetate (Otic Domeboro) [Astringent/Antiinfective]

Uses: *Otitis externa* **Action:** Antiinfective **Dose:** 4–6 gtt in ear(s) q2–3h **Caution:** [C, ?] **Contra:** Perforated tympanic membranes **Disp:** 2% otic soln **SE:** Local irritation **NIPE:** Burning w/ instillation or irrigation

Acetylcysteine (Acetadote, Mucomyst) [Mucolytic/Amino Acid Derivative]

Uses: *Mucolytic, antidote to APAP hepatotox * adjuvant Rx for chronic bronchopulmonary Dzs w/ CF;* **Action:** Splits disulfide linkages between mucoprotein molecular complexes; protects liver by restoring glutathione in APAP OD **Dose:** *Adults & Peds. Nebulizer:* 3–5 mL of 20% soln diluted w/ equal vol of H_2O or NS tid–qid. *Antidote:* PO or NG: 140 mg/load load, then 70 mg/kg q4h for 17 doses. (Dilute 1:3 in carbonated beverage or orange juice) *Acetadote:* load 150 mg/kg over 15 min, then 50 mg/kg over 4h, then 100 mg/kg over 16 h **Caution:** [C, ?] **Disp:** Soln inhaled and oral 10%, 20%; Acetadote IV soln 20% SG **SE:** Bronchospasm (inhal), N/V, drowsiness; anaphylactoid Rxns w/ IV **Notes:** Activated charcoal adsorbs acetylcysteine if given PO for APAP ingestion; start Rx for APAP overdose w/in 6–8 h **Interactions:** Discolors rubber, Fe, Cu, Ag; incompatible w/ multiple antibiotics—administer drugs separately **Labs:** Monitor ABGs & pulse oximetry w/ bronchospasm **NIPE:** Inform pt of ↑ productive cough, clear airway before aerosol administration, ↑ fluids to liquefy secretions, unpleasant odor will disappear & may cause N/V

Acitretin (Soriatane) [Retinoid] **WARNING:** Must not be used by females who are pregnant or intend to become pregnant during therapy or for up to 3 y following D/C of therapy; EtOH must not be ingested during therapy or for 2 mo following cessation of therapy; do not donate blood for 3 y following cessation **Uses:** *Severe psoriasis*; *other keratinization disorders (lichen planus, etc) **Action:** Retinoid-like activity **Dose:** 25–50 mg/d PO, w/ main meal; ↑ if no response by 4 wk to 75 mg/d **Caution:** [X, –] Renal/hepatic impair; in women of reproductive potential **Contra:** See Warning **Disp:** Caps 10, 25 mg **SE:** Cheilitis, skin peeling, alopecia, pruritus, rash, arthralgia, GI upset, photosensitivity, thrombocytosis, hypertriglyceridemia **Notes:** Follow LFTs and lipids; response often takes 2–3 mo; pt agreement/informed consent prior to use **Interactions:** ↑ ½ life w/ EtOH use, ↑ hepatotoxicity w/ MTX, ↓ effects OF progestin-only contraceptives **Labs:** Monitor LFTs, lipids, FBS, HbA1c **NIPE:** Use effective contraception; ⊘ donate blood for 3 y after Rx, teach pt S/Sxs pancreatitis

Acyclovir (Zovirax) [Antiviral/Synthetic Purine Nucleoside] **Uses:** *Herpes simplex & zoster Infxns* **Action:** Interferes w/ viral DNA synthesis **Dose:** *Adults.* PO: Initial genital herpes: 200 mg PO q4h while awake, 5 caps/d × 10 d or 400 mg PO tid × 7–10 d. *Chronic suppression:* 400 mg PO bid. *Intermittent Rx:* As for initial Rx, except treat for 5 d, or 800 mg PO bid at prodrome. *Herpes zoster:* 800 mg PO 5×/d for 7–10 d. *IV:* 5–10 mg/kg/dose IV q8h. *Topical: Initial herpes genitalis:* Apply q3h (6 times/d) for 7 d. *Peds.* 5–10 mg/kg/dose IV or PO q8h or 750 mg/m²/24 h ÷ q8h. *Chickenpox:* 20 mg/kg/dose PO qid; ↓ w/ CrCl <50 mL/min **Caution:** [B (PO & IV), C (topical), +] **Disp:** Caps 200 mg; tabs 400, 800 mg; susp 200 mg/5 mL; inj 500 mg/vial; 1000, injection soln 25 mg/mL, 50 mg/mL; oint 5% and cream 5% **SE:** Dizziness, lethargy, confusion, rash, inflammation at IV site **Notes:** PO better than topical for herpes genitalis **Interactions:** ↑ CNS SE w/ MTX & zidovudine, ↑ blood levels w/ probenecid **Labs:** Monitor BUN, SCr, LFTs, CBC **NIPE:** Start immediately w/ Sxs, ↑ hydration w/ IV dose, ↑ risk cervical cancer w/ genital herpes, ↑ length of Rx in immunocompromised pts

Adalimumab (Humira) [Antirheumatic/TNF Alpha Blocker] **WARNING:** Cases of TB have been observed; check TB skin test prior to use; Hepatitis B reactivation has also occurred **Uses:** *Moderate–severe RA w/ an inadequate response to one or more DMARDs* **Action:** TNF-α inhibitor **Dose:** 40 mg SQ qowk; may ↑ 40 mg qwk if not on MTX **Caution:** [B, ?/–] Serious Infxns & sepsis reported **Disp:** Prefilled 0.8 mL (40 mg) syringe **SE:** Inj site Rxns, serious Infxns, neurologic events, malignancies **Notes:** Refrigerate prefilled syringe, rotate inj sites, OK w/ other DMARDs **Interactions:** ↑ Effects w/ MTX **Labs:** May ↑ lipids, alkaline phosphatase **NIPE:** ⊘ exposure to infection; ⊘ admin live-virus vaccines

Adefovir (Hepsera) [Antiviral/Acyclic Nucleotide Analogue] **WARNING:** Acute exacerbations of hepatitis may occur following D/C therapy (monitor LFTs); chronic use may lead to nephrotox especially in pts w/ underlying renal impair (monitor renal Fxn); HIV resistance may emerge; lactic acidosis & severe hepatomegaly w/ steatosis reported when used alone or in combo w/ other antiretrovirals **Uses:** *Chronic active hepatitis B virus* **Action:** Nucleotide analog **Dose:** CrCl > 50 mL/min: 10 mg PO qd; CrCl 20–49 mL/min: 10 mg PO q48h; CrCl 10–19 mL/min: 10 mg PO q72h; HD: 10 mg PO q7d postdialysis; adjust w/ CrCl < 50 mL/min **Caution:** [C, –] **Disp:** Tabs 10 mg **SE:** Asthenia, HA, abdominal pain; see Warning **Interactions:** See Warning **Labs:** LFTs, BUN, creatinine, creatine kinase, amylase **NIPE:** Effects on fetus & baby not known—⊘ breastfeed; use barrier contraception

Adenosine (Adenocard) [Antiarrhythmic/Nucleoside] Uses: *PSVT;* including associated w/ WPW **Action:** Class IV antiarrhythmic; slows AV node conduction **Dose:** *Adults.* 6 mg IV bolus; may repeat in 1–2 min; max 12 mg IV. *Peds.* 0.05 mg/kg IV bolus; may repeat q1-2 min to 0.25 mg/kg max **Caution:** [C, ?] **Contra:** 2nd- or 3rd-degree AV block or SSS (w/o pacemaker); recent MI or cerebral hemorrhage **Disp:** Inj 3 mg/mL **SE:** Facial flushing, HA, dyspnea, chest pressure, ↓ BP **Notes:** Doses >12 mg not OK; can cause momentary asystole when administered; **Interactions:** ↓ Effects w/ theophylline, caffeine, guarana; ↑ effects w/ dipyridamole; ↑ risk OF hypotension & chest pain w/ nicotine; ↑ risk OF bradycardia w/ BBs; ↑ risk OF heart block w/ carbamazepine; ↑ risk OF ventricular fibrillation w/ digitalis glycosides **Labs:** Monitor ECG during administration **NIPE:** Monitor BP & pulse during therapy, monitor resp status—↑ risk of bronchospasm in asthmatics, discard unused or unclear soln

Albumin (Albuminar, Buminate, Albutein) [Plasma Volume Expander] Uses: *Plasma volume expansion for shock* (eg, burns, hemorrhage) **Action:** Maint of plasma colloid oncotic pressure **Dose:** *Adults.* Initial 25 g IV; subsequent dose based on response; 250 g/48h max. *Peds.* 0.5–1 g/kg/dose; inf at 0.05–0.1 g/min **Caution:** [C, ?] Severe anemia; cardiac, renal, or hepatic insuff due to added protein load & possible hypovolemia **Contra:** Cardiac failure **Disp:** Soln 5%, 25% **SE:** Chills, fever, CHF, tachycardia, ↓ BP, hypervolemia **Notes:** Contains 130–160 mEq Na+/L; may precipitate pulmonary edema **Interactions:** Atypical Rxns w/ ACEI—withhold 24 h prior to plasma administration **Labs:** ↑ Alkaline phosphatase; monitor Hmg, Hct, electrolytes, serum protein **NIPE:** Monitor BP & DC if hypotensive, monitor intake & output, admin to all blood types

Albuterol (Proventil, Ventolin, Volmax) [Bronchodilator/ Adrenergic] Uses: *Asthma; prevent exercise-induced bronchospasm* **Action:** β-adrenergic sympathomimetic bronchodilator; relaxes bronchial smooth muscle **Dose:** *Adults.* Inhaler: 2 inhal q4–6h PRN; 1 Rotacap inhal q4–6h. *PO:* 2–4 mg PO tid-qid. *Neb:* 1.25–5 mg (0.25–1 mL of 0.5% soln in 2–3 mL of NS) tid-qid. *Peds.* Inhaler: 2 inhal q4–6h. *PO:* 0.1–0.2 mg/kg/dose PO; max 2–4 mg PO tid; *Neb:* 0.05 mg/kg (max 2.5 mg) in 2–3 mL of NS tid-qid **Caution:** [C, +] **Disp:** Tabs 2, 4 mg; XR tabs 4, 8 mg; syrup 2 mg/5 mL; 90 mcg/dose met-dose inhaler; soln for neb 0.083, 0.5% **SE:** Palpitations, tachycardia, nervousness, GI upset **Interactions:** ↑ Effects w/ other sympathomimetics; ↑ CV effects w/ MAOI, TCA, inhaled anesthetics; ↓ effects w/ BBs; ↓ effectiveness OF insulin, oral hypoglycemics, digoxin **Labs:** Transient ↑ in serum glucose after inhalation; transient ↓ K+ after inhalation **NIPE:** Monitor HR, BP, ABGs, s&s bronchospasm & CNS stimulation; instruct on use of inhaler, must use as 1st inhaler, & rinse mouth after use

Albuterol & Ipratropium (Combivent) [Bronchodilator/Adrenergic, Anticholinergic]
Uses: *COPD* **Action:** Combo of β-adrenergic bronchodilator & quaternary anticholinergic **Dose:** 2 inhal qid; neb 3 mL q 6 h **Caution:** [C, +] **Contra:** Allergy to peanut/soybean **Disp:** Met-dose inhaler, 18 mcg ipratropium/103 mcg albuterol/puff; nebulization soln (DuoNeb) Ipratropium 0.5 mg Albuterol 2.5 mg/3 mL **SE:** Palpitations, tachycardia, nervousness, GI upset, dizziness, blurred vision **Interactions:** ↑ Effects w/ anticholinergics, including ophthalmic meds; ↓ effects w/ herb jaborandi tree, pill-bearing spurge **NIPE:** See Albuterol; may cause transient blurred vision/irritation or urinary changes

Aldesleukin [IL-2] (Proleukin) [Immunomodulator/Antineoplastic]
WARNING: Use restricted to pts w/ nl pulmonary & cardiac Fxn **Uses:** *Metastatic RCC, melanoma* **Action:** Acts via IL-2 receptor; numerous immunomodulatory effects **Dose:** 600,000 IU/kg q8h × 14 doses (FDA-approved dose/schedule for RCC). Multiple cont inf & alternate schedules (including "high dose" using 24×10^6 IU/m² IV q8h on days 1–5 & 12–16) **Caution:** [C, ?/–] **Contra:** Organ allografts **Disp:** Powder for reconstitution 22×10^6 IU, when reconstituted 18 million int units/mL = 1.1 mg/mL **SE:** Flu-like syndrome (malaise, fever, chills), N/V/D, ↑ bilirubin; capillary leak syndrome w/ ↓ BP, pulmonary edema, fluid retention, & weight gain; renal & mild hematologic tox (anemia, thrombocytopenia, leukopenia) & secondary eosinophilia; cardiac tox (ischemia, atrial arrhythmias); neurologic tox (CNS depression, somnolence, rarely coma, delirium). Pruritic rashes, urticaria, & erythroderma common. **Notes:** Cont inf less likely to cause severe ↓ BP & fluid retention **Interactions:** May ↑ toxicity OF cardiotoxic, hepatotoxic, myelotoxic, & nephrotoxic drugs; ↓ hypotension w/ antihypertensive drugs; ↓ effects w/ corticosteroids; acute Rxn w/ iodinated contrast media up to several months after inf; CNS effects w/ psychotropics **Labs:** May cause ↑ alkaline phosphatase, bilirubin, BUN, SCr, LFTs **NIPE:** Thoroughly explain serious SE of drug & that some SE are expected; ⊘ EtOH, NSAIDs, ASA

Alefacept (Amevive) [Antipsoriatic/Immunosuppressive]
WARNING: Must monitor CD4 before each dose; w/hold if <250; D/C if <250 × 1 month **Uses:** *Moderate/severe chronic plaque psoriasis* **Action:** Fusion protein inhibitor **Dose:** 7.5 mg IV or 15 mg IM once weekly × 12 wk **Caution:** [B, ?/–] PRG registry; associated w/ serious Infxn **Contra:** Lymphopenia **Disp:** 7.5-, 15-mg vials **SE:** Pharyngitis, myalgia, inj site Rxn, malignancy **Notes:** IV or IM different formulations; may repeat course 12 wk later if CD4 OK **Interactions:** No studies performed **Labs:** Monitor WBCs, CD4+ T lymphocyte counts **NIPE:** ↑ Risk of infection; ⊘ exposure to infections; inj site inflammation; rotate sites

Alendronate (Fosamax, Fosamax Plus D) [Antiosteoporotic]
Uses: *Rx & prevention of osteoporosis, Rx of steroid-induced osteoporosis & Paget Dz* **Action:** ↓ nl & abnormal bone resorption **Dose:** *Osteoporosis: Rx:* 10 mg/d PO or 70 mg qwk; Fosamax plus D 1 tab qwk. *Steroid-induced osteoporosis: Rx:* 5 mg/d PO. *Prevention:* 5 mg/d PO or 35 mg qwk. *Paget Dz:* 40 mg/d PO **Caution:** [C, ?] Not OK if CrCl <35 mL/min, w/NSAID use **Contra:** Esophageal anomalies, inability to sit/stand upright for 30 min, ↓ Ca^{2+} **Disp:** Tabs 5, 10, 35, 40, 70 mg, soln 70 mg/75 mL, Fosamax plus D Alendronate 70 mg and cholecalciferol 2800 int units **SE:** GI disturbances, HA, pain, jaw osteonecrosis (w/ dental procedures, chemo) **Notes:** Take 1st thing in AM w/ H$_2$O (8 oz) > 30 min before 1st food/beverage of the day. Do not lie down for 30 min after. Ca^{2+} & vitamin D supl necessary for regular tab **Interactions:** ↓ Absorption w/ antacids, Ca suppls, Fe, food; ↑ risk of upper GI bleed w/ ASA & NSAIDs **Labs:** May cause transient ↑ serum Ca & phosphate **NIPE:** Adequate Ca & vitamin D suppl needed, ↓ weight-bearing activity, ↓ smoking, EtOH use

Alfentanil (Alfenta) [Narcotic Analgesic] [C-II]
Uses: *Adjunct in the maint of anesthesia; analgesia* **Action:** Short-acting narcotic analgesic **Dose:** *Adults & Peds >12 y.* 3–75 mcg/kg (IBW) IV inf; total depends on duration of procedure **Caution:** [C, +/–] ↑ ICP, resp depression **Disp:** Inj 500 mcg/mL **SE:** Bradycardia, ↓ BP arrhythmias, peripheral vasodilation, ↑ ICP, drowsiness, resp depression **Interactions:** ↓ Effect w/ phenothiazines; ↑ effects w/ BBs, CNS depressants, erythromycin **NIPE:** Monitor HR, BP, resp rate

Alfuzosin (Uroxatral) [Selective Alpha Adrenergic Antagonist]
WARNING: May prolong QTc interval **Uses:** *BPH* **Action:** α-Blocker **Dose:** 10 mg PO daily immediately after the same meal **Caution:** [B, –] **Contra:** w/ CYP3A4 inhibitors; moderate–severe hepatic impair **Disp:** Tabs 10 mg **SE:** Postural ↓ BP, dizziness, HA, fatigue **Notes:** XR tablet—do not cut or crush; fewest reports of ejaculatory disorders compared w/ other drugs in class **Interactions:** ↑ Effects w/ atenolol, azole antifungals, cimetidine, ritonavir; ↑ effects OF antihypertensives **NIPE:** Not indicated for use in women or children; take w/ food; ↑ risk of postural hypotension; ⊘ take other meds that prolong QT interval

Alginic Acid + Aluminum Hydroxide & Magnesium Trisilicate (Gaviscon) [Antacid] [OTC]
Uses: *Heartburn*; pain from hiatal hernia **Action:** Protective layer blocks gastric acid **Dose:** 2–4 tabs or 15–30 mL PO qid followed by H$_2$O; **Caution:** [B, –] Avoid in renal impair or Na$^+$-restricted diet **Disp:** Tabs, susp **SE:** D, constipation **Interactions:** ↓ Absorption of tetracyclines

Alglucosidase alfa (Myozyme) [Recombinant Acid Alpha-glucosidase]
WARNING: Life-threatening anaphylactic Rxns have occurred w/ infusion; appropriate medical support measures should be immediately available **Uses:** *Rx Pompe DZ* **Action:** Recombinant acid alpha-glucosidase; degrades glycogen in lysosomes **Dose:** 20 mg/kg IV q 2 wks over 4 h (see labeling

for details) **Caution:** [B,?/–] Illness at time of inf may ↑ inf Rxns **Disp:** Powder 50 mg/vial **SE:** Hypersensitivity, fever, rash, D, V, gastroenteritis, pneumonia, URI, cough, respiratory distress, inf Rxns, cardiorespiratory failure, cardiac arrhythmia w/ general anesthesia

Allopurinol (Zyloprim, Lopurin, Aloprim) [Xanthine Oxidase Inhibitor] Uses: *Gout, hyperuricemia of malignancy, uric acid urolithiasis* **Action:** Xanthine oxidase inhibitor; ↓ uric acid production **Dose:** *Adults.* PO: Initial 100 mg/d; usual 300 mg/d; max 800 mg/d. *IV:* 200–400 mg/m^2/d (max 600 mg/24 h); take after meal w/ plenty of fluid *Peds.* Only for hyperuricemia of malignancy if <10 y: 10 mg/kg/24 h PO or 200 mg/m^2/d IV ÷ q6–8h (max 600 mg/24 h); ↓ in renal impair **Caution:** [C, M] **Disp:** Tabs 100, 300 mg; inj 500 mg/30 mL (Aloprim) **SE:** Skin rash, N/V, renal impair, angioedema **Notes:** Aggravates acute gout; begin after acute attack resolves; IV dose of 6 mg/mL final conc as single daily inf or ÷ 6-, 8-, or 12-h intervals **Interactions:** ↑ Effect OF theophylline, oral anticoagulants; ↑ hypersensitivity Rxns w/ ACEIs, thiazide diuretics; ↑ risk of rash w/ ampicillin/amoxicillin; ↑ bone marrow depression w/ cyclophosphamide, azathioprine, mercaptopurine; ↓ effects w/ EtOH **Labs:** ↑ Alkaline phosphatase, bilirubin, LFTs **NIPE:** ↑ fluids to 2–3 L/day, take pc, may ↑ drowsiness

Almotriptan (Axert) [Serotonin 5-HT1 Receptor Agonist] See Table 11

Alosetron (Lotronex) [Selective 5-HT3 Receptor Antagonist] **WARNING:** Serious GI side effects, some fatal, including ischemic colitis reported. May be prescribed only through participation in the prescribing program for Lotronex **Uses:** *Severe diarrhea-predominant IBS in women who fail conventional therapy* **Action:** Selective 5-HT$_3$ receptor antagonist **Dose:** *Adults.* 1 mg PO qd × 4 wk; titrate to 1 mg bid max; D/C after 4 wk at max dose if Sxs not controlled **Caution:** [B, ?/–] **Contra:** Hx chronic/severe constipation, GI obstruction, strictures, toxic megacolon, GI perforation, adhesions, ischemic colitis, Crohn Dz, ulcerative colitis, diverticulitis, thrombophlebitis, or hypercoagulable state. **Disp:** Tabs 0.5, 1 mg **SE:** Constipation, abdominal pain, nausea **Notes:** D/C immediately if constipation or Sxs of ischemic colitis develop; pt must sign informed consent prior to use "patient–health provider agreement" **Interactions:** ↑ Risk constipation w/ other drugs that ↓ GI motility, inhibits *N*-acetyltransferase & may influence metabolism of INH, procainamide, hydralazine **NIPE:** Administer w/o regard to food, eval effectiveness >4 w

Alpha₁-Protease Inhibitor (Prolastin) [Alpha Protease Inhibitor Replacement/Respiratory agent] Uses: *α₁-Antitrypsin deficiency*; panacinar emphysema **Action:** Replace human α₁-protease inhibitor **Dose:** 60 mg/kg IV once/wk **Caution:** [C, ?] **Contra:** Selective IgA deficiencies w/ known IgA antibodies **Disp:** Inj 500 mg/20 mL, 1000 mg/40 mL powder for inj **SE:** Fever, dizziness, flu-like Sxs, allergic Rxns **NIPE:** Infuse over 30 min, ⊘ mix w/ other drugs, use w/in 3 h of reconstitution

Alprazolam (Xanax, Niravam) [Anxiolytic/Benzodiazepine] [C-IV]

Uses: *Anxiety & panic disorders,* anxiety w/ depression Action: Benzodiazepine; antianxiety agent Dose: *Anxiety:* Initial, 0.25–0.5 mg tid; ↑ to a max of 4 mg/d in ÷ doses. *Panic:* Initial, 0.5 mg tid; may gradually ↑ to response; ↓ in elderly, debilitated, & hepatic impair Caution: [D, –] Contra: NA glaucoma, concomitant itra-/ketoconazole Disp: Tabs 0.25, 0.5, 1, 2 mg; Xanax XR 0.5, 1, 2, 3 mg; Niravam (orally disintegrating tabs) 0.25, 0.5, 1, 2 mg; soln 1 mg/mL SE: Drowsiness, fatigue, irritability, memory impair, sexual dysfunction Notes: Avoid abrupt D/C after prolonged use Interactions: ↑ CNS depression w/ EtOH, other CNS depressants, narcotics, MAOIs, anesthetics, antihistamines, theophylline, & herbs: kava kava, valerian; ↑ effect w/ oral contraceptives, cimetidine, INH, disulfiram, omeprazole, valproic acid, ciprofloxacin, erythromycin, clarithromycin, phenytoin, verapamil, grapefruit juice; ↑ risk OF ketoconazole, itraconazole, & digitalis toxicity, ↓ effectiveness OF levodopa; ↓ effect w/ carbamazepine, rifampin, rifabutin, barbiturates, cigarette smoking Labs: ↑ Alkaline phosphatase, may cause ↓ Hct & neutropenia NIPE: Monitor for resp depression

Alprostadil [Prostaglandin E₁] (Prostin VR) [Prostaglandin]

Uses: *Conditions where blood flow must be maintained in ductus arteriosus* sustain pulmonary/systemic circulation until surgery (eg, pulmonary atresia/stenosis, tricuspid atresia, transposition, severe tetralogy of Fallot) Action: Vasodilator, plt inhibitor; ductus arteriosus smooth muscle is especially sensitive Dose: 0.05 mcg/kg/min IV; ↓ to lowest that maintains response Caution: [X, –] Contra: Neonatal resp distress syndrome Disp: Inj 500 mcg/mL SE: Cutaneous vasodilation, Sz-like activity, jitteriness, ↑ temp, ↓ Ca^{2+}, apnea, thrombocytopenia, ↓ BP; may cause apnea Notes: Keep intubation kit at bedside Interactions: ↑ Effects OF anticoagulants & antihypertensives, ↓ effects OF cyclosporine Labs: ↑ fibrinogen NIPE: Dilute drug before administration, refrigerate & discard >24 h, apnea & bradycardia indicates drug overdose, central line preferred, flushing indicates catheter malposition

Alprostadil, Intracavernosal (Caverject, Edex) [Prostaglandin/GU agent]

Uses: *Erectile dysfunction* Action: Relaxes smooth muscles, dilates cavernosal arteries, ↑ lacunar spaces and blood entrapment by compressing venules against tunica Caution: [X, –] Contra: Predisposition to priapism (eg, sickle cell); penile deformities/implants; men in whom sexual activity is inadvisable Disp: *Caverject:* 5, 10, 20, 40 mcg vials ± diluent syringes. *Caverject Impulse:* Self-contained syringe (29 gauge) 10 & 20 mcg. *Edex:* 10, 20, 40 mcg cartridges SE: Local pain w/ injection Notes: Counsel about priapism, penile fibrosis, & hematoma risks, titrate w/ Obs Interactions: ↑ Effects OF anticoagulants & antihypertensives, ↓ effects OF cyclosporine Labs: ↑ Fibrinogen NIPE: Vaginal itching and burning in female partners, ⊘ inj >3×/wk or closer than 24 h/dose

Alprostadil, Urethral Suppository (Muse) [Prostaglandin/GU agent]

Uses: *Erectile dysfunction* Action: Urethral mucosal

absorption; vasodilator, smooth muscle relaxant of corpus cavernosa **Dose:** 125–1000 mcg system 5–10 min prior to sexual activity; titrate at health provider's office **Caution:** [X, –] **Contra:** Predisposition to priapism (eg, sickle cell) penile deformities/implants; men in whom sexual activity is inadvisable **Disp:** 125, 250, 500, 1000 mcg w/ a transurethral delivery system **SE:** ↓ BP, dizziness, syncope, penile/testicular pain, urethral burning/bleeding, priapism **Notes:** Supervision, titrate w/ Obs **Interactions:** ↑ Effects OF anticoagulants & antihypertensives, ↓ effects OF cyclosporine **Labs:** ↓ Fibrinogen; **NIPE:** No more than 2 supp/24 h, urinate prior to use

Alteplase, Recombinant [tPA] (Activase) [Thrombolytic Enzyme]   **Uses:** *AMI, PE, acute ischemic stroke, & CV cath occlusion* **Action:** Thrombolytic; binds to fibrin in the thrombus, initiates fibrinolysis **Dose:** *AMI & PE:* 100 mg IV over 3 h (10 mg over 2 min, then 50 mg over 1 h, then 40 mg over 2 h). *Stroke:* 0.9 mg/kg (max 90 mg) inf over 60 min. *Cath occlusion:* 10–29 kg 1 mg/mL; = 30 kg 2 mg/mL **Caution:** [C, ?] **Contra:** Active internal bleeding; uncontrolled HTN (systolic BP = > 185 mm Hg/diastolic = > 110 mm Hg); recent (w/in 3 mo) CVA, GI bleed, trauma, surgery, prolonged external cardiac massage; intracranial neoplasm, suspected aortic dissection, AVM/aneurysm/subarachnoid hemorrhage, bleeding/hemostatic defects, Sz at the time of stroke **Disp:** Powder for inj 50, 100 mg **SE:** Bleeding, bruising (eg, venipuncture sites), ↓ BP **Notes:** Give heparin to prevent reocclusion; in AMI, doses of >150 mg associated w/ intracranial bleeding **Interactions:** ↑ Risk of bleeding w/ heparin, ASA, NSAIDs, abciximab, dipyridamole, eptifibatide, tirofiban; ↓ effects w/ nitroglycerine **Labs:** ↓ Fibrinogen **NIPE:** Compress venipuncture site at least 30 min, monitor PT/PTT, bed rest during inf

Altretamine (Hexalen) [Antineoplastic/Alkylating Agent]   **Uses:** *Epithelial ovarian CA* **Action:** Unknown; cytotoxic agent, unknown alkylating agent; ↓ nucleotide incorporation into DNA/RNA **Dose:** 260 mg/m²/d in 4 ÷ doses for 14–21 d of a 28-d Rx cycle; dose ↑ to 150 mg/m²/d for 14 d in multiagent regimens (Per protocols); after meals and at bedtime **Caution:** [D, ?/–]. **Contra:** Preexisting BM depression or neurologic tox **Disp:** Caps 50 mg **SE:** V/D, cramps; neurologic (peripheral neuropathy, CNS depression); minimally myelosuppressive **Interactions:** ↑ Effect w/ phenobarbital, ↑ antibody response w/ live virus vaccines, ↑ risk of toxicity w/ cimetidine & hypotension w/ MAOIs, ↑ bone marrow depression w/ radiation **Labs:** ↑ Alkaline phosphatase, BUN, & SCr **NIPE:** Use barrier contraception, take w/ food, monitor CBC

Aluminum Hydroxide (Amphojel, AlternaGEL) [OTC] [Antacid/Aluminum salt]   **Uses:** *Relief of heartburn, upset or sour stomach, or acid indigestion*; supl to Rx of hyperphosphatemia **Action:** Neutralizes gastric acid; binds PO₄⁻² **Dose:** *Adults.* 10-30 mL or 300–1200 mg PO q4–6h. *Peds.* 5–15 mL PO q4–6h or 50–150 mg/kg/24 h PO q4–6h (hyperphosphatemia) **Caution:** [C, ?] **Disp:** Tabs 300, 600 mg; chew tabs 500 mg; susp 320, 600 mg/5 mL **SE:** constipation **Notes:** OK in renal failure **Interactions:** ↓ Absorption & effects OF allopurinol, benzodiazepines, corticosteroids, chloroquine, cimetidine, digoxin, INH, phenytoin, quinolones, ranitidine, tetracycline **Labs:** ↑ Serum gastrin, ↓ serum phosphate **NIPE:** Separate other drug administration by 2 h, ↑ effectiveness of liquid form

Aluminum Hydroxide + Magnesium Carbonate (Gaviscon Extra Strength, Liquid) [OTC] [Antacid/aluminum & magnesium salts] Uses: *Relief of heartburn, acid indigestion* **Action:** Neutralizes gastric acid **Dose:** *Adults.* 15–30 mL PO pc & hs. *Peds.* 5–15 mL PO qid or PRN; avoid in renal impair **Caution:** ↑ Mg²⁺ (w/ renal insuff) [C, ?] **Disp:** Liq w/ aluminum hydroxide 95 mg + magnesium carbonate 358 mg/15 mL; Extra Strength liq AlOH 254 mg/Mg carbonate 237 mg/15 mL; chew tabs AlOH 160 mg/Mg carb 105 mg **SE:** Constipation, D **Notes:** Doses qid are best given pc & hs; may affect absorption of some drugs **Interactions:** In addition to Al hydroxide ↓ effects OF histamine blockers, hydantoins, nitrofurantoin, phenothiazines, ticlopidine, ↑ effects OF quinidine, sulfonylureas **NIPE:** ⊘ Concurrent drug use & separate by 2–3 h, ↑ fiber

Aluminum Hydroxide + Magnesium Hydroxide (Maalox) [OTC] [Antacid/aluminum & magnesium salts] Uses: *Hyperacidity* (peptic ulcer, hiatal hernia, etc) **Action:** Neutralizes gastric acid **Dose:** *Adults.* 10–20 mL or 2–4 tabs PO qid or PRN. *Peds.* 5–15 mL PO qid or PRN **Caution:** [C, ?] **Disp:** Tabs, susp **SE:** May cause ↑ Mg²⁺ in renal insuff, constipation, D **Notes:** Doses qid best given pc & hs **Interactions:** In addition to Al hydroxide, ↓ effects OF digoxin, quinolines, phenytoin, Fe suppl, and ketoconazole **NIPE:** ⊘ Concurrent drug use; separate by 2 h

Aluminum Hydroxide + Magnesium Hydroxide & Simethicone (Mylanta, Mylanta II, Maalox Plus) [OTC] [Antacid/aluminum & magnesium salts] Uses: *Hyperacidity w/ bloating* **Action:** Neutralizes gastric acid & defoaming **Dose:** *Adults.* 10–20 mL or 2–4 tabs PO qid or PRN. *Peds.* 5–15 mL PO qid or PRN; avoid in renal impair **Caution:** [C, ?] **Disp:** Tabs, susp, liquid **SE:** ↑ Mg²⁺ in renal insuff, D, constipation **Notes:** Mylanta II contains 2X aluminum & magnesium hydroxide of Mylanta; may affect absorption of some drugs **Interactions:** In addition to Al hydroxide, ↓ effects OF digoxin, quinolones, phenytoin, Fe suppl, and ketoconazole **NIPE:** ⊘ Concurrent drug use; separate by 2 h

Aluminum Hydroxide + Magnesium Trisilicate (Gaviscon, Regular Strength) [OTC] [Antacid/aluminum & magnesium salts] Uses: *Relief of heartburn, upset or sour stomach, or acid indigestion* **Action:** Neutralizes gastric acid **Dose:** Chew 2–4 tabs qid; avoid in renal impair **Caution:** [C, ?] **Contra:** Mg²⁺, sensitivity **Disp:** *Gaviscon:* Aluminum hydroxide 80 mg & magnesium trisilicate 20 mg; **SE:** ↑ Mg²⁺ in renal insuff, constipation, D **Notes:** May affect absorption of some drugs **Interactions:** In addition to Al hydroxide, ↓ effects OF digoxin, quinolines, phenytoin, Fe suppl, and ketoconazole **NIPE:** ⊘ Concurrent drug use; separate by 2 h

Amantadine (Symmetrel) [Antiviral, Antiparkinsonian]

Uses: *Rx or prophylaxis influenza A, parkinsonism, & drug-induced EPS (Note: Do not use for Influenza A in the US due to increased resistance)* **Action:** Prevents release of infectious viral nucleic acid into host cell; releases dopamine from intact dopaminergic terminals **Dose:** *Adults.* Influenza A: 200 mg/d PO or 100 mg PO bid. *Parkinsonism:* 100 mg PO qd–bid. *Peds.* 1–9 y: 4.4–8.8 mg/kg/24 h to 150 mg/24 h max % doses daily–bid. *10–12 y:* 100–200 mg/d in 1–2 % doses; ↓ in renal impair **Caution:** [C, M] **Disp:** Caps 100 mg; tabs 100 mg; soln 50 mg/5 mL **SE:** Orthostatic ↓ BP, edema, insomnia, depression, irritability, hallucinations, dream abnormalities **Interactions:** ↑ Effects w/ HCTZ, triamterene, amiloride, pheasant's eye herb, scopolia root, benztropine **Labs:** ↑ BUN, SCr, CPK, alkaline phosphatase, bilirubin, LDH, AST, ALT **NIPE:** ⊘ Discontinue abruptly, take at least 4 h before sleep if insomnia occurs, eval for mental status changes, take w/ meals, ⊘ EtOH

Amifostine (Ethyol) [Antidote]

Uses: *Xerostomia prophylaxis during RT (head, neck, ovarian, non-small-cell lung CA). ↓ renal tox associated w/ repeated administration of cisplatin* **Action:** Prodrug, dephosphorylated by alkaline phosphatase to active thiol metabolite **Dose:** 910 mg/m²/d 15-min IV inf 30 min prior to chemo **Caution:** [C, +/–] **Disp:** 500 mg vials powder, reconstitute in sterile NS **SE:** Transient ↓ BP (>60%), N/V, flushing w/ hot or cold chills, dizziness, ↓ Ca²⁺, somnolence, sneezing. **Notes:** Does not reduce the effectiveness of cyclophosphamide plus cisplatin chemo **Interactions:** ↑ Effects w/ antihypertensives **Labs:** ↓ Calcium levels **NIPE:** Monitor BP, ensure adequate hydration, infuse over 15 min w/pt supine

Amikacin (Amikin) [Antibiotic/Aminoglycoside]

Uses: *Serious gram(–) bacterial Infxns* & mycobacteria **Action:** Aminoglycoside; ↓ protein synthesis *Spectrum:* Good gram(–) bacterial coverage: *Pseudomonas* sp; *Mycobacterium* sp **Dose:** *Adults & Peds.* 5–7.5 mg/kg/dose q 8 h, once daily: 15—20 mg/kg q 24 h based on renal Fxn; % interval w/ renal impair. *Neonates <1200 g, 0–4 wk:* 7.5 mg/kg/dose q12h–18h. *Postnatal age <7 d, 1200–2000 g:* 7.5 mg/kg/dose q12h; *>2000 g:* 10 mg/kg/dose q12h. *Postnatal age >7 d, 1200–2000 g:* 7 mg/kg/dose q8h; *>2000 g:* 7.5–10 mg/kg/dose q8h **Caution:** [C, +/–] avoid use w/ diuretics **Disp:** Inj 50 mg/mL, 250 mg/mL **SE:** Nephro/oto/neurotox; **Notes:** May be effective in gram(–) bacteria resistant to gentamicin & tobramycin; monitor renal Fxn & levels for dosage adjustments; (Table 2) **Interactions:** ↑ Risk OF ototoxicity and nephrotoxicity w/ acyclovir, amphotericin B, cephalosporins, cisplatin, loop diuretics, methoxyflurane, polymyxin B, vancomycin; ↑ neuromuscular blocking effect w/muscle relaxants & anesthetics **Labs:** ↑ BUN, SCr, AST, ALT, serum alkaline phosphatase, bilirubin, LDH **NIPE:** ↑ Fluid consumption

Amiloride (Midamor) [Potassium Sparing Diuretic]

Uses: *HTN, CHF, & thiazide-induced ↓ K⁺* **Action:** K⁺-sparing diuretic; interferes w/K+/Na+ exchange in distal tubule **Dose:** *Adults.* 5–10 mg PO daily. *Peds.* 0.625 mg/kg/d; ↓ in renal impair **Caution:** [B, ?] **Contra:** ↑ K+, SCr > 1.5, BUN > 30 **Disp:** Tabs 5 mg **SE:** ↑ K+ possible; HA, dizziness, dehydration, impotence **Notes:** monitor K+; **Interactions:** ↑ Risk OF hyperkalemia w/ ACE-I, K-sparing diuretics, NSAIDs, & K salt substitutes; ↑ effects OF Li, digoxin, antihypertensives, amantadine; ↑ risk OF hypokalemia w/ licorice **NIPE:** Take w/ food, I&O, daily weights, ⊘ salt substitutes, bananas, & oranges

Aminocaproic Acid (Amicar) [Antithrombotic Agent] Uses: *Excessive bleeding from systemic hyperfibrinolysis & urinary fibrinolysis* **Action:** ↓ fibrinolysis via inhibition of TPA substances **Dose:** *Adults.* 5 g IV or PO (1st hr) followed by 1—1.25 g/h IV or PO (max dose/d: 30 g) *Peds.* 100 mg/kg IV (1st h) then 1 g/m²/h; max 18 g/m²/d; ↓ in renal failure **Caution:** [C, ?] Upper urinary tract bleeding **Contra:** DIC **Disp:** Tabs 500 mg, 1000 mg; syrup 250 mg/mL; inj 250 mg/mL **SE:** ↓ BP, bradycardia, dizziness, HA, fatigue, rash, GI disturbance, ↓ plt Fxn **Notes:** Administer for 8 h or until bleeding controlled; not for upper urinary tract bleeding **Interactions:** ↑ Coagulation w/ estrogens & oral contraceptives **Labs:** ↑ K+ levels, false ↑ urine amino acids **NIPE:** Creatine kinase monitoring w/ long-term use, eval for thrombophlebitis & difficulty urinating

Amino-Cerv pH 5.5 Cream [Cervical Hydrating Agent] Uses: *Mild cervicitis,* postpartum cervicitis/cervical tears, postcauterization, postcryosurgery, & postconization **Action:** Hydrating agent; removes excess keratin in hyperkeratotic conditions **Dose:** 1 Applicatorful intravag hs for 2–4 wk **Caution:** [C, ?] Use in viral skin Infxn **Disp:** Vaginal cream **SE:** Transient stinging, local irritation **Notes:** AKA carbamide or urea; contains 8.34% urea, 0.5% sodium propionate, 0.83% methionine, 0.35% cystine, 0.83% inositol, & benzalkonium chloride

Aminoglutethimide (Cytadren) [Adrenal Steroid Inhibitor] Uses: *Cushing syndrome* Adrenocortical carcinoma, * breast CA & CAP **Action:** ↓ adrenal steroidogenesis & conversion of androgens to estrogens **Dose:** 750–1500 mg/d in divided doses w/ hydrocortisone 20–40 mg/d; ↓ in renal insuff **Caution:** [D, ?] **Disp:** Tabs 250 mg **SE:** Adrenal insuff ("medical adrenalectomy"), hypothyroidism, masculinization, ↓ BP, vomiting, rare hepatotox, rash, myalgia, fever **Interactions:** ↓ Effects w/ dexamethasone & hydrocortisone, ↓ effects OF warfarin, theophylline, medroxyprogesterone **NIPE:** Masculinization reversible after DC drug, ⊘ PRG

Aminophylline [Bronchodilator/Xanthine Derivative] Uses: *Asthma, COPD* & bronchospasm **Action:** Relaxes smooth muscle (bronchi, pulmonary vessels); stimulates diaphragm **Dose:** *Adults.* Acute asthma: Load 6 mg/kg IV, then 0.4–0.9 mg/kg/h IV cont inf. *Chronic asthma:* 24 mg/kg/24 h PO or PR % q6h. *Peds.* Load 6 mg/kg IV, then 1 mg/kg/h IV cont inf; ↓ in hepatic insuff & w/ certain drugs (macrolide & quinolone antibiotics, cimetidine, & propranolol) **Caution:** [C, +] Uncontrolled arrhythmias/Sz disorder, hyperthyroidism, peptic ulcers **Disp:** Tabs 100, 200 mg; soln 105 mg/5 mL, 90 mg/5 mL; supp 250, 500 mg; inj

25 mg/mL **SE:** N/V, irritability, tachycardia, ventricular arrhythmias, Szs **Notes:** Individualize dosage; follow levels (as theophylline, Table 2); aminophylline ↓ Effects OF Li, phenytoin, adenosine; ↓ effects w/ phenobarbital, aminoglutethamide, barbiturates, rifampin, ritonavir, thyroid meds; ↑ effects w/ cimetidine, ciprofloxacin, erythromycin, INH, oral contraceptives, verapamil, tobacco, charcoal-broiled foods, St. John's wort **Labs:** ↑ Uric acid levels, falsely ↑ levels w/ furosemide, probenecid, acetaminophen, coffee, tea, cola, chocolate **NIPE:** ⊘ Chew or crush time-released capsules & take on empty stomach, immediate release can be taken w/ food, ↑ fluids 2 L/d, tobacco ↓ drug elimination

Amiodarone (Cordarone, Pacerone) [Ventricular Antiarrhythmic]

Uses: *Recurrent VF or hemodynamically unstable VT,* supraventricular arrhythmias, AF **Action:** Class III antiarrhythmic Table 12) **Dose:** *Adults.* Ventricular arrhythmias: IV: 15 mg/min for 10 min, then 1 mg/min for 6 h, then maint 0.5 mg/min cont. inf or *PO:* Load: 800–1600 mg/d PO for 1–3 wk. Maint: 600–800 mg/d PO for 1 mo, then 200–400 mg/d. *Supraventricular arrhythmias: IV:* 300 mg IV over 1 h, then 20 mg/kg for 24 h, then 600 mg PO qd for 1 wk, then maint 100–400 mg qd or *PO:* Load: 600–800 mg/d PO for 1–4 wk. Maint: Gradually ↓ to 100–400 mg q day. *Peds.* 10–15 mg/kg/24 h ÷ q12h PO for 7–10 d, then 5 mg/kg/24 h ÷ q12h or daily (infants/neonates require higher loading); ↓ in liver insuff **Caution:** [D, –] **Contra:** Sinus node dysfunction, 2nd- or 3rd-degree AV block, sinus bradycardia (w/o pacemaker) **Disp:** Tabs 100, 200, 400 mg; inj 50 mg/mL **SE:** Pulmonary fibrosis, exacerbation of arrhythmias, prolongs QT interval; CHF, hypo-/hyperthyroidism, ↑ LFTs, liver failure, corneal microdeposits, optic neuropathy/neuritis, peripheral neuropathy, photosensitivity **Notes:** Half-life 53 d; IV conc of >0.2 mg/mL via a central catheter; may require ↓ digoxin dose and warfarin dose **Interactions:** ↑ Serum levels OF digoxin, quinidine, procainamide, flecainide, phenytoin, warfarin, theophylline, cyclosporine; ↑ levels w/ cimetidine, indinavir, ritonavir; ↓ levels w/ cholestyramine, rifampin, St. John's wort; ↑ cardiac effects w/ BBs, CCB **Labs:** ↑ T_4 & RT_3, ANA titer, ↓ T_3 **NIPE:** Monitor cardiac rhythm, BP, LFTs, thyroid Fxn, ophthalmologic exam; ↑ photosensitivity—use sunscreen; take w/ food

Amitriptyline (Elavil) [Antidepressant/TCA]

WARNING: Antidepressants may (up) risk of suicidality; consider risks and benefits of use. Monitor patients closely **Uses:** * Depression,* peripheral neuropathy, chronic pain, tension HAs **Action:** TCA; ↓ reuptake of serotonin & norepinephrine by presynaptic neurons **Dose:** *Adults.* Initial, 30–50 mg PO hs; may ↑ to 300 mg hs. *Peds.* Not OK <12 y unless for chronic pain; initial 0.1 mg/kg PO hs, ↑ over 2–3 wk to 0.5–2 mg/kg PO hs; taper when D/C **Caution:** [D, +/–] NA glaucoma, hepatic impair **Contra:** W/ MAOIs, during acute MI recovery **Disp:** Tabs 10, 25, 50, 75, 100, 150 mg; inj 10 mg/mL **SE:** Strong anticholinergic SEs; OD may be fatal; urine retention, sedation, ECG changes, photosensitivity **Interactions:** ↓ Effects w/ carbamazepine, phenobarbital, rifampin, cholestyramine, colestipol, tobacco; ↑ effects w/ cimetidine, quinidine, indinavir, ritonavir, CNS depressants, SSRIs, haloperidol, oral contraceptives, BBs, phenothiazines, EtOH, evening primrose oil; ↑ effects OF amphetamines, anticholinergics, epinephrine, hypoglycemics, phenylephrine **Labs:** ↑ Glucose, false ↑ carbamazepine levels **NIPE:** ↑ Photosensitivity—use sunscreen, appetite, & craving for sweets, ⊘ DC abruptly, may turn urine blue-green

Amlodipine (Norvasc) [Antihypertensive, Antianginal/CCB]
Uses: *HTN, stable or unstable angina* **Action:** CCB; relaxes coronary vascular smooth muscle **Dose:** 2.5–10 mg/d PO; Ø w/ hepatic impair **Caution:** [C, ?] **Disp:** Tabs 2.5, 5, 10 mg **SE:** Peripheral edema, HA, palpitations, flushing **Notes:** Take w/o regard to meals **Interactions:** ↑ Effect OF hypotension w/ antihypertensives, fentanyl, nitrates quinidine, ETOH, grapefruit juice; ↑ risk OF neurotoxicity w/ lithium; ↓ effects w/ NSAIDs **Labs:** Monitor bun, creatinine, LFTs

Amlodipine/Atorvastatin (Caduet) [Antianginal, Antihypertensive, Antilipemic/CCB, HMG-CoA reductase inhibitor]
Uses: * HTN, chronic stable/vasospastic angina, control cholesterol & triglycerides* **Action:** CCB & HMG-CoA reductase inhibitor **Dose:** Amlodipine 2.5–10 mg w/ Atorvastatin 10–80 mg PO qd **Caution:** [X, –] use w/ patients w/ CHF **Contra:** Active liver Dz, ↑ serum transaminases **Disp:** Tabs amlodipine/atorvastatin: 2.5/10, 2.5/20, 2.5/40, 5/10, 5/20, 5/40, 5/80, 10/10, 10/20, 10/40, 10/80 mg **SE:** Peripheral edema, HA, palpitations, flushing, myopathy, arthralgia, myalgia, GI upset Interactions: ↑ Hypotension w/ fentanyl, nitrates, EtOH, quinidine, other antihypertensives, grapefruit juice; ↑ effects w/ diltiazem, erythromycin, H_2 blockers, proton pump inhibitors, quinidine; ↓ effects w/ NSAIDs, barbiturates, rifampin **Labs:** Monitor LFTs and CPK **NIPE:** ⊘ DC abruptly, ↑ photosensitivity—use sunscreen; rare risk of rhabdomyolysis

Amlodipine Besylate/Benazepril Hydrochloride (Lotrel) [Antianginal, Antihypertensive/CCB, ACEI] Uses: HTN Action: CCB relaxes coronary vascular smooth muscle, ACEI suppresses rennin-angiotensin-aldosterone system **Dose:** Amlodipine besylate 2.5–10 mg/ Benazepril hydrochloride 10–40 mg PO OD titrate dose upward; CrCl < 30 mL/min not recommended **Caution:** [C (1st tri), D (2nd & 3rd tri), –] **Contra:** Angioedema **Disp:** Amlodipine besylate/benazepril hydrochloride caps 2.5/10, 5/10, 5/20, 5/40, 10/20, 10/40 **SE:** Peripheral edema, HA, palpitations, flushing, dizziness, ↑ K^+, nonproductive cough **Interactions:** ↑ Effect OF hypotension w/ antihypertensives, capsaicin, fentanyl, nitrates, quinidine, ETOH, grapefruit juice; ↑ risk OF neurotoxicity w/ lithium; ↑ effects OF insulin, Li; ↑ risk OF hyperkalemia w/ trimethoprim & K-sparing diuretics; ↓ effects w/ NSAIDs, ASA **Labs:** Monitor bun, creatinine, K^+, LFTs; ↓ hemoglobin; ECG changes; **NIPE:** ⊘ use for initial treatment of HTN; higher incidence of angioedema in AA; persistent cough and/or taste changes may develop; ⊘ PRG, DC if angioedema

Ammonium Aluminum Sulfate [Alum] [GU Astringent] [OTC]
Uses: *Hemorrhagic cystitis when saline bladder irrigation fails* **Action:**

Astringent **Dose:** 1–2% soln w/ constant NS bladder irrigation **Caution:** [+/–] **Disp:** Powder for reconstitution **SE:** Encephalopathy possible; can precipitate & occlude catheters **Labs:** Obtain aluminum levels, especially in renal insuff; **NIPE:** Safe to use w/o anesthesia & w/ vesicoureteral reflux

Amoxicillin (Amoxil, Polymox) [Antibiotic/Aminopenicillin] **Uses:** **Ear, nose, & throat, lower resp, skin, urinary tract Infxns resulting from susceptible gram(+) bacteria * endocarditis prophylaxis **Action:** β-Lactam antibiotic; ↓ cell wall synthesis *Spectrum:* Gram(+) (*Strep* sp, *Enterococcus* sp); some gram(–) (*H. influenzae, E. coli, N. gonorrhoeae H. pylori,* & *P. mirabilis)* **Dose:** *Adults.* 250–500 mg PO tid or 500–875 mg bid. *Peds.* 25–100 mg/kg/24 h PO ÷ q8h. 200–400 mg PO bid (equivalent to 125–250 mg tid); ↓ in renal impair **Caution:** [B, +] **Disp:** Caps 250, 500 mg; chew tabs 125, 200, 250, 400 mg; susp 50 mg/mL, 125, 200, 250, & 400 mg/5 mL; tabs 500, 875 mg **SE:** D; skin rash common **Notes:** Cross hypersensitivity w/ PCN; many strains of *E. coli*-resistant **Interactions:** ↑ Effects OF warfarin, ↑ effects w/ probenecid, disulfiram, ↑ risk of rash w/ allopurinol, ↓ effects OF oral contraceptives, ↓ effects w/ tetracyclines, chloramphenicol **Labs:** ↑ Serum alkaline phosphatase, LDH, LFTs, false + direct Coombs test **NIPE:** Space meds over 24/h, eval for superinfection, use barrier contraception

Amoxicillin & Clavulanic Acid (Augmentin, Augmentin 600 ES, Augmentin XR) [Antibiotic/Aminopenicillin, Beta-lactamase Inhibitor] **Uses:** **Ear, lower resp, sinus, urinary tract, skin Infxns caused by β-lactamase-producing *H. influenzae, S. aureus,* & *E. coli** **Action:** Combo β-lactam antibiotic & β-lactamase inhibitor. *Spectrum:* Gram(+) same as amox alone, MSSA; gram(–) as w/ amox alone, β-lactamase-producing *H. influenzae, Klebsiella* sp, *M. catarrhalis* **Dose:** *Adults.* 250–500 mg PO q8h or 875 mg q12h; XR 2000 mg PO Q12H. *Peds.* 20–40 mg/kg/d as amoxicillin PO ÷ q8h or 45 mg/kg/d ÷ q12h; ↓ in renal impair; take w/ food **Caution:** [B, ?] **Disp** (as amoxicillin/clavulanic acid): Tabs 250/125, 500/125, 875/125 mg; chew tabs 125/31.25, 200/28.5, 250/62.5, 400/57 mg; susp 125/31.25, 250/62.5, 200/28.5, 400/57 mg/5 mL; susp: ES 600/42.9 mg/5 mL; XR tab 1000/62.5 mg **SE:** Abdominal discomfort, N/V/D, allergic Rxn, vaginitis **Notes:** Do not substitute two 250-mg tabs for one 500-mg tab (OD of clavulanic acid) **Interactions:** ↑ Effects OF warfarin, ↑ effects w/ probenecid, disulfiram, ↑ risk of rash w/ allopurinol, ↓ effects OF oral contraceptives, ↓ effects w/ tetracyclines, chloramphenicol **Labs:** ↑ Serum alkaline phosphatase, LDH, LFTs, false + direct Coombs' test **NIPE:** Space meds over 24/h, eval for superinfection, use barrier contraception

Amphotericin B (Amphocin) [Antifungal] **Uses:** **Severe, systemic fungal Infxns; oral & cutaneous candidiasis** **Action:** Binds ergosterol in the fungal membrane to alter permeability **Dose:** *Adults & Peds. Test dose:* 1 mg IV in adults or 0.1 mg/kg to 1 mg IV in children; then 0.25–1.5 mg/kg/24 h IV over 2–6 h (range 25–50 mg/d or qod). Total dose varies w/ indication. *PO:* 1 mL qid. *Topical:*

Apply bid–qid for 1–4 wk depending on Infxn; ↓ in renal impair **Caution:** [B, ?] **Disp:** Powder for inj 50 mg/vial; PO susp 100 mg/mL; cream, lotion, oint 3% **SE:** K⁺/Mg²⁺ from renal wasting; anaphylaxis reported HA, fever, chills, nephrotoxicity, (dn) BP, anemia **Notes:** Monitor renal Cr/LFTs; pretreatment w/ APAP & antihistamines (Benadryl) minimizes adverse IV effects (eg, fever, chills)) **Interactions:** ↑ Nephrotoxic effects w/ antineoplastics, cyclosporine, furosemide, vancomycin, aminoglycosides, ↑ hypokalemia w/ corticosteroids, skeletal muscle relaxants **Labs:** ↑ Serum bilirubin, serum cholesterol **NIPE:** Monitor CNS effects & ⊘ take hs; topical cream discolors skin

Amphotericin B Cholesteryl (Amphotec) [Antifungal]
Uses: *Aspergillosis in pts intolerant or refractory to conventional amphotericin B,* systemic candidiasis **Action:** Binds sterols in the cell membrane, alters permeability **Dose:** *Adults & Peds.* Test dose 1.6–8.3 mg, over 15–20 min, then 3–4 mg/kg/d; 1 mg/kg/h inf; ↓ in renal insuff **Caution:** [B, ?] **Disp:** Powder for inj 50 mg, 100 mg/vial **SE:** Anaphylaxis reported; fever, chills, HA, ↓ K⁺, ↓ Mg²⁺, nephrotox, ↓ BP, anemia **Notes:** Do not use in-line filter; monitor LFT & electrolytes **Interactions:** See Amphotericin B

Amphotericin B Lipid Complex (Abelcet) [Antifungal]
Uses: *Refractory invasive fungal Infxn in pts intolerant to conventional amphotericin B* **Action:** Binds cell membrane sterols, alters permeability **Dose:** *Adults & Peds.* 5 mg/kg/d IV single daily dose; 2.5 mg/kg/h inf **Caution:** [B, ?] **Disp:** Inj 5 mg/mL **SE:** Anaphylaxis reported; fever, chills, HA, ↓ K⁺, ↓ Mg²⁺, nephrotox, ↓ BP, anemia **Notes:** Filter soln w/5-micron filter needle; do not mix in electrolyte-containing solns; if inf >2 h, manually mix bag **Interactions:** See Amphotericin B

Amphotericin B Liposomal (AmBisome) [Antifungal]
Uses: *Refractory invasive fungal Infxn in pts intolerant to conventional amphotericin B, cryptococcal meningitis in HIV, empiric Rx for febrile neutropenia, visceral leishmaniasis* **Action:** Binds to sterols in cell membrane, changes membrane permeability **Dose:** *Adults & Peds.* 3–6 mg/kg/d inf 60–120 min; ↓ in renal insuff **Caution:** [B, ?] **Disp:** Powder for inj 50 mg **SE:** Anaphylaxis reported; fever, chills, HA, ↓ K⁺, ↓ Mg²⁺ nephrotox, ↓ BP, anemia **Notes:** Use no less than 1-micron filter **Interactions:** See Amphotericin B

Ampicillin (Amcill, Omnipen) [Antibiotic/Aminopenicillin]
Uses: *Resp, GU, or GI tract Infxns, meningitis due to gram(–) & gram(+) bacteria; endocarditis prophylaxis* **Action:** β-Lactam antibiotic; ↓ cell wall synthesis. **Spectrum:** Gram(+) (*Streptococcus* sp, *Staphylococcus* sp, *Listeria*); gram(–) (*Klebsiella* sp, *E. coli, H. influenzae, P. mirabilis, Shigella* sp, *Salmonella* sp) **Dose:** *Adults.* 500 mg-2 g IM or IV q6h or 250–500 mg PO q6h. *Peds.* Neonates <7 d: 50–100 mg/kg/24 h IV ÷ q8h. *Term infants:* 75–150 mg/kg/24 h ÷ q6–8h IV or PO. *Children >1 mo:* 100–200 mg/kg/24 h ÷ q4–6h IM or IV; 50–100 mg/kg/24 h ÷ q6h PO up to 250 mg/dose. *Meningitis:* 200–400 mg/kg/24 h ÷ q4–6h IV; ↓ in renal impair; take on empty stomach **Caution:** [B, M] Cross-hypersensitivity

w/ PCN **Disp:** Caps 250, 500 mg; susp 100 mg/mL (reconstituted as drops); 125 mg/5 mL, 250 mg/5 mL, 500 mg/5 mL; powder for inj 125 mg, 250 mg, 500 mg, 1 g, 2 g, 10 g/vial **SE:** D, skin rash, allergic Rxn **Notes:** Many strains of *E. coli*-resistant **Interactions:** ↓ Effects OF oral contraceptives & atenolol, ↑ effects w/ chloramphenicol, erythromycin, tetracycline, & food; ↓ effects OF anticoagulants & MTX; ↑ risk of rash w/ allopurinal; ↑ effects w/ probenecid & disulfiram **Labs:** ↑ LFTs, serum protein, serum theophylline, serum uric acid; ↓ serum estrogen, serum cholesterol, serum folate; false + direct Coombs' test, urine glucose, & urine amino acids **NIPE:** Take on empty stomach & around the clock; may cause candidal vaginitis; use barrier contraception

Ampicillin–Sulbactam (Unasyn) [Antibiotic/Aminopenicillin & Beta-lactamase Inhibitor]

Uses: *Gynecologic, intraabdominal, skin Infxns caused by β-lactamase-producing strains of *S. aureus, Enterococcus, H. influenzae, P. mirabilis,* & *Bacteroides* sp* **Action:** Combo β-lactam antibiotic & a β-lactamase inhibitor. *Spectrum:* Gram(+) & gram(–) as above *also Enterobacter, Acinetobacter, Bacteroides* **Dose:** *Adults.* 1.5–3 g IM or IV q6h. *Peds.* 100-200 mg ampicillin/kg/d (150–300 mg Unasyn) q6h; ↓ in renal failure **Caution:** [B, M] **Disp:** Powder for inj 1.5, 3.0 g/vial, 15 g bulk package **SE:** Allergy Rxns, rash, D, pain at injection site **Notes:** A 2:1 ratio ampicillin:sulbactam Interactions: See Ampicillin

Amprenavir (Agenerase) [Antiviral/HIV Protease Inhibitor]

WARNING: PO soln contra in children <4 y (potential tox from large volume of polypropylene glycol in formulation) **Uses:** *HIV Infxn* **Action:** Protease inhibitor; prevents maturation to mature virus **Dose:** *Adults.* 1200 mg bid. *Peds.* 20 mg/kg bid or 15 mg/kg tid up to 2400 mg/d **Caution:** [C, ?] CDC recommends HIV-infected mothers not breast-feed (risk of HIV transmission); Hx sulfonamides allergy **Contra:** CYP450 3A4 substrates (ergot derivatives, midazolam, triazolam, etc); soln < 4 y, PRG, hepatic or renal failure, disulfiram, or metronidazole **Disp:** Caps 50, 150 mg; soln 15 mg/mL **SE:** Life-threatening rash, hyperglycemia, hypertriglyceridemia, fat redistribution, N/V/D, depression **Notes:** Caps & soln contain vitamin E exceeding RDA; avoid high-fat meals; many drug interactions **Interactions:** ↑ Effects w/ abacavir, cimetidine, delavirdine, indinavir, itraconazole, ketoconazole, macrolides, ritonavir, zidovudine, grapefruit juice; ↑ effects OF cisapride, clozapine, ergotamine, loratadine, nelfinavir, dapsone, pimozide, rifabutin, saquinavir, sildenafil, terfenadine, triazolam, warfarin, zidovudine, HMG-CoA reductase inhibitors; ↓ effects w/ antacids, barbiturates, carbamazepine, nevirapine, phenytoin, rifampin, St. John's wort, high-fat food; ↓ effects OF oral contraceptives **Labs:** ↑ Serum glucose, cholesterol, & triglyceride levels **NIPE:** Use barrier contraception, may take w/ food other than high-fat food, ⊘ take vitamin E

Anakinra (Kineret) [Antirheumatic/Immunomodulator]

WARNING: Associated w/ ↑ incidence of serious Infxn; D/C w/ serious Infxn

Uses: *Reduce signs & Sxs of moderate/severe active RA, failed 1 or more DMARD* Action: Human IL-1 receptor antagonist Dose: 100 mg SQ qd Caution: [B, ?] Contra: Allergy to *E. coli*-derived proteins, active Infxn, <18 y Disp: 100-mg prefilled syringes SE: Neutropenia especially when used w/ TNF-blocking agents, inj site Rxn, Infxn Interactions: ↓ Effects OF immunizations; ↑ risk OF infections if combined w/ TNF-blocking drugs Labs: ↓ WBCs, plts, absolute neutrophil count NIPE: Store drug in refrigerator, ⊘ light exposure, & discard any unused portion; ⊘ use soln if discolored or has particulate matter

Anastrozole (Arimidex) [Antineoplastic/Nonsteroidal Aromatase Inhibitor] Uses: *Breast CA: postmenopausal w/ metastatic breast CA, adjuvant Rx of postmenopausal w/ early hormone-receptor(+) breast CA* Action: Selective nonsteroidal aromatase inhibitor, ↓ circ estradiol Dose: 1 mg/d Caution: [D, ?] Contra: PRG Disp.: Tabs 1 mg SE: May ↑ cholesterol; D, HTN, flushing, ↑ bone & tumor pain, HA, somnolence Notes: No effect on adrenal corticosteroids or aldosterone Interactions: None noted Labs: ↑ GTT, LFTs, alkaline phosphatase, total & LDL cholesterol NIPE: May ↓ fertility & cause fetal damage, eval for pain & administer adequate analgesia, may cause vaginal bleeding first few weeks

Anidulafungin (Eraxis) [Glucan Synthesis Inhibitor] Uses: *Candidemia, esophageal candidiasis, and other Candida Infxn (peritonitis, intra-abdominal abscess)* Action: Echinocandin; ↓ cell wall synthesis *Spectrum: C. albicans, C. glabrata, C. parapsilosis, and C. tropicalis* Dose: Candidemia, others: 200 mg IV (times) 1, then 100 mg IV daily (Tx 14 days after last + culture); Esophageal candidiasis: 100 mg IV (times) 1, then 50 mg IV daily (Tx >14 d and 7 d after resolution of Sx); 1.1 mg/min max inf rate Caution: [C, ?/-] Contra: Echinocandin hypersensitivity Disp: Powder 50 mg/vial SE: Histamine-mediated infusion Rxns (urticaria, flushing, pruritus, rash, hypotension, dyspnea), fever, N/V/D, hypokalemia, HA, hepatitis, worsening hepatic failure Labs: ↑ LFTs, NIPE: ↓ inf rate to <1.1 mg/min w/ inf Rxns

Anistreplase (Eminase) [Antithrombotic Agent] Uses: *AMI* Action: Thrombolytic; activates conversion of plasminogen to plasmin, ↑ thrombolysis Dose: 30 units IV over 2–5 min Caution: [C, ?] Contra: Active internal bleeding, Hx CVA, recent (<2 mo) intracranial or intraspinal surgery/trauma, intracranial neoplasm, AVM, aneurysm, bleeding diathesis, severe uncontrolled HTN Disp: Vials w/30 units SE: Bleeding, ↓ BP, hematoma Notes: Ineffective if readministered >5 d after the previous dose of anistreplase or streptokinase, or streptococcal Infxn (production of antistreptokinase Ab) Interactions: ↑ Risk OF hemorrhage w/ warfarin, oral anticoagulants, ASA, NSAIDs, dipyridamole; ↓ effectiveness w/ aminocaproic acid Labs: ↓ Plasminogen & fibrinogen, ↑ transaminase level, thrombin time, APTT & PT NIPE: Store powder in refrigerator & use w/in 30 min of reconstitution, initiate therapy ASAP after MI, monitor S/Sxs internal bleeding

Anthralin (Anthra-Derm) [Keratolytic Dermatologic Agent]
Uses: *Psoriasis* **Action:** Keratolytic **Dose:** Apply qd **Caution:** [C, ?] **Contra:** Acutely inflamed psoriatic eruptions, erythroderma **Disp:** Cream, oint 0.1, 0.25, 0.4, 0.5, 1% **SE:** Irritation; hair/fingernails/skin discoloration **Interactions:** ↑ Toxicity if used immediately after long-term topical corticosteroid therapy **NIPE:** May stain fabric; external use only; ⊘ sunlight-medicated areas

Antihemophilic Factor [AHF, Factor VIII] (Monoclate) [Antihemophilic]
Uses: *Classic hemophilia A, von Willebrand Dz* **Action:** Provides factor VIII needed to convert prothrombin to thrombin **Dose:** *Adults & Peds.* 1 AHF unit/kg ↑ factor VIII level ≈2%. Units required = (kg) (desired factor VIII ↑ as % nl) × (0.5). Prevent spontaneous hemorrhage = 5% nl. Hemostasis after trauma/surgery = 30% nl. Head injuries, major surgery, or bleeding = 80–100% nl. **Caution:** [C, ?] **Disp:** Check each vial for units contained **SE:** Rash, fever, HA, chills, N/V Notes: Determine pt's % of nl factor VIII before dosing **Interactions:** None **Labs:** Monitor CBC & direct Coombs' test **NIPE:** ⊘ ASA, immunize against Hep B, DC if tachycardic

Antithymocyte Globulin [ATG] (ATGAM) [Immunosuppressive Agent]
Uses: *RX allograft rejection in transplant Pts* **Action:** Reduces the number of circulating, thymus-dependent lymphocytes **Dose:** 10–15 mg/kg **Caution:** [C, ?/–] **Contra:** ⊘ Use w/ a Hx of severe systemic Rxn to other equine gamma globulin prep **Disp.:** Inj 50 mg/mL **SE:** Thrombocytopenia, leukopenia Notes: DC if severe thrombocytopenia/leucopenia **Interactions:** ↑ Risk of infection w/ antineoplastics, corticosteroids, cyclosporines **Labs:** Baseline hematopoietic function & periodically during drug therapy **NIPE:** Refrigerate & keep out of light, reconstitute at room temperature, soln stable for 4 h after reconstitution, 1st dose infused over 6 h

Apomorphine (Apokyn) [Antiparkinsonian/Dopamine Agonist]
WARNING: Do not administer IV **Uses:** *Acute, intermittent hypomobility ("off") episodes of Parkinson Dz* **Action:** Dopamine agonist **Dose:** *Adults.* 0.2-mL SQ test dose under medical supervision; if BP OK, initial 0.2 mL SQ during "off" periods; only 1 dose per "off" period; requires careful titration; 0.6 mL max single doses; use w/ antiemetic; ↓ in renal impair **Caution:** [C, +/–] Avoid EtOH; antihypertensives, vasodilators, cardio or cerebrovascular Dz, hepatic impair **Contra:** 5HT3 antagonists, sulfite allergy **Disp:** Inj 10 mg/mL, 3-mL pen cartridges; 2-mL amp **SE:** Emesis, syncope, QT prolongation, orthostatic ↓ BP, somnolence, ischemia, injection site Rxn, abuse potential, dyskinesia, fibrotic conditions, priapism Notes: Daytime somnolence may limit activities; trimethobenzamide 300 mg tid PO or other non-5HT3 antagonist antiemetic given 3 d prior to & up to 2 mo following initiation **Interactions:** ↑ Risk of hypotension w/ alosetron, dolasetron, granisetron, ondansetron, palonosetron **Labs:** ECG--monitor for prolongation of QT interval **NIPE:** Start antiemetic 3 d before therapy and for 2 mo after therapy ends

Apraclonidine (Iopidine) [Alpha-adrenergic Agonist/Glaucoma agent] Uses: *Glaucoma, postop intraocular HTN* Action: α₂-adrenergic agonist Dose: 1–2 gtt of 0.5% tid Caution: [C, ?] Contra: MAOI use Disp: 0.5, 1% soln SE: Ocular irritation, lethargy, xerostomia Interactions: ↓ Intraocular pressure w/ pilocarpine or topical BBs NIPE: Monitor CV status of pts w/ CAD, potential for dizziness

Aprepitant (Emend) [Centrally Acting Antiemetic] Uses: *Prevents N/V assoc w/ emetogenic CA chemo (eg, cisplatin) (use in combo w/ other antiemetics)* Action: Substance P/neurokinin 1(NK₁) receptor antagonist Dose: 125 mg PO day 1, 1 h before chemo, then 80 mg PO q AM on days 2 & 3 Caution: [B, ?/–]; substrate & moderate inhibitor of CYP3A4; inducer of CYP2C9 (Table 13) Contra: use w/ pimozide Disp: Caps 80, 125 mg SE: Fatigue, asthenia, hiccups Notes: ↓ Effectiveness of PO contraceptives; ↓ effect of warfarin Interactions: ↑ Effects w/clarithromycin, diltiazem, itraconazole, ketoconazole, nefazodone, nelfinavir, ritonavir, troleandomycin; ↑effects OF alprazolam, astemizole, cisapride, dexamethasone, methylprednisolone, midazolam, pimozide, terfenadine, triazolam, and chemotherapeutic agents, eg, docetaxel, etoposide, ifosfamide, imatinib, irinotecan, paclitaxel, vinblastine, vincristine, vinorelbine; ↓ effects w/ paroxetine, rifampin; ↓ effects OF oral contraceptives, paroxetine, phenytoin, tolbutamide, warfarin Labs: ↑ ALT, AST, BUN, alkaline phosphatase, leukocytes NIPE: Use barrier contraception, take w/o regard to food

Aprotinin (Trasylol) [Antithrombotic Agent] Uses: *↓/Prevents blood loss during CABG* Action: Protease inhibitor, antifibrinolytic Dose: 1-mL IV test dose. *High dose:* 2 million KIU load, 2 million KIU to prime pump, then 500,000 KIU/h until surgery ends. *Low dose:* 1 million KIU load, 1 million KIU to prime pump, then 250,000 KIU/h until surgery ends; 7 million KIU max total Caution: [B, ?] Thromboembolic Dz requiring anticoagulants or blood factor administration Disp: Inj 1.4 mg/mL (10,000 KIU/mL) SE: AF, MI, heart failure, dyspnea, postop renal dysfunction Notes: 1000/KIU = 0.14 mg of aprotinin Interactions: ↑ Clotting time w/ heparin; ↓effects of fibrinolytics, captopril Labs: Monitor aPTT, ACT, CBC, BUN, creatinine NIPE: Monitor cardiac and pulmonary status during inf

Ardeparin (Normiflo) [Anticoagulant] Uses: *Prevents DVT/PE following knee replacement* Action: LMW heparin Dose: 35–50 units/kg SQ q12h. Begin day of surgery, continue up to 14 d Caution: [C, ?] ↓ Renal Fxn Contra: Active hemorrhage; allergy to pork products Disp: Inj 5000, 10,000 IU/0.5 mL SE: Bleeding, bruising, thrombocytopenia, pain at inj site, ↑ serum transaminases Notes: Lab monitoring usually not necessary

Argatroban (Acova) [Anticoagulant] Uses: *Prevent/Treat thrombosis in HIT, PCI in pts w/ risk of HIT* Action: Anticoagulant, direct thrombin inhibitor Dose: 2 mcg/kg/min IV; adjust until aPTT 1.5–3× baseline not to exceed 100 s; 10 mcg/kg/min max; ↓ in hepatic impair Caution: [B, ?] Avoid PO anticoagulants, ↑ bleeding risk; avoid use w/ thrombolytics Contra: Overt major bleed

Disp: Inj 100 mg/mL **SE:** AF, cardiac arrest, cerebrovascular disorder, ↓ BP, VT, N/V/D, sepsis, cough, renal tox, ↓ Hgb **Notes:** Steady State 1-3h **Interactions:** ↑ Risk OF bleeding w/ anticoagulants, feverfew, garlic, ginger, ginkgo, ↑ risk OF intracranial bleed w/ thrombolytics **Labs:** ↑ aPTT, PT, INR, ACT, thrombin time **NIPE:** Report ↑ bruising & bleeding, ⊘ breast-feed

Aripiprazole (Abilify) [Antipsychotic/Psychotropic] WARNING: Increased mortality in elderly with dementia-related psychosis Uses:
Schizophrenia **Action:** Dopamine & serotonin antagonist **Dose:** *Adults.* 10–15 mg PO qd; ↓ dose w/ CYP3A4 or CYP2D6 inhibitors (Table 13); ↑ dose w/ inducer of CYP3A4 **Caution:** [C, –] **Disp:** Tabs 2, 5, 10, 15, 20, 30 mg; soln 1 mg/ml **SE:** Neuroleptic malignant syndrome, tardive dyskinesia, orthostatic ↓ BP, cognitive & motor impair, hyperglycemia **Interactions:** ↑ Effects w/ ketoconazole, quinidine, fluoxetine, paroxetine, ↓ effects w/ carbamazepine **NIPE:** ⊘ Breast-feed, consume EtOH, or use during PRG; use barrier contraception; ↑ fluid intake

Artificial Tears (Tears Naturale) [Ocular Lubricant] [OTC]
Uses: *Dry eyes* **Action:** Ocular lubricant **Dose:** 1–2 gtt tid–qid **Disp:** OTC soln

L-Asparaginase (Elspar, Oncaspar) [Antineoplastic] Uses:
ALL (in combo w/ other agents) **Action:** Protein synthesis inhibitor **Dose:** 500–20,000 IU/m²/d for 1-14 d (Per protocols) bd]**Caution:** [C, ?] **Contra:** Active/Hx pancreatitis **Disp:** Inj 10,000 IU **SE:** Allergy 20–35% (from urticaria to anaphylaxis test dose recommended); rare GI tox (mild nausea/anorexia, pancreatitis) **Interactions:** ↑ Effects w/ prednisone, vincristine; ↓ effects OF MTX, sulfonylureas, insulin **Labs:** ↓ T₄ & T₄-binding globulin, serum albumin, total cholesterol, plasma fibrinogen; ↑ BUN, glucose, uric acid, LFTs, alkaline phosphatase **NIPE:** ↑ Fluid intake, monitor for bleeding, monitor I&O and weight, ⊘ EtOH or ASA

Aspirin (Bayer, Ecotrin, St. Joseph's) [OTC] [Antipyretic, Analgesic/Salicylate] Uses:
Angina, CABG, PTCA, carotid endarterectomy, ischemic stroke, TIA, MI, arthritis, pain, HA, *fever,* inflammation, Kawasaki Dz **Action:** Prostaglandin inhibitor **Dose:** *Adults.* Pain, fever: 325–650 mg q4–6h PO or PR. *RA:* 3–6 g/d PO in ÷ doses. *Plt inhibitor:* 81–325 mg PO qd. *Prevent MI:* 81–325 mg PO qd. *Peds.* Antipyretic: 10–15 mg/kg/dose PO or PR q4h up to 80 mg/kg/24 h. *RA:* 60–100 mg/kg/24 h PO ÷ q4–6h (keep levels between 15 & 30 mg/dL); avoid w/ CrCl <10 mL/min, severe liver Dz **Caution:** [C, M] Use linked to Reye syndrome; avoid w/ viral illness in children **Contra:** Allergy to ASA, chickenpox/flu Sxs, syndrome of nasal polyps, asthma, rhinitis **Disp:** Tabs 325, 500 mg; chew tabs 81 mg; EC tabs 81, 162, 325, 500, 650, 975 mg; SR tabs 650, 800 mg; effervescent tabs 325, 500 mg; supp 125, 200, 300, 600 mg **SE:** GI upset & erosion **Notes:** D/C 1 wk prior to surgery to ↓ bleeding; avoid/limit EtOH **Interactions:** ↑ Effects w/ anticoagulants, ammonium chloride, antibiotics, ascorbic acid, furosemide, methionine, nizatidine, NSAIDs, verapamil, EtOH, feverfew, garlic, ginkgo biloba, horse chestnut, kelparee (black-tang), prickly ash, red clover; ↓ effects w/ antacids, activated charcoal, corticosteroids,

griseofulvin, $NaHCO_3$, ginseng, food; ↑ effects OF ACEI, hypoglycemics, insulin, Li, MTX, phenytoin, sulfonamides, valproic acid; ↓ effects OF BBs, probenecid, spironolactone, sulfinpyrazone **Labs:** False – results of urinary glucose & urinary ketone tests, serum albumin, total serum phenytoin, T_3 & T_4 **NIPE:** Chronic ASA use may result in ↓ folic acid, Fe-deficiency anemia, & hypernatremia; ⊘ foods ↑ salicylate, eg curry powder, paprika, licorice, prunes, raisins, tea; take ASA w/ food or milk; report S/Sxs bleeding/GI pain/ringing in ears

Aspirin & Butalbital Compound (Fiorinal) [Analgesic & Barbiturate] [C-III]
Uses: *Tension HA,* pain **Action:** Combo barbiturate & analgesic **Dose:** 1–2 PO q4h PRN, max 6 tabs/d; avoid w/ CrCl <10 mL/min & severe liver Dz **Caution:** [C (D if prolonged use or high doses at term), ?] **Contra:** ASA allergy, GI ulceration, bleeding disorder, porphyria, syndrome of nasal polyps, angioedema, & bronchospasm to NSAIDs **Disp:** Caps (Fiorgen PF, Fiorinal) Tabs (Fiorinal, Lanorinal): ASA 325 mg/butalbital 50 mg/caffeine 40 mg **SE:** Drowsiness, dizziness, GI upset, ulceration, bleeding **Notes:** Butalbital habit-forming; avoid or limit EtOH intake See Aspirin **Additional Interactions:** ↑ Effect OF benzodiazepines, CNS depressants, chloramphenicol, methylphenidate, propoxyphene, valproic acid; ↓ effects OF BBs, corticosteroids, chloramphenicol, cyclosporines, doxycycline, griseofulvin, haloperidol, oral contraceptives, phenothiazines, quinidine, TCAs, theophylline, warfarin **NIPE:** Use barrier contraception, ⊘ EtOH

Aspirin + Butalbital, Caffeine, & Codeine (Fiorinal + Codeine) [Narcotic Analgesic] [C-III]
Uses: Mild *pain*, HA, especially when associated w/ stress **Action:** Sedative analgesic, narcotic analgesic **Dose:** 1–2 tabs (caps) PO q4–6h PRN **Caution:** [D, ?] **Contra:** Allergy to ASA and codeine **Disp:** Cap/tab contains 325 mg ASA, 40 mg caffeine, 50 mg of butalbital, 30 mg of codeine **SE:** Drowsiness, dizziness, GI upset, ulceration, bleeding; avoid or limit ETOH. See Aspirin + Butalbital **Additional Interactions:** ↑ Effects w/ narcotic analgesics, MAOIs, neuromuscular blockers, ↓ effects w/ tobacco smoking; ↑ effects OF digitoxin, phenytoin, rifampin; ↑ resp & CNS depression w/ cimetidine **Labs:** ↑ Plasma amylase & lipase **NIPE:** May cause constipation, ↑ fluids & fiber, take w/ milk to ↓ GI distress

Aspirin + Codeine (Empirin No. 3,4) [Narcotic Analgesic] [C-III]
Uses: Mild to *moderate pain* **Action:** Combined effects of ASA & codeine **Dose:** *Adults.* 1–2 tabs PO q4–6h PRN. *Peds.* ASA 10 mg/kg/dose; codeine 0.5–1 mg/kg/dose q4h **Caution:** [D, M] **Contra:** Allergy to ASA/codeine, PUD, bleeding, anticoagulant Rx, children w/ chickenpox or flu Sxs **Disp:** Tabs 325 mg of ASA & codeine (Codeine in No. 3 = 30 mg, No. 4 = 60 mg) **SE:** Drowsiness, dizziness, GI upset, ulceration, bleeding See Aspirin. **Additional Interactions:** ↑ Effects w/ narcotic analgesics, MAOIs, neuromuscular blockers, ↓ effects w/ tobacco smoking; ↑ effects OF digitoxin, phenytoin, rifampin; ↑ resp & CNS depression w/ cimetidine **Labs:** ↑ Plasma amylase & lipase **NIPE:** May cause constipation, ↑ fluids & fiber, take w/ milk to ↓ GI distress

Atazanavir (Reyataz) [Antiretroviral/HIV-1 Protease Inhibitor] WARNING: Hyperbilirubinemia may require drug D/C Uses: ***HIV-1 Infxn*** Action: Protease inhibitor Dose: 400 mg PO qd w/ food; when given w/ efavirenz 600 mg, administer atazanavir 300 mg + ritonavir 100 mg once/d; separate doses from buffered didanosine administration; ↓ in hepatic impair Caution: [B, –]; ↑ levels of statins, sildenafil, antiarrhythmics, warfarin, cyclosporine, TCAs; atazanavir ↓ by St. John's wort Contra: Use w/midazolam, triazolam, ergots, cisapride, pimozide Disp: Caps 100, 150, 200 mg SE: HA, N/V/D, rash, abdominal pain, DM, photosensitivity, ↑ PR interval Notes: May have iris adverse effect on cholesterol Interactions: ↑ Effects w/ amprenavir, clarithromycin, indinavir, lamivudine, lopinavir, ritonavir, saquinavir, stavudine, tenofovir, zalcitabine, zidovudine; ↑ effects OF amiodarone, atorvastatin, CCBs, clarithromycin, cyclosporine, diltiazem, irinotecan, lidocaine, lovastatin, oral contraceptives, rifabutin, quinidine, saquinavir, sildenafil, simvastatin, sirolimus, tacrolimus, TCAs, warfarin; ↓ effects w/ antacids, antimycobacterials, efavirenz, esomeprazole, H₂ receptor antagonists, lansoprazole, omeprazole, rifampin, St. John's wort Labs: ↑ ALT, AST, total bilirubin, amylase, lipase, serum glucose, ↓ Hgb, neutrophils NIPE: Take w/ food; will not cure HIV or ↓ risk of transmission; use barrier contraception; ↑ risk of skin and/or scleral yellowing

Atenolol (Tenormin) [Antihypertensive, Antianginal/Beta Blocker] Uses: ***HTN, angina, MI*** Action: Competitively blocks β-adrenergic receptors, β₁ Dose: HTN & angina: 50–100 mg/d PO. AMI: 5 mg IV ×2 over 10 min, then 50 mg PO bid if tolerated; ↓ in renal impair Caution: [D, M] DM, bronchospasm; abrupt D/C can exacerbate angina & ↑ MI risk Contra: Bradycardia, cardiogenic shock, cardiac failure, 2nd- or 3rd-degree AV block Disp: Tabs 25, 50, 100 mg; inj 5 mg/10 mL SE: Bradycardia, ↓ BP, 2nd- or 3rd-degree AV block, dizziness, fatigue Interactions: ↑ Effects w/ other antihypertensives especially diltiazem & verapamil, nitrates, EtOH; ↑ bradycardia w/ adenosine, digitalis glycosides, dipyridamole, physostigmine, tacrine; ↓ effects w/ ampicillin, antacids, NSAIDs, salicylates; ↑ effects OF lidocaine; ↓ effects OF dopamine, glucagons, insulin, sulfonylureas Labs: ↑ ANA titers, BUN, glucose, serum lipoprotein, K⁺, triglyceride, uric acid levels; ↓ HDL NIPE: May mask S/Sxs hypoglycemia, may ↑ sensitivity to cold, may ↑ depression, wheezing, orthostatic hypotension

Atenolol & Chlorthalidone (Tenoretic) [Antihypertensive, Antianginal/Beta Blocker & Diuretic] Uses: ***HTN*** Action: β-adrenergic blockade w/ diuretic Dose: 50–100 mg/d PO; ↓ in renal impair Caution: [D, M] DM, bronchospasm Contra: See atenolol; anuria, sulfonamide cross-sensitivity Disp: Tenoretic 50: Atenolol 50 mg/chlorthalidone 25 mg; Tenoretic 100: Atenolol 100 mg/chlorthalidone 25 mg SE: Bradycardia, ↓ BP, 2nd- or 3rd-degree AV block, dizziness, fatigue, ↓ K⁺, photosensitivity See Atenolol. Additional Interactions: ↑ Effects w/ other antihypertensives; ↓ effects w/ cholestyramine, NSAIDs; ↑ effects OF Li, digoxin, ↓ effects OF sulfonylureas

Labs: False ↓ urine esriol; ↑ CPK, serum ammonia, amylase, Ca²⁺, Cl⁻, cholesterol, glucose; ↓ serum Cl⁻, Mg²⁺, K⁺, Na⁻ **NIPE:** Take in AM to prevent nocturia, use sunblock >SPF 15, monitor S/Sxs gout

Atomoxetine (Strattera) [ADHD/Selective Norepinephrine Reuptake Inhibitor] WARNING: Severe liver injury may occur in rare cases. D/C w/ jaundice or (up) LFTs

Uses: * ADHD* **Action:** Selective norepinephrine reuptake inhibitor **Dose:** *Adults & children >70 kg.* 40 mg × 3 days, ↑ to 80–100 mg ÷ daily-bid. *Peds < 70 kg.* 0.5 mg/kg × 3 d, then ↑ 1.2 mg/kg max daily or bid **Caution:** [C, ? /–] **Contra:** NA glaucoma, use w/ or w/in 2 wk of D/C w MAOI **Disp:** Caps 10, 18, 25, 40, 60 mg **SE:** ↑ BP, tachycardia, weight loss, sexual dysfunction **Notes:** ↓ dose w/ hepatic insuff, ↓ in combo w/ inhibitors of CYP2D6 (Table 13)

Atorvastatin (Lipitor) [Antilipemic/HMG-CoA Reductase Inhibitor]

Uses: *↑ cholesterol & triglycerides* **Action:** HMG-CoA reductase inhibitor **Dose:** Initial 10 mg/d, may ↑ to 80 mg/d **Caution:** [X, –] **Contra:** Active liver Dz, unexplained ↑ of LFTs **Disp:** Tabs 10, 20, 40, 80 mg **SE:** Myopathy, HA, arthralgia, myalgia, GI upset **Notes:** monitor LFTs; instruct patient to report unusual muscle pain or weakness **Interactions:** ↑ Effects w/ azole antifungals, erythromycin, nefazodone, protease inhibitors, grapefruit juice; ↓ effects w/ antacids, bile acid sequestrants; ↑ effects OF digoxin, levothyroxine, oral contraceptives **Labs:** ↑ LFTs, CPK, ↓ lipid levels **NIPE:** ⊘ EtOH, breast-feeding, or while PRG

Atovaquone (Mepron) [Antiprotozoal]

Uses: *Rx & prevention PCP* **Action:** ↓ nucleic acid & ATP synthesis **Dose:** *Rx:* 750 mg PO bid for 21 d. *Prevention:* 1500 mg PO once/d (w/ meals) **Caution:** [C, ?] **Disp:** Suspension 750 mg/5 mL **SE:** Fever, HA, anxiety, insomnia, rash, N/V **Interactions:** ↓ Effects w/ metoclopramide, rifabutin, rifampin, tetracycline **NIPE:** ↑ Absorption w/ meal esp ↑ fat, monitor LFTs w/ long-term use

Atovaquone/Proguanil (Malarone) [Antimalarial]

Uses: *Prevention or Rx P. falciparum malaria* **Action:** Antimalarial **Dose:** *Adults: Prevention:* 1 tab PO 2 d before, during, & 7 d after leaving endemic region; *Rx:* 4 tabs PO single dose qd ×3 d. *Peds.* See insert **Caution:** [C, ?] **Contra:** CrCl < 30 mL/min **Disp:** Tab atovaquone 250 mg/proguanil 100 mg; peds 62.5/25 mg **SE:** HA, fever, myalgia. See Atovaquone

Atracurium (Tracrium) [Skeletal Muscle Relaxant]

Uses: *Anesthesia adjunct to facilitate ET intubation* **Action:** Nondepolarizing neuromuscular blocker **Dose:** *Adults & Peds.* 0.4-0.5 mg/kg IV bolus, then 0.08–0.1 mg/kg q20–45 min PRN **Caution:** [C, ?] **Disp:** Inj 10 mg/mL **SE:** Flushing **Notes:** Pt must be intubated & on controlled ventilation; use adequate amounts of sedation & analgesia **Interactions:** ↑ Effects w/ general anesthetics, aminoglycosides, bacitracin, BBs, β agonists, clindamycin, CCBs, diuretics, lidocaine, Li, Mg sulfate, narcotic analgesics, procainamide, quinidine, succinylcholine, trimethaphan, verapamil; ↓ effects w/ Ca, carbamazepine, phenytoin, theophylline, caffeine **Labs:**

Monitor BUN, creatinine, LFTs **NIPE:** Drug does not affect consciousness or pain, inability to speak until drug wears off

Atropine [Antiarrhythmic/Anticholinergic]

Uses: *Preanesthetic; symptomatic bradycardia & asystole* **Action:** Antimuscarinic agent; blocks acetylcholine at parasympathetic sites **Dose: Adults.** ECC: 0.5–1 mg IV q3–5min. *Preanesthetic:* 0.3–0.6 mg IM. **Peds.** ECC: 0.01–0.03 mg/kg IV q2–5min, max 1 mg, min dose 0.1 mg. *Preanesthetic:* 0.01 mg/kg/dose SC/IV (max 0.4 mg) **Caution:** [C, +] **Contra:** Glaucoma **Disp:** Tabs 0.3, 0.4, 0.6 mg; inj 0.05, 0.1, 0.3, 0.4, 0.5, 0.8, 1 mg/mL; ophth sol 0.5, 1, 2%; ophth oint 1% **SE:** Blurred vision, urinary retention, constipation, dried mucous membranes **Interactions:** ↑ Effects w/ amantadine, antihistamines, disopyramide, procainamide, quinidine, TCA, thiazides, betel palm, squaw vine; ↓ effects w/ antacids, levodopa; ↓ effects of phenothiazines **Labs:** ↓ Gastric motility & emptying may effect results of upper GI series **NIPE:** Monitor I&O, ↑ fluids & oral hygiene, wear dark glasses to ↓ photophobia

Azathioprine (Imuran) [Immunosuppressant]

Uses: *Adjunct to prevent renal transplant rejection, RA,* SLE **Action:** Immunosuppressive; antagonizes purine metabolism **Dose: Adults & Peds.** 1–3 mg/kg/d IV or PO (↓ w/ renal insuff) **Caution:** [D, ?] **Contra:** PRG **Disp:** Tabs 50 mg; inj 100 mg powder for reconstitution. **SE:** GI intolerance, fever, chills, leukopenia, thrombocytopenia; chronic use may ↑ neoplasia **Notes:** Handle inj w/ cytotoxic precautions; interaction w/ allopurinol; do not administer live vaccines to a pt taking azathioprine **Interactions:** ↑ Effects w/ allopurinol; ↑ effects OF antineoplastic drugs, cyclosporine, myelosuppressive drugs, MTX; ↑ risk OF severe leucopenia w/ ACEI; ↓ effects OF nondepolarizing neuromuscular blocking drugs, warfarin **Labs:** Monitor BUN, creatinine, CBC, LFTs during therapy **NIPE:** ⊘ PRG, breast-feeding, immunizations, take w/ or pc

Azelastine (Astelin, Optivar) [Antihistamine]

Uses: *Allergic rhinitis (rhinorrhea, sneezing, nasal pruritus); allergic conjunctivitis* **Action:** Histamine H_1-receptor antagonist **Dose:** *Nasal:* 2 sprays/nostril bid. *Ophth:* 1 gt into each affected eye bid **Caution:** [C, ?/–] **Contra:** Component sensitivity **Disp:** Nasal 137 mcg/spray; ophth soln 0.05% **SE:** Somnolence, bitter taste **Interactions:** ↑ Effects w/ cimetidine; ↑ effects OF EtOH, CNS depressants **Labs:** ↑ AST, ↓ skin reactions to antigen skin tests **NIPE:** Systemically absorbed; clear nares before admin; prime pump before use

Azithromycin (Zithromax) [Antibiotic/Macrolide]

Uses: *Community-acquired pneumonia, pharyngitis, otitis media, skin Infxns, nongonococcal urethritis, & PID; Rx & prevention of MAC in HIV* **Action:** Macrolide antibiotic; ↓ protein synthesis. *Spectrum: Chlamydia, H. ducreyi, H. influenzae, Legionella, M. catarrhalis, M. pneumoniae, M. hominis, N. gonorrhoeae, S. aureus, S. agalactiae, S. pneumoniae, S. pyogenes* **Dose: Adults.** PO: Resp tract Infxns: 500 mg day 1, then 250 mg/d PO × 4 d 500 mg/d PO × 3 days; or 2 g PO × 1. *Nongonococcal urethritis:* 1 g PO single dose. *Prevention of MAC:* 1200 mg PO once/wk. *IV:*

500 mg ×2 d, then 500 mg PO ×7–10 d. *Peds.* Otitis media: 10 mg/kg PO day 1, then 5 mg/kg/d days 2–5. *Pharyngitis:* 12 mg/kg/d PO ×5 d (take susp on an empty stomach; tabs may be taken w/wo food) **Caution:** [B, +] **Disp:** Tabs 250, 500, 600 mg; Z-Pack (5-day); Tri-Pak (500-mg tabs × 3); susp 1-g; single-dose packet; Zmax XR suspension (2 gm); susp 100, 200 mg/5 mL; inj 500 mg powder for re-constitution; **SE:** GI upset **Interactions:** ↓ Effects w/ Al- & Mg-containing antacids, atovaquone, food (suspension); ↑ effects OF alfentanil, barbiturates, bromocriptine, carbamazepine, cyclosporine, digoxin, disopyramide, ergot alka-loids, phenytoin, pimozide, terfenadine, theophylline, triazolam, warfarin; ↓ effects OF penicillins **Labs:** May ↑ serum bilirubin, alkaline phosphatase, BUN, creati-nine, CPK, glucose, K^+, LFTs, LDH, PT; may ↓ WBC, plt count, serum folate **NIPE:** Monitor S/Sxs superinfection, use sunscreen & protective clothing

Aztreonam (Azactam) [Antibiotic/Monobactam] Uses: *Aero-bic gram(–) UTIs, lower resp, intraabdominal, skin, gynecologic Infxns & sep-ticemia* **Action:** Monobactam. ↓ Cell wall synthesis. *Spectrum:* Gram(–) (*Pseudomonas, E. coli, Klebsiella, H. influenzae, Serratia, Proteus, Enterobacter, Citrobacter*) **Dose:** *Adults.* 1–2 g IV/IM q6–12h. *Peds.* Premature: 30 mg/kg/dose IV q12h. *Term & children:* 30 mg/kg/dose q6–8h; ↓ in renal impair **Caution:** [B, +] **Disp:** Inj (soln), 1 g, 2 g ; Inj powder for reconstitution 500 mg, 1 gm, **SE:** N/V/D, rash, pain at injection site **Notes:** No gram(+) or anaerobic activity; OK in PCN-allergic pts **Interactions:** ↑ Effects w/ probenecid, aminoglycosides, β-lac-tam antibiotics; ↓ effects w/ cefoxitin, chloramphenicol, imipenem **Labs:** ↑ LFTs, alkaline phosphatase, SCr, PT, PTT, & + Coombs' test **NIPE:** Monitor S/Sxs su-perinfection, taste changes w/ IV administration

Bacitracin, Ophthalmic (AK-Tracin Ophthalmic); Bacitracin & Polymyxin B, Ophthalmic (AK Poly Bac Ophthalmic, Polysporin Ophthalmic); Bacitracin, Neomycin, & Poly-mixin B, Ophthalmic (AK Spore Ophthalmic, Neosporin Ophthalmic); Bacitracin, Neomycin, Polymyxin B, & Hydrocortisone, Ophthalmic (AK Spore HC Ophthalmic, Cortisporin Ophthalmic) [antibiotic] Uses: *Steroid-responsive in-flammatory ocular conditions* **Action:** Topical antibiotic w/antiinflammatory **Dose:** Apply q3–4h into conjunctival sac **Caution:** [C, ?] **Contra:** Viral, mycobac-terial, fungal eye Infxn **Disp:** See Bacitracin, Topical equivalents, below **Interac-tions:** ↑ Effects w/ neuromuscular blocking agents, anesthetics, nephrotoxic drugs **NIPE:** May cause blurred vision

Bacitracin, Topical (Baciguent); Bacitracin & Polymyxin B, Topical (Polysporin); Bacitracin, Neomycin, & Polymyxin B, Topical (Neosporin Ointment); Bacitracin, Neomycin, Polymyxin B, & Hydrocortisone, Topical (Cortisporin); Baci-tracin, Neomycin, Polymyxin B, & Lidocaine, Topical (Clomycin) [Antibiotic] Uses: Prevent/Rx of *minor skin Infxns* **Action:**

Topical antibiotic w/ added components (antiinflammatory & analgesic) **Dose:** Apply sparingly bid-qid **Caution:** [C, ?] **Disp:** Bacitracin 500 U/g oint; Bacitracin 500 U/polymyxin B sulfate 10,000 U/g oint & powder; Bacitracin 400 U/neomycin 3.5 mg/polymyxin B 5000 U/g oint; Bacitracin 400 U/neomycin 3.5 mg/polymyxin B/10,000 U/hydrocortisone 10 mg/g oint; Bacitracin 500 U/neomycin 3.5 mg/polymyxin B 5000 U/lidocaine 40 mg/g oint. Notes: Systemic & irrigation forms available, but not generally used due to potential tox

Baclofen (Lioresal) [Skeletal Muscle Relaxant] Uses: *Spasticity due to severe chronic disorders (eg, MS, ALS, or spinal cord lesions),* trigeminal neuralgia, hiccups **Action:** Centrally acting skeletal muscle relaxant; ↓ transmission of both monosynaptic & polysynaptic cord reflexes **Dose:** *Adults.* Initial, 5 mg PO tid; ↑ q3d to effect; max 80 mg/d. *Intrathecal:* via implantable pump *Peds.* 2–7 y: 10–15 mg/d ÷ q8h; titrate, max 40 mg/d. >8 y: Max 60 mg/d. *IT:* via implantable pump; ↓ in renal impair; w/ food or milk **Caution:** [C, +] Epilepsy, neuropsychiatric disturbances; withdrawal may occur w/ abrupt D/C **Disp:** Tabs 10, 20 mg; IT inj 50 mcg/mL, 10 mg/20 mL, 10 mg/5 mL **SE:** Dizziness, drowsiness, insomnia, ataxia, weakness, ↓ BP **Interactions:** ↑ CNS depression w/ CNS depressants, MAOIs, EtOH, antihistamines, opioid analgesics, sedatives, hypnotics; ↑ effects OF antihypertensives, clindamycin, guanabenz; ↑ risk of resp paralysis & renal failure w/ aminoglycosides **Labs:** ↑ Serum glucose, AST, ammonia, alkaline phosphatase; ↓ bilirubin **NIPE:** Take oral meds w/ food

Balsalazide (Colazal) [Anti-inflammatory] Uses: *Ulcerative colitis* **Action:** 5-ASA derivative, antiinflammatory, ↓ leukotriene synthesis **Dose:** 2.25 g (3 caps) tid ×8-12 wk **Caution:** [B, ?] Severe renal/hepatic failure **Contra:** Mesalamine or salicylates hypersensitivity **Disp:** Caps 750 mg **SE:** Dizziness, HA, nausea, agranulocytosis, pancytopenia, renal impair, allergic Rxns **Notes:** Daily dose of 6.75 g = to 2.4 g mesalamine **Interactions:** Oral antibiotics may interfere w/ mesalamine release in the colon **Labs:** ↑ Bilirubin, CPK, LFTs, LDH, plasma fibrinogen; ↓ Ca²⁺, K⁺, protein **NIPE:** ⊘ if ASA allergy, take w/ food & swallow capsule whole

Basiliximab (Simulect) [Immunosuppressant] Uses: *Prevent acute transplant rejection* **Action:** IL-2 receptor antagonists **Dose:** *Adults.* 20 mg IV 2 h before transplant, then 20 mg IV 4 d posttransplant. *Peds.* 12 mg/m² ↑ to max of 20 mg 2 h prior to transplant; the same dose IV 4 d posttransplant **Caution:** [B, ?/–] **Contra:** Hypersensitivity to Murine proteins **Disp:** Inj: powder for reconstitution 10, 20 mg **SE:** Edema, HTN, HA, dizziness, fever, pain, Infxn, GI effects, electrolyte disturbances **Notes:** Murine/human MoAb **Interactions:** May ↑ immunosuppression w/ other immunosuppressive drugs **Labs:** ↑ Serum cholesterol, BUN, creatinine, uric acid; ↓ serum Mg phosphate, plts; ↑ or ↓ in Hgb, Hct, serum glucose, K⁺, Ca²⁺ **NIPE:** Monitor for infection, hypersensitivity Rxns, IV dose over 20–30 min

BCG [Bacillus Calmette-Guérin] (TheraCys, Tice BCG) [Antineoplastic, Antituberculotic] Uses: *Bladder carcinoma (superficial),*

TB prophylaxis **Action:** Immunomodulator **Dose:** Bladder CA, 1 vial prepared & instilled in bladder for 2 h. Repeat once/wk for 6 wk; then 1 treatment at 3, 6, 12, 18, & 24 mo after initial therapy **Caution:** [C, ?] Asthma, do not administer w/traumatic catheterization or UTI **Contra:** Immunosuppression, UTI, steroid use, acute illness, fever of unknown origin **Disp:** Inj 81 mg ($10.5 \pm 8.7 \times 10^8$ CFU/vial) (TheraCys), 50 mg ($1–8 \times 10^8$ CFU/vial) (Tice BCG) **SE:** *Intravesical:* Hematuria, urinary frequency, dysuria, bacterial UTI, rare BCG sepsis **Notes:** Routine US adult BCG immunization not rec; occasionally used in high-risk children who are PPD (–) & cannot take INH **Interactions:** ↓ Effects w/ antimicrobials, immunosuppressives, radiation **Labs:** Prior BCG may cause false + PPD **NIPE:** Monitor for S/Sxs systemic infection, report persistent pain on urination or blood in urine

Becaplermin (Regranex Gel) [Growth Factor]
Uses: Adjunct to local wound care w/*diabetic foot ulcers* **Action:** Recombinant PDGF, enhances granulation tissue **Dose:** Based on lesion; 1½-in. ribbon from 2-g tube, ⅔-in. ribbon from 7.5- or 15-g tube/in.^{2} of ulcer; apply & cover w/moist gauze; rinse after 12h; do not reapply; repeat in 12 h **Caution:** [C, ?] **Contra:** Neoplasm/or active site Infxn **Disp:** 0.01% gel in 2-, 7.5-, 15-g tubes **SE:** Erythema, local pain **Notes:** Use w/ good wound care; wound must be vascularized **Interactions:** None known **NIPE:** Dosage recalculated q1–2wk

Beclomethasone (Beconase, Vancenase Nasal Inhaler) [Anti-inflammatory/Corticosteroid]
Uses: *Allergic rhinitis* refractory to antihistamines & decongestants; *nasal polyps* **Action:** Inhaled steroid **Dose:** *Adults.* 1 spray intranasal bid-qid. *Aqueous inhal:* 1–2 sprays/nostril bid. *Peds 6–12 y.* 1 spray intranasal tid **Caution:** [C, ?] **Disp:** Nasal met-dose inhaler **SE:** Local irritation, burning, epistaxis **Notes:** Nasal spray delivers 42 mcg/dose & 84 mcg/dose **Interactions:** None noted **NIPE:** Prior use of decongestant nasal gtt if edema or secretions, may take several days for full steroid effect

Beclomethasone (QVAR) [Antiasthmatic/Synthetic Corticosteroid]
Uses: Chronic *asthma* **Action:** Inhaled corticosteroid **Dose:** *Adults & Peds.* 1–4 inhal bid (Rinse mouth/throat after) **Caution:** [C, ?] **Contra:** Acute asthma **Disp:** PO met-dose inhaler; 40, 80 mcg/inhal **SE:** HA, cough, hoarseness, oral candidiasis **Notes:** Not effective for acute asthma **Interactions:** None noted **NIPE:** Use inhaled bronchodilator prior to inhaled steroid, rinse mouth after inhaled steroid

Belladonna & Opium Suppositories (B & O Supprettes) [Antispasmodic, Analgesic] [C-II]
Uses: *Bladder spasms; moderate/severe pain* **Action:** Antispasmodic, analgesic **Dose:** 1 supp PR q6h PRN; 15A = 30 mg powdered opium/16.2 mg belladonna extract; 16A = 60 mg powdered opium/16.2 mg belladonna extract **Caution:** [C, ?] **Disp:** Supp 15A, 16A **SE:** Anticholinergic (sedation, urinary retention, constipation) **Interactions:** ↑ Effects w/ CNS depressants, TCAs; ↓ effects w/ phenothiazines **Labs:** ↑ LFTs **NIPE:** ⊘ Refrigerate, moisten finger & supp before insertion, may cause blurred vision

Benazepril (Lotensin) [Antihypertensive/ACEI] Uses: *HTN,* DN, CHF **Action:** ACE inhibitor **Dose:** 10–40 mg/d PO **Caution:** [C (1st tri), D (2nd & 3rd tri), +] **Contra:** Angioedema, Hx edema **Disp:** Tabs 5, 10, 20, 40 mg **SE:** Symptomatic ↓ BP w/ diuretics; dizziness, HA, ↓ K⁺, nonproductive cough **Interactions:** ↑ Effects w/ α-blockers, diuretics, capsaicin; ↓ effects w/ NSAIDs, ASA; ↑ effects OF insulin, Li; ↑ risk OF hyperkalemia w/ trimethoprim & K-sparing diuretics **Labs:** ↑ BUN, SCr, K⁺; ↓ hemoglobin; ECG changes **NIPE:** Persistent cough and/or taste changes may develop, ⊘ PRG, DC if angioedema

Benzocaine & Antipyrine (Auralgan) [Otic Anesthetic] Uses: *Analgesia in severe otitis media* **Action:** Anesthetic w/ local decongestant **Dose:** Fill ear & insert a moist cotton plug; repeat 1–2 h PRN **Caution:** [C, ?] **Contra:** w/ perforated eardrum **Disp:** Soln **SE:** Local irritation **Interactions:** May ↓ effects of sulfonamides

Benzonatate (Tessalon Perles) [Antitussive] Uses: Symptomatic relief of *cough* **Action:** Anesthetizes the stretch receptors in the resp passages **Dose:** *Adults & Peds >10 y.* 100 mg PO tid **Caution:** [C, ?] **Disp:** Caps 100, 200 mg **SE:** Sedation, dizziness, GI upset **Notes:** Do not chew or puncture the caps **Interactions:** ↑ CNS depression w/ antihistamines, EtOH, hypnotics, opioids, sedatives **NIPE:** ↑ Fluid intake to liquefy secretions

Benztropine (Cogentin) [Antiparkinsonian/Anticholinergic] Uses: *Parkinsonism & drug-induced extrapyramidal disorders* **Action:** Partially blocks striatal cholinergic receptors **Dose:** *Adults.* 0.5–6 mg PO, IM, or IV in ÷ doses/d. *Peds >3 y.* 0.02–0.05 mg/kg/dose 1–2/d **Caution:** [C, ?] **Contra:** <3 y **Disp:** Tabs 0.5, 1, 2 mg; inj 1 mg/mL **SE:** Anticholinergic side effects **Notes:** Physostigmine 1–2 mg SC/IV to reverse severe Sxs **Interactions:** ↑ Sedation and depressant effects w/ EtOH & CNS depressants; ↑ anticholinergic effects w/ antihistamines, phenothiazines, quinidine, disopyramide, TCAs, MAOIs; ↑ effect OF digoxin; ↓ effect OF levodopa; ↓ effects w/ antacids and antidiarrheal drugs **NIPE:** May ↑ susceptibility to heat stroke, take w/ meals to avoid GI upset

Beractant (Survanta) [Lung Surfactant] Uses: *Prevention & Rx of RDS in premature infants* **Action:** Replaces pulmonary surfactant **Dose:** 100 mg/kg via ET tube; may repeat 3× q6h; max 4 doses/48 h **Disp:** Susp 25 mg of phospholipid/mL **SE:** Transient bradycardia, desaturation, apnea **Notes:** Administer via 4-quadrant method **Interactions:** None noted **NIPE:** ↑ Risk OF nosocomial sepsis after Rx w/ this drug

Betaxolol (Kerlone) [Antihypertensive/Beta Blocker] Uses: *HTN* **Action:** Competitively blocks β-adrenergic receptors, β₁ **Caution:** [C (1st tri), D (2nd or 3rd tri), +/–] **Contra:** Sinus bradycardia, AV conduction abnormalities, cardiac failure **Dose:** 10–20 mg/d **Disp:** Tabs 10, 20 mg **SE:** Dizziness, HA, bradycardia, edema, CHF **Interactions:** ↑ Effects w/ anticholinergics, verapamil, general anesthetics; ↓ effects w/ thyroid drugs, amphetamine, cocaine, ephedrine, epinephrine, norepinephrine, phenylephrine, pseudoephedrine, NSAIDs; ↑ effects

OF insulin, digitalis glycosides; ↓ effects OF theophylline, dopamine, glucagon
Labs: ↑ BUN, serum lipoprotein, glucose, K⁺, triglyceride, uric acid, ANA titers
NIPE: May ↑ sensitivity to cold, ⊘ DC abruptly]

Betaxolol, Ophthalmic (Betoptic) [Beta Blocker] Uses: Glaucoma **Action:** Competitively blocks β-adrenergic receptors, β₁ **Dose:** 1–2 gtt bid **Caution:** [C (1st tri), D (2nd or 3rd tri), ?/–] **Disp:** Soln 0.5%; susp 0.25% **SE:** Local irritation, photophobia; See Betaxolol + **NIPE:** Use sunglasses to ⊘ exposure, may cause photophobia, review installation procedures

Bethanechol (Urecholine, Duvoid, others) [Urinary Tract Stimulant/Cholinergic Agonist] Uses: *Neurogenic bladder atony w/ retention,* acute *postop* & postpartum functional *(nonobstructive)* urinary retention* **Action:** Stimulates cholinergic smooth muscle receptors in bladder & GI tract **Dose:** *Adults.* 10–50 mg PO tid–qid or 2.5–5 mg SQ tid–qid & PRN. *Peds.* 0.6 mg/kg/24 h PO ÷ tid–qid or 0.15–2 mg/kg/d SQ ÷ 3–4× (take on empty stomach) **Caution:** [C, ?/–] **Contra:** BOO, PUD, epilepsy, hyperthyroidism, bradycardia, COPD, AV conduction defects, parkinsonism ↓ BP, vasomotor instability **Disp:** Tabs 5, 10, 25, 50 mg; inj 5 mg/mL **SE:** Abdominal cramps, D, salivation, ↓ BP **Notes:** Do not use IM/IV **Interactions:** ↑ Effects w/ BBs, tacrine, cholinesterase inhibitors; ↓ effects w/ atropine, anticholinergic drugs, procainamide, quinidine, epinephrine **Labs:** ↑ In serum AST, ALT, amylase, lipase, bilirubin **NIPE:** May cause blurred vision, monitor I&O, take on empty stomach

Bevacizumab (Avastin) [Antineoplastic/Monoclonal Antibody] WARNING: Associated w/ GI perforation, wound dehiscence, & fatal hemoptysis Uses: * Metastatic Colorectal carcinoma, w/ 5-FU* Nonsquamous NSCLC w/ paclitaxel and carboplatin **Action:** Vascular endothelial GF inhibitor **Dose:** *Adults.* 5 mg/kg IV q14d; 1st dose over 90 min; 2nd over 60 min, 3rd over 30 min if tolerated **Caution:** [C, –] Do not use w/in 28 d of surgery if time for separation of drug & anticipated surgical procedures is unknown; D/C if serious adverse events **Disp:** 100 mg/4 mL, 400 mg/16 mL vials **SE:** Wound dehiscence, GI perforation, hemoptysis, hemorrhage, HTN, proteinuria, CHF, inf Rxns, D, leucopenia, thromboembolism **Labs:** Monitor for ↑ BP & proteinuria

Bicalutamide (Casodex) [Antiandrogen/Hormone] Uses: *Advanced CAP (metastatic)* (w/ GnRH agonists [eg, leuprolide, goserelin]) **Action:** Nonsteroidal antiandrogen **Dose:** 50 mg/d **Caution:** [X, ?] **Contra:** Women **Disp:** Caps 50 mg **SE:** Hot flashes, loss of libido, impotence, D/N/V, gynecomastia, & LFT elevation **Interactions:** ↑ Effects OF anticoagulants, TCAs, phenothiazides; ↓ effects OF antipsychotic drugs **Labs:** ↑ LFTs, alkaline phosphatase, bilirubin, BUN, creatinine; ↓ Hgb, WBCs **NIPE:** Monitor PSA, may experience hair loss

Bicarbonate (See Sodium Bicarbonate, page 245)

Bisacodyl (Dulcolax) [Stimulant Laxative] [OTC] Uses: *Constipation; preop bowel prep* **Action:** Stimulates peristalsis **Dose:** *Adults.* 5–15 mg PO or 10 mg PR PRN. *Peds.* <2 y: 5 mg PR PRN. >2 y: 5 mg PO or 10 mg PR

PRN (do not chew tabs or give w/in 1 h of antacids or milk) **Caution:** [B, ?] **Contra:** Acute abdomen or bowel obstruction, appendicitis, gastroenteritis **Disp:** EC tabs 5 mg; DR Tab 5 mg; supp 10 mg **SE:** Abdominal cramps, proctitis, & inflammation w/ suppositories **Interactions:** Antacids & milk ↑ dissolution OF enteric coating causing abdominal irritation **Labs:** False ↓ urine glucose **NIPE:** ↑ Fluid intake & high-fiber foods, ⊘ take w/ milk or antacids

Bismuth Subsalicylate (Pepto-Bismol) [OTC] [Antidiarrheal/Adsorbent]
Uses: Indigestion, nausea, & *D;* combo for Rx of *H. pylori* Infxn* **Action:** Antisecretory & antiinflammatory effects **Dose: Adults.** 2 tabs or 30 mL PO PRN (max 8 doses/24 h). **Peds.** 3–6 y: ⅓ tab or 5 mL PO PRN (max 8 doses/24 h). 6–9 y: ⅔ tab or 10 mL PO PRN (max 8 doses/24 h). 9–12 y: 1 tab or 15 mL PO PRN (max 8 doses/24 h) **Caution:** [C, D (3rd tri), –] Avoid in renal failure **Contra:** Influenza or chickenpox (↑ risk of Reye syndrome), ASA allergy **Disp:** Chew tabs 262 mg; Caplets 262 mg, liq 262, 524 mg/15 mL **SE:** May turn tongue & stools black **Interactions:** ↑ Effects OF ASA, MTX, valproic acid; ↓ effects of tetracyclines, quinolones, probenecid; ↓ effects w/ corticosteroids **Labs:** False ↑ uric acid, AST; may interfere w/ GI tract x-rays; ↓ K⁺, T_3, & T_4 **NIPE:** May darken tongue & stool, chew tab, ⊘ swallow whole

Bisoprolol (Zebeta) [Antihypertensive/Beta Blocker]
Uses: *HTN* **Action:** Competitively blocks $β_1$-adrenergic receptors **Dose:** 5–10 mg/d (max dose 20 mg/d); ↓ in renal impair **Caution:** [C (D 2nd & 3rd tri), +/–] **Contra:** Sinus bradycardia, AV conduction abnormalities, cardiac failure **Disp:** Tabs 5, 10 mg **SE:** Fatigue, lethargy, HA, bradycardia, edema, CHF **Notes:** Not dialyzed **Interactions:** ↑ Bradycardia w/ adenosine, amiodarone, digoxin, dipyridamole, neostigmine, physostigmine, tacrine; ↑ effects w/ cimetidine, fluoxetine, prazosin; ↓ effects w/ NSAIDs, rifampin; ↓ effects of theophylline, glucagon **Labs:** ↑ T_4, cholesterol, glucose, triglycerides, uric acid; ↓ HDL **NIPE:** ⊘ DC abruptly, may mask S/Sxs hypoglycemia, take w/o regard to food

Bitolterol (Tornalate) [Bronchodilator]
Uses: Prophylaxis & Rx of *asthma* & reversible bronchospasm **Action:** Sympathomimetic bronchodilator; stimulates pulmonary $β_2$-adrenergic receptors **Dose: Adults & Peds >12 y.** 2 inhal q8h **Caution:** [C, ?] **Disp:** Aerosol 0.8% SE: Dizziness, nervousness, trembling, HTN, palpitations **Interactions:** ↑ Cardiac effects OF theophylline; ↑ hypokalemia w/ furosemide; ↑ effects w/ other β-adrenergic bronchodilators, MAOIs, TCAs, inhaled anesthetics; ↓ effects w/ β-adrenergic blockers; **Labs:** ↑ AST, ↓ plts, WBCs, proteinuria **NIPE:** Wait 15 min after use of this drug before using an adrenocorticoid inhaler. Shake inhaler well before use

Bivalirudin (Angiomax) [Anticoagulant/Direct Thrombin Inhibitor]
Uses: *Anticoagulant w/ ASA in unstable angina undergoing PTCA, PCI or in pts undergoing PCI w/ or at risk of HIT/HITTS* ** **Action:** Anticoagulant, thrombin inhibitor **Dose:** 0.75 mg/kg IV bolus, then 1.75 mg/kg/h for duration of procedure and up to 4 h post; check ACT 5 min after bolus, may repeat 0.3

mg/kg bolus if necessary (give w/ aspirin 300–325 mg/d; start pre-PTCA) **Caution:** [B, ?] **Contra:** Major bleeding **Disp:** Powder 250 mg for inj **SE:** Bleeding, back pain, nausea, HA **Interactions:** ↑ Cardiac effects OF theophylline; ↑ hypokalemia w/ furosemide; ↑ effects w/ other β-adrenergic bronchodilators, MAOIs, TCAs, inhaled anesthetics; ↓ effects w/ β-adrenergic blockers; **Labs:** ↑ AST, ↓ plts, WBCs, proteinuria **NIPE:** Wait 15 min after use of this drug before using an adrenocorticoid inhaler. Shake inhaler well before use

Bleomycin Sulfate (Blenoxane) [Antineoplastic/Antibiotic]

Uses: *Testis CA; Hodgkin Dz & NHLs; cutaneous lymphomas; & squamous cell CA (head & neck, larynx, cervix, skin, penis); sclerosing agent for malignant pleural effusion* **Action:** Induces breakage (scission) of DNA **Dose:** (Per protocols); ↓ in renal impair **Caution:** [D, ?] Severe pulmonary Dz **Disp:** Inj powder for reconstitution 15, 30 units **SE:** Hyperpigmentation (skin staining) & allergy (rash to anaphylaxis); fever in 50%; lung tox (idiosyncratic & dose related); pneumonitis may progress to fibrosis; Raynaud phenomenon. **N/V Notes:** Test dose 1 mg (U) OK, especially in lymphoma pts; lung tox w/ total dose >400 mg (U) **Interactions:** ↑ Effects w/ cisplatin & other antineoplastic drugs; ↓ effects OF digoxin & phenytoin **Labs:** Monitor CBC, LFTs, BUN, creatinine; pulmonary Fxn tests **NIPE:** ⊘ Immunizations, breast-feeding; use contraception method

Bortezomib (Velcade) [Antineoplastic/Proteosome Inhibitor]

WARNING: May worsen preexisting neuropathy **Uses:** *Progression of multiple myeloma despite one previous Rxs* **Action:** Proteasome inhibitor **Dose:** 1.3 mg/m^2 bolus IV 2×/wk × 2 wk, w/ 10-day rest period (= 1 cycle); ↓ dose w/hematologic tox, neuropathy **Caution:** [D, ?/–] **Disp:** 3.5-mg vial **SE:** Asthenia, GI upset, anorexia, dyspnea, HA, orthostatic ↓ BP, edema, insomnia, dizziness, rash, pyrexia, arthralgia, neuropathy **Interactions:** ↑ Risk OF peripheral neuropathy and/or hypotension w/ amiodarone, antivirals, INH, nitrofurantoin, statins **Labs:** Monitor for ↑ uric acid, ↓ K$^+$, Ca^{2+}, neutrophils, plts **NIPE:** ⊘ PRG or breast-feeding; use contraception; caution w/ driving due to fatigue/dizziness; ↑ fluids if C/O N/V

Brimonidine (Alphagan) [Alpha Agonist/Glaucoma Agent]

Uses: *Open-angle glaucoma, ocular HTN* **Action:** α$_2$-adrenergic agonist **Dose:** 1 gtt in eye(s) tid (wait 15 min to insert contacts) **Caution:** [B, ?] **Contra:** MAOI therapy **Disp:** 0.2% soln **SE:** Local irritation, HA, fatigue **Interactions:** ↑ Effects OF antihypertensives, BBs, cardiac glycosides, CNS depressants; ↓ effects w/ TCAs **NIPE:** ⊘ EtOH, insert soft contact lenses 15 + min after drug use

Brinzolamide (Azopt) [Carbonic Anhydrase Inhibitor/Glaucoma Agent]

Uses: *Open-angle glaucoma, ocular HTN* **Action:** Carbonic anhydrase inhibitor **Dose:** 1 gt in eye(s) tid **Caution:** [C, ?] **Disp.:** 1% susp **SE:** Blurred vision, dry eye, blepharitis, taste disturbance **Interactions:** ↑ Effects w/ oral carbonic anhydrase inhibitors **Labs:** Check LFTs, BUN, creatinine **NIPE:** ⊘ Use drug if ↓ renal & hepatic studies or allergies to sulfonamides; shake well before use; insert soft contact lenses 15 + min after drug use; wait 10 min before use of other topical ophthalmic drugs

Bromocriptine (Parlodel) [Antiparkinson/Dopamine Receptor Agonist]
Uses: *Parkinson Dz, hyperprolactinemia, acromegaly, pituitary tumors* Action: Direct-acting on the striatal dopamine receptors; ↓ prolactin secretion Dose: Initial, 1.25 mg PO bid; titrate to effect, w/food Caution: [C, ?] Contra: Severe ischemic heart Dz or PVD Disp: Tabs 2.5 mg; caps 5 mg SE: ↓ BP, Raynaud phenomenon, dizziness, nausea, hallucinations Interactions: ↑ Effects w/ erythromycin, fluvoxamine, nefazodone, sympathomimetics; ↓ effects w/ phenothiazines, antipsychotics; Labs: ↑ BUN, AST, ALT, CPK, alkaline phosphatase, uric acid NIPE: ◯ Breast-feeding, PRG, oral contraceptives; drug may cause intolerance to EtOH, return of menses & suppression of galactorrhea may take 6–8 wk

Budesonide (Rhinocort, Pulmicort) [Anti-inflammatory/Glucocorticoid]
Uses: *Allergic & nonallergic rhinitis, asthma* Action: Steroid Dose: Adults: Intranasal: 1–4 sprays/nostril/d; Turbuhaler 1–4 inhal bid; Peds: intranasal 1–2 sprays/nostril/d; Turbuhaler 1–2 inhal bid, Respules: 0.25–0.5 mg QD or bid (Rinse mouth after PO use) Caution: [C, ?/–] Disp: Met-dose Turbuhaler, 200 mcg/inhalation; Respules 0.25 mg/mL, 0.5 mL; Rhinocort Aqua 32 mcg/spray SE: HA, cough, hoarseness, Candida Infxn, epistaxis Interactions: ↑ Effects w/ ketoconazole, itraconazole, ritonavir, indinavir, saquinavir, erythromycin, and grapefruit juice NIPE: Shake inhaler well before use, rinse mouth & wash inhaler after use, swallow capsules whole, ◯ exposure chickenpox or measles.

Bumetanide (Bumex) [Diuretic/Loop]
Uses: *Edema from CHF, hepatic cirrhosis, & renal Dz* Action: Loop diuretic; ↓ reabsorption of Na⁺ & Cl⁻, in the ascending loop of Henle & the distal tubule Dose: Adults. 0.5–2 mg/d PO; 0.5–1 mg IV/IM q8–24h (max 10 mg/d) for PO and IV. Peds. 0.015–0.1 mg/kg/d PO, q6–24h Caution: [D, ?] Contra: Anuria, hepatic coma, severe electrolyte depletion Disp: Tabs 0.5, 1, 2 mg; inj 0.25 mg/mL SE: ↓ K⁺, ↓ Na⁺, ↑ creatinine, ↑ uric acid, dizziness, ototox Notes: Monitor fluid & electrolytes Interactions: ↑ Effects w/ antihypertensives, thiazides, nitrates, clofibrate; ↑ effects OF Li, warfarin, thrombolytic drugs, anticoagulants; ↑ K⁺ loss w/ carbenoxolone, corticosteroids, terbutaline; ↑ ototoxicity w/ aminoglycosides, cisplatin; ↓ effects w/ cholestyramine, colestipol, NSAIDs, probenecid, barbiturates, phenytoin Labs: ↑ T₄, T₃, BUN, serum glucose, creatinine uric acid; ↓ serum K⁺, Ca²⁺, Mg²⁺ NIPE: Take drug w/ food, take early to prevent nocturia, daily weights

Bupivacaine (Marcaine) [Anesthetic]
Uses: *Local, regional, & spinal anesthesia, local & regional analgesia* Action: Local anesthetic Dose: Adults & Peds. Dose-dependent on procedure (ie, tissue vascularity, depth of anesthesia, etc) (Table 3) Caution: [C, ?] Contra: Severe bleeding, ↓ BP, shock & arrhythmias, local Infxns at anesthesia site, septicemia Disp: Inj 0.25, 0.5, 0.75%

SE: ↓ BP, bradycardia, dizziness, anxiety **Interactions:** ↑ Effects w/ BBs, hyaluronidase, ergot-type oxytocics, MAOI, TCAs, phenothiazines, vasopressors, CNS depressants; ↓ effects w/ chloroprocaine **NIPE:** Anesthetized area has temporary loss of sensation & Fxn

Buprenorphine (Buprenex) [Analgesic/Opioid Agonist-Antagonist] [C-V] Uses: *Moderate/severe pain* **Action:** Opiate agonist–antagonist **Dose:** 0.3–0.6 mg IM or slow IV push q6h PRN **Caution:** [C, ?/–] **Disp:** 0.3 mg/mL **SE:** Sedation, ↓ BP, resp depression **Notes:** withdrawal if opioid-dependent **Interactions:** ↑ Effects of resp & CNS depression w/ EtOH, opiates, benzodiazepines, TCAs, MAOIs, other CNS depressants **Labs:** ↑ Serum amylase and lipase **NIPE:** ⊘ EtOH & other CNS depressants

Bupropion (Wellbutrin, Wellbutrin SR, Wellbutrin XL, Zyban) [Antidepressant/Smoking Cessation/Aminoketone]
WARNING: Closely monitor for worsening depression or emergence of suicidality **Uses:** *Depression, adjunct to smoking cessation* **Action:** Weak inhibitor of neuronal uptake of serotonin & norepinephrine; ↓ neuronal dopamine reuptake **Dose:** *Depression:* 100–450 mg/d ÷ bid–tid; SR 100–200 mg bid; XL 150–300 mg qd. *Smoking cessation:* 150 mg/d × 3 d, then 150 mg bid ×8–12 wk; ↓ in renal/hepatic impair **Caution:** [B, ?/–] **Contra:** Sz disorder, Hx anorexia nervosa or bulimia, MAOI, abrupt D/C of EtOH or sedatives **Disp:** Tabs 75, 100 mg; SR tabs 100, 150, 200 mg; XL tabs 150, 300 mg; Zyban 150 mg tabs **SE:** Associated w/ Szs; agitation, insomnia, HA, tachycardia **Notes:** Avoid EtOH & other CNS depressants **Interactions:** ↑ Effects w/ cimetidine, levodopa, MAOIs; ↑ risk of Szs w/ EtOH, phenothiazines, antidepressants, theophylline, TCAs, or abrupt withdrawal of corticosteroids, benzodiazepines **Labs:** ↑ Prolactin level **NIPE:** Drug may cause Szs, take 3–4 wk for full effect, ⊘ EtOH or abrupt DC

Buspirone (BuSpar) [Anxiolytic] WARNING: Closely monitor for worsening depression or emergence of suicidality **Uses:** Short-term relief of *anxiety* **Action:** Antianxiety; antagonizes CNS serotonin receptors **Dose:** Initial: 7.5 mg PO bid; ↑ by 5 mg q 2—3 days to effect; usual 20—30 mg/d; max 60 mg/d; ↓ w/severe hepatic/renal insuff **Caution:** [B, ?/–] **Disp:** Tabs divide dose 5, 7.5, 10, 15, 30 mg **SE:** Drowsiness, dizziness; HA, N **Notes:** No abuse potential or physical/psychologic dependence **Interactions:** ↑ Effects w/ erythromycin, clarithromycin, itraconazole, ketoconazole, diltiazem, verapamil, grapefruit juice; ↓ effects w/ carbamazepine, rifampin, phenytoin, dexamethasone, phenobarbital, fluoxetine **Labs:** ↑ AST, ALT, growth hormone, prolactin **NIPE:** ↑ Sedation w/ EtOH, therapeutic effects may take up to 4 wk

Busulfan (Myleran, Busulfex) [Antineoplastic/Alkylating Drug] Uses: *CML.* preparative regimens for allogeneic & ABMT in high doses **Action:** Alkylating agent **Dose:** (Per protocol) **Caution:** [D, ?] **Disp:** Tabs 2 mg, inj 60 mg/10 mL **SE:** Myelosuppression, pulmonary fibrosis, nausea (w/ high-dose), gynecomastia, adrenal insuff, & skin hyperpigmentation **Interactions:**

↑ Effects w/ acetaminophen; ↑ bone-marrow suppression w/ antineoplastic drugs & radiation therapy; ↑ uric acid levels w/ probenecid & sulfinpyrazone; ↓ effects w/ itraconazole, phenytoin **Labs:** ↑ Uric acid; monitor CBC, LFTs **NIPE:** ⊘ Immunizations, PRG, breast-feeding; ↑ fluids; use barrier contraception; ↑ risk of hair loss, rash, darkened skin pigment; ↑ susceptibility to infection

Butorphanol (Stadol) [Analgesic/Opioid Agonist-Antagonist] [C-IV]
Uses: *Anesthesia adjunct, pain* & migraine HA **Action:** Opiate agonist–antagonist w/ central analgesic actions **Dose:** 1–4 mg IM or IV q3–4h PRN. *HA:* 1 spray in 1 nostril; may repeat ×1 if pain not relieved in 60–90 min; ↓ in renal impair **Caution:** [C (D if high doses or prolonged periods at term), +] **Disp:** Inj 2 mg/mL; nasal spray 10 mg/mL **SE:** Drowsiness, dizziness, nasal congestion **Notes:** May induce withdrawal in opioid dependency **Interactions:** ↑ Effects w/ EtOH, antihistamines, cimetidine, CNS depressants, phenothiazines, barbiturates, skeletal-muscle relaxants, MAOIs; ↓ effects OF opioids **Labs:** ↑ Serum amylase & lipase **NIPE:** ⊘ EtOH or other CNS depressants

Calcipotriene (Dovonex) [Keratolytic]
Uses: *Plaque psoriasis* **Action:** Keratolytic **Dose:** Apply bid **Caution:** [C, ?] **Contra:** ↑ Ca^{2+}; vitamin D tox; do not apply to face **Disp:** Cream; oint; soln 0.005% **SE:** Skin irritation, dermatitis **Interactions:** None noted **Labs:** Monitor serum Ca **NIPE:** Wash hands after application or wear gloves to apply, DC drug if ↑ Ca

Calcitonin (Cibacalcin, Miacalcin) [Hypocalcemic, Bone Resorption Inhibitor/Thyroid Hormone]
Uses: *Paget Dz of bone, ↑ Ca^{2+},* osteogenesis imperfecta, *postmenopausal osteoporosis* **Action:** Polypeptide hormone **Dose:** *Paget Dz salmon form:* 100 units/d IM/SC initial, 50 units/d or 50–100 units q1–3d maint. *↑ Ca^{2+} salmon calcitonin:* 4 units/kg IM/SC q12h; ↑ to 8 units/kg q12h, max q6h. *Osteoporosis salmon calcitonin:* 100 units/d IM/SQ; intranasal 200 units = 1 nasal spray/d **Caution:** [C, ?] **Disp:** Spray, nasal 200 units/activation; inj, salmon 200 units/mL (2 mL) **SE:** Facial flushing, nausea, injection site edema, nasal irritation, polyuria **Notes:** For nasal spray alternate nostrils daily. **Interactions:** Prior treatment w/alendronate, risedronate, etidronate, or pamidronate may ↓ effects of calcitonin **Labs:** ↓ Serum Li; monitor serum calcium and alkaline phosphatase **NIPE:** Allergy skin test prior to use; flushing > inj is transient; nausea > inj will < w/ continued treatment

Calcitriol (Rocaltrol, Calcijex) [Antihypocalcemic/Vitamin D Analog]
Uses: *Reduction of ↑ PTH levels, ↓ Ca^{2+} on dialysis* **Action:** 1,25-Dihydroxycholecalciferol (vitamin D analog) **Dose:** **Adults.** Renal failure: 0.25 mcg/d PO, ↑ 0.25 mcg/d q4–6wk PRN; 0.5 mcg 3×/wk IV, ↑ PRN. *Hyperparathyroidism:* 0.5–2 mcg/d. **Peds.** Renal failure: 15 ng/kg/d, ↑ PRN; maint 30–60 ng/kg/d. *Hyperparathyroidism:* <5 y, 0.25–0.75 mcg/d. >6 y, 0.5–2 mcg/d **Caution:** [C, ?] **Contra:** ↑ Ca^{2+}; vitamin D tox **Disp:** Inj 1, 2 mcg/mL (in 1-mL); caps 0.25, 0.5 mcg, sol 1 mcg/mL **SE:** ↑ Ca^{2+} possible **Notes:** Monitor to keep Ca^{2+} WNL **Interactions:** ↑ Effect w/ thiazide diuretics; ↓ effect w/ cholestyramine,

colestipol **Labs:** ↑ Ca^{2+}, cholesterol, Mg^{2+}, BUN, AST, ALT; ↓ alkaline phosphatase; **NIPE:** ⊘ Mg-containing antacids or suppls

Calcium Acetate (PhosLo) [Calcium supplement, Antiarrhythmic/Mineral, Electrolyte] Uses: *ESRD-associated hyperphosphatemia* **Action:** Ca^{2+} supl w/o aluminum to ↓ PO_4^{-} **Dose:** 2–4 tabs PO w/ meals **Caution:** [C, ?] **Contra:** ↑ Ca^{2+} **Disp:** Gelcap 667 mg; Inj 0.5 meq/mL **SE:** Can ↑ Ca^{2+}, hypophosphatemia, constipation **Notes:** Monitor Ca^{2+} **Interactions:** ↑ Effects OF quinidine; ↓ effects w/ large intake of dietary fiber, spinach, rhubarb; ↓ effects OF atenolol, CCB, etidronate, tetracyclines, fluoroquinolones, phenytoin, Fe salts **Labs:** ↑ Ca^{2+}; ↓ Mg^{2+} **NIPE:** ⊘ EtOH, caffeine, tobacco; separate Ca suppls and other meds by 1–2 h

Calcium Carbonate (Tums, Alka-Mints) [OTC] [Antacid, Calcium Supplement/Mineral, Electrolyte] Uses: *Hyperacidity associated w/ peptic ulcer Dz, hiatal hernia,* etc **Action:** Neutralizes gastric acid **Dose:** 500 mg–2 g PO PRN; ↓ in renal impair **Caution:** [C, ?] **Disp:** Chew tabs 350, 420, 500, 550, 750, 850 mg; susp **SE:** ↑ Ca^{2+}, hypophosphatemia, constipation **Interactions:** ↓ Effect OF tetracyclines, fluoroquinolones, Fe salts, and ASA; ↓ Ca absorption w/ high intake of dietary fiber **Labs:** ↑ Ca^{2+}, ↓ Mg^{2+} **NIPE:** ↑ Fluids, may cause constipation, ⊘ EtOH, caffeine, tobacco; separate Ca suppls and other meds by 1–2 h, chew tablet well

Calcium Glubionate (Neo-Calglucon) [OTC] [Calcium Supplement, Anti-Arrhythmic/Mineral, Electrolyte] Uses: *Rx & prevent calcium deficiency* **Action:** Ca^{2+} supl **Dose:** *Adults.* 6–18 g/d ÷ doses. *Peds.* 600–2000 mg/kg/d ÷ qid (9 g/d max); ↓ in renal impair **Caution:** [C, ?] **Contra:** ↑ Ca^{2+} **Disp:** OTC syrup 1.8 g/5 mL = Ca 115 mg/5 mL **SE:** ↑ Ca^{2+}, hypophosphatemia, constipation **Interactions:** ↑ Effects OF quinidine; ↓ effect of tetracyclines; ↓ Ca absorption w/ high intake of dietary fiber; **Labs:** ↑ Ca^{2+}, ↓ Mg^{2+} **NIPE:** ⊘ EtOH, caffeine, tobacco, separate Ca suppls and other meds by 1–2 h, chew tab well

Calcium Salts (Chloride, Gluconate, Gluceptate) [Calcium Supplement, Anti-Arrhythmic/Mineral, Electrolyte] Uses: *Ca^{2+} replacement,* VF, Ca^{2+} blocker tox, Mg^{2+} intox, tetany, *hyperphosphatemia in ESRD* **Action:** Ca^{2+} supl/replacement **Dose:** *Adults.* Replacement: 1–2 g/d PO. *Cardiac emergencies:* CaCl 0.5–1 g IV q 10 min or Ca gluconate 1–2 g IV q 10 min. *Tetany:* 1 g CaCl over 10–30 min; repeat in 6 h PRN. *Peds.* Replacement: 200–500 mg/kg/24 h PO or IV ÷ qid. *Cardiac emergency:* 100 mg/kg/dose IV gluconate salt q 10 min. *Tetany:* 10 mg/kg CaCl over 5–10 min; repeat in 6 h or use inf (200 mg/kg/d max). *Adult & Peds.* ↓ Ca^{2+} due to citrated blood inf: 0.45 mEq Ca/100 mL citrated blood inf (↓ in renal impair) **Caution:** [C, ?] **Contra:** ↑ Ca^{2+} **Disp:** CaCl inj 10% = 100 mg/mL = 27.2 mg/mL = 10-mEq amp; Ca gluconate inj 10% = 100 mg/mL = Ca 9 mg/mL; tabs 500 mg = 45 mg Ca, 650 mg = 58.5 mg Ca, 975 mg = 87.75 mg Ca, 1 g = 90 mg Ca; Ca gluceptate inj 220 mg/mL = 18 mg/mL Ca **SE:** Bradycardia, cardiac arrhythmias, ↑ Ca^{2+} **Notes:** CaCl 270 mg (13.6 mEq) elemental Ca/g, & calcium gluconate 90 mg (4.5 mEq) Ca/g. *RDA for Ca:* Adults = 800 mg/d; Peds = <6 mo 360 mg/d, 6 mo–1 y 540 mg/d, 1–10 y 800 mg/d, 10–18 y 1200 mg/d **Interactions:** ↑ Effects OF quinidine and digitalis; ↓ effects OF tetracyclines, quinolones, verapamil, CCBs, Fe salts, ASA, atenolol; ↓ Ca absorption w/ high intake of dietary fiber **Labs:** ↑ Ca^{2+}, Mg^{2+} **NIPE:** ⊘ EtOH, caffeine, tobacco; separate Ca suppls and other meds by 1–2 h, chew tablet well

Calfactant (Infasurf) [RDS Agent/Surfactant] **Uses:** *Prevention & Rx of RSD in infants* **Action:** Exogenous pulmonary surfactant **Dose:** 3 mL/kg instilled into lungs. Can retreat for a total of 3 doses given 12 h apart **Caution:** [?, ?] **Disp:** Intratracheal susp 35 mg/mL **SE:** Monitor for cyanosis, airway obstruction, bradycardia during administration **Interactions:** None noted **NIPE:** ⊘ Reconstitute, dilute, or shake vial; refrigerate & keep away from light; no need to warm soln prior to use

Candesartan (Atacand) [Antihypertensive/ARB] **Uses:** *HTN,* DN, CHF **Action:** Angiotensin II receptor antagonist **Dose:** 4-32 mg/d (usual 16 mg/d) **Caution:** [X, –] **Contra:** Primary hyperaldosteronism; bilateral renal artery stenosis **Disp:** Tabs 4, 8, 16, 32 mg **SE:** Dizziness, HA, flushing, angioedema **Interactions:** ↑ Effects w/ cimetidine; ↑ risk of hyperkalemia w/ amiloride, spironolactone, triamterene, K suppls; ↑ effects OF Li; ↓ effects w/ phenobarbital, rifampin **Labs:** ↑ Creatine phosphatase; monitor for albuminuria, hyperglycemia, triglyceridemia, uricemia. **NIPE:** ⊘ Breast-feeding or PRG, use barrier contraception, may take 4–6 wk for full effect, adequate fluid intake, take w/o regard to food

Capsaicin (Capsin, Zostrix, others) [Topical Anesthetic/ Analgesic] [OTC] **Uses:** Pain due to *postherpetic neuralgia,* chronic neuralgia, *arthritis,* diabetic neuropathy,* postop pain, psoriasis, intractable pruritus **Action:** Topical analgesic **Dose:** Apply tid–qid **Caution:** [?, ?] **Disp:** OTC creams; gel; lotions; roll-ons **SE:** Local irritation, neurotox, cough **Interactions:** May ↑ cough w/ ACEIs **NIPE:** External use only, ⊘ contact w/ eyes or broken/irritated skin, apply w/ gloves, transient stinging/burning

Captopril (Capoten, others) [Antihypertensive/ACEI] **Uses:** *HTN, CHF, MI,* LVD, DN **Action:** ACE inhibitor **Dose:** *Adults.* HTN: Initial, 25 mg PO bid–tid; ↑ to maint q1–2wk by 25-mg increments/dose (max 450 mg/d) to effect. *CHF:* Initial, 6.25–12.5 mg PO tid; titrate PRN *LVD:* 50 mg PO tid. *DN:* 25 mg PO tid. *Peds.* Infants <2 mo: 0.05–0.5 mg/kg/dose PO q8–24h. *Children:* Initial, 0.3–0.5 mg/kg/dose PO tid; ↑ to 6 mg/kg/d max (1 h before meals) **Caution:** [C (1st tri); D (2nd & 3rd tri); unknown effects in renal impair +] **Contra:** Hx angioedema **Disp:** Tabs 12.5, 25, 50, 100 mg **SE:** Rash, proteinuria, cough, ↑ K^+ **Interactions:** ↑ Effects w/ antihypertensives, diuretics, nitrates, probenecid, black catechu; ↓ effects w/ antacids, ASA, NSAIDs, food; ↑ effects OF digoxin, insulin, oral hypoglycemics, Li **Labs:** False + urine acetone; may ↑ urine protein, serum

BUN, creatinine, K^+, prolactin, LFTs; may ↓ FBS **NIPE:** ⊘ PRG, breast-feeding, K-sparing diuretics; take w/o food, may take 2 wk for full therapeutic effect

Carbamazepine (Tegretol XR, carbatrol, Epitol) [Anticonvulsant/Analgesic]

WARNING: Aplastic anemia & agranulocytosis have been reported w/carbamazepine **Uses:** *Epilepsy, trigeminal neuralgia,* EtOH withdrawal **Action:** Anticonvulsant **Dose:** *Adults.* Initial, 200 mg PO bid; or 100 mg 4 times/day q susp; ↑ by 200 mg/d; usual 800–1200 mg/d ÷ doses. *Peds.* <6 y: 5 mg/kg/d, ↑ to 10–20 mg/kg/d ÷ in 2–4 doses. *6–12 y:* Initial, 100 mg PO bid or 10 mg/kg/24 h PO ÷ qd–bid; ↑ to maint 20–30 mg/kg/24 h ÷ tid–qid; ↓ in renal impair (take w/ food) **Caution:** [D, +] **Contra:** MAOI use, Hx BM suppression **Disp:** Tabs 200 mg; chew tabs 100 mg; XR tabs 100, 200, 400 mg; Caps ER 100, 200, 300 mg; susp 100 mg/5 mL **SE:** Drowsiness, dizziness, blurred vision, N/V, rash, ↓ Na^+, leukopenia, agranulocytosis **Notes:** Monitor CBC & serum levels (Table 2), generic products not interchangeable **Interactions:** ↑ Effects w/ cimetidine, clarithromycin, danazol, diltiazem, felbamate, fluconazole, fluoxetine, fluvoxamine, INH, itraconazole, ketoconazole, macrolides, metronidazole, propoxyphene, protease inhibitors, valproic acid, verapamil, grapefruit juice; ↑ effects OF Li, MAOIs; ↓ effects w/ phenobarbital, phenytoin, primidone, plantain; ↓ effects OF benzodiazepines, corticosteroids, cyclosporine, doxycycline, felbamate, haloperidol, oral contraceptives, phenytoin, theophylline, thyroid hormones, TCAs, warfarin **Labs:** ↑ BUN, LFTs, bilirubin, alkaline phosphatase; ↓ Ca^{2+}, T_3, T_4, Na; false—PRG test & uric acid **NIPE:** Take w/ food, may cause photosensitivity—use sunscreen, use barrier contraception, abrupt withdrawal may cause Szs, ⊘ breast-feeding or PRG

Carbidopa/Levodopa (Sinemet, Parcopa) [Antiparkinsonian]

Uses: *Parkinson Dz* **Action:** ↑ CNS dopamine levels **Dose:** 25/100 mg bid–qid; ↑ as needed (max 200/2000 mg/d) **Caution:** [C, ?] **Contra:** NA glaucoma, suspicious skin lesion (may activate melanoma),melanoma, MAOI use **Disp:** Tabs (mg carbidopa/mg levodopa) 10/100, 25/100, 25/250; tabs SR (mg carbidopa/mg levodopa) 25/100, 50/200 **SE:** Psychiatric disturbances, orthostatic ↓ BP, dyskinesias, cardiac arrhythmias **Interactions:** ↑ Effects w/ antacids; ↓ effects w/ anticonvulsants, benzodiazepines, haloperidol, Fe, methionine, papaverine, phenothiazines, phenytoin, pyridoxine, spiramycin, tacrine, thioxanthenes, high protein food **Labs:** ↑ Urine amino acids, serum acid phosphatase, aspartate aminotransferase; ↓ serum bilirubin, BUN, creatinine, glucose, uric acid **NIPE:** Darkened urine & sweat may result, ⊘ crush or chew sustained release tabs, take w/o food

Carboplatin (Paraplatin) [Antineoplastic/Alkylating Agent]

Uses: *Ovarian, lung, head & neck, testicular, urothelial,* & brain *CA, NHL* & allogeneic & ABMT in high doses **Action:** DNA cross-linker; forms DNA-platinum adducts **Dose:** 360 mg/m² (ovarian carcinoma); AUC dosing 4–7 mg/mL (Culvert formula): mg = AUC × [25 + calculated GFR]); adjust based on pretreatment plt count, CrCl, & BSA (Egorin formula); up to 1500 mg/m² used in ABMT setting (Per protocols) **Caution:** [D, ?] **Contra:** Severe BM suppression, excessive bleeding **Disp:** Inj 50, 150, 450 mg **SE:** Myelosuppression, N/V/D, nephrotox, hematuria, neurotox, ↑ LFTs **Notes:** Physiologic dosing based on either Culvert or Egorin formula allows ↑ doses w/ ↓ tox **Interactions:** ↑ Myelosuppression w/ myelosuppressive drugs; ↑ hemotologic effects w/ bone-marrow suppressants; ↑ bleeding w/ ASA; ↑ nephrotoxicity w/ nephrotoxic drugs; ↓ effects OF phenytoin; ↓ effects w/ food and w/ Al **Labs:** ↓ Mg²⁺, K⁺, Na⁺, Ca²⁺; ↑ LFTs **NIPE:** ⊘ Use w/ Al needles or IV administration sets, PRG, breast-feeding; antiemetics prior to admin may prevent N/V, maintain adequate food & fluid intake

Carisoprodol (Soma) [Skeletal Muscle Relaxant] Uses: *Adjunct to sleep & physical therapy to relieve painful musculoskeletal conditions* **Action:** Centrally acting muscle relaxant **Dose:** 350 mg PO tid–qid **Caution:** [C, M] Tolerance may result; w/ renal/hepatic impair **Contra:** Allergy to meprobamate; acute intermittent porphyria **Disp:** Tabs 350 mg **SE:** CNS depression, drowsiness, dizziness, tachycardia **Notes:** Avoid EtOH & other CNS depressants; available in combo w/ ASA or codeine. **Interactions:** ↑ Effects w/ CNS depressants, phenothiazines, EtOH **NIPE:** ⊘ Breast-feeding, take w/ food if GI upset

Carmustine [BCNU] (BiCNU, Gliadel) [Antineoplastic, Alkylating Agent] Uses: *Primary brain tumors, melanoma, Hodgkin lymphoma & NHLs, multiple myeloma, & induction for allogeneic & ABMT in high doses; adjunct to surgery in pts w/ recurrent glioblastoma* **Action:** Alkylating agent; nitrosourea forms DNA cross-links to inhibit DNA **Dose:** 150–200 mg/m² q6–8wk single or ÷ dose qd inj over 2 d; 20–65 mg/m² q4–6wk; 300–900 mg/m² in BMT (Per protocols); ↓ in hepatic impair **Caution:** [D, ?] ↓ WBC, RBC, plt counts, renal/hepatic impair **Contra:** Myelosuppression, PRG **Disp:** Inj 100 mg/vial; wafer: 7.7 mg **SE:** ↓ BP, N/V, myelosuppression (WBC & plt), phlebitis, facial flushing, hepatic/renal dysfunction, pulmonary fibrosis, optic neuroretinitis; hematologic tox may persist 4–6 wk after dose **Notes:** Do not give course more frequently than q6wk (cumulative tox); baseline PFTs OK **Interactions:** ↑ Bleeding w/ ASA, anticoagulants; ↑ hepatic dysfunction w/ etoposide; ↑ myelosuppression w/ cimetidine; ↑ suppression OF bone marrow w/ radiation or additional antineoplastics; ↓ effects OF phenytoin, digoxin; ↓ pulmonary Fxn **Labs:** ↑ AST, alkaline phosphatase, bilirubin; monitor CBC, plts, LFTs, PFTs **NIPE:** ⊘ PRG, breast-feeding, exposure to infections, ASA products

Carteolol (Cartrol, Ocupress Ophthalmic) [Beta Blocker/ Glaucoma Agent] Uses: *HTN, ↑ intraocular pressure, chronic open-angle glaucoma* **Action:** Blocks β-adrenergic receptors (β₁, β₂), mild ISA **Dose:** PO 2.5–5 mg/d; ophth 1 gt in eye(s) bid; ↓ in renal impair **Caution:** [C (1st tri); D (2nd & 3rd tri), ?/–] Cardiac failure, asthma **Contra:** Sinus bradycardia; heart block >1st degree; bronchospasm **Disp:** Tabs 2.5, 5 mg; ophth soln 1% **SE:** Drowsiness, sexual dysfunction, bradycardia, edema, CHF; *ocular:* conjunctival hyperemia, anisocoria, keratitis, eye pain **Notes:** No value in CHF **Interactions:**

↑ Effects w/ amiodarone, adenosine, barbiturates, CCBs, digoxin, dipyridamole, fluoxetine, rifampin, tacrine, nitrates, EtOH; ↑ α-adrenergic effects w/ amphetamines, cocaine, ephedrine, epinephrine, phenylephrine; ↑ effects OF theophylline; ↓ effects w/ antacids, NSAIDs, thyroid drugs, clonidine; ↓ effects OF hypoglycemics, theophylline, dopamine **Labs:** ↑ BUN, uric acid, K⁺, serum lipoprotein, triglycerides, glucose, ANA titers **NIPE:** Ophthalmic drug may cause photophobia & risk of burning; may ↑ cold sensitivity, mental confusion

Carvedilol (Coreg) [Antihypertensive/Alpha1 & Beta Blocker] Uses: *HTN, CHF, MI* Action: Blocks adrenergic receptors, β₁, β₂, α Dose: *HTN:* 6.25–12.5 mg bid. *CHF:* 3.125–25 mg bid; w/ food to minimize ↓ BP **Caution:** [C (1st tri); D (2nd & 3rd tri), ?/–] Bradycardia, asthma, diabetes **Contra:** Decompensated cardiac failure, 2nd-/3rd-degree heart block, SSS, severe hepatic impair **Disp:** Tabs 3.125, 6.25, 12.5, 25 mg **SE:** Dizziness, fatigue, hyperglycemia, bradycardia, edema, hypercholesterolemia **Notes:** Do not D/C abruptly; ↑ digoxin levels **Interactions:** ↑ Effects w/ cimetidine, clonidine, MAOIs, reserpine, verapamil, fluoxetine, paroxetine; ↑ effects OF digoxin, hypoglycemics, cyclosporine, CCBs; ↓ effects w/ rifampin, NSAIDs; **Labs:** ↑ LFTs, K⁺, triglycerides, uric acid, BUN, creatinine, alkaline phosphatase; ↓ HDL **NIPE:** Food slows absorption, may cause dry eyes w/ contact lenses

Caspofungin (Cancidas) [Antifungal] Uses: *Invasive aspergillosis refractory/intolerant to standard therapy, esophageal candidiasis* Action: An echinocandin; ↓ fungal cell wall synthesis; highest activity in regions of active cell growth **Dose:** 70 mg IV load day 1, 50 mg/d IV; slow inf; ↓ in hepatic impair **Caution:** [C, ?/–] Do not use w/ cyclosporine; not studied as initial therapy **Contra:** Allergy to any component **Disp:** Inj 50, 70 mg **SE:** Fever, HA, N/V, thrombophlebitis at site; ↑ LFTs **Notes:** Monitor during inf; limited experience beyond 2 wk of therapy **Interactions:** ↑ Effects w/ cyclosporine; ↓ effects w/ carbamazepine, dexamethasone, efavirenz, nelfinavir, nevirapine, phenytoin, rifampin; ↓ effects OF tacrolimus **Labs:** ↑ LFTs, serum alkaline phosphatase, eosinophils, PT, urine protein & RBCs; ↓ K⁺, albumin, WBCs, Hgb, Hct, plts, neutrophils; **NIPE:** Infuse slowly over 1 h & ⊘ mix w/ other drugs

Cefaclor (Ceclor, Raniclor) [Antibiotic/Cephalosporin–2nd-gen] Uses: *Bacterial Infxns of the upper & lower resp tract, skin, bone, urinary tract, abdomen, gynecologic system* Action: 2nd-gen cephalosporin; ↓ cell wall synthesis. *Spectrum:* More gram(–) activity than 1st-gen cephalosporins; effective against gram(+) (S. aureu) good gram(–) coverage against *Haemophilus influenzae)* **Dose:** *Adults.* 250–500 mg PO tid; XR 375–500 mg bid. *Peds.* 20–40 mg/kg/d PO ÷ 8–12h; ↓ renal impair **Caution:** [B, +] **Contra:** Cephalosporin allergy **Disp:** Caps 250, 500 mg; Chew tabs 125, 187, 250, 375 mg; susp 125, 187, 250, 375 mg/5 mL **SE:** D, rash, eosinophilia, ↑ transaminases **Interactions:** ↑ Bleeding w/ anticoagulants; ↑ nephrotoxicity w/ aminoglycosides, loop diuretics; ↑ effects w/ probenecid; ↓ effects w/ antacids, chloramphenicol **Labs:** + Direct

Coombs' test; ↑ LFTs, alkaline phosphatase, bilirubin, LDH, BUN, creatinine; false + of serum or UCr, false + urine glucose **NIPE:** Food w/ ER tabs ↑ absorption, monitor for superinfection, ⊘ breast-feeding

Cefadroxil (Duricef) [Antibiotic/Cephalosporin–1st-gen]

Uses: *Infxns of skin, bone, upper & lower resp tract, urinary tract* **Action:** 1st-gen cephalosporin; ↓ cell wall synthesis. *Spectrum:* Good gram(+) coverage, (group A β-hemolytic *Strep, Staph*); gram(−) (*E. coli, Proteus, Klebsiella*) **Dose:** *Adults.* 1–2 g/d PO, 2 ÷ doses *Peds.* 30 mg/kg/d ÷ bid; ↓ in renal impair **Caution:** [B, +] **Contra:** Cephalosporin allergy **Disp:** Caps 500 mg; tabs 1 g; susp 250, 500 mg/5 mL **SE:** N/V/D, rash, eosinophilia, ↑ transaminases **Interactions:** ↑ Bleeding w/ anticoagulants; ↑ nephrotoxicity w/ aminoglycosides, loop diuretics; ↓ effects w/ probenecid; ↓ effects w/ antacids, chloramphenicol **Labs:** + Direct Coombs' test; ↑ LFTs, alkaline phosphatase, bilirubin, LDH, BUN, creatinine; false + of serum or UCr, false + urine glucose **NIPE:** Food w/ ER tabs ↑ absorption, monitor for superinfection, ⊘ breast-feeding; give w/o regard to food

Cefazolin (Ancef, Kefzol) [Antibiotic/Cephalosporin–1st-gen]

Uses: * Infxns of skin, bone, upper & lower resp tract, urinary tract* **Action:** 1st-gen cephalosporin; ↓ cell wall synthesis. *Spectrum:* Good coverage gram(+) bacilli & cocci, (*Strep, Staph* (except *Enterococcus*); some gram(−) (*E. coli, Proteus, Klebsiella*) **Dose:** *Adults.* 1–2 g IV q8h *Peds.* 25–100 mg/kg/d IV ÷ q6–8h; ↓ in renal impair **Caution:** [B, +] **Contra:** Cephalosporin allergy **Disp:** Premixed infusion 500 mg, 1 g, **Inj:** 500 mg, 1, 10, 20 g **SE:** D, rash, eosinophilia, elevated transaminases, pain at inj site **Notes:** Widely used for surgical prophylaxis **Interactions:** ↑ Bleeding w/ anticoagulants; ↑ nephrotoxicity w/ aminoglycosides, loop diuretics; ↓ effects w/ probenecid; ↓ effects w/ antacids, chloramphenicol **Labs:** + Direct Coombs' test; ↑ LFTs, alkaline phosphatase, bilirubin, LDH, BUN, creatinine; false + of serum or UCr, false + urine glucose **NIPE:** Food w/ ER tabs ↑ absorption, monitor for superinfection, ⊘ breast-feeding; monitor renal Fxn, I&O

Cefdinir (Omnicef) [Antibiotic/Cephalosporin–3rd-gen]

Uses: *Infxns of the resp tract, skin, bone, & urinary tract* **Action:** 3rd-gen cephalosporin; ↓ cell wall synthesis *Spectrum:* Active against wide range of gram(+) & gram(−) organisms; more active than cefaclor & cephalexin against *Streptococcus, Staphylococcus;* active against some anaerobes **Dose:** *Adults.* 300 mg PO bid or 600 mg/d PO. *Peds.* 7 mg/kg PO bid or 14 mg/kg/d PO; ↓ in renal impair **Caution:** [B, +] In PCN-sensitive pts, serum sickness–like Rxns reported **Contra:** Hypersensitivity to cephalosporins **Disp:** Caps 300 mg; susp 125, 250 mg/5 mL **SE:** Anaphylaxis, D, rare pseudomembranous colitis **Interactions:** ↑ Bleeding w/ anticoagulants; ↑ nephrotoxicity w/ aminoglycosides, loop diuretics; ↓ effects w/ probenecid; ↓ effects w/ antacids, chloramphenicol; ↓ effects w/ Fe suppls **Labs:** + Direct Coombs' test; ↑ LFTs, alkaline phosphatase, bilirubin, LDH, BUN, creatinine; false + of serum or UCr, false + urine glucose **NIPE:** Food w/ ER tabs

↑ absorption, monitor for superinfection, ⊘ breast-feeding; stools may initially turn red in color, sucrose in suspension

Cefditoren (Spectracef) [Antibiotic/Cephalosporin—3rd-gen]
Uses: *Acute exacerbations of chronic bronchitis, pharyngitis, tonsillitis; skin Infxns* **Action:** 3rd-gen cephalosporin; ↓ cell wall synthesis. *Spectrum:* Good gram(+) (*Strep & Staph*); gram(–) (*Haemophilus influenzae & Moraxella catarrhalis*) **Dose:** *Adults & Peds >12 y.* Skin: 200 mg PO bid × 10 days. *Chronic bronchitis, pharyngitis, tonsillitis:* 400 mg PO bid × 10 days; avoid antacids w/in 2 h; take w/ meals; ↓ in renal impair **Caution:** [B, ?] Renal/hepatic impair **Contra:** Cephalosporin/PCN allergy, milk protein, or carnitine deficiency **Disp:** 200-mg tabs **SE:** HA, N/V/D, colitis, nephrotox, hepatic dysfunction, Stevens-Johnson syndrome, toxic epidermal necrolysis, allergy Rxns **Notes:** Causes renal excretion of carnitine; tablets contain milk protein **Interactions:** ↑ Bleeding w/ anticoagulants; ↑ nephrotoxicity w/ aminoglycosides, loop diuretics; ↑ effects w/ probenecid; ↓ effects w/ antacids, chloramphenicol **Labs:** + Direct Coombs' test; ↑ LFTs, alkaline phosphatase, bilirubin, LDH, BUN, creatinine; false + of serum or UCr, false + urine glucose **NIPE:** Food w/ ER tabs ↑ absorption, monitor for superinfection, ⊘ breast-feeding, sensitive to milk protein; monitor for Sz activity

Cefepime (Maxipime) [Antibiotic/Cephalosporin—4th-gen]
Uses: *UTI, pneumonia, febrile neutropenia, skin/soft tissue Infxns* **Action:** 4th-gen cephalosporin; ↓ cell wall synthesis. *Spectrum:* gram(+) *S. pneumoniae, S. aureus,* gram(–) *K. pneumoniae, E. coli, P. aeruginosa, & Enterobacter* sp **Dose:** *Adults.* 1–2 g IV q12h. *Peds.* 50 mg/kg q8h for febrile neutropenia; 50 mg/kg bid for skin/soft tissue Infxns; ↓ in renal impair **Caution:** [B, +] **Contra:** Cephalosporin allergy **Disp:** Inj 500 mg, 1, 2 g **SE:** Rash, pruritus, N/V/D, fever, HA, (+) Coombs' test w/o hemolysis **Notes:** Administered as IM or IV **Interactions:** ↑ Bleeding w/ anticoagulants; ↑ nephrotoxicity w/ aminoglycosides, loop diuretics; ↑ effects w/ probenecid; ↓ effects w/ antacids, chloramphenicol; ↓ effects OF oral contraceptives **Labs:** + Direct Coombs' test; ↑ LFTs, alkaline phosphatase, bilirubin, LDH, BUN, creatinine; false + of serum or UCr, false + urine glucose **NIPE:** Food w/ ER tabs ↑ absorption, monitor for superinfection, ⊘ breast-feeding or use EtOH w/ drug or w/in 3 d of taking drug

Cefixime (Suprax) [Antibiotic/Cephalosporin—3rd-gen]
Uses: *Infxns of the resp tract, skin, bone, & urinary tract* **Action:** 3rd-gen cephalosporin; ↓ cell wall synthesis. *Spectrum: S. pneumoniae, S. pyogenes, H. influenzae,* & enterobacteria. **Dose:** *Adults.* 400 mg PO qd–bid. *Peds.* 8 mg/kg/d PO ÷ qd–bid; ↓ in renal impair **Caution:** [B, +] **Contra:** Cephalosporin allergy **Disp:** Tabs 200, 400 mg; Susp 100 mg/5 mL **SE:** N/V/D, flatulence, & abdominal pain **Notes:** Monitor renal & hepatic Fxn; use susp for otitis media **Interactions:** ↑ Bleeding w/ anticoagulants; ↑ nephrotoxicity w/ aminoglycosides, loop diuretics; ↑ effects w/ probenecid; ↓ effects w/ antacids, chloramphenicol; ↓ effects OF oral contraceptives **Labs:** + Direct Coombs' test; ↑ LFTs, alkaline phosphatase,

bilirubin, LDH, BUN, creatinine; false + of serum or UCr, false + urine glucose **NIPE:** Food w/ ER tabs ↑ absorption, monitor for superinfection, ⊘ breast-feeding

Cefmetazole (Zefazone) [Antibiotic/Cephalosporin−2nd-gen]

Uses: *Rx Infxns of the upper & lower resp tract, skin, bone, urinary tract, abdomen, & gynecologic system* **Action:** 2nd-gen cephalosporin; ↓ cell wall synthesis. *Spectrum:* Gram(+) against *S. aureus;* gram(−) activity & some anaerobic activity; use in mixed aerobic−anaerobic Infxns where *Bacteroides fragilis* likely **Dose:** *Adults.* 2 g IV q6−12h; ↓ in renal impair **Caution:** [B, +] **Contra:** Cephalosporin allergy **Disp:** Inj 1, 2 g **SE:** Eosinophilia, leukopenia, N/V/D, ↑ LFTs, bleeding risk, rash, pseudomembranous colitis, disulfram Rxn **Notes:** safety not established in children **Interactions:** ↑ Bleeding w/ anticoagulants; ↑ nephrotoxicity w/ aminoglycosides, loop diuretics; ↑ effects w/ probenecid; ↓ effects w/ antacids, chloramphenicol **Labs:** + Direct Coombs' test; ↑ LFTs, alkaline phosphatase, bilirubin, LDH, BUN, creatinine; false + of serum or UCr, false + urine glucose **NIPE:** Food w/ ER tabs ↑ absorption, monitor for superinfection, ⊘ breast-feeding or use EtOH w/ drug or w/in 3 d of taking drug

Cefonicid (Monocid) [Antibiotic/Cephalosporin−2nd-gen]

Uses: *Rx bacterial Infxns (resp tract, skin, bone & joint, urinary tract, gynecologic, sepsis)* **Action:** 2nd-gen cephalosporin; ↓ bacterial cell wall synthesis. *Spectrum:* Gram(+) including MSSA & many streptococci; gram(−) bacilli including *E. coli, Klebsiella, P. mirabilis, H. influenzae,* & *Moraxella* **Dose:** 0.5−2 g/24 h IM/IV; ↓ in renal impair **Caution:** [B, +] **Contra:** Cephalosporin allergy **Disp:** Powder for inj 500 mg, 1 g, 10 g **SE:** D, rash, ↑ plts, eosinophilia, ↑ transaminases **Interactions:** ↑ Bleeding w/ anticoagulants; ↑ nephrotoxicity w/ aminoglycosides, loop diuretics; ↑ effects w/ probenecid; ↓ effects w/ antacids, chloramphenicol **Labs:** + Direct Coombs' test; ↑ LFTs, alkaline phosphatase, bilirubin, LDH, BUN, creatinine; false + of serum or UCr, false + urine glucose **NIPE:** Food w/ ER tabs ↑ absorption, monitor for superinfection, ⊘ breast-feeding

Cefoperazone (Cefobid) [Antibiotic/Cephalosporin−3rd-gen]

Uses: *Rx Infxns of the resp, skin, urinary tract, sepsis* **Action:** 3rd-gen cephalosporin; ↓ bacterial cell wall synthesis. *Spectrum:* Gram(−) (eg, *E. coli, Klebsiella*); variable against *Streptococcus* & *Staphylococcus* sp; active *P. aeruginosa* < ceftazidime **Dose:** *Adults.* 2−4 g/d IM/IV ÷ q 8−12h (12 g/d max). *Peds.* (not approved) 100−150 mg/kg/d IM/IV ÷ bid-tid (12 g/d max); ↓ in renal/hepatic impair **Caution:** [B, +] May ↑ risk of bleeding **Contra:** Cephalosporin allergy **Disp:** Powder for inj 1, 2, 10 g **SE:** D, rash, eosinophilia, ↑ LFTs, hypoprothrombinemia, & bleeding (due to MTT side chain) **Notes:** May interfere w/ warfarin **Interactions:** ↑ Bleeding w/ anticoagulants; ↑ nephrotoxicity w/ aminoglycosides, loop diuretics; ↑ effects w/ probenecid; ↓ effects w/ antacids, chloramphenicol **Labs:** + Direct Coombs' test; ↑ LFTs, alkaline phosphatase, bilirubin, LDH, BUN, creatinine; false + of serum or UCr, false + urine glucose **NIPE:** Food w/ ER tabs ↑ absorption, monitor for superinfection, ⊘ breast-feeding or use EtOH w/ drug or w/in 3 d of taking drug

Cefotaxime (Claforan) [Antibiotic/Cephalosporin—3rd-gen]
Uses: *Rx Infxns of resp tract, skin, bone, urinary tract, meningitis, sepsis* **Action:** 3rd-gen cephalosporin; ↓ cell wall synthesis. *Spectrum:* Most gram(–) (not *Pseudomonas*), some gram(+) cocci (not *Enterococcus*); many PCN-resistant pneumococci **Dose:** *Adults.* 1–2 g IV q4–12h. *Peds.* 50–200 mg/kg/d IV ÷ q 4–12h; ↓ dose renal/hepatic impair **Caution:** [B, +] Arrhythmia associated w/ rapid inj; caution in colitis **Contra:** Cephalosporin allergy **Disp:** Powder for inj 500 mg, 1, 2, 10, 20 g **SE:** D, rash, pruritus, colitis, eosinophilia, ↑ transaminases **Interactions:** ↑ Bleeding w/ anticoagulants; ↑ nephrotoxicity w/ aminoglycosides, loop diuretics; ↑ effects w/ probenecid; ↓ effects w/ antacids, chloramphenicol **Labs:** + Direct Coombs' test; ↑ LFTs, alkaline phosphatase, bilirubin, LDH, BUN, creatinine; false + of serum or UCr, false + urine glucose **NIPE:** Food w/ ER tabs ↑ absorption, monitor for superinfection, ⊘ breast-feeding or use EtOH w/ drug or w/in 3 d of taking drug

Cefotetan (Cefotan) [Antibiotic/Cephalosporin—2nd-gen]
Uses: *Rx Infxns of the upper & lower resp tract, skin, bone, urinary tract, abdomen, & gynecologic system* **Action:** 2nd-gen cephalosporin; ↓ cell wall synthesis. *Spectrum:* Less active against gram(+); anaerobes including *B. fragilis;* gram(–), including *E. coli, Klebsiella,* & *Proteus* **Dose:** *Adults.* 1–2 g IV q12h. *Peds.* 20–40 mg/kg/d IV ÷ q12h; ↓ in renal impair **Caution:** [B, +] May ↑ bleeding risk; in those Hx of PCN allergies **Contra:** Cephalosporin allergy **Disp:** Powder for inj 1, 2, 10 g **SE:** D, rash, eosinophilia, ↑ transaminases, hypoprothrombinemia, & bleeding (due to MTT side chain) **Notes:** Caution w/ other nephrotoxic drugs; may interfere w/ warfarin **Interactions:** ↑ Bleeding w/ anticoagulants; ↑ nephrotoxicity w/ aminoglycosides, loop diuretics; ↑ effects w/ probenecid; ↓ effects w/ antacids, chloramphenicol **Labs:** + Direct Coombs' test; ↑ LFTs, alkaline phosphatase, bilirubin, LDH, BUN, creatinine; false + of serum or UCr, false + urine glucose **NIPE:** Food w/ ER tabs ↑ absorption, monitor for superinfection, ⊘ breast-feeding or use EtOH w/ drug or w/in 3 d of taking drug

Cefoxitin (Mefoxin) [Antibiotic/Cephalosporin—2nd-gen]
Uses: *Rx Infxns of the upper & lower resp tract, skin, bone, urinary tract, abdomen, & gynecologic system* **Action:** 2nd-gen cephalosporin; ↓ cell wall synthesis. *Spectrum:* Good gram(–) against enteric bacilli (ie, *E. coli, Klebsiella,* & *Proteus*); anaerobic activity against *B. fragilis* **Dose:** *Adults.* 1–2 mg IV q6–8h. *Peds.* 80–160 mg/kg/d ÷ q4–6h; ↓ in renal impair **Caution:** [B, +] **Contra:** Cephalosporin allergy **Disp:** Powder for inj 1, 2, 10 g **SE:** D, rash, eosinophilia, ↑ transaminases **Interactions:** ↑ Bleeding w/ anticoagulants; ↑ nephrotoxicity w/ aminoglycosides, loop diuretics; ↑ effects w/ probenecid; ↓ effects w/ antacids, chloramphenicol **Labs:** + Direct Coombs' test; ↑ LFTs, alkaline phosphatase, bilirubin, LDH, BUN, creatinine; false + of serum or UCr, false + urine glucose **NIPE:** Food w/ ER tabs ↑ absorption, monitor for superinfection, ⊘ breast-feeding

Cefpodoxime (Vantin) [Antibiotic/Cephalosporin—3rd-gen]
Uses: *Rx resp, skin, & urinary tract Infxns* **Action:** 3rd-gen cephalosporin;

↓ cell wall synthesis. *Spectrum:* S. pneumoniae or non-β-lactamase-producing *H. influenzae;* acute uncomplicated *N. gonorrhoeae;* some uncomplicated gram(–) *(E. coli, Klebsiella, Proteus)* **Dose:** *Adults.* 200–400 mg PO q12h. *Peds.* 10 mg/kg/d PO ÷ bid; ↓ in renal impair, take w/ food **Caution:** [B, +] **Contra:** Cephalosporin allergy **Disp:** Tabs 100, 200 mg; susp 50, 100 mg/5 mL **SE:** D, rash, HA, eosinophilia, elevated transaminases **Notes:** Drug interactions w/ agents that ↑ gastric pH **Interactions:** ↑ Bleeding w/ anticoagulants; ↑ nephrotoxicity w/ aminoglycosides, loop diuretics; ↑ effects w/ probenecid; ↓ effects w/ antacids, chloramphenicol **Labs:** + Direct Coombs' test; ↑ LFTs, alkaline phosphatase, bilirubin, LDH, BUN, creatinine; false + of serum or UCr, false + urine glucose **NIPE:** Food w/ ER tabs ↑ absorption, monitor for superinfection, ⊘ breast-feeding. See Cefaclor. **Additional Interactions:** ↑ Effects if taken w/ food

Cefprozil (Cefzil) [Antibiotic/Cephalosporin–2nd-gen] Uses:
Rx resp tract, skin, & urinary tract Infxns **Action:** 2nd-gen cephalosporin; ↓ cell wall synthesis. *Spectrum:* Active against MSSA, strep, & gram(–) bacilli *(E. coli, Klebsiella, P. mirabilis, H. influenzae, Moraxella)* **Dose:** *Adults.* 250–500 mg PO daily–bid. *Peds.* 7.5–15 mg/kg/d PO ÷ bid; ↓ in renal impair **Caution:** [B, +] **Contra:** Cephalosporin allergy **Disp:** Tabs 250, 500 mg; susp 125, 250 mg/5 mL **SE:** D, dizziness, rash, eosinophilia, ↑ transaminases **Notes:** Use higher doses for otitis & pneumonia **Interactions:** ↑ Bleeding w/ anticoagulants; ↑ nephrotoxicity w/ aminoglycosides, loop diuretics; ↑ effects w/ probenecid; ↓ effects w/ antacids, chloramphenicol **Labs:** + Direct Coombs' test; ↑ LFTs, alkaline phosphatase, bilirubin, LDH, BUN, creatinine; false + of serum or UCr, false + urine glucose **NIPE:** Food w/ ER tabs ↑ absorption, monitor for superinfection, ⊘ breast-feeding

Ceftazidime (Fortaz, Ceptaz, Tazidime, Tazicef) [Antibiotic/Cephalosporin–3rd-gen] Uses:
Rx resp tract, skin, bone, urinary tract Infxns, meningitis, & septicemia **Action:** 3rd-gen cephalosporin; ↓ cell wall synthesis. *Spectrum:* P. aeruginosa sp, good gram(–) activity **Dose:** *Adults.* 500–2 g IV q8–12h. *Peds.* 30–50 mg/kg/dose IV q8h; ↓ in renal impair **Caution:** [B, +] **Contra:** Cephalosporin allergy **Disp:** Powder for inj 500 mg, 1, 2, 6 g **SE:** D, rash, eosinophilia, ↑ transaminases **Interactions:** ↑ Bleeding w/ anticoagulants; ↑ nephrotoxicity w/ aminoglycosides, loop diuretics; ↑ effects w/ probenecid; ↓ effects w/ antacids, chloramphenicol **Labs:** + Direct Coombs' test; ↑ LFTs, alkaline phosphatase, bilirubin, LDH, BUN, creatinine; false + of serum or UCr, false + urine glucose **NIPE:** Food w/ ER tabs ↑ absorption, monitor for superinfection, ⊘ breast-feeding or use EtOH w/in 3 d of taking drug

Ceftibuten (Cedax) [Antibiotic/Cephalosporin–3rd-gen]
Uses: *Rx resp tract, skin, urinary tract Infxns & otitis media* **Action:** 3rd-gen cephalosporin; ↓ cell wall synthesis. *Spectrum:* H. influenzae & M. catarrhalis; weak against *S. pneumoniae* **Dose:** *Adults.* 400 mg/d PO. *Peds.* 9 mg/kg/d PO; ↓ in renal impair; take on empty stomach **Caution:** [B, +] **Contra:** Cephalosporin allergy **Disp:** Caps 400 mg; susp 90 mg/5 mL **SE:** D, rash, eosinophilia, ↑ transami-

nases **Interactions:** ↑ Bleeding w/ anticoagulants; ↑ nephrotoxicity w/ aminogly-cosides, loop diuretics; ↑ effects w/ probenecid; ↓ effects w/ antacids, chloram-phenicol **Labs:** + Direct Coombs' test; ↑ LFTs, alkaline phosphatase, bilirubin, LDH, BUN, creatinine; false + of serum or UCr, false + urine glucose **NIPE:** Food w/ ER tabs ↑ absorption, monitor for superinfection, ⊘ breast-feeding or use EtOH w/in 3 d of taking drug

Ceftizoxime (Cefizox) [Antibiotic/Cephalosporin−3rd-gen]

Uses: *Rx resp tract, skin, bone, & urinary tract Infxns, meningitis, septicemia* **Action:** 3rd-gen cephalosporin; ↓ cell wall synthesis. *Spectrum:* Good gram(-) bacilli (not *Pseudomonas*), some gram(+) cocci (not *Enterococcus*), & some anaer-obes **Dose:** *Adults.* 1–2 g IV q8–12h. *Peds.* 150–200 mg/kg/d IV ÷ q6–8h; ↓ in renal impair **Caution:** [B, +] **Contra:** Cephalosporin allergy **Disp:** Inj 1, 2, 10 g **SE:** D, fever, rash, eosinophilia, thrombocytosis, ↑ transaminases **Interactions:** ↑ Bleeding w/ anticoagulants; ↑ nephrotoxicity w/ aminoglycosides, loop diuret-ics; ↑ effects w/ probenecid; ↓ effects w/ antacids, chloramphenicol **Labs:** + Direct Coombs' test; ↑ LFTs, alkaline phosphatase, bilirubin, LDH, BUN, creatinine; false + of serum or UCr, false + urine glucose **NIPE:** Food w/ ER tabs ↑ absorp-tion, monitor for superinfection, ⊘ breast-feeding

Ceftriaxone (Rocephin) [Antibiotic/Cephalosporin−3rd-gen]

Uses: *Resp tract (pneumonia), skin, bone, urinary tract Infxns, meningitis, & sep-ticemia;* **Action:** 3rd-gen cephalosporin; ↓ cell wall synthesis. *Spectrum:* Moder-ate gram(+); excellent against β-lactamase producers **Dose:** *Adults.* 1–2 g IV q12–24h. *Peds.* 50–100 mg/kg/d IV ÷ q12–24h; ↓ in renal impair **Caution:** [B, +] **Contra:** Cephalosporin allergy; hyperbilirubinemic neonates (displaces bilirubin from binding sites) **Disp:** Powder for inj 500 mg, 1, 2, 10 g **SE:** D, rash, leukopenia, thrombocytosis, eosinophilia, ↑ transaminases **Interactions:** ↑ Bleed-ing w/ anticoagulants; ↑ nephrotoxicity w/ aminoglycosides, loop diuretics; ↑ ef-fects w/ probenecid; ↓ effects w/ antacids, chloramphenicol **Labs:** + Direct Coombs' test; ↑ LFTs, alkaline phosphatase, bilirubin, LDH, BUN, creatinine; false + of serum or UCr, false + urine glucose **NIPE:** Food w/ ER tabs ↑ absorp-tion, monitor for superinfection, ⊘ breast-feeding or use EtOH w/in 3 d of taking drug (NR) mix w/ other antimicrobials

Cefuroxime (Ceftin [PO], Zinacef [parenteral]) [Antibiotic/Cephalosporin−2nd-gen]

Uses: *Upper & lower resp tract, skin, bone, urinary tract, abdomen, gynecologic Infxns* **Action:** 2nd-gen cephalosporin; ↓ cell wall synthesis *Spectrum:* Staphylococci, group B streptococci, *H. influenzae, E. coli, Enterobacter, Salmonella, & Klebsiella* **Dose:** *Adults.* 750 mg–1.5 g IV q8h or 250–500 mg PO bid. *Peds.* 100–150 mg/kg/d IV ÷ q8h or 20–30 mg/kg/d PO ÷ bid; ↓ in renal impair; take w/ food **Caution:** [B, +] **Contra:** Cephalosporin allergy **Disp:** Tabs 125, 250, 500 mg; susp 125, 250 mg/5 mL; powder for inj 750 mg, 1.5, 7.5 g **SE:** D, rash, eosinophilia, ↑ LFTs **Notes:** Cefuroxime film-coated tablets & PO susp not bioequivalent; do not substitute on a mg/mg basis; IV crosses blood–brain barrier **Interactions:** ↑ Bleeding w/ anticoagulants; ↑ nephrotoxicity w/ aminoglycosides, loop diuretics; ↑ effects w/ probenecid; ↓ effects w/ antacids, chloramphenicol **Labs:** + Direct Coombs' test; ↑ LFTs, alkaline phosphatase, bilirubin, LDH, BUN, creatinine; false + of serum or UCr, false + urine glucose **NIPE:** Food w/ ER tabs ↑ absorption, monitor for superinfection, ⊘ breast-feeding or use EtOH w/ drug or w/in 3 d of taking drug, food will ↓ GI distress & ↑ absorption, swallow tabs whole

Celecoxib (Celebrex) [Anti-inflammatory/COX-2 Inhibitor]

WARNING: ↑ Risk of serious CV thrombotic events, MI & stroke, which can be fatal; ↑ risk of serious GI adverse events including bleeding, ulceration, & perforation of the stomach or intestines, which can be fatal. **Uses:** *Osteoarthritis & RA, ankylosing spondylitis*; acute pain, primary dysmenorrhea; preventive in familial adenomatous polyposis **Action:** NSAID; ↓ the COX-2 pathway **Dose:** 100–200 mg/d or bid; FAP: 400 mg po bid; ↓ in hepatic impair; take w/ food/milk **Caution:** [C/D (3rd tri), ?] Caution in renal impair **Contra:** Allergy to sulfonamides, periop CABG **Disp:** Caps 100, 200, 400 mg **SE:** see Warning; GI upset, HTN, edema, renal failure, HA **Notes:** Watch for Sxs of GI bleeding; no effect on plt/bleeding time; can affect drugs metabolized by P-450 pathway **Interactions:** ↑ Effects w/ fluconazole; ↑ effects OF Li; ↑ risks OF GI upset &/or bleeding w/ ASA, NSAIDs, warfarin, EtOH; ↓ effects w/ Al- & Mg-containing antacids, ↓ effects of thiazide diuretics, loop diuretics, ACEIs **Labs:** ↑ LFTs, BUN, creatinine, CPK, alkaline phosphatase; monitor for hypercholesterolemia, hyperglycemia, hypokalemia, hypophosphatemia, albuminuria, hematuria **NIPE:** Take w/ food if GI distress

Cephalexin (Keflex, Keftab, Pranixine Disperdose) [Antibiotic/Cephalosporin–1st-gen]

Uses: *Skin, bone, upper/lower resp tract, urinary tract Infxns* **Action:** 1st-gen cephalosporin; ↓ cell wall synthesis. *Spectrum: Strep, Staph, E. coli, Proteus, Klebsiella* **Dose:** *Adults.* 250–500 mg PO qid. *Peds.* 25–100 mg/kg/d PO ÷ qid; ↓ in renal impair; (on empty stomach) **Caution:** [B, +] **Contra:** Cephalosporin allergy **Disp:** Caps 250, 500 mg; tabs for oral susp 125, 250mg; susp 125, 250 mg/5 mL **SE:** D, rash, eosinophilia, ↑ LFTs **Interactions:** ↑ Bleeding w/ anticoagulants; ↑ nephrotoxicity w/ aminoglycosides, loop diuretics; ↑ effects w/ probenecid; ↓ effects w/ antacids, chloramphenicol **Labs:** + Direct Coombs' test; ↑ LFTs, alkaline phosphatase, bilirubin, LDH, BUN, creatinine; false + of serum or UCr, false + urine glucose **NIPE:** Food w/ ER tabs ↑ absorption, monitor for superinfection, ⊘ breast-feeding

Cephradine (Velosef) [Antibiotic/Cephalosporin–1st-gen]

Uses: *Respiratory, GU, GI, skin, soft tissue, bone, & joint Infxns* **Action:** 1st-gen cephalosporin; ↓ cell wall synthesis. *Spectrum:* Gram(+) bacilli & cocci (not *Enterococcus*); some gram(−) bacilli (*E. coli, Proteus, & Klebsiella*) **Dose:** *Adults.* 250–500 mg q6–12h (8 g/d max); *Peds.* 25–100 mg/kg/d ÷ bid–qid (4 g/d max); ↓ in renal impair **Caution:** [B, +] **Contra:** Cephalosporin allergy **Disp:** Caps: 250, 500 mg; powder for susp 125, 250 mg/5 mL, inj **SE:** Rash, eosinophilia, ↑ LFTs, N/V/D **Interactions:** ↑ Bleeding w/ anticoagulants; ↑ nephrotoxicity w/ aminoglycosides, loop diuretics; ↑ effects w/ probenecid; ↓ effects w/ antacids, chloramphenicol **Labs:** + Direct Coombs' test; ↑ LFTs, alkaline phosphatase, bilirubin, LDH, BUN, creatinine; false + of serum or UCr, false + urine glucose **NIPE:** Food w/ ER tabs ↑ absorption, monitor for superinfection, ⊘ breast-feeding or use EtOH w/ drug or w/in 3 d of taking drug, ⊘ take w/ any other antibiotic, take w/ food

Cetirizine (Zyrtec, Zyrtec D) [Antihistamine] **Uses:** *Allergic rhinitis & other allergic Sxs including urticaria* **Action:** Nonsedating antihistamine **Dose:** *Adults & Children >6 y.* 5–10 mg/d; Zyrtec D 5/20 mg PO bid whole **Peds.** 6–11 mo: 2.5 mg qd. *12–23 mo:* 2.5 mg qd–bid; ↓ in renal/hepatic impair **Caution:** [B, ?/–] Elderly & nursing mothers; >10 mg/d may cause drowsiness **Contra:** Allergy to cetirizine, hydroxyzine **Disp:** Tabs 5, 10 mg; Chew Tabs 5, 10 mg; syrup 5 mg/5 mL; Zyrtec D: tabs 5/120 mg (cetirizine/pseudoephedrine) **SE:** HA, drowsiness, xerostomia **Notes:** Can cause sedation **Interactions:** ↑ Effects w/ anticholinergics, CNS depressants, theophylline, EtOH **Labs:** May cause false – w/ allergy skin tests **NIPE:** ⊘ take w/ EtOH or CNS depressants

Cetuximab (Erbitux) [EGFR Antagonist/Recombinant Monoclonal Antibody] **WARNING:** Severe inf Rxns including rapid onset of airway obstruction (bronchospasm, stridor, hoarseness), urticaria, & hypotension. Permanent D/C is required. **Uses:** EGFR-expressing metastatic colorectal CA w/wo irinotecan, unresectable head/neck SCC w/RT; monotherapy in met head/neck cancer* **Action:** Human/mouse recombinant MoAb; binds EGFR, ↓ tumor cell growth **Dose:** Per protocol; load 400 mg/m² IV over 2 h; 250 mg/m² given over 1 h × 1 wk **Caution:** [C, –] **Disp:** Inj 100 mg/ 50 mL **SE:** Acneform rash, asthenia/malaise, N/V/D, abdominal pain, alopecia, inf Rxn, dermatologic tox, interstitial lung disease, fever, sepsis, dehydration, kidney failure, PE **Notes:** Assess tumor for EGFR before Rx; pretreat w/ diphenhydramine; w/ mild SE ↓ inf rate by 50%; limit sun exposure **NIPE:** Monitor for infusion reactions for 1 h after infusion; During first 2 wks observe for skin toxicity

Charcoal, Activated (Suporbar, Actidose, Liqui-Char) [Adsorbent] **Uses:** *Emergency Rx in poisoning by most drugs & chemicals (see Contra)* **Action:** Adsorbent detoxicant **Dose:** Give w/ 70% sorbitol (2 mL/kg); repeated use of sorbitol not OK **Adults.** Acute intox: 30–100 g/dose. *GI dialysis:* 20–50 g q6h for 1–2 d. **Peds 1–12 y.** Acute intox: 1–2 g/kg/dose. *GI dialysis:* 5–10 g/dose q4–8h **Caution:** [C, ?] May cause vomiting (hazardous in petroleum distillate & caustic ingestions); do not mix w/ dairy **Contra:** Not effective for cyanide, mineral acids, caustic alkalis, organic solvents, iron, EtOH, methanol poisoning, Li; do not use sorbitol in pts w/ fructose intolerance **Disp:** Powder, liq, caps **SE:** Some liq dosage forms in sorbitol base (a cathartic); V/D, black stools, constipation **Notes:** Charcoal w/ sorbitol not OK in children < 1 y; monitor for ↓ K⁺ & Mg²⁺; protect airway in lethargic or comatose pts **Interactions:** ↓ Effects if taken w/ ice cream, milk, or sherbet; ↓ effects OF digoxin & absorption of other oral meds, ↓ effects OF syrup of ipecac **NIPE:** Most effective if given w/in 30 min of acute poisoning, only give to conscious patients

Chloral Hydrate (Aquachloral, Supprettes) [C-IV] [Sedative/Hypnotic/CNS Depressant]

Uses: *Short-term nocturnal & preop sedation* **Action:** Sedative hypnotic; active metabolite trichloroethanol **Dose:** *Adults.* Hypnotic: 500 mg–1 g PO or PR 30 min hs or before procedure. *Sedative:* 250 mg PO or PR tid. *Peds.* Hypnotic: 20–50 mg/kg/24 h PO or PR 30 min hs or before procedure. *Sedative:* 5–15 mg/kg/dose q8h; avoid w/ CrCl <50 mL/min or severe hepatic impair **Caution:** [C, +] Porphyria & neonates **Contra:** Allergy to components; severe renal, hepatic or cardiac Dz **Disp:** Caps 500 mg; syrup 250, 500 mg/5 mL; supp 324, 648 mg **SE:** GI irritation, drowsiness, ataxia, dizziness, nightmares, rash **Notes:** May accumulate; tolerance may develop >2 wk; taper dose; mix syrup in H$_2$O or fruit juice; avoid EtOH & CNS depressants **Interactions:** ↑ Effects w/ antihistamines, barbiturates, paraldehyde, CNS depressants, opioid analgesics, EtOH; ↑ effects OF anticoagulants **Labs:** False + of urine glucose, may interfere w/ tests for catecholamines and urinary 17-hydroxycorticosteroids **NIPE:** ⊘ Take w/ EtOH, CNS depressants; ⊘ chew or crush capsules

Chlorambucil (Leukeran) [Antineoplastic/Alkylating Agent]

Uses: *CLL, Hodgkin Dz, Waldenström macroglobulinemia* **Action:** Alkylating agent **Dose:** 0.1–0.2 mg/kg/d for 3–6 wk or 0.4 mg/kg/dose q2wk (Per protocol) **Caution:** [D, ?] Sz disorder & BM suppression; affects human fertility **Contra:** Previous resistance; alkylating agent allergy **Disp:** Tabs 2 mg **SE:** Myelosuppression, CNS stimulation, N/V, drug fever, skin rash, chromosomal damage can cause secondary leukemias, alveolar dysplasia, pulmonary fibrosis, hepatotox **Notes:** Monitor LFTs, CBC, leukocyte counts, plts, serum uric acid; ↓ initial dosage if pt has received radiation therapy **Interactions:** ↑ Bone marrow suppression w/ antineoplastic drugs and immunosuppressants; ↑ risk OF bleeding w/ ASA, anticoagulants **Labs:** ↑ Urine and serum uric acid, ALT, alkaline phosphatase **NIPE:** ⊘ PRG, breast-feeding, infection; ↑ fluids to 2–3 L/d; monitor lab work periodically & CBC w/ differential weekly during drug use, may cause hair loss

Chlordiazepoxide (Librium, Mitran, Libritabs) [Anxiolytic, Sedative/Hypnotic/Benzodiazepine] [C-IV]

Uses: *Anxiety, tension, EtOH withdrawal,* & preop apprehension **Action:** Benzodiazepine; antianxiety agent **Dose:** *Adults.* Mild anxiety: 5–10 mg PO tid–qid or PRN. *Severe anxiety:* 25–50 mg IM, IV, or PO q6–8h or PRN. *EtOH withdrawal:* 50–100 mg IM or IV; repeat in 2–4 h if needed, up to 300 mg in 24 h; gradually taper daily dose. *Peds >6 y.* 0.5 mg/kg/24 h PO or IM ÷ q6–8h; ↓ in renal impair, elderly **Caution:** [D, ?] Resp depression, CNS impair, Hx of drug dependence; avoid in hepatic impair **Contra:** Preexisting CNS depression **Disp:** Caps 5, 10, 25 mg; inj 100 mg **SE:** Drowsiness, CP, rash, fatigue, memory impair, xerostomia, weight gain **Notes:** Erratic IM absorption **Interactions:** ↑ Effects w/ antidepressants, antihistamines, anticonvulsants, barbiturates, general anesthetics, MAOIs, narcotics, phenothiazines cimetidine, disulfiram, fluconazole, itraconazole, ketoconazole, oral contraceptives, INH, metoprolol, propoxyphene, propranolol, valproic acid, EtOH, grapefruit juice, kava kava, valerian; ↑ effects of digoxin, phenytoin; ↓ effects w/ aminophylline, antacids, carbamazepine, theophylline, rifampin, rifabutin, tobacco; ↓ effects OF levodopa **Labs:** ↑ LFTs, alkaline phosphatase, bilirubin, triglycerides; false ↑ urine 5-HIAA, urine 17-ketosteroids; false + urine PRG test; false ↓ urine 17 ketogenic steroids; ⊘ HDL **NIPE:** ⊘ EtOH, PRG, breast-feeding; risk of photosensitivity—use sunscreen, orthostatic hypotension, tachycardia

Chlorothiazide (Diuril) [Antihypertensive/Thiazide Diuretic]

Uses: *HTN, edema* **Action:** Thiazide diuretic **Dose:** *Adults.* 500 mg–1 g PO daily–bid; 100–500 mg/d IV (for edema only). *Peds >6 mo.* 20–30 mg/kg/24 h PO ÷ bid; 4 mg/kg/d IV **Caution:** [D, +] **Contra:** Cross-sensitivity to thiazides/sulfonamides, anuria **Disp:** Tabs 250, 500 mg; susp 250 mg/5 mL; inj 500 mg/vial **SE:** ↓ K⁺, Na⁺, dizziness, hyperglycemia, hyperuricemia, hyperlipidemia, photosensitivity **Notes:** Do not administer inj IM or SQ; May be taken w/ food/milk; take early in the day to avoid nocturia; use sunblock; monitor electrolytes **Interactions:** ↑ Effects w/ ACEI, amphotericin B, corticosteroids; ↑ effects OF diazoxide, Li, MTX; ↓ effects w/ colestipol, cholestyramine, NSAIDs; ↓ effects OF hypoglycemics **Labs:** ↑ CPK, ammonia, amylase, Ca²⁺, Cl⁻, cholesterol, glucose, Mg²⁺, K⁺, Na⁺, uric acid **NIPE:** Monitor for gout, hyperglycemia, photosensitivity—use sunscreen, I&O, weight

Chlorpheniramine (Chlor-Trimeton, others [OTC]) [Antihistamine]

Uses: *Allergic Rxns; common cold* **Action:** Antihistamine **Dose:** *Adults.* 4 mg PO q4–6h or 8–12 mg PO bid of SR **Peds.** 0.35 mg/kg/24 h PO ÷ q4–6h or 0.2 mg/kg/24 h SR **Caution:** [C, ?/–] BOO; NA glaucoma; hepatic insuff **Contra:** Allergy **Disp:** Tabs 4 mg; chew tabs 2 mg; SR tabs 8, 12 mg; syrup 2 mg/5 mL; inj 10, 100 mg/mL **SE:** Anticholinergic SE & sedation common, postural ↓ BP, QT changes, extrapyramidal Rxns, photosensitivity **Interactions:** ↑ Effects w/ other CNS depressants, EtOH, opioids, sedatives, MAOIs, atropine, haloperidol, phenothiazines, quinidine, disopyramide; ↑ effects OF epinephrine; ↓ effects OF heparin, sulfonylureas **Labs:** False – w/ allergy testing **NIPE:** Stop drug 4 d prior to allergy testing, take w/ food if GI distress

Chlorpromazine (Thorazine) [Antipsychotic, Antiemetic/Phenothiazine]

Uses: *Psychotic disorders, N/V,* apprehension, intractable hiccups **Action:** Phenothiazine antipsychotic; antiemetic **Dose:** *Adults.* Psychosis: 10–25 mg PO or PR bid-tid (usual 30–800 mg/d in ÷ doses). *Severe Sxs:* 25 mg IM/IV initial; may repeat in 1–4 h; then 25–50 mg PO or PR tid. *Hiccups:* 25–50 mg PO bid–tid. *Children >6 mo.* Psychosis & N/V: 0.5–1 mg/kg/dose PO q4–6h or IM/IV q6–8h; **Caution:** [C, ?/–] Safety in children <6 mo not established; avoid in severe hepatic impair; Szs; BM suppression **Contra:** Cross-sensitivity w/ phenothiazines; NA glaucoma **Disp:** Tabs 10, 25, 50, 100, 200 mg; SR caps 30, 75, 150 mg; syrup 10 mg/5 mL; conc 100 mg/mL; supp 100 mg; inj 25 mg/mL **SE:** Extrapyramidal SE & sedation; α-adrenergic blocking properties; ↓ BP; prolongs QT interval **Notes:** Do not D/C abruptly; dilute PO conc in 2–4 oz of liq **Interactions:** ↑ Effects w/ amodiaquine, chloroquine, sulfadoxine-pyrimethamine, antidepressants, narcotic analgesics, propranolol, quinidine, BBs, MAOIs, TCAs, EtOH, kava kava; ↑ effects OF anticholinergics, centrally acting antihypertensives, propranolol, valproic acid; ↓ effects w/ antacids, antidiarrheals, barbiturates, Li, tobacco; ↓ effects OF anticonvulsants, guanethidine, levodopa, Li, warfarin **Labs:** False + for amylase, phenylketonuria, urine bilirubin, urine protein, uroporphyrins, urobilinogen, PRG test; ↑ plasma cholesterol **NIPE:** Risk of photosensitivity—use sunscreen & tardive dyskinesia, take w/ food if GI upset, may darken urine

Chlorpropamide (Diabinese) [Hypoglycemic/Sulfonylurea]
Uses: *Type 2 DM* **Action:** Sulfonylurea; ↑ pancreatic insulin release; ↑ peripheral insulin sensitivity; ↓ hepatic glucose output **Dose:** 100–500 mg/d; w/ food **Caution:** [C, ?/–] CrCl < 50 mL/min; ↓ in hepatic impair **Contra:** Cross-sensitivity w/ sulfonamides **Disp:** Tabs 100, 250 mg **SE:** HA, dizziness, rash, photosensitivity, hypoglycemia, SIADH **Notes:** Avoid EtOH (disulfiram-like Rxn) **Interactions:** ↑ Effects w/ ASA, NSAIDs, anticoagulants, BBs, chloramphenicol, guanethidine, insulin, MAOIs, phenytoin, probenecid, rifampin, sulfonamides, EtOH, juniper berries, ginseng, garlic, fenugreek, coriander, dandelion root, celery, bitter melon, ginkgo biloba; ↑ effects OF anticoagulants, phenytoin, ASA, NSAIDs; ↓ effects w/ diazoxide, thiazide diuretics **Labs:** False ↑ serum Ca

Chlorthalidone (Hygroton, others) [Antihypertensive/Thiazide Diuretic]
Uses: *HTN* **Action:** Thiazide diuretic **Dose:** *Adults.* 50–100 mg PO daily. *Peds.* (Not approved) 2 mg/kg/dose PO 3×/wk or 1–2 mg/kg/d PO; ↓ in renal impair **Caution:** [D, +] **Contra:** Cross-sensitivity w/ thiazides or sulfonamides; anuria **Disp:** Tabs 15, 25, 50, 100 mg **SE:** ↓ K⁺, dizziness, photosensitivity, hyperglycemia, hyperuricemia, sexual dysfunction **Interactions:** ↑ Effects w/ ACEIs, diazoxide; ↑ effects OF digoxin, Li, MTX; ↓ effects w/ cholestyramine, colestipol, NSAIDs; ↓ effects of hypoglycemics; ↓ K⁺ w/ amphotericin B, carbenoxolone, corticosteroids **Labs:** ↑ CPK, amylase, Ca²⁺, Cl⁻, cholesterol, glucose, uric acid; ↓ Cl⁻, Mg²⁺, K⁺, Na⁺ **NIPE:** May take w/ food, and milk, take early in day, use sunscreen

Chlorzoxazone (Paraflex, Parafon Forte DSC, others) [Skeletal Muscle Relaxant]
Uses: *Adjunct to rest & physical therapy to relieve discomfort associated w/ acute, painful musculoskeletal conditions* **Action:** Centrally acting skeletal muscle relaxant **Dose:** *Adults.* 250–500 mg PO tid–qid. *Peds.* 20 mg/kg/d in 3–4 ÷ doses **Caution:** [C, ?] Avoid EtOH & CNS depressants **Contra:** Severe liver Dz **Disp:** Tabs 250, 500 mg; caps 250, 500 mg **SE:** Drowsiness, tachycardia, dizziness, hepatotox, angioedema **Interactions:** ↑ Effects W/ antihistamines, CNS depressants, MAOIs, TCAs, opioids, EtOH, watercress **Labs:** Monitor LFTs **NIPE:** Urine may turn reddish purple or orange

Cholecalciferol [Vitamin D₃] (Delta D) [Vitamin/Dietary Supl] Uses: Dietary supl to Rx vitamin D deficiency **Action:** Enhances intestinal Ca^{2+} absorption **Dose:** 400–1000 IU/d PO **Caution:** [A (D doses above the RDA), +] **Contra:** ↑ Ca^{2+}, hypervitaminosis, allergy **Disp:** Tabs 400, 1000 IU **SE:** Vitamin D tox (renal failure, HTN, psychosis) **Notes:** 1 mg cholecalciferol = 40,000 IU vitamin D activity **Interactions:** ↑ Risk OF arrhythmias w/ cardiac glycosides; ↓ effects w/ cholestyramine, colestipol, mineral oil, orlistat, Phenobarbital, phenytoin; **Labs:** ↑ bun, calcium, cholesterol, creatinine, LFTs, urine urea; **NIPE:** Vitamin D is fat soluble; mineral oil interferes with Vit D absorption; Vit D needed for calcium absorption;

Cholestyramine (Questran, Prevalite, LoCHOLEST) [Antilipemic, Bile Acid Sequestrant] Uses: *Hypercholesterolemia; Rx pruritus associated w/ partial biliary obstruction; diarrhea associated w/ excess fecal bile acids* **Action:** Binds intestinal bile acids, forms insoluble complexes **Dose:** *Adults.* Individualize: 4 g/d–bid (↑ to max 24 g/d & 6 doses/d). *Peds.* 240 mg/kg/d in 3 ÷ doses **Caution:** [C, ?] Constipation, phenylketonuria **Contra:** Complete biliary obstruction; hypolipoproteinemia types III, IV, V **Disp:** 4 g of cholestyramine resin/9 g powder; w/ aspartame: 4 g resin/5 g powder **SE:** Constipation, abdominal pain, bloating, HA, rash **Notes:** OD may result in GI obstruction; mix 4 gm in 2–6 oz of noncarbonated beverage; take other meds 1–2 h before or 6 h after **Interactions:** ↓ Effects OF acetaminophen, amiodarone, anticoagulants, ASA, cardiac glycosides, clindamycin, corticosteroids, diclofenac, fat-soluble vitamins, gemfibrozil, glipizide, Fe salts, MTX, methyldopa, nicotinic acid, penicillins, phenobarbital, phenytoin, propranolol, thiazide diuretics, tetracyclines, thyroid drugs, troglitazone, warfarin **Labs:** ↑ LFTs, PT, P, Cl, alkaline phosphatase, ↓ serum Ca^{2+}, Na^+, K^+, cholesterol **NIPE:** ↑ fluids, take other drugs 1 h before or 6 h after

Ciclopirox (Loprox, Penlac) [Antifungal] Uses: *Tinea pedis, tinea cruris, tinea corporis, cutaneous candidiasis, tinea versicolor* **Action:** Antifungal antibiotic in vitro cellular depletion of essential substrates &/or ions **Dose:** *Adults & Peds >10 y.* Massage into affected area bid; Onychomycosis: apply to nails QD, with removal every 7 d **Caution:** [B, ?] **Contra:** Component sensitivity **Disp:** Cream, gel, lotion 1%, topical sus 0.77%, shampoo 1%, nail lacquer 8% **SE:** Pruritus, local irritation, burning **Notes:** D/C if irritation occurs; avoid dressings; gel best for athletes foot **Interactions:** None noted **NIPE:** Nail lacquer may take 6 mo to see improvement, cream/gel/lotion see improvement by 4 wk

Cidofovir (Vistide) [Antiviral] WARNING: Renal impair is the major tox. Follow administration instructions Uses: *CMV retinitis in pts w/ HIV* **Action:** Selective inhibition of viral DNA synthesis **Dose:** *Rx:* 5 mg/kg IV over 1 h once/wk for 2 wk w/ probenecid. *Maint:* 5 mg/kg IV once/2 wk w/ probenecid. *Probenecid:* 2 g PO 3 h prior to cidofovir, then 1 g PO at 2 h & 8 h after cidofovir; ↓ in renal impair **Caution:** [C, –] SCr >1.5 mg/dL or CrCl = 55 mL/min or urine protein >100 mg/dL; w/ other nephrotoxic drugs **Contra:** Probenecid or sulfa allergy **Disp:** Inj 75 mg/mL **SE:** Renal tox, chills, fever, HA, N/V/D, thrombocytopenia, neutropenia **Notes:** Hydrate w/ NS prior to each inf **Interactions:** ↑ Nephrotoxicity w/ aminoglycosides, amphotericin B, foscarnet, IV pentamidine, NSAIDs, vancomycin; ↑ effects w/ zidovudine **Labs:** ↑ SCr, BUN, alkaline phosphatase, LFTs, urine protein, WBCs; monitor for hematuria, glycosuria, hypocalcemia, hyperglycemia, hypokalemia, hyperlipidemia **NIPE:** Coadminister oral probenecid w/ each dose, possible hair loss

Cilostazol (Pletal) [Antiplatelet, Arterial Vasodilator/Phosphodiesterase Inhibitor]

Uses: *Reduce Sxs of intermittent claudication* **Action:** Phosphodiesterase III inhibitor; ↑s cAMP in plts & blood vessels, vasodilation & inhibit plt aggregation **Dose:** 100 mg PO bid, ½ h before or 2 h after breakfast & dinner **Caution:** [C, +/–] ↓ dose when used w/ other drugs that inhibit CYP3A4 & CYP2C19 **Contra:** CHF **Disp:** Tabs 50, 100 mg **SE:** HA, palpitation, D **Interactions:** ↑ Effects w/ diltiazem, macrolides, omeprazole, fluconazole, itraconazole, ketoconazole, sertraline, grapefruit juice; ↑ effects OF ASA; ↓ effects w/ cigarette smoking; **Labs:** ↑ BUN/creatinine, ↓ Hgb, Hct **NIPE:** Take on empty stomach; may take up to 12 wk to ↓ cramping pain; may cause dizziness

Cimetidine (Tagamet, Tagamet HB, Tagamet DS OTC) [OTC] [Antiulcerative/H₂-receptor Antagonist]

Uses: *Duodenal ulcer; ulcer prophylaxis in hypersecretory states, (eg, trauma, burns); & GERD* **Action:** H₂ receptor antagonist **Dose:** *Adults.* Active ulcer: 2400 mg/d IV cont inf or 300 mg IV q6h; 400 mg PO bid or 800 mg hs. *Maint:* 400 mg PO hs. *GERD:* 800–600 mg PO q6h; maint 800 mg PO hs. *Peds.* Infants: 10–20 mg/kg/24 h PO or IV ÷ q6–12h. *Children:* 20–40 mg/kg/24 h PO or IV ÷ q6h; ↑ interval w/ renal insuff; ↓ dose in the elderly **Caution:** [B, +] Many drug interactions (P-450 system) **Contra:** Component sensitivity **Disp:** Tabs 200, 300, 400, 800 mg; liq 300 mg/5 mL; inj 300 mg/2 mL **SE:** Dizziness, HA, agitation, thrombocytopenia, gynecomastia **Notes:** Take 1 h before or 2 h after antacids; avoid EtOH **Interactions:** ↑ Effects OF benzodiazepines, disulfiram, flecainide, INH, lidocaine, oral contraceptives, sulfonylureas, warfarin, theophylline, phenytoin, metronidazole, triamterene, procainamide, quinidine, propranolol, diazepam, nifedipine, TCAs, procainamide, tacrine, carbamazepine, valproic acid, xanthines; ↓ effects w/ antacids, tobacco; ↓ effects OF digoxin, ketoconazole, cefpodoxime, indomethacin, tetracyclines **Labs:** ↑ Creatinine, LFTs, false + hemoccult **NIPE:** Take w/ meals, monitor for gynecomastia, breast pain, impotence

Cinacalcet (Sensipar) [Hyperparathyroidism Agent]

Uses: *Secondary hyperparathyroidism in CRF; ↑ Ca²⁺ in parathyroid carcinoma* **Action:** ↓ PTH by ↑ calcium-sensing receptor sensitivity **Dose:** *Secondary hyperparathyroidism:* 30 mg PO daily. *Parathyroid carcinoma:* 30 mg PO bid; titrate q2–4wk based on calcium & PTH levels; swallow whole; take w/ food **Caution:** [C, ?/–] Dose adjust w/ addition/deletion of CYP3A4 inhibitors (Table 13) **Disp:**

Tabs 30, 60, 90 mg **SE:** N/V/D, myalgia, dizziness, ↓ Ca^{2+}, PO_4^{-2}, PTH **Labs:** Monitor serum Ca and serum P **NIPE:** Must take drug with vitamin D and/or phosphate binders

Ciprofloxacin (Cipro, Proquin XR) [Antibiotic/Fluoroquinolone]

Uses: *Rx lower resp tract, sinuses, skin & skin structure, bone/joints, & UT Infxns including prostatitis* **Action:** Quinolone antibiotic; ↓ DNA gyrase. *Spectrum:* Broadspectrum gram(+) & gram(−) aerobics; little against *Strep;* good *Pseudomonas, E. coli, B. fragilis, P. mirabilis, K. pneumoniae, Campylobacter jejuni,* or *Shigella* **Dose:** *Adults.* 250–750 mg PO q12h; XR 500–1000 mg PO q24h; or 200–400 mg IV q12h; ↓ in renal impair **Caution:** [C, ?/−] Children <18 y **Contra:** Component sensitivity **Disp:** Tabs 100, 250, 500, 750 mg; Tabs XR 500, 1000 mg; susp 5 g/100 mL, 10 g/100 mL; inj 200, 400 mg **SE:** Restlessness, N/V/D, rash, ruptured tendons, ↑ LFTs **Notes:** Avoid antacids; reduce/restrict caffeine intake; interactions w/ theophylline, caffeine, sucralfate, warfarin, antacids **Interactions:** ↑ Effects w/ probenecid; ↑ effects OF diazepam, theophylline, caffeine, metoprolol, propranolol, phenytoin, warfarin; ↓ effects w/ antacids, didanosine, Fe salts, Mg, sucralfate, Na bicarbonate, Zn **Labs:** ↑ LFTs, alkaline phosphatase, serum bilirubin, LDH, BUN, SCr, amylase, uric acid, K^+, PT, triglycerides, cholesterol; ↓ Hmg, Hct; **NIPE:** ⊘ give to children <18 y, ↑ fluids to 2–3 L/d, may cause photosensitivity—use sunscreen

Ciprofloxacin, Ophthalmic (Ciloxan) [Antibiotic/Fluoroquinolone Opht Agent]

Uses: *Rx & prevention of ocular Infxns (conjunctivitis, blepharitis, corneal abrasions)* **Action:** Quinolone antibiotic; ↓ DNA gyrase **Dose:** 1–2 gtt in eye(s) q2h while awake for 2 d, then 1–2 gtt q4h while awake for 5 d; Oint ½" ribbon in eye tid times 2 days, then bid times 5 days **Caution:** [C, ?/−] **Contra:** Component sensitivity **Disp:** Soln 3.5 mg/mL; oint 35 g **SE:** Local irritation **Interactions:** None reported **NIPE:** Limited systemic absorption

Ciprofloxacin, Otic (Cipro HC Otic) [Antibiotic/Fluoroquinolone Otic Agent]

Uses: *Otitis externa* **Action:** Quinolone antibiotic; ↓ DNA gyrase **Dose:** *Adult & Peds >1 mo.* 1–2 gtt in ear(s) bid for 7 d **Caution:** [C, ?/−] **Contra:** Perforated tympanic membrane, viral Infxns of the external canal **Disp:** Susp ciprofloxacin 0.2% & hydrocortisone 1% **SE:** HA, pruritus **NIPE:** w/ diabetics, first-choice therapy for otitis externa

Cisplatin (Platinol, Platinol AQ) [Antineoplastic/Alkylating Agent]

Uses: *Testicular, small-cell & non-small-cell lung, bladder, ovarian, breast, head & neck, & penile CAs; osteosarcoma; ped brain tumors* **Action:** DNA-binding; denatures double helix; intrastrand cross-linking **Dose:** 10–20 mg/m²/d for 5 d q3wk; 50–120 mg/m² q3–4wk; (Per protocols); ↓ in renal impair **Caution:** [D, −] Cumulative renal tox may be severe; monitor Mg^{2+}, electrolytes before & w/in 48 h after cisplatin **Contra:** Allergy to platinum-containing compounds; preexisting renal insuff, myelosuppression, hearing impair **Disp:** Inj 1 mg/mL **SE:** Allergic Rxns, N/V, nephrotox (worse w/administration of other nephrotoxic drugs; minimize by NS inf & mannitol diuresis, high-frequency hearing loss in 30%, peripheral "stocking glove"-type neuropathy, cardiotox (ST-, T-wave changes), ↓ Mg^{2+}, mild myelosuppression, hepatotox; renal impair dose-related & cumulative **Notes:** Give taxanes before platinum derivatives **Interactions:** ↑ Effects OF antineoplastic drugs and radiation therapy; ↑ ototoxicity w/ loop diuretics; ↑ nephrotoxicity w/ aminoglycosides, amphotericin B, vancomycin; ↓ effects w/ Na thiosulfate; ↓ effects OF phenytoin **Labs:** ↑ BUN, creatinine, serum bilirubin, AST; ↓ Ca^{2+}, Mg^{2+}, phosphate, Na^+, K^+ **NIPE:** Drug ineffective w/ Al needles or equipment, may cause infertility, ⊘ immunizations

Citalopram (Celexa) [Antidepressant/SSRI]
WARNING: Closely monitor for worsening depression or emergence of suicidality, particularly in ped pts **Uses:** *Depression* **Action:** SSRI **Dose:** Initial 20 mg/d, may ↑ to 40 mg/d; ↓ in elderly & hepatic/renal insuff **Caution:** [C, +/–] Hx of mania, Szs & pts at risk for suicide **Contra:** MOAI or w/in 14 d of MAOI use **Disp:** Tabs 10, 20, 40 mg; Soln 10 mg/5 mL **SE:** Somnolence, insomnia, anxiety, xerostomia, diaphoresis, sexual dysfunction **Notes:** May cause ↓ Na^+/SIADH **Interactions:** ↑ Effects w/ azole antifungals, cimetidine, Li, macrolides, EtOH; ↑ effects OF BBs, carbamazepine, warfarin; ↓ effects w/ carbamazepine; ↓ effects OF phenytoin; may cause fatal Rxn w/ MAOIs **Labs:** ↑ LFTs, alkaline phosphatase **NIPE:** ⊘ PRG, breast-feeding, use barrier contraception

Cladribine (Leustatin) [Antineoplastic Agent]
Uses: *HCL, CLL, NHLs, progressive MS* **Action:** Induces DNA strand breakage; interferes w/ DNA repair/synthesis; purine nucleoside analog **Dose:** 0.09–0.1 mg/kg/d cont IV inf for 1–7 d (Per protocols) **Caution:** [D, ?/–] Causes neutropenia & Infxn **Contra:** Component sensitivity **Disp:** Inj 1 mg/mL **SE:** Myelosuppression, T-lymphocyte suppression may be prolonged (26–34 wk), fever in 46% (May cause tumor lysis), Infxns (especially lung & IV sites), rash (50%), HA, fatigue **Notes:** Consider prophylactic allopurinol; **Interactions:** ↑ Risk of bleeding w/ anticoagulants, NSAIDs, salicylates, ↑ risk OF nephrotoxicity w/ amphotericin B; **Labs:** Monitor CBC, LFTs, SCr **NIPE:** ⊘ PRG, breast-feeding

Clarithromycin (Biaxin, Biaxin XL) [Antibiotic/Macrolide]
Uses: *Upper/lower resp tract, skin/skin structure Infxns, H. pylori Infxns, & Infxns caused by nontuberculosis (atypical) Mycobacterium; prevention of MAC Infxns in HIV-Infxn* **Action:** Macrolide antibiotic, ↓ protein synthesis. *Spectrum: H. influenzae, M. catarrhalis, S. pneumoniae, Mycoplasma pneumoniae, H. pylori* **Dose:** *Adults.* 250–500 mg PO bid or 1000 mg (2 × 500 mg XR tab)/d. *Mycobacterium:* 500–1000 mg PO bid. *Peds >9 mo.* 7.5 mg/kg/dose PO bid; ↓ in renal/hepatic impair **Caution:** [C, ?] Antibiotic-associated colitis; rare QT prolongation & ventricular arrhythmias, including torsades de pointes **Contra:** Allergy to macrolides; combo w/ ranitidine in pts w/ Hx of porphyria or CrCl < 25 mL/min **Disp:** Tabs 250, 500 mg; susp 125, 250 mg/5 mL; 500 mg XR tab **SE:** Prolongs QT interval, causes metallic taste, N/D, abdominal pain, HA, rash **Notes:** Multiple

drug interactions, ↑ theophylline & carbamazepine levels; do not refrigerate suspension **Interactions:** ↑ Effects w/ amprenavir, indinavir, nelfinavir, ritonavir; ↑ effects OF atorvastatin, buspirone, clozapine, colchicine, diazepam, felodipine, itraconazole, lovastatin, simvastatin, methylprednisolone, theophylline, phenytoin, quinidine, digoxin, carbamazepine, triazolam, warfarin, ergotamine, alprazolam, valproic acid; ↓ effects w/ EtOH; ↓ effects OF penicillin, zafirlukast **Labs:** ↑ Serum AST, ALT, GTT, alkaline phosphatase, LDH, total bilirubin, BUN, creatinine, PT; ↓ WBC **NIPE:** May take w/ food

Clemastine Fumarate (Tavist, Dayhist-1) [OTC] [Antihistamine]

Uses: *Allergic rhinitis & Sxs of urticaria* **Action:** Antihistamine **Dose:** *Adults & Peds >12 y.* 1.34 mg bid–2.68 mg tid; max 8.04 mg/d *<12 y.* 0.4 mg PO bid **Caution:** [C, M] BOO **Contra:** NA glaucoma **Disp:** Tabs 1.34, 2.68 mg; syrup 0.67 mg/5 mL **SE:** Drowsiness, dyscoordination, epigastric distress, urinary retention **Notes:** Avoid EtOH **Interactions:** ↑ Effects w/ CNS depressants, MAOIs, EtOH; ↓ effects OF heparin, sulfonylureas

Clindamycin (Cleocin, Cleocin-T, others) [Antibiotic/Lincomycin Derivative]

Uses: *Rx aerobic & anaerobic Infxns; topical for severe acne & vaginal Infxns* **Action:** Bacteriostatic; interferes w/ protein synthesis. **Spectrum:** Streptococci, pneumococci, staphylococci, & gram(+) & gram(−) anaerobes; no activity against gram(−) aerobes & bacterial vaginosis **Dose:** *Adults.* PO: 150–450 mg PO q6–8h. *IV:* 300–600 mg IV q6h or 900 mg IV q8h. *Vaginal:* 1 applicator hs for 7 d. *Topical:* Apply 1% gel, lotion, or soln bid. *Peds.* Neonates: (Avoid use; contains benzyl alcohol) 10–15 mg/kg/24 h ÷ q8–12h. *Children >1 mo:* 10–30 mg/kg/24 h ÷ q6–8h, to a max of 1.8 g/d PO or 4.8 g/d IV. *Topical:* Apply 1%, gel, lotion, or soln bid; ↓ in severe hepatic impair **Caution:** [B, +] Can cause fatal colitis **Contra:** Hx pseudomembranous colitis **Disp:** Caps 75, 150, 300 mg; susp 75 mg/5 mL; inj 300 mg/2 mL; vaginal cream 2%; topical sol 1%, gel 1%, lotion 1%, vaginal supp 100 mg **SE:** Diarrhea may be pseudomembranous colitis caused by *C. difficile*, rash, ↑ LFTs **Notes:** D/C drug w/diarrhea, evaluate for *C. difficile* **Interactions:** ↑ Effects OF neuromuscular blockage w/ tubocurarine, pancuronium; ↓ effects w/ erythromycin, kaolin, foods w/ sodium cyclamate **Labs:** Monitor CBC, LFTs, BUN, creatinine; false ↑ serum theophylline **NIPE:** ⊘ Intercourse, tampons, douches while using vaginal cream; take oral meds w/ 8 oz water

Clofarabine (Clolar DS) [Antimetabolite]

Uses: Rx relapsed/refractory ALL after at least 2 regimens in children 1–21 y **Action:** Antimetabolite; ↓ ribonucleotide reductase w/ false nucleotide base-inhibiting DNA synthesis **Dose:** 52 mg/m^2 IV over 2 h qd × 5 d (repeat q2–6wk); Per protocol **Caution:** [D, −] **Disp:** Inj 20 mg/20 mL **SE:** N/V/D, anemia, leukopenia, thrombocytopenia, neutropenia, Infxn **Notes:** Monitor for tumor lysis syndrome & systemic inflammatory response syndrome (SIRS)/capillary leak syndrome **Labs:** ↑ AST, ALT; **NIPE:** Pts at risk for tumor lysis syndrome—monitor serum uric acid, phosphate, calcium & creatinine bid for 2–3 days after starting chemotherapy

Clonazepam (Klonopin) [C-IV] [Anticonvulsant/Benzodiazepine] **Uses:** *Lennox–Gastaut syndrome, akinetic & myoclonic Szs, absence Szs, panic attacks,* restless legs syndrome, neuralgia, parkinsonian dysarthria, bipolar disorder **Action:** Benzodiazepine; anticonvulsant **Dose:** *Adults.* 1.5 mg/d PO in 3 ÷ doses; ↑ by 0.5–1 mg/d q3d PRN up to 20 mg/d. *Peds.* 0.01–0.03 mg/kg/24 h PO ÷ tid; ↑ to 0.1–0.2 mg/kg/24 h ÷ tid; avoid abrupt withdrawal **Caution:** [D, M] Elderly pts, resp Dz, CNS depression, severe hepatic impair, NA glaucoma **Contra:** Severe liver Dz, acute NA glaucoma **Disp:** Tabs 0.5, 1, 2 mg; Oral disintegrating tabs 0.125, 0.25, 0.5, 1, 2 mg **SE:** CNS side effects, including drowsiness, dizziness, ataxia, memory impair **Notes:** Can cause retrograde amnesia; CYP3A4 substrate **Interactions:** ↑ Effects w/ anticonvulsants, antihistamines, cimetidine, ciprofloxacin, clarithromycin, clozapine, CNS depressants, diltiazem, disulfiram, digoxin, erythromycin, fluconazole, fluoxetine, INH, itraconazole, ketoconazole, labetalol, levodopa, metoprolol, opioids, ritonavir, valproic acid, verapamil, EtOH, kava kava, valerian; ↑ effects OF phenytoin; ↓ effects w/ barbiturates, carbamazepine, phenytoin, rifampin, rifabutin; ↓ effects OF levodopa **NIPE:** ⊘ DC abruptly

Clonidine, Oral (Catapres) [Antihypertensive/Centrally Acting Sympatholytic] **Uses:** *HTN*; opioid, EtOH, & tobacco withdrawal **Action:** Centrally acting α-adrenergic stimulant **Dose:** *Adults.* 0.1 mg PO bid adjust daily by 0.1- to 0.2-mg increments (max 2.4 mg/d). *Peds.* 5–10 mcg/kg/d ÷ q8–12h (max 0.9 mg/d); ↓ in renal impair **Caution:** [C, +/–] Avoid w/ β-blocker; withdraw slowly **Contra:** Component sensitivity **Disp:** Tabs 0.1, 0.2, 0.3 mg **SE:** Drowsiness, orthostatic ↓ BP, xerostomia, constipation, bradycardia, dizziness **Notes:** More effective for HTN if combined w/ diuretics

Clonidine, Transdermal (Catapres TTS) [Antihypertensive/Centrally Acting Sympatholytic] **Uses:** *HTN* **Action:** Centrally acting α-adrenergic stimulant **Dose:** Apply 1 patch q7d to hairless area (upper arm/torso); titrate to effect; ↓ in severe renal impair; **Caution:** [C, +/–] Avoid w/ β-blocker, withdraw slowly **Contra:** Component sensitivity **Disp:** TTS-1, TTS-2, TTS-3 (delivers 0.1, 0.2, 0.3 mg, respectively, of clonidine/d for 1 wk) **SE:** Drowsiness, orthostatic ↓ BP, xerostomia, constipation, bradycardia **Notes:** Do not D/C or withdraw (rebound HTN); Doses >2 TTS-3 usually not associated w/ ↑ efficacy; steady state in 2–3 d **Interactions:** ↑ Effects w/ BBs, neuroleptics, nitroprusside, EtOH; ↑ effects OF barbiturates; ↓ effects w/ MAOIs, TCAs, tolazoline, antidepressants, prazosin, capsicum; ↓ effects OF levodopa **Labs:** ↑ Glucose, phosphatase, CPK **NIPE:** Tolerance develops w/ long-term use

Clopidogrel (Plavix) [Antiplatelet] **Uses:** *Reduction of atherosclerotic events* **Action:** ↓ Plt aggregation **Dose:** 75 mg/d; 300 mg PO (times) 1 dose can be used to load pts **Caution:** [B, ?] Active bleeding; risk of bleeding from trauma & other causes; TTP; liver Dz **Contra:** Active bleeding; intracranial bleeding **Disp:** Tabs 75 mg **SE:** Prolongs bleeding time, GI intolerance, HA, dizziness, rash, thrombocytopenia, leukopenia **Notes:** Plt aggregation returns to baseline ≅5 d after D/C; plt transfusion reverses effects acutely; **Interactions:** ↑ Risk of GI bleed w/ ASA, NSAIDs, heparin, warfarin, feverfew, garlic, ginger, ginkgo biloba; ↑ effects OF phenytoin, tamoxifen, tolbutamide **Labs:** ↑ LFTs; ↓ plts, neutrophils **NIPE:** DC drug 1 wk prior to surgery

Clorazepate (Tranxene) [C-IV] [Anxiolytic, Anticonvulsant, Sedative/Hypnotic/Benzodiazepine] Uses: *Acute anxiety disorders, acute EtOH withdrawal Sxs, adjunctive therapy in partial Szs* **Action:** Benzodiazepine; antianxiety agent **Dose:** *Adults.* 15–60 mg/d PO single or ÷ doses. *Elderly & debilitated pts:* Initial 7.5–15 mg/d in ÷ doses. *EtOH withdrawal:* Day 1: Initial 30 mg; then 30–60 mg in ÷ doses; Day 2: 45–90 mg in ÷ doses; Day 3: 22.5–45 mg in ÷ doses; Day 4: 15–30 mg in ÷ doses. *Peds.* 3.75–7.5 mg/dose bid to 60 mg/d max ÷ bid–tid **Caution:** [D, ?/–] elderly; Hx depression **Contra:** Not OK for <9 y of age; NA glaucoma **Disp:** Tabs 3.75, 7.5, 15 mg; Tabs-SD (once-daily) 11.25, 22.5 mg **SE:** CNS depressant effects (drowsiness, dizziness, ataxia, memory impair), ↓ BP **Notes:** Monitor pts w/ renal/hepatic impair (drug may accumulate); may cause dependence **Interactions:** ↑ Effects w/ antidepressants, antihistamines, barbiturates, MAOIs, narcotics, phenothiazines, cimetidine, disulfiram, EtOH; ↓ effects OF levodopa; ↓ effects w/ ginkgo, tobacco **Labs:** ↓ Hct, abnormal LFTs, BUN, creatinine **NIPE:** ⊘ DC abruptly

Clotrimazole (Lotrimin, Mycelex, others) [OTC] [Antifungal] Uses: *Candidiasis & tinea Infxns* **Action:** Antifungal; alters cell wall permeability. *Spectrum:* Oropharyngeal candidiasis, dermatophytes, superficial mycoses, cutaneous candidosis, & vulvovaginal candidiasis **Dose:** *PO: Prophylaxis:* One troche dissolved in mouth tid *Rx:* One troche dissolved in mouth 5 ×/d for 14 d. *Vaginal 1% Cream:* 1 applicatorful hs for 7 d. *2% Cream:* 1 applicatorful hs for 3 d *Tabs:* 100 mg vaginally hs for 7 d or 200 mg (2 tabs) vaginally hs for 3 d or 500-mg tabs vaginally hs once. *Topical:* Apply bid for 10–14 d **Caution:** [B, (C if PO), ?] Not for systemic fungal Infxn; safety in children <3 y not established **Contra:** Allergy to any component **Disp:** 1% cream; soln; lotion; troche 10 mg; vaginal tabs 100, 500 mg; vaginal cream 1%, 2% **SE:** *Topical:* Local irritation; *PO:* N/V, ↑ LFTs **Notes:** PO prophylaxis used for immunosuppressed pts **Interactions:** ↑ Effects of cyclosporine, tacrolimus; ↓ effects of spermicides

Clotrimazole & Betamethasone (Lotrisone) [Antifungal, Anti-inflammatory] Uses: *Fungal skin Infxns* **Action:** Imidazole antifungal & antiinflammatory. *Spectrum:* Tinea pedis, cruris, & corpora **Dose:** *Pts ≥17 y.* Apply & massage into area bid for 2–4 wk **Caution:** [C, ?] Varicella Infxn **Contra:** Children <12 y **Disp:** Cream 15, 45 g; lotion 30 mL **SE:** Local irritation, rash **Notes:** Not for diaper dermatitis or under occlusive dressings

Clozapine (Clozaril) [Antipsychotic] WARNING: Myocarditis, agranulocytosis, Szs, & orthostatic ↓ BP associated w/ clozapine; ↑ mortality in elderly w/ dementia-related psychosis Uses: *Refractory severe schizophrenia*;

childhood psychosis **Action:** "Atypical" TCA **Dose:** 25 mg daily–bid initial; ↑ to 300–450 mg/d over 2 wk. Maintain at lowest dose possible; do not D/C abruptly **Caution:** [B, +/–] Monitor for psychosis & cholinergic rebound **Contra:** Uncontrolled epilepsy; comatose state; WBC <\<=}3500 cells/mm³ before Rx or <3000 cells/mm³ during Rx **Disp:** Tabs 25, 100 mg **SE:** Tachycardia, drowsiness, weight gain, constipation, incontinence, rash, Szs, CNS stimulation, hyperglycemia **Notes:** Benign, self-limiting temperature elevations may occur during the 1st 3 wk of Rx, weekly CBC mandatory 1st 6 mo, then qowk **Interactions:** ↑ Effects w/ clarithromycin, cimetidine, erythromycin, fluoxetine, paroxetine, quinidine, sertraline; ↑ depressant effects w/ CNS depressants, EtOH; ↑ effects OF digoxin, warfarin; ↓ effects w/ carbamazepine, phenytoin, primidone, phenobarbital, valproic acid, St. John's wort, nutmeg, caffeine; ↓ effects OF phenytoin **Labs:** Monitor WBCs **NIPE:** ↑ Risk of developing agranulocytosis

Cocaine [C-II] [Narcotic analgesic]

Uses: *Topical anesthetic for mucous membranes* **Action:** Narcotic analgesic, local vasoconstrictor **Dose:** Apply lowest amount of topical soln that provides relief; 1 mg/kg max **Caution:** [C, ?] **Contra:** PRG **Disp:** Topical soln & viscous preparations 4–10%; powder **SE:** CNS stimulation, nervousness, loss of taste/smell, chronic rhinitis **Notes:** Use only on mucous membranes of the PO, laryngeal, & nasal cavities; do not use on extensive areas of broken skin **Interactions:** ↑ Effects w/ MAOIs, ↑ risk of HTN & arrhythmias w/ epinephrine

Codeine [C-II] [Analgesic, Antitussive/Opioid]

Uses: *Mild–moderate pain; symptomatic relief of cough* **Action:** Narcotic analgesic; depresses cough reflex **Dose:** *Adults. Analgesic:* 15–60 mg PO or IM q/d PRN. *Antitussive:* 10–20 mg PO q4h PRN; max 120 mg/d. *Peds. Analgesic:* 0.5–1 mg/kg/dose PO q4–6h PRN. *Antitussive:* 1–1.5 mg/kg/24 h PO ÷ q4h; max 30 mg/24 h; ↓ in renal/hepatic impair **Caution:** [C, (D if prolonged use or high doses at term), +] **Contra:** Component sensitivity **Disp:** Tabs 15, 30, 60 mg; soln 15 mg/5 mL; inj 15, 30 mg/mL **SE:** Drowsiness, constipation **Notes:** Usually combined w/ APAP for pain or w/ agents (eg, terpin hydrate) as an antitussive; 120 mg IM = 10 mg IM morphine **Interactions:** ↑ CNS depression w/ CNS depressants, antidepressants, MAOIs, TCAs, barbiturates, benzodiazepines, muscle relaxants, phenothiazines, cimetidine, antihistamines, sedatives, EtOH; ↑ effects OF digitoxin, phenytoin, rifampin; ↓ effects w/ nalbuphine, pentazocine, tobacco **Labs:** False ↑ amylase, lipase, ↑ urine morphine

Colchicine [Antigout Agent]

Uses: *Acute gouty arthritis & prevention of recurrences; familial Mediterranean fever*; primary biliary cirrhosis **Action:** ↓ migration of leukocytes; ↓ leukocyte lactic acid production **Dose:** *Initial:* 0.5–1.2 mg PO, then 0.5–0.6 mg q1–2h until relief or GI SE develop (max 8 mg/d); do not repeat for 3 d. *IV:* 1–3 mg, then 0.5 mg q6h until relief (max 4 mg/d); do not repeat for 7 d. *Prophylaxis:* PO: 0.5–0.6 mg/d or 3–4 d/wk; ↓ renal impair; caution in elderly **Caution:** [D, +] In elderly **Contra:** Serious renal, GI, hepatic, or cardiac disorders; blood dyscrasias **Disp:** Tabs 0.6 mg; inj 1 mg/2 mL **SE:** N/V/D, abdominal pain, BM suppression, hepatotox; severe local irritation can occur following SQ/IM **Notes:** Colchicine 1–2 mg IV w/in 24–48 h of an acute attack diagnostic/therapeutic in monoarticular arthritis **Interactions:** ↑ GI effects w/ NSAIDs; ↑ effects OF sympathomimetics, CNS depressants, bone marrow depressants, radiation therapy; ↓ effects OF vitamin B₁₂ **Labs:** Monitor CBC, BUN, creatinine; false + urine Hgb & RBCs **NIPE:** ⊘ EtOH

Colesevelam (WelChol) [Antilipemic/Bile Acid Sequestrant]
Uses: *Reduction of LDL & total cholesterol alone or in combo w/ an HMG-CoA reductase inhibitor* **Action:** Bile acid sequestrant **Dose:** 3 tabs PO bid w/ meals **Caution:** [B, ?] Severe GI motility disorders; safety & efficacy not established in peds **Contra:** Bowel obstruction **Disp:** Tabs 625 mg **SE:** Constipation, dyspepsia, myalgia, weakness **Notes:** May ↓ absorption of fat-soluble vitamins **Interactions:** ↓ Effects OF verapamil **Labs:** Monitor lipids **NIPE:** Take w/ food and liquid

Colestipol (Colestid) [Antilipemic/Bile Acid Sequestrant]
Uses: *Adjunct to ↓ serum cholesterol in primary hypercholesterolemia* **Action:** Binds intestinal bile acids to form insoluble complex **Dose:** Granules: 5–30 g/d ÷ 2–4 doses; tabs: 2–16 g/d daily–bid **Caution:** [C, ?] Avoid w/ high triglycerides, GI dysfunction **Contra:** Bowel obstruction **Disp:** Tabs 1 g; granules 5, 7.5, 300, 450, 500 g **SE:** Constipation, abdominal pain, bloating, HA **Notes:** Do not use dry powder; mix w/ beverages, soups, cereals, etc; may ↓ absorption of other medications; may ↓ absorption of fat-soluble vitamins **Interactions:** ↓ Absorption OF numerous drugs especially anticoagulants, cardiac glycosides, digitoxin, digoxin, phenobarbital, penicillin G, tetracycline, thiazide diuretics, thyroid drugs **Labs:** ↓ Serum cholesterol, ↑ PT **NIPE:** Take other meds 1 h before or 4 h after colestipol

Conivaptan HCL (Vaprisol) [Vasopressin Receptor Antagonist]
Uses: Euvolemic hyponatremia **Action:** Dual arginine vasopressin V₁ₐ /V₂ receptor antagonist **Dose:** 20 mg IV ¥ 1 over 30 min, then 20 mg cont IV inf over 24 h; 20 mg/d cont IV inf for 1–3 more d; may ↑ to 40 mg/d if Na⁺ not responding; 4 d max use; use large vein, change site q 24 h **Caution:** [C; ?/–] Rapid ↑ Na⁺ (>12 mEq/L/24 h) may cause osmotic demyelination syndrome; impaired renal/hepatic fxn; CYP3A4 inhibitor **Contra:** Hypovolemic hyponatremia; w/CYP3A4 inhibitors (Table 13) **Disp:** Ampule 20 mg/4 mL **SE:** Infusion site Rxns, HA, N/V/D, constipation, thirst, dry mouth, pyrexia, pollakiuria, polyuria, Infxn **Labs:** may ↑ digoxin level; ↓ K⁺; monitor Na⁺; D/C w/ very rapid ↑ Na⁺; **NIPE:** Monitor volume and neurologic status; mix only w/ 5% dextrose

Cortisone   See Steroids, Tables 4 & 5
Cromolyn Sodium (Intal, NasalCrom, Opticrom) [Anti-asthmatic/mast cell stabilizer] **Uses:** *Adjunct to the Rx of asthma; prevent exercise-induced asthma; allergic rhinitis; ophth allergic manifestations*; food allergy **Action:** Antiasthmatic; mast cell stabilizer **Dose:** *Adults & Children >12 y.* Inhal: 20 mg (as powder in caps) inhaled qid or met-dose inhaler 2 puffs qid. *PO:*

200 mg qid 15–20 min ac, up to 400 mg qid. *Nasal instillation:* Spray once in each nostril 2–6x/d. *Ophth:* 1–2 gtt in each eye 4–6x/d. **Peds.** Inhal: 2 puffs qid of met-dose inhaler. *PO: Infants <2 y:* (not OK) 20 mg/kg/d in 4 ÷ doses. *2–12 y:* 100 mg qid ac **Caution:** [B, ?] **Contra:** Acute asthmatic attacks **Disp:** PO conc 100 mg/5 mL; soln for neb 20 mg/2 mL; met-dose inhaler; nasal soln 40 mg/mL; ophth soln 4% **SE:** Unpleasant taste, hoarseness, coughing **Notes:** No benefit in acute Rx; 2–4 wk for maximal effect in perennial allergic disorders **Interactions:** None noted **Labs:** Monitor pulmonary Fxn tests

Cyanocobalamin [Vitamin B$_{12}$] [Vitamin B/Dietary Supl]

Uses: *Pernicious anemia & other vitamin B$_{12}$ deficiency states; ↑ requirements due to PRG; thyrotoxicosis; liver or kidney Dz* **Action:** Dietary vitamin B$_{12}$ supl **Dose: Adults.** 100 mcg IM or SQ qd for 5–10 d, then 100 mcg IM 2×/wk for 1 mo, then 100 mcg IM monthly. **Peds.** 100 mcg/d IM or SQ for 5–10 d, then 30–50 mcg IM q4wk **Caution:** [A (C if dose exceeds RDA), +] **Contra:** Allergy to cobalt; hereditary optic nerve atrophy; Leber Dz **Disp:** Tabs 50, 100, 250, 500, 1000, 2500 mcg; inj 100, 1000 mcg/mL; gel 500 mcg/0.1 mL **SE:** Itching, D, HA, anxiety **Notes:** PO absorption erratic, altered by many drugs & not recommended; for use w/ hyperalimentation **Interactions:** ↓ Effects w/ aminosalicylic acid, chloramphenicol, cholestyramine, cimetidine, colchicines, neomycin, amino salicylate, EtOH **Labs:** Antibiotics, MRX, pyrimethamine invalidate blood assays of vitamin B$_{12}$ and folic acid

Cyclobenzaprine (Flexeril) [Skeletal Muscle Relaxant/TCI]

Uses: *Relief of muscle spasm* **Action:** Centrally acting skeletal muscle relaxant; reduces tonic somatic motor activity **Dose:** 10 mg PO bid–qid (2–3 wk max) **Caution:** [B, ?] Shares the toxic potential of the TCAs; urinary hesitancy or angle-closure glaucoma **Contra:** Do not use concomitantly or w/in 14 d of MAOIs; hyperthyroidism; heart failure; arrhythmias **Disp.:** Tabs 5, 7.5, 10 mg **SE:** Sedation & anticholinergic effects **Notes:** May inhibit mental alertness or physical coordination **Interactions:** ↑ Effects of CNS depression w/ CNS depressants, TCAs, barbiturates, EtOH; ↑ risk of HTN & convulsions w/ MAOIs **NIPE:** ↑ Fluids & fiber for constipation

Cyclopentolate ophthalmic (Cyclogyl) [Anticholinergic]/Cycloplegic mydriatic agent]

Uses: *Diagnostic procedures requiring cycloplegia & mydriasis* **Action:** Cycloplegic & mydriatic agent (can last up to 24 h); anticholinergic inhibits iris sphincter and ciliary body **Dose: Adults.** 1 gtt in eye 40–50 min preprocedure, may repeat (times) 1 in 5–10 min as adult, children 0.5–1.0%; infants use 0.5% **Caution:** [C] [may cause late-term fetal anoxia/brady-cardia, +/–], premature infants HTN, Down synd, elderly **Contra:** Narrow-angle glaucoma **Caution:** [C] [may cause late-term fetal anoxia/bradycardia, +/–], premature infants HTN, Down synd, elderly **Contra:** Narrow-angle glaucoma **Disp:** Ophth soln 0.5, 1, 2% **SE:** SE: Tearing, HA, irritation, eye pain, photophobia, arrhythmia, tremor, ↑ IOP, confusion **Note:** Compress lacrimal sac for several min after dose; heavily pigmented irises may require ↑ strength; peak 25–75 min, cycloplegia 6–24 h, mydriasis up to 24 h; **Interactions:** ↓ Effects OF carbachol, cholinesterase inhibitors, pilocarpine **NIPE:** Burning sensation when instilled

Cyclopentolate with Phenylephrine (Cyclomydril) [Anticholinergic/Cycloplegic mydriatic, α-Adrenergic agonist]
Uses: *Action:* Cycloplegic mydriatic, α-adrenergic agonist w/ anticholinergic to inhibit iris sphincter **Dose:** 1 gtt in eye q 5–10 min (max 3 doses) 40–50 min preprocedure **Caution:** [C] [may cause late-term fetal anoxia/bradycardia, +/–] HTN, w/elderly w/CAD **Contra:** Narrow-angle glaucoma **Disp:** Ophth soln Cyclopentolate 0.2%/phlenphrine 1% (2, 5 mL) **SE:** Tearing, HA, irritation, eye pain, photophobia, arrhythmia, tremor **NIPE:** Compress lacrimal sac for several min after dose; heavily pigmented irises may require ↑ strength; peak 25–75 min, cycloplegia 6–24 h, mydriasis up to 24 h

Cyclophosphamide (Cytoxan, Neosar) [Antineoplastic/Alkylating Agent] **Uses:** *Hodgkin Dz & NHLs; multiple myeloma; small-cell lung, breast, & ovarian CAs; mycosis fungoides; neuroblastoma; retinoblastoma; acute leukemias; & allogeneic & ABMT in high doses; severe rheumatologic disorders* **Action:** Converted to acrolein & phosphoramide mustard, the active alkylating moieties **Dose:** 500–1500 mg/m² as single dose at 2–4-wk intervals; 1.8 g/m² to 160 mg/kg (or ≅12 g/m² in a 75-kg individual) in the BMT setting (Per protocols); adjust in renal/hepatic impair **Caution:** [D, ?] w/ BM suppression **Contra:** Component sensitivity **Disp:** Tabs 25, 50 mg; inj 500 mg, 1g, 2g **SE:** Myelosuppression (leukopenia & thrombocytopenia); hemorrhagic cystitis, SIADH, alopecia, anorexia; N/V; hepatotox & rarely interstitial pneumonitis; irreversible testicular atrophy possible; cardiotox rare; 2nd malignancies (bladder CA & ALL); cumulative risk 3.5% at 8 y, 10.7% at 12 y **Notes:** Hemorrhagic cystitis prophylaxis: continuous bladder irrigation & mesna uroprotection; encourage hydration, long-term bladder CA screening **Interactions:** ↑ Effects w/ allopurinol, cimetidine, phenobarbital, rifampin; ↑ effects OF succinylcholine, warfarin; ↓ effects OF digoxin **Labs:** May inhibit + Rxns to skin tests for PPD, risk of false + Pap smear results **NIPE:** May cause sterility, hair loss, ⊘ PRG, breast-feeding, immunizations

Cyclosporine (Sandimmune, NeOral, Gengraf) [Immunosuppressant/Antibiotic] **Uses:** *Organ rejection in kidney, liver, heart, & BMT w/ steroids; RA; psoriasis;* **Action:** Immunosuppressant; reversible inhibition of immunocompetent lymphocytes **Dose:** *Adults & Peds.* PO: 15 mg/kg/d 12 h pretransplant; after 2 wk, taper by 5 mg/wk to 5–10 mg/kg/d. *IV:* If NPO, give ⅓ PO dose IV; ↓ in renal/hepatic impair **Caution:** [C, ?] Dose-related risk of nephrotox/hepatotox; live, attenuated vaccines may be less effective **Contra:** Abnormal renal Fxn; uncontrolled HTN **Disp:** Caps 25, 50, 100 mg; PO soln 100 mg/mL; inj 50 mg/mL **SE:** May ↑ BUN & creatinine & mimic transplant rejection;

HTN; HA; hirsutism **Notes:** Administer in glass container; many drug interactions; NeOral & Sandimmune not interchangeable; interaction w/ St. John's wort. Follow levels (Table 2) **Interactions:** ↑ Effects w/ azole antifungals, allopurinol, amiodarone, anabolic steroids, CCBs, cimetidine, chloroquine, clarithromycin, clonidine, diltiazem, macrolides, metoclopramide, NSAIDs, oral contraceptives, ticlopidine, grapefruit juice; ↑ nephrotoxicity w/ aminoglycosides, amphotericin B, acyclovir, colchicine, enalapril, ranitidine, sulfonamides; ↑ risk OF digoxin toxicity; ↑ risk of hyperkalemia w/ diuretics, ACEIs; ↓ effects w/ barbiturates, carbamazepine, INH, nafcillin, pyrazinamide, phenytoin, rifampin, sulfonamides, St. John's wort, alfalfa sprouts, astragalus, echinacea, licorice; ↓ effects OF immunizations **Labs:** ↑ SCr, BUN, total bilirubin, K⁺, alkaline phosphatase, lipids **Notes:** Monitor for hyperglycemia, hyperkalemia, hyperuricemia, risk of photosensitivity—use sunscreen

Cyclosporine ophthalmic (Restasis) [Immunosuppressant/ Anti-inflammatory] **Uses:** ↑ Tear production suppressed due to ocular inflammation * **Action:** Immune modulator, antiinflammatory **Dose:** 1 gtt bid each eye 12 h apart. OK w/ artificial tears, allow 15 min between **Caution:** [C, –] **Contra:** Ocular Infxn, component allergy **Disp:** Single-use vial 0.05% **SE:** Ocular burning/hyperemia **Notes:** Mix vial well
NIPE: ⊘ children < 16 years; may insert contact lenses 15 min after installation;

Cyproheptadine (Periactin) [Antihistamine, Antipruritic] **Uses:** *Allergic Rxns; itching* **Action:** Phenothiazine antihistamine; serotonin antagonist **Dose:** **Adults.** 4–20 mg PO ÷ q8h; max 0.5 mg/kg/d. **Peds.** 2–6 y: 2 mg bid–tid (max 12 mg/24 h). 7–14 y: 4 mg bid–tid; ↓ in hepatic impair **Caution:** [B, ?] BPH **Contra:** Neonates or <2 y; NA glaucoma; BOO; acute asthma; GI obstruction **Disp:** Tabs 4 mg; syrup 2 mg/5 mL **SE:** Anticholinergic, drowsiness, **Notes:** May stimulate appetite **Interactions:** ↑ Effects w/ CNS depressants, MAOIs, EtOH; ↓ effects OF epinephrine, fluoxetine **Labs:** False – skin testing; false + urine TCA assay; ↑ serum amylase, prolactin; ↓ FBS **NIPE:** ↑ Risk photosensitivity—use sunscreen, take w/ food if GI distress

Cytarabine [ARA-C] (Cytosar-U) [Antineoplastic/Antimetabolite] **Uses:** *Acute leukemias, CML, NHL; IT for leukemic meningitis or prophylaxis* **Action:** Antimetabolite; interferes w/ DNA synthesis **Dose:** 100–150 mg/m²/d for 5–10 d (low dose); 3 g/m² q12h for 8–12 doses (high dose); 1 mg/kg 1–2/wk (SQ maint regimens); 5–70 mg/m² up to 3/wk IT (Per protocols); ↓ in renal/hepatic impair **Caution:** [D, ?] w/ marked BM suppression, ↓ dosage by ↓ the number of days of administration **Contra:** Component sensitivity **Disp:** Inj 100, 500 mg, 1, 2 g **SE:** Myelosuppression, N/V/D, stomatitis, flu-like syndrome, rash on palms/soles, hepatic dysfunction, cerebellar dysfunction, noncardiogenic pulmonary edema, neuropathy **Notes:** Little use in solid tumors; tox of high-dose regimens (conjunctivitis) ameliorated by corticosteroid ophth soln **Interactions:** ↑ Effects w/ alkylating drugs and radiation therapy; ↓ effects OF digoxin, gentam-

icin, MTX, flucytosine **Labs:** ↑ Uric acid, monitor CBC, BUN, creatinine, LFTs **NIPE:** ⊘ EtOH, NSAIDs, ASA, PRG, breast-feeding, immunizations

Cytarabine Liposome (DepoCyt) [Antimetabolite] **Uses:** *Lymphomatous meningitis* **Action:** Antimetabolite; interferes w/ DNA synthesis **Dose:** 50 mg IT q14d for 5 doses, then 50 mg IT q28d for 4 doses; use dexamethasone prophylaxis **Caution:** [D, ?] May cause neurotox; blockage to CSF flow may ↑ the risk of neurotox; use in peds not established **Contra:** Active meningeal Infxn **Disp:** IT inj 50 mg/5 mL **SE:** Neck pain/rigidity, HA, confusion, somnolence, fever, back pain, N/V, edema, neutropenia, thrombocytopenia, anemia **Notes:** Cytarabine liposomes are similar in microscopic appearance to WBCs; caution in interpreting CSF studies **Interactions:** None noted, perhaps because of limited systemic exposure **Labs:** May interfere w/ CSF interpretation **NIPE:** ⊘ PRG, use contraception

Cytomegalovirus Immune Globulin [CMV-IG IV] (CytoGam) [Immune Globulin] **Uses:** *Attenuation of primary CMV Dz associated w/ transplantation* **Action:** Exogenous IgG antibodies to CMV **Dose:** 150 mg/kg/dose w/in 72 h of transplant, for 16 wk posttransplant; see insert for dosing schedule **Caution:** [C, ?] Anaphylactic Rxns; renal dysfunction **Contra:** Allergy to immunoglobulins; immunoglobulin A deficiency **Disp:** Inj 50 mg/mL **SE:** Flushing, N/V, muscle cramps, wheezing, HA, fever **Notes:** IV use only; administer by separate line; do not shake **Interactions:** ↓ Effects OF live virus vaccines **NIPE:** Admin immunizations at least 3 mo after CMV-IG

Dacarbazine (DTIC) [Antineoplastic/Alkylating Agent] **Uses:** *Melanoma, Hodgkin Dz, sarcoma* **Action:** Alkylating agent; antimetabolite as a purine precursor; ↓ protein synthesis, RNA, & especially DNA **Dose:** 2–4.5 mg/kg/d for 10 consecutive d or 250 mg/m²/d for 5 d (Per protocols); ↓ in renal impair **Caution:** [C, ?] In BM suppression; renal/hepatic impair **Contra:** Component sensitivity **Disp:** Inj 100, 200 mg **SE:** Myelosuppression, severe N/V, hepatotox, flu-like syndrome, ↓ BP, photosensitivity, alopecia, facial flushing, facial paresthesias, urticaria, phlebitis at inj site **Notes:** Avoid extravasation **Interactions:** ↑ Effects w/ amphotericin B, anticoagulants, ASA, bone-marrow suppressants; ↑ effects OF phenobarbital, phenytoin **Labs:** ↑ AST, ALT **NIPE:** Risk of photosensitivity—use sunscreen, hair loss, infection

Daclizumab (Zenapax) [Immunosuppressant] **Uses:** *Prevent acute organ rejection* **Action:** IL-2 receptor antagonist **Dose:** 1 mg/kg/dose IV; 1st dose pretransplant, then 4 doses 14 d apart posttransplant **Caution:** [C, ?] **Contra:** Component sensitivity **Disp:** Inj 5 mg/mL **SE:** Hyperglycemia, edema, HTN, ↓ BP, constipation, HA, dizziness, anxiety, nephrotox, pulmonary edema, pain **Notes:** Administer w/in 4 h of preparation **Interactions:** ⊘ Echinacea **NIPE:** ⊘ Immunizations, infections, ↑ fluid intake

Dactinomycin (Cosmegen) [Antineoplastic/Antibiotic] **Uses:** *Choriocarcinoma, Wilms' tumor, Kaposi sarcoma, Ewing sarcoma, rhabdomyosarcoma, testicular CA* **Action:** DNA intercalating agent **Dose:** 0.5 mg/d for 5 d; 2 mg/wk for 3 consecutive wk; 15 mcg/kg or 0.45 mg/m²/d (max 0.5 mg) for 5 d q3–8wk in ped sarcoma (Per protocols); ↓ in renal impair **Caution:** [C, ?] **Contra:** w/ concurrent or recent chickenpox or herpes zoster; infants <6 mo **Disp:** Inj 0.5 mg **SE:** Myelo-/immunosuppression, severe N/V, alopecia, acne, hyperpigmentation, radiation recall phenomenon, tissue damage w/ extravasation, hepatotoxin **Interactions:** ↑ Effects OF bone marrow suppressants, radiation therapy; ↓ effects OF vitamin K **Labs:** ↑ Uric acid; monitor CBC w/ differential & plts, LFTs, BUN, creatinine **NIPE:** ⊘ PRG, breast-feeding; risk of irreversible infertility, reversible hair loss, ↑ fluids to 2–3 L/d

Dalteparin (Fragmin) [Anticoagulant/Low Molecular Wt. Heparin]

Uses: *Unstable angina, non-Q-wave MI, prevention of ischemic complications due to clot formation in pts on concurrent ASA, prevention & Rx of DVT following surgery* **Action:** LMW heparin **Dose:** *Angina/MI:* 120 IU/kg (max 10,000 IU) SQ q12h w/ ASA. *DVT prophylaxis:* 2500–5000 IU SC 1–2 h preop, then qd for 5–10 d. *Systemic anticoagulation:* 200 IU/kg/d SQ or 100 IU/kg bid SQ; caution in renal/hepatic impair **Caution:** [B, ?] in renal/hepatic impair, active hemorrhage, cerebrovascular Dz, cerebral aneurysm, severe uncontrolled HTN **Contra:** HIT; allergy to pork products; **Disp:** Inj 2500 IU (16 mg/0.2 mL), 5000 IU (32 mg/0.2 mL), 10,000 IU (64 mg/mL) **SE:** Bleeding, pain at inj site, thrombocytopenia **Notes:** Predictable antithrombotic effects eliminate need for lab monitoring; not for IM/IV use **Interactions:** ↑ Bleeding w/ oral anticoagulants, plt inhibitors, penicillins, cephalosporins, garlic, ginger, ginkgo biloba, ginseng, chamomile, vitamin E **Labs:** ↑ AST, ALT, monitor CBC and plts **NIPE:** ⊘ Give PO or IM; give deep SC

Dantrolene (Dantrium) [Skeletal Muscle Relaxant]

Uses: *Rx clinical spasticity due to upper motor neuron disorders, (eg, spinal cord injuries, strokes, CP, MS); malignant hyperthermia* **Action:** Skeletal muscle relaxant **Dose:** *Adults.* Spasticity: Initial, 25 mg PO daily; ↑ 25 mg to effect to 100 mg max PO qid PRN. *Peds.* Initial, 0.5 mg/kg/dose bid; ↑ by 0.5 mg/kg to effect, to 3 mg/kg/dose max qid PRN. *Adults & Peds.* Malignant hyperthermia: Rx: Continuous rapid IV , start 1 mg/kg until Sxs subside or 10 mg/kg is reached. *Postcrisis follow-up:* 4–8 mg/kg/d in 3–4 ÷ doses for 1–3 d to prevent recurrence **Caution:** [C, ?] Impaired cardiac/pulmonary Fxn **Contra:** Active hepatic Dz; where spasticity needed to maintain posture or balance **Disp:** Caps 25, 50, 100 mg; powder for inj 20 mg/vial **SE:** Hepatotox w/↑ LFTs, drowsiness, dizziness, rash, muscle weakness, pleural effusion w/ pericarditis, D, blurred vision, hepatitis **Notes:** Monitor LFTs; avoid sunlight/EtOH/CNS depressants **Interactions:** ↑ effects w/ CNS depressants, antihistamines, opioids, EtOH; ↑ risk of hepatotoxicity w/ estrogens; ↑ risk of CV collapse & ventricular fib w/ CCBs; ↓ plasma protein binding w/ clofibrate, warfarin **Labs:** ↑ AST, ALT, alkaline phosphatase, LDH, BUN, total serum bilirubin **NIPE:** ↑ Risk of photosensitivity—use sunscreen

Dapsone (Avlosulfon) [Antileprotic, Antimalarial] Uses: *Rx & prevent PCP; toxoplasmosis prophylaxis; leprosy* **Action:** Unknown; bactericidal **Dose:** *Adults.* PCP prophylaxis 50–100 mg/d PO; Rx PCP 100 mg/d PO w/ TMP 15–20 mg/kg/d for 21 d. *Peds.* Prophylaxis of PCP 1–2 mg/kg/24 h PO daily; max 100 mg/d **Caution:** [C, +] G6PD deficiency; severe anemia **Contra:** Component sensitivity **Disp:** Tabs 25, 100 mg **SE:** Hemolysis, methemoglobinemia, agranulocytosis, rash, cholestatic jaundice **Notes:** Absorption ↑ by an acidic environment; for leprosy, combine w/ rifampin & other agents **Interactions:** ↑ Effects w/ probenecid, trimethoprim; ↓ effects w/ activated charcoal, rifampin **Labs:** Monitor CBC, LFTs **NIPE:** ↑ Risk of photosensitivity—use sunscreen

Daptomycin (Cubicin) [Antibiotic] Uses: *Complicated skin/skin structure Infxns due to gram(+) organisms* **Action:** Cyclic lipopeptide, causes rapid membrane depolarization & bacterial death *Spectrum: Staphylococcus aureus* (including MRSA), *Streptococcus pyogenes, S. agalactiae, S. dysgalactiae* subsp *Equisimilis* & *Enterococcus faecalis* (vancomycin-susceptible strains only) **Dose:** 4 mg/kg IV daily × 7–14 d (over 30 min); w/ CrCl < 30 mL/min/dialysis: 4 mg/kg q48h **Caution:** [B, ?] w/HMG-CoA inhibitors **Disp:** Inj 250, 500 mg/10 mL **SE:** Constipation, N/V/D, HA, rash, site Rxn, muscle pain/weakness, edema, cellulitis, ↑ hyperglycemia, ↑ alkaline phosphatase, cough, back pain, abdominal pain, ↓ K⁺, anxiety, chest pain, sore throat, cardiac failure, confusion, Candida Infxns **Notes:** Monitor CPK weekly; Consider D/C stopping HMG-CoA reductase inhibitors (↑ myopathy risk) **Interactions:** ↑ effects OF anticoagulants; ↓ effects OF tobramycin; ↓ effects w/ tobramycin; Labs: monitor CPK, LFTs, PT, INR; ↑ alkaline phosphatase, CPK, LFTs; ↓ hmg, hct, K⁺; **NIPE:** Monitor for pseudomembranous colitis; safety & efficacy not established in pts < 18 years

Darbepoetin Alfa (Aranesp) [Antianemic] Uses: *Anemia associated w/ CRF* **Action:** ↑ Erythropoiesis, recombinant erythropoietin variant **Dose:** 0.45 mcg/kg single IV or SQ qwk; titrate, do not exceed target Hgb of 12 g/dL; see insert to convert from Epogen **Caution:** [C, ?] May ↑ risk of CV &/or neurologic SE in renal failure; HTN; w/ Hx Szs **Contra:** Uncontrolled HTN, component allergy **Disp:** 25, 40, 60, 100 mcg/mL, in polysorbate or albumin excipient **SE:** May ↑ risk of cardiac events, CP, hypo/hypertension, N/V/D, myalgia, arthralgia, dizziness, edema, fatigue, fever, ↑ risk Infxn **Notes:** Longer ½-life than Epogen; weekly CBC until stable **Interactions:** None noted **Labs:** Monitor CBC w/ differential & plts, BUN, creatinine, serum P, K⁺, Fe stores **NIPE:** Monitor BP & for Sz activity, shaking vial inactivates drug

Darifenacin (Enablex) [Antispasmodic/Anticholinergic] Uses: OAB, urinary antispasmodic, **Action:** Muscarinic receptor antagonist **Dose:** 7.5 mg/d PO; 15 mg/d max (7.5 mg/d w/ moderate hepatic impair or w/ CYP3A4 inhibitors) w/ drugs metabolized by CYP2D (Table 13); swallow whole **Caution:** [C, ?/–] **Contra:** Urinary/gastric retention, uncontrolled NA glaucoma **Disp:** Tabs ER 7.5 mg, 15 mg **SE:** Xerostomia/eyes, constipation, dyspepsia, abdominal pain, retention, abnormal vision, dizziness, asthenia **Interactions:** ↑ effects w/ clarithromycin, itraconazole, ketaconazole, ritonavir, nelfinavir, ↑ effects of flecainide, TCAs, thioridazine; **Labs:** monitor LFTs; **NIPE:** take w/ or w/o food & swallow whole; drug will relieve symptoms but not treat cause

Daunorubicin (Daunomycin, Cerubicin) [Antineoplastic]
WARNING: Cardiac Fxn should be monitored due to potential risk for cardiac tox & CHF **Uses:** Acute leukemias **Action:** DNA intercalating agent; ↓ topoisomerase II; generates oxygen free radicals **Dose:** 45–60 mg/m²/d for 3 consecutive d; 25 mg/m²/wk (Per protocols); ↓ in renal/hepatic impair **Caution:** [D, ?] **Contra:** Component sensitivity **Disp:** Inj 20, 50 mg **SE:** Myelosuppression, mucositis, N/V, alopecia, radiation recall phenomenon, hepatotox (hyperbilirubinemia), tissue necrosis w/ extravasation, cardiotox (1–2% CHF risk w/ 550 mg/m² cumulative dose) **Notes:** Prevent cardiotox w/ dexrazoxane (when pt received > 300mg/m² of daunorubicin cum dose); administer allopurinol prior to Rx to prevent hyperuricemia **Interactions:** ↑ Risk of cardiotoxicity w/ cyclophosphamide; ↑ myelosuppression w/ antineoplastic agents; ↓ response to live virus vaccines **Labs:** ↑ Serum alkaline phosphatase, bilirubin, AST, monitor uric acid, CBC, LFTs **NIPE:** ASA, NSAIDs, EtOH, PRG, breast-feeding; immunizations; risk of hair loss

Decitabine (Dacogen) **Uses:** *MDS* **Action:** Inhibits DNA methyltransferase **Dose:** 15 mg/m² cont inf over 3 h; repeat q 8 h (times) 3 days; repeat cycle q 6 wk, min 4 cycles; delay Tx and ↓ dose if inadequate hematologic recovery at 6 wk (see label protocol) **Caution:** [D, ?/-]; renal/hepatic impair **Disp:** Powder 50 mg/vial SE: Neutropenia, febrile neutropenia, thrombocytopenia, anemia, leukopenia, petechiae, N/V/D, constipation, stomatitis, dyspepsia, cough, fever, fatigue, hyperglycemia, Infxn **Labs:** ↑ LFTs, bili, glucose; check CBC and plt before each cycle and prn **NIPE:** May premedicate w/anti-emetic; ∅ pregnancy; males should not father a child during or 2 months after use

Delavirdine (Rescriptor) [Antiretroviral/NNRTI] **Uses:** *HIV Infxn* **Action:** Nonnucleoside RT inhibitor **Dose:** 400 mg PO tid **Caution:** [C, ?] CDC recommends HIV-infected mothers not breast-feed due to risk of HIV transmission; w/renal/hepatic impair **Contra:** Use w/ drugs dependent on CYP3A for clearance (Table 13) **Disp:** Tabs 100, 200 mg **SE:** HA, fatigue, rash, ↑ transaminases, N/V/D **Notes:** Avoid antacids; ↓ cytochrome P-450 enzymes; numerous drug interactions; monitor LFTs **Interactions:** ↑ Effects w/fluoxetine; (up) benzodiazepines, cisapride, clarithromycin, dapsone, ergotamines, indinavir, lovastatin, midazolam, nifedipine, quinidine, ritonavir, simvastatin, terfenadine, triazolam; ↓ effects w/ antacids, barbiturates, carbamazepine, cimetidine, famotidine, lansoprazole, nizatidine, phenobarbital, phenytoin, ranitidine, rifabutin, rifampin; ↓ effects OF didanosine **Labs:** ↑ AST, ALT, ↓ neutrophil counts **NIPE:** Take w/o regard to food

Deferasirox (Exjade) [Iron Chelator] **Uses:** *Chronic iron overload due to transfusion in patients >2 yrs* **Action:** Oral iron chelator **Dose:** Initial:

20 mg/kg PO/d; adjust by 5–10 mg/kg q 3–6 mo based on monthly ferritin; 30 mg/kg/d max; on empty stomach 30 min before food; dissolve in water, orange, apple juice (< 1 gm/3.5 oz; >1 gm in 7 oz); drink immediately; resuspend residue and swallow; do not chew, swallow whole tabs or take w/ Al-containing antacids **Caution:** [B, ?/–] **Disp:** Tabs for oral susp 125, 250, 500 mg **SE:** N/V/D, abdominal pain, skin rash, HA, fever, cough, Infxn, hearing loss, dizziness, cataracts, retinal disorders, ↑ IOP, lens opacities, dizziness **Labs:** ↑ Cr, LFTs; monthly Cr, urine protein, and LFTs **NIPE:** Dose to nearest whole tablet; auditory and ophthalmic testing initially and q 12 mo

Demeclocycline (Declomycin) [Antibiotic] Uses: SIADH **Action:** Antibiotic, antagonizes ADH action on renal tubules **Dose:** 300–600 mg PO q12h on empty stomach; ↓ in renal failure; avoid antacids **Caution:** [D, +] Avoid in hepatic/renal impair & children **Contra:** Allergy to tetracyclines **Disp:** Tabs 150, 300 mg **SE:** D, abdominal cramps, photosensitivity, DI **Interactions:** Effects OF digoxin, anticoagulants; ↓ effects w/ antacids, Bi salts, Fe, Na bicarbonate, barbiturates, carbamazepine, hydantoins, food; ↓ effects OF oral contraceptives, penicillin **Labs:** False − urine glucose; monitor CBC, LFTs, BUN, creatinine **NIPE:** Risk of photosensitivity—use sunscreen & avoid sunlight

Desipramine (Norpramin) [Antidepressant/TCA] WARNING: Closely monitor for worsening depression or emergence of suicidality Uses: *Endogenous depression,* chronic pain, & peripheral neuropathy **Action:** TCA; ↑ synaptic concentration of serotonin or norepinephrine in CNS **Dose:** 100–200 mg/d single or ÷ doses; usually a single hs dose (max 300 mg/d) **Caution:** [C, ?/–] CV Dz, Sz disorder, hypothyroidism **Contra:** Use of MAOIs w/in 14 d; during recovery phase of MI **Disp:** Tabs 10, 25, 50, 75, 100, 150 mg; caps 25, 50 mg **SE:** Anticholinergic (blurred vision, urinary retention, xerostomia); orthostatic ↓ BP; prolongs QT interval, arrhythmias **Notes:** Numerous drug interactions; may cause urine to turn blue-green urine; avoid sunlight **Interactions:** ↑ Effects w/ cimetidine, diltiazem, fluoxetine, indinavir, MAOIs, paroxetine, propoxyphene, quinidine, ritonavir ranitidine, EtOH, grapefruit juice; ↑ effects OF Li, sulfonylureas; ↓ effects w/ barbiturates, carbamazepine rifampin, tobacco **NIPE:** Full effect of drug may take 4 wk, risk of photosensitivity—use sunscreen

Desloratadine (Clarinex) [Antihistamine/Selective H₁-receptor antagonist] Uses: *Symptoms of seasonal & perennial allergic rhinitis; chronic idiopathic urticaria* **Action:** active metabolite of Claritin, H₁-antihistamine, blocks inflammatory mediators **Dose:** *Adults & Peds >12 y.* 5 mg PO qd; in hepatic/renal impair 5 mg PO qod **Caution:** [C, ?/–] RediTabs contain phenylalanine; safety not established for <12 y **Disp:** Tabs & Reditabs (rapid dissolving) 5 mg **SE:** Allergy, anaphylaxis, somnolence, HA, dizziness, fatigue, pharyngitis, xerostomia, nausea, dyspepsia, myalgia **Labs:** ↑ bilirubin **NIPE:** Take w/o regard to food

Desmopressin (DDAVP, Stimate) [Antidiuretic/Hormone] Uses: *DI (intranasal & parenteral); bleeding due to uremia, hemophilia A, & type

I von Willebrand Dz (parenteral), nocturnal enuresis* **Action:** Synthetic analog of vasopressin, a naturally occurring human ADH; ↑ factor VIII **Dose:** *DI: Intranasal: Adults.* 0.1–0.4 mL (10–40 mcg/d in 1–3 ÷ doses. *Peds 3 mo–12 y.* 0.05–0.3 mL/d in 1 or 2 doses. *Parenteral: Adults.* 0.5–1 mL (2–4 mcg/d in 2 ÷ doses); if converting from nasal to parenteral, use ¹⁄₁₀ nasal dose. *PO: Adults.* 0.05 mg bid; ↑ to max of 1.2 mg. *Hemophilia A & von Willebrand Dz (type I): Adults & Peds >10 kg.* 0.3 mcg/kg in 50 mL NS, inf over 15–30 min. *Peds <10 kg.* As above w/ dilution to 10 mL w/ NS. *Nocturnal enuresis: Peds >6 y.* 20 mcg intranasally hs **Caution:** [B, M] Avoid overhydration **Contra:** Hemophilia B; severe classic von Willebrand Dz; pts w/ factor VIII antibodies **Disp:** Tabs 0.1, 0.2 mg; inj 4, 15 mcg/mL; nasal soln 0.1, 1.5 mg/mL **SE:** Facial flushing, HA, dizziness, vulval pain, nasal congestion, pain at inj site; ↓ Na⁺, H₂O intox **Notes:** In very young & old pts, ↓ fluid intake to avoid H₂O intox & ↓ ↓ Na⁺ **Interactions:** ↑ Antidiuretic effects w/ carbamazepine, chlorpropamide, clofibrate; ↑ effects OF vasopressors; ↓ antidiuretic effects w/ demeclocycline, Li, norepinephrine **NIPE:** Monitor I&O, ⊘ EtOH, overhydration

Dexamethasone, Nasal (Dexacort Phosphate Turbinaire) [Anti-inflammatory, Immunosuppressant/Glucocorticoid]

Uses: *Chronic nasal inflammation or allergic rhinitis* **Action:** Antiinflammatory corticosteroid **Dose:** *Adult & Peds >12 y.* 2 sprays/nostril bid–tid, max 12 sprays/d. *Peds 6–12 y.* 1–2 sprays/nostril bid, max 8 sprays/d **Caution:** [C, ?] **Contra:** Untreated Infxn **Disp:** Aerosol, 84 mcg/activation **SE:** Local irritation **NIPE:** Use decongestant nose gtt 1st if nasal congestion

Dexamethasone, Ophthalmic (AK-Dex Ophthalmic, Decadron Ophthalmic) [Anti-inflammatory, Immunosuppressant/Glucocorticoid]

Uses: *Inflammatory or allergic conjunctivitis* **Action:** Antiinflammatory corticosteroid **Dose:** Instill 1–2 gtt tid–qid **Caution:** [C, ?/–] **Contra:** Active untreated bacterial, viral, & fungal eye Infxns **Disp:** Susp & soln 0.1%; oint 0.05% **SE:** Long-term use associated w/ cataracts **NIPE:** Eval intraocular pressure and lens if prolonged use

Dexamethasone Systemic, Topical (Decadron) [Anti-inflammatory, Immunosuppressant/Glucocorticoid]

See Steroids, Systemic, Table 4 & 5, pages 308–309 **Interactions:** ↑ effects w/ cyclosporine, estrogens, oral contraceptives, macrolides; ↑ effects OF cyclosporine; ↓ effects w/ aminoglutethimide, antacids, barbiturates, carbamazepine, cholestyramine, colestipol, phenytoin, phenobarbital, rifampin; ↓ effects OF anticoagulants, hypoglycemics, INH, toxoids, salicylates, vaccines **Labs:** False − allergy skin tests **NIPE:** ⊘ Vaccines, breast-feeding, use on broken skin

Dexpanthenol (Ilopan-Choline PO, Ilopan) [Cholinergic]

Uses: *Minimize paralytic ileus, Rx postop distention* **Action:** Cholinergic agent **Dose:** *Adults.* Relief of gas: 2–3 tabs PO tid. *Prevent postop ileus:* 250–500 mg IM stat, repeat in 2 h, then q6h PRN. *Ileus:* 500 mg IM stat, repeat in 2 h, followed by doses q6h, PRN **Caution:** [C, ?] **Contra:** Hemophilia, mechanical obstruction **Disp:** Inj; tabs 50 mg; cream **SE:** GI cramps **NIPE:** Monitor BP during IV administration

Dexrazoxane (Zinecard) [Chelating Agent]
Uses: *Prevent anthracycline-induced (eg, doxorubicin) cardiomyopathy* **Action:** Chelates heavy metals; binds intracellular iron & prevents anthracycline-induced free radicals **Dose:** 10:1 ratio dexrazoxane:doxorubicin 30 min prior to each dose **Caution:** [C, ?] **Contra:** Component sensitivity **Disp:** Inj powder 250, 500 mg (10 mg/mL) **SE:** Myelosuppression (especially leukopenia), fever, Infxn, stomatitis, alopecia, N/V/D; mild ↑ transaminase, pain at inj site **Interactions:** ↑ Length of muscle relaxation w/ succinylcholine

Dextran 40 (Rheomacrodex) [Plasma Volume Expander]
Uses: *Shock, prophylaxis of DVT & thromboembolism, adjunct in peripheral vascular surgery* **Action:** Expands plasma volume; ↓ blood viscosity **Dose:** *Shock:* 10 mL/kg inf rapidly; 20 mL/kg max in the 1st 24 h; beyond 24 h 10 mL/kg max; D/C after 5 d. *Prophylaxis of DVT & thromboembolism:* 10 mL/kg IV day of surgery, then 500 mL/d IV for 2–3 d, then 500 mL IV q2–3d based on risk for up to 2 wk **Caution:** [C, ?] Inf Rxns; pts receiving corticosteroids **Contra:** Major hemostatic defects; cardiac decompensation; renal Dz w/ severe oliguria/anuria **Disp:** 10% dextran 40 in 0.9% NaCl or 5% dextrose **SE:** Allergy/anaphylactoid Rxn (observe during 1st min of inf), arthralgia, cutaneous Rxns, ↓ BP, fever **Notes:** Monitor Cr & electrolytes; pts should be well hydrated **Interactions:** ↑ Bleeding times w/ antiplt agents or anticoagulants **Labs:** False ↑ serum glucose, urinary protein, bilirubin assays, & total protein assays **NIPE:** Draw blood before administration of drug, pt should be well hydrated prior to inf

Dextromethorphan (Mediquell, Benylin DM, PediaCare 1, others) [OTC] [Antitussive]
Uses: *Controlling nonproductive cough* **Action:** Suppresses medullary cough center **Dose:** *Adults.* 10–30 mg PO q4h PRN (max 120 mg/24 h). *Peds.* 7 mo–1 y: 2–4 mg q6–8h. *2–6 y:* 2.5–7.5 mg q4–8h (max 30 mg/24 h). *7–12 y:* 5–10 mg q4–8h (max 60 mg/24h) **Caution:** [C, ?/–] Not for persistent or chronic cough **Disp:** Caps 30 mg; lozenges 2.5, 5, 7.5, 15 mg; syrup 15 mg/15 mL, 10 mg/5 mL; liq 10 mg/15 mL, 3.5, 7.5, 15 mg/5 mL; sustained-action liq 30 mg/5 mL **SE:** GI disturbances **Notes:** Found in combo OTC products w/ guaifenesin **Interactions:** ↑ Effects w/ amiodarone, fluoxetine, quinidine, terbinafine; ↑ risk of serotonin syndrome w/ sibutramine, MAOIs; ↑ CNS depression w/ antihistamines, antidepressants, sedative, opioids, EtOH **NIPE:** ↑ Fluids, humidity to environment, stop MAOIs for 2 wk before administering drug

Dezocine (Dalgan) [Narcotic Analgesic]
Uses: *Moderate–severe pain* **Action:** Narcotic agonist–antagonist **Dose:** 5–20 mg IM or 2.5–10 mg IV q2–4h PRN; ↓ in renal impair **Caution:** [C, ?] **Contra:** Pts <18 y **Disp:** Inj 5, 10, 15 mg/mL **SE:** Sedation, dizziness, vertigo, N/V, inj site Rxn **Notes:** Withdrawal possible in narcotic dependency **Interactions:** ↑ Effects w/ CNS depressants, ⊘ MAOIs **NIPE:** ↑ Resp depression greatest 1st h after admin

Diazepam (Valium) [Anxiolytic, Skeletal Muscle Relaxant, Anticonvulsant, Sedative/Hypnotic/Benzodiazepine] [C-IV]

Uses: *Anxiety, EtOH withdrawal, muscle spasm, status epilepticus, panic disorders, amnesia, preop sedation* **Action:** Benzodiazepine **Dose:** *Adults.* Status epilepticus: 5–10 mg q10–20 min to 30 mg max in 8-h period. *Anxiety, muscle spasm:* 2–10 mg PO bid–qid or IM/IV q3–4h PRN. *Preop:* 5–10 mg PO or IM 20–30 min or IV just prior to procedure. *EtOH withdrawal:* Initial 2–5 mg IV, then 5–10 mg q5–10 min, 100 mg in 1 h max. May require up to 1000 mg in 24-h period for severe withdrawal. Titrate to agitation; avoid excessive sedation; may lead to aspiration or resp arrest. **Peds.** Status epilepticus: <5 y: 0.05–0.3 mg/kg/dose IV q15–30 min up to a max of 5 mg. >5 y: Give up to max of 10 mg. *Sedation, muscle relaxation:* 0.04–0.3 mg/kg/dose q2–4 h IM or IV to max of 0.6 mg/kg in 8 h, or 0.12–0.8 mg/kg/24 h PO ÷ tid–qid; ↓ in hepatic impair **Caution:** [D, ?/–] **Contra:** Coma, CNS depression, resp depression, NA glaucoma, severe uncontrolled pain, PRG **Disp:** Tabs 2, 5, 10 mg; soln 1, 5 mg/mL; inj 5 mg/mL; rectal gel 5 mg/mL **SE:** Sedation, amnesia, bradycardia, ↓ BP, rash, ↓ resp rate **Notes:** Do not exceed 5 mg/min IV in adults or 1–2 mg/min in peds because resp arrest possible; IM absorption erratic; avoid abrupt D/C **Interactions:** ↑ Effects w/ antihistamines, azole antifungals, BBs, CNS depressants, cimetidine, ciprofloxin, disulfiram, INH, oral contraceptives, omeprazole, phenytoin, valproic acid, verapamil, EtOH, kava kava, valerian; ↑ effects OF digoxin, diuretics; ↓ effects w/ barbiturates, carbamazepine, theophylline, ranitidine, tobacco; ↓ effects OF haloperidol, levodopa **Labs:** False − urine glucose; monitor LFTs, BUN, creatinine, CBC w/ long-term drug use **NIPE:** Risk ↑ Sz activity

Diazoxide (Hyperstat, Proglycem) [Antihypertensive/Peripheral Vasodilator]

Uses: *Hypoglycemia due to hyperinsulinism (Proglycem); hypertensive crisis (Hyperstat)* **Action:** ↓ Pancreatic insulin release; antihypertensive **Dose:** *Hypertensive crisis:* 1–3 mg/kg IV (150 mg max in single inj); repeat in 5–15 min until BP controlled; repeat every 4–24 h; monitor BP closely. *Hypoglycemia:* **Adults & Peds.** 3–8 mg/kg/24 h PO ÷ q8–12h. *Neonates.* 8–15 mg/kg/24 h ÷ in 3 equal doses; maint 8–10 mg/kg/24 h PO in 2–3 equal doses **Caution:** [C, ?] ↓ effect w/ phenytoin; ↑ effect w/ diuretics, warfarin **Contra:** Allergy to thiazides or other sulfonamide-containing products; HTN associated w/ aortic coarctation, AV shunt, or pheochromocytoma **Disp:** Inj 15 mg/mL; caps 50 mg; PO susp 50 mg/mL **SE:** Hyperglycemia, ↓ BP, dizziness, Na+ & H2O retention, N/V, weakness **Notes:** Can give false-negative insulin response to glucagons; treat extravasation w/ warm compress **Interactions:** ↑ Effects w/ carboplatin, cisplatin, diuretics, phenothiazines; ↑ effects OF anticoagulants; ↓ effects w/ sulfonylureas; ↓ effects OF phenytoin, sulfonylureas **Labs:** ↑ Serum uric acid, AST, alkaline phosphatase, false − response to glucagon **NIPE:** Daily weights, ↑ reversible body hair growth

Dibucaine (Nupercainal) [Topical Anesthetic]

Uses: *Hemorrhoids & minor skin conditions* **Action:** Topical anesthetic **Dose:** Insert PR w/ applicator bid & after each bowel movement; apply sparingly to skin **Caution:** [C, ?] **Contra:** Component sensitivity **Disp:** 1% Oint w/ rectal applicator; 0.5% cream **SE:** Local irritation, rash **Interactions:** None noted

Diclofenac (Cataflam, Voltaren) [Antiarthritic, Anti-inflammatory/NSAID]

WARNING: May ↑ risk of cardiovascular events & GI bleeding **Uses:** *Arthritis & pain* **Action:** NSAID **Dose:** 50–75 mg PO bid; w/ food or milk **Caution:** [B (D 3rd tri or near delivery), ?] CHF, HTN, renal/hepatic dysfunction, & Hx PUD **Contra:** Allergy to NSAIDs or aspirin; porphyria **Disp:** Tabs 50 mg; tabs DR 25, 50, 75, 100 mg; XR tabs 100 mg; ophthal soln 0.1% **SE:** Abdominal cramps, heartburn, GI ulceration, rash, interstitial nephritis **Notes:** Watch for GI bleed **Interactions:** ↑ Risk of bleeding w/ feverfew, garlic, ginger, ginkgo biloba; ↑ effects OF digoxin, MTX, cyclosporine, Li, insulin, sulfonylureas, K-sparing diuretics, warfarin; ↓ effects w/ ASA; ↓ effects OF thiazide diuretics, furosemide, BBs **Labs:** ↑ LFTs, serum glucose & cortisol, ↓ serum uric acid; **NIPE:** Risk of photosensitivity—use sunscreen, monitor LFTs, CBC, BUN, creatinine, take w/ food, ⊘ crush tablets

Dicloxacillin (Dynapen, Dycill) [Antibiotic/Penicillin]

Uses: *Rx of pneumonia, skin & soft tissue Infxns, & osteomyelitis caused by penicillinase-producing staphylococci* **Action:** Bactericidal; ↓ cell wall synthesis. *Spectrum: S. aureus & Strep* **Dose:** *Adults.* 250–500 mg qid **Peds** *<40 kg.* 12.5–25 mg/kg/d ÷ qid; take on empty stomach **Caution:** [B, ?] **Contra:** Component or PCN sensitivity **Disp:** Caps 125, 250, 500 mg; soln 62.5 mg/5 mL **SE:** N/D; abdominal pain **Notes:** Monitor PTT if pt on warfarin **Interactions:** ↑ Effects w/ disulfiram, probenecid; ↑ effects OF MRX; ↓ effects w/ macrolides, tetracyclines, food; ↓ effects OF oral contraceptives, warfarin **Labs:** False ↑ nafcillin level, urine & serum proteins, uric acid **NIPE:** Take w/ water

Dicyclomine (Bentyl) [Antimuscarinic, GI Antispasmodic/Anticholinergic]

Uses: *Functional IBSs* **Action:** Smooth muscle relaxant **Dose:** *Adults.* 20 mg PO qid; ↑ to 160 mg/d max or 20 mg IM q6h **Peds.** Infants >6 mo: 5 mg/dose tid–qid. *Children:* 10 mg/dose tid–qid **Caution:** [B, –] **Contra:** Infants < 6 mo, NA glaucoma, MyG, severe UC, BOO **Disp.:** Caps 10, 20 mg; tabs 20 mg; syrup 10 mg/5 mL; inj 10 mg/mL **SE:** Anticholinergic SE's may limit dose **Notes:** Take 30–60 min before meal; **Interactions:** ↑ Anticholinergic effects w/ anticholinergics, antihistamines, amantadine, MAOIs, TCAs, phenothiazines; ↑ effects OF atenolol, digoxin; ↓ effects w/ antacids; ↓ effects OF haloperidol, ketoconazole, levodopa, phenothiazines **NIPE:** ⊘ EtOH, CNS depressant; adequate hydration

Didanosine [ddI] (Videx) [Antiretroviral, NRTI]

WARNING: Allergy manifested as fever, rash, fatigue, GI/resp Sxs reported; stop drug immediately & do not rechallenge; lactic acidosis & hepatomegaly/steatosis reported **Uses:** *HIV Infxn in zidovudine-intolerant pts* **Action:** Nucleoside antiretroviral agent **Dose:** *Adults.* >60 kg: 400 mg/d PO or 200 mg PO bid. *<60 kg:* 250 mg/d

PO or 125 mg PO bid; adults should take 2 tabs/administration. **Peds.** Dose by following table; ↓ in renal impair:

BSA (m²)	Tablets (mg)	Powder (mg)
1.1–1.4	100 bid	125 bid
0.8–1	75 bid	94 bid
0.5–0.7	50 bid	62 bid
<0.4	25 bid	31 bid

Caution: [B, –] CDC recommends HIV-infected mothers not breast-feed due to risk of HIV transmission **Contra:** Component sensitivity **Disp:** Chew tabs 25, 50, 100, 150, 200 mg; powder packets 100, 167, 250, 375 mg; powder for soln 2, 4 g **SE:** Pancreatitis, peripheral neuropathy, D, HA **Notes:** Do not take w/ meals; thoroughly chew tablets, do not mix w/ fruit juice or other acidic beverages; reconstitute powder w/ H_2O **Interactions:** ↑ Effects w/ allopurinol, ganciclovir; ↓ effects w/ methadone, food; ↑ risk of pancreatitis w/ thiazide diuretics, IV pentamidine, EtOH; ↓ effects OF azole antifungals, dapsone, delavirdine, ganciclovir, indinavir, quinolines, ranitidine, tetracyclines **Labs:** ↑ LFTs, uric acid, amylase, lipase, triglycerides **NIPE:** May cause hyperglycemia, take w/o food, chew or crush tabs

Diflunisal (Dolobid) [Analgesic, Antipyretic, Anti-inflammatory/NSAID] WARNING: May ↑ risk of cardiovascular events & GI bleeding **Uses:** *Mild–moderate pain; osteoarthritis* **Action:** NSAID **Dose:** *Pain:* 500 mg PO bid. *Osteoarthritis:* 500–1500 mg PO in 2–3 ÷ doses; ↓ in renal impair, take w/ food/milk **Caution:** [C (D 3rd tri or near delivery), ?] CHF, HTN, renal/hepatic dysfunction, & Hx PUD. **Contra:** Allergy to NSAIDs or aspirin, active GI bleed **Disp:** Tabs 250, 500 mg **SE:** May ↑ bleeding time; HA, abdominal cramps, heartburn, GI ulceration, rash, interstitial nephritis, fluid retention **Interactions:** ↑ Effects w/ probenecid; ↑ effects OF acetaminophen, anticoagulants, digoxin, HCTZ, indomethacin, Li, MTX, phenytoin, sulfonamides, sulfonylureas; ↓ effects w/ antacids, ASA; ↓ effects OF furosemide **Labs:** ↑ Salicylate levels, PT, ↓ uric acid, T_3, T_4 **NIPE:** Take w/ food, ⊘ chew or crush tabs

Digoxin (Lanoxin, Lanoxicaps) [Antiarrhythmic/Cardiac Glycoside] **Uses:** *CHF, AF & flutter, & PAT* **Action:** Positive inotrope; ↑ AV node refractory period **Dose:** **Adults.** PO digitalization: 0.5–0.75 mg PO, then 0.25 mg PO q6–8 h to total 1–1.5 mg. *IV or IM digitalization:* 0.25–0.5 mg IM or IV, then 0.25 mg q4–6 h to total ≅1 mg. *Daily maint:* 0.125–0.5 mg/d PO, IM, or IV (average daily dose 0.125–0.25 mg). **Peds.** Preterm infants: Digitalization: 30 mcg/kg PO or 25 mcg/kg IV; give ½ of dose initial, then ¼ of dose at 8–12-h intervals for 2 doses. *Maint:* 5–7.5 mcg/kg/24 h PO or 4–6 mcg/ kg/24 h IV ÷

q12 h. *Term infants: Digitalization:* 25–35 mcg/kg PO or 20–30 mcg/kg IV; give ½ the initial dose, then ⅓ of dose at 8–12 h. *Maint:* 6–10 mcg/kg/24 h PO or 5–8 mcg/kg/24 h ÷ q12 h. *1 mo–2 y: Digitalization:* 35–60 mcg/kg PO or 30–50 mcg/kg IV; give ½ the initial dose, then ⅓ dose at 8–12-h intervals for 2 doses. *Maint:* 10–15 mcg/kg/24 h PO or 7.5–15 mcg/kg/24 h IV ÷ q12 h. *2–10 y: Digitalization:* 30–40 mcg/kg PO or 25 mcg/kg IV; give ½ initial dose, then ⅓ of the dose at 8–12-h intervals for 2 doses. *Maint:* 8–10 mcg/kg/24 h PO or 6–8 mcg/kg/24 h IV ÷ q12 h. *7–10 y:* Same as for adults; ↓ in renal impair, **Caution:** [C, +] **Contra** AV block; idiopathic hypertrophic subaortic stenosis; constrictive pericarditis **Disp:** Caps 0.05, 0.1, 0.2 mg; tabs 0.125, 0.25, 0.5 mg; elixir 0.05 mg/mL; inj 0.1, 0.25 mg/mL **SE:** Can cause heart block; ↓ K⁺ potentiates tox; N/V, HA, fatigue, visual disturbances (yellow-green halos around lights), cardiac arrhythmias **Notes:** Multiple drug interactions; IM inj painful, has erratic absorption & should not be used; follow serum levels (Table 2). **Interactions:** ↑ Effects w/ alprazolam, amiodarone, azole antifungals, BBs, carvedilol, cyclosporine, corticosteroids, diltiazem, diuretics, erythromycin, NSAIDs, quinidine, spironolactone, tetracyclines, verapamil, goldenseal, hawthorn, licorice, quinine, Siberian ginseng; ↓ effects w/ charcoal, cholestyramine, cisapride, neomycin, rifampin, sucralfate, thyroid hormones, psyllium, St. John's wort **Labs:** ↓ PT, monitor serum electrolytes, LFTs, BUN, creatinine **NIPE:** Different bioavailability in various brands

Digoxin Immune Fab (Digibind) [Cardiac Glycoside Antidote]

Uses: *Life-threatening digoxin intox* **Action:** Antigen-binding fragments bind & inactivate digoxin **Dose:** *Adults & Peds.* Based on serum level & pt's weight; see charts provided w/ drug **Caution:** [C, ?] **Contra:** Allergy to sheep products **Disp:** Inj 38–40 mg/vial **SE:** Worsening of cardiac output or CHF, ↓ K⁺, facial swelling, & redness **Notes:** Each vial binds ≅ 0.6 mg of digoxin; renal failure may require redosing in several days **Interactions:** ↓ Effects OF cardiac glycosides **NIPE:** Will take up to 1 wk for accurate serum digoxin levels after use of Digibind

Diltiazem (Cardizem, Cardizem CD, Cardizem SR, Cartia XT, Dilacor XR, Diltia XT, Tiamate, Tiazac) [Antianginal/CCB]

Uses: *Angina, prevention of reinfarction, HTN, AF or flutter, & PAT* **Action:** CCB **Dose:** *PO:* Initial, 30 mg PO qid; ↑ to 180–360 mg/d in 3–4 ÷ doses PRN. *SR:* 60–120 mg PO bid; ↑ to 360 mg/d max. *CD or XR:* 120–360 mg/d (max 480 mg/d). *IV:* 0.25 mg/kg IV bolus over 2 min; may repeat in 15 min at 0.35 mg/kg; begin inf of 5–15 mg/h **Caution:** [C, +] ↑ effect w/ amiodarone, cimetidine, fentanyl, lithium, cyclosporine, digoxin, β-blockers, cisapride, theophylline **Contra:** SSS, AV block, ↓ BP, AMI, pulmonary congestion **Disp:** *Cardizem CD:* Caps 120, 180, 240, 300, 360 mg; *Cardizem SR:* caps 60, 90, 120 mg; *Cardizem:* Tabs 30, 60, 90, 120 mg; *Cartia XT:* Caps 120, 180, 240, 300 mg; *Dilacor XR:* Caps 180, 240 mg; *Diltia XT:* Caps 120, 180, 240 mg; *Tiazac:* Caps 120, 180, 240, 300, 360, 420 mg; *Tiamate (XR):* Tabs 120, 180, 240 mg; inj 5 mg/mL **SE:** Gingival hyperplasia, bradycardia, AV block, ECG abnormalities, peripheral edema, dizziness, HA **Notes:** Cardizem CD, Dilacor XR, & Tiazac not interchangeable **Interactions:** ↑ Effects w/ α-blockers, azole antifungals, BBs, erythromycin, H_2 receptor antagonists, nitroprusside, quinidine, EtOH, grapefruit juice; ↑ effects OF carbamazepine, cyclosporine, digitalis glycosides, quinidine, phenytoin, prazosin, theophylline, TCAs; ↓ effects w/ NSAIDs, phenobarbital, rifampin **Labs:** False ↑ urine ketones, ↑ LFTs, BUN, creatinine **NIPE:** ⊘ Chew or crush SR or ER preps, risk of photosensitivity—use sunscreen

Dimenhydrinate (Dramamine, others) [Antiemetic/Antivertigo/Anticholinergic] **Uses:** *Prevention & Rx of N/V, dizziness, or vertigo of motion sickness* **Action:** Antiemetic **Dose:** *Adults.* 50–100 mg PO q4–6 h, max 400 mg/d; 50 mg IM/IV PRN. *Peds.* 2–6 yrs: 12.5–25 mg q6–8 h max 75 mg/day, *6–12 yrs:* 25–50 mg q6–8 h max 150 mg/d; 1.25 mg/kg or 37.5/mg/m² IM q6 h 300 mg/day max **Caution:** [B, ?] **Contra:** Component sensitivity **Disp:** Tabs 50 mg; chew tabs 50 mg; liq 12.5 mg/4 mL, 12.5 mg/5 mL, 15.62 mg/5 mL; inj 50 mg/mL **SE:** Anticholinergic side effects **Interactions:** ↑ Effects w/ CNS depressants, antihistamines, opioids, quinidine, MAOIs, TCAs, EtOH **Labs:** False ↓ allergy skin tests **NIPE:** ⊘ Drug 72 h prior to allergy skin testing, take before motion sickness occurs

Dimethyl Sulfoxide [DMSO] (Rimso 50) [GU Agent] **Uses:** *Interstitial cystitis* **Action:** Unknown **Dose:** Intravesical, 50 mL, retain for 15 min; repeat q2wk until relief **Caution:** [C, ?] **Contra:** Component sensitivity **Disp:** 50% & 100% soln **SE:** Cystitis, eosinophilia, GI, & taste disturbance **Interactions:** ↓ Effects OF sulindac **Labs:** Monitor CBC, LFTs, BUN, creatinine levels **NIPE:** ↑ Taste & smell of garlic

Dinoprostone (Cervidil Vaginal Insert, Prepidil Vaginal Gel) [Prostaglandin/Abortifacient] **Uses:** *Induce labor; terminate PRG (12–20 wk); evacuate uterus in missed abortion or fetal death* **Action:** prostaglandin, changes consistency, dilatation, & effacement of the cervix; induces uterine contraction **Dose:** *Gel:* 0.5 mg; if no cervical/uterine response, repeat 0.5 mg q6h (max 24-h dose 1.5 mg). *Vaginal insert:* 1 insert (10 mg = 0.3 mg dinoprostone/h over 12 h); remove w/ onset of labor or 12 h after insertion. *Vaginal supp:* 20 mg repeated every 3–5 h; adjust PRN supp: 1 high in vagina, repeat at 3–5-h intervals until abortion (240 mg max) **Caution:** [X, ?] **Contra:** Ruptured membranes, allergy to prostaglandins, placenta previa or unexplained vaginal bleeding during PRG, when oxytocic drugs contraindicated or if prolonged uterine contractions are inappropriate (Hx C-section, presence of cephalopelvic disproportion, etc) **Disp:** *Endocervical gel:* 0.5 mg in 3-g syringes (each package contains a 10-mm & 20-mm shielded catheter) *Vaginal gel:* 0.5 mg/3 g *Vaginal supp:* 20 mg *Vaginal insert, CR:* 0.3 mg/h **SE:** N/V/D, dizziness, flushing, HA, fever **Interactions:** ↑ Effects OF oxytocics, ↓ effects w/ large amts ETOH **NIPE:** Pt supine after insertion of supp or gel up to ½ h

Diphenhydramine (Benadryl) [Antihistamine/Antitussive/Antiemetic] [OTC] Uses: *Rx & prevent allergic Rxns, motion sickness, potentiate narcotics, sedation, cough suppression, & Rx of extrapyramidal Rxns* Action: Antihistamine, antiemetic Dose: *Adults.* 25–50 mg PO, IV, or IM bid–tid. *Peds.* 5 mg/kg/24 h PO or IM ÷ q6h (max 300 mg/d); ↑ dosing interval in moderate–severe renal failure Caution: [B, –] Contra: Do not use in acute asthma attack Disp: Tabs & caps 25, 50 mg; chew tabs 12.5 mg; elixir 12.5 mg/5 mL; syrup 12.5 mg/5 mL; liq 6.25 mg/5 mL, 12.5 mg/5 mL; inj 50 mg/mL SE: Anticholinergic side effects (xerostomia, urinary retention, sedation) Interactions: ↑ Effects w/ CNS depressants, antihistamines, opioids, MAOIs, TCAs, EtOH; ↑ effects OF metoprolol Labs: ↓ Response to allergy skin testing NIPE: ↑ Risk of photosensitivity—use sunscreen

Diphenoxylate + Atropine (Lomotil) [C-V] [Opioid Antidiarrheal] Uses: *D* Action: Constipating meperidine congener, reduces GI motility Dose: *Adults.* Initial, 5 mg PO tid–qid until under control, then 2.5–5.5 mg PO bid. *Peds >2 y:* 0.3–0.4 mg/kg/24 h (of diphenoxylate) bid–qid Caution: [C, +] Contra: Obstructive jaundice, diarrhea due to bacterial Infxn; children <2 y Disp: Tabs 2.5 mg of diphenoxylate/0.025 mg of atropine; liq 2.5 mg diphenoxylate/0.025 mg atropine/5 mL SE: Drowsiness, dizziness, blurred vision, urinary retention, constipation Interactions: ↑ Effects w/ CNS depressants, opioids, EtOH, ↑ risk HTN crisis w/ MAOIs NIPE: ↓ Effectiveness w/ diarrhea caused by antibiotics

Diphtheria, Tetanus Toxoids, & Acellular pertussis adsorbed, Hepatitis B (Recombinant), & Inactivated Poliovirus Vaccine [IPV] combined (Pediarix) [Vaccine, inactivated] Uses: *Vaccine against diphtheria, tetanus, pertussis, HBV, polio (types 1, 2, 3) as a 3-dose primary series in infants & children <7, born to HBsAg–mothers* Actions: Active immunization Dose: *Infants:* Three 0.5-mL doses IM, at 6–8-wk intervals, start at 2 mo; child given 1 dose of hep B vaccine, same; previously vaccinated w/ one or more doses IPV, use to complete series Caution: [C, N/A] Contra: If HbsAG+ mother, adults, children >7 y, immunosuppressed, allergy to yeast, neomycin, or polymyxin B, Hx allergy to any component, encephalopathy, or progressive neurologic disorders; caution in bleeding disorders. Disp: Single-dose vials 0.5 mL SE: Drowsiness, restlessness, fever, fussiness, ↓ appetite, nodule redness, pain/swelling at inj site Notes: Give IM only Interactions: ↓ Effects w/ immunosuppressants, corticosteroids

Dipivefrin (Propine) [Alpha Adrenergic Agonist/Glaucoma Agent] Uses: *Open-angle glaucoma* Action: α-Adrenergic agonist Dose: 1 gtt into eye q12h Caution: [B, ?] Contra: Closed-angle glaucoma Disp: 0.1% soln SE: HA, local irritation, blurred vision, photophobia, HTN Interactions: ↑ Effects w/ BBs, ophthalmic anhydrase inhibitors, osmotic drugs, sympathomimetics, ↑ risk of cardiac arrhythmias w/ digoxin, TCAs NIPE: Discard discolored solutions

Dipyridamole (Persantine) [Coronary Vasodilator/Platelet Aggregation Inhibitor] Uses: *Prevent postop thromboembolic disorders often in combo w/ ASA or warfarin (eg, CABG, vascular graft); w/ warfarin after artificial heart valve; chronic angina; w/ ASA to prevent coronary artery thrombosis; dipyridamole IV used in place of exercise stress test for CAD* **Action:** Anti-plt activity; coronary vasodilator **Dose:** *Adults.* 75–100 mg PO tid–qid; stress test 0.14 mg/kg/min (max 60 mg over 4 min). *Peds >12 y.* 3–6 mg/kg/d divided tid (safety/efficacy not established) **Caution:** [B, ?/–] Caution w/ other drugs that affect coagulation **Contra:** Component sensitivity **Disp:** Tabs 25, 50, 75 mg; inj 5 mg/mL **SE:** HA, ↓ BP, nausea, abdominal distress, flushing rash, dyspnea **Notes:** IV use can worsen angina **Interactions:** ↑ Effects w/ anticoagulants, heparin, evening primrose oil, feverfew, garlic, ginger, ginkgo biloba, ginseng, grapeseed extract; ↑ effects OF adenosine; ↑ bradycardia w/ BBs; ↓ effects w/ aminophylline **NIPE:** ⊘ EtOH or tobacco because of vasoconstriction effects; + effects may take several mo

Dipyridamole & Aspirin (Aggrenox) [Platelet Aggregation Inhibitor] Uses: *↓ Reinfarction after MI; prevent occlusion after CABG; ↓ risk of stroke* **Action:** ↓ Plt aggregation (both agents) **Dose:** 1 cap PO bid **Caution:** [C, ?] **Contra:** Ulcers, bleeding diathesis **Disp:** Dipyridamole (XR) 200 mg/aspirin 25 mg **SE:** ASA component: allergic Rxns, skin Rxns, ulcers/GI bleed, bronchospasm; dipyridamole component: dizziness, HA, rash **Interactions:** ↑ risk of GI bleed w/ ETOH, NSAIDs; ↑ effects OF acetazolamide, adenosine, anticoagulants, methotrexate, oral hypoglycemics; ↓ effects OF ACEIs, BB, cholinesterase inhibitors, diuretics **NIPE:** Swallow capsule whole

Dirithromycin (Dynabac) [antibiotic, macrolide] Uses: *Bronchitis, community-acquired pneumonia, & skin & skin structure Infxns* **Action:** Macrolide antibiotic. *Spectrum: M. catarrhalis, Streptococcus pneumoniae, Legionella, H. influenzae, S. pyogenes, S. aureus* **Dose:** 500 mg/d PO; w/ food; swallow whole **Caution:** [C, M] **Contra:** w/ pimozide **Disp:** Tabs 250 mg **SE:** Abdominal discomfort, HA, rash, ↑ K⁺ **NIPE:** Evaluate for macrolide sensitivity; take with food and swallow tablet whole

Disopyramide (Norpace, NAPamide) [Antiarrhythmic] Uses: *Suppression & prevention of VT* **Action:** Class 1A antiarrhythmic **Dose:** *Adults.* 400–800 mg/d ÷ q6h for regular & q12h for SR. *Peds.* <1 y: 10–30 mg/kg/24 h PO (÷ qid). *1–4 y:* 10–20 mg/kg/24 h PO (÷ qid). *4–12 y:* 10–15 mg/kg/24 h PO (÷ qid). *12–18 y:* 6–15 mg/kg/24 h PO (÷ qid); ↓ in renal/hepatic impair **Caution:** [C, +] **Contra:** AV block, cardiogenic shock **Disp:** Caps 100, 150 mg; SR caps 100, 150 mg **SE:** Anticholinergic SEs; negative inotrope, may induce CHF **Notes:** Check Drug Levels, (Table 2). **Interactions:** ↑ Effects w/ cimetidine, clarithromycin, erythromycin, quinidine; ↑ effects OF digoxin, hypoglycemics, insulin, warfarin; ↑ risk of arrhythmias w/ pimozide; ↓ effects w/ barbiturates, phenytoin, phenobarbital, rifampin **Labs:** ↑ LFTs, lipids, BUN, creatinine; ↓ serum glucose, Hmg, Hct **NIPE:** Risk of photosensitivity—use sunscreen, daily weights

Dobutamine (Dobutrex) [Vasopressor/Adrenergic Beta-1 Agonist] Uses: *Short-term use in cardiac decompensation secondary to depressed contractility* **Action:** Positive inotrope **Dose:** *Adults & Peds.* Cont IV inf of 2.5–15 mcg/kg/min; rarely, 40 mcg/kg/min may be required; titrate to response **Caution:** [C, ?] **Contra:** Sensitivity to sulfites, idiopathic hypertrophic subaortic stenosis **Disp:** Inj 250 mg/20 mL **SE:** Chest pain, HTN, dyspnea **Notes:** Monitor PWP & cardiac output if possible; check ECG for ↑ heart rate, ectopic activity; follow BP **Interactions:** ↑ Effects w/ furazolidone, methyldopa, MAOIs, TCAs; ↓ effects w/ BBs, NaHCO₃; ↓ effects OF guanethidine **Labs:** ↓ K; **NIPE:** Eval for adequate hydration; monitor I&O, cardiac output, ECG, BP during inf

Docetaxel (Taxotere) [Antineoplastic] Uses: *Breast (anthracycline-resistant), ovarian, lung, & prostate CAs,* **Action:** Antimitotic agent; promotes microtubular aggregation; semisynthetic taxoid **Dose:** 100 mg/m² over 1 h IV q3wk (Per protocols); start dexamethasone 8 mg bid prior & continue for 3–4 d; ↓ dose w/ ↑ bilirubin levels **Caution:** [D, –] **Contra:** Component sensitivity **Disp:** Inj 20, 40, 80 mg/mL **SE:** Myelosuppression, neuropathy, N/V, alopecia, fluid retention syndrome; cumulative doses of 300–400 mg/m² w/o steroid prep & posttreatment & 600–800 mg/m² w/ steroid prep; allergy possible, but rare w/ steroid prep **Interactions:** ↑ Effects w/ cyclosporine, ketoconazole, erythromycin, terfenidine **Labs:** ↑ AST, ALT, alkaline phosphatase **NIPE:** ↑ Fluids to 2–3 L/d, ↑ risk of hair loss, ↑ susceptibility to infection, urine may become reddish-brown

Docusate Calcium (Surfak)/Docusate Potassium (Dialose)/ Docusate Sodium (DOSS, Colace) [Emollient Laxative/Fecal Softener] Uses: *Constipation; adjunct to painful anorectal conditions (hemorrhoids)* **Action:** Stool softener **Dose:** *Adults.* 50–500 mg PO ÷ daily–qid. *Peds. Infants–3 y:* 10–40 mg/24 h ÷ daily–qid. *3–6 y:* 20–60 mg/24 h ÷ qd–qid. *6–12 y:* 40–120 mg/24 h ÷ daily–qid **Caution:** [C, ?] **Contra:** Concomitant use of mineral oil; intestinal obstruction, acute abdominal pain, N/V **Disp:** *Ca:* Caps 50, 240 mg. *K:* Caps 100, 240 mg. *Na:* Caps 50, 100 mg; syrup 50, 60 mg/15 mL; liq 150 mg/15 mL; soln 50 mg/mL **SE:** rare abdominal cramping, D; **Notes:** Take w/ full glass of H₂O; no laxative action ; do not use >1 wk **Interactions:** ↑ Absorption OF mineral oil **Labs:** ↓ K⁺ Cl **NIPE:** Short-term use, take w/ juices or milk to mask bitter taste

Dofetilide (Tikosyn) [Antiarrhythmic] WARNING: To minimize the risk of induced arrhythmia, pts initiated or reinitiated on Tikosyn should be placed for a minimum of 3 d in a facility that can provide calculations of CrCl, continuous ECG monitoring, & cardiac resuscitation **Uses:** *Maintain normal sinus rhythm in AF/A flutter after conversion* **Action:** Type III antiarrhythmic **Dose:** 125–500 mcg PO bid based on CrCl & QTc (see insert) **Caution:** [C, –] **Contra:** Baseline QTc is > 440 ms (500 ms w/ ventricular conduction abnormalities) or CrCl < 20 mL/min; concomitant use of verapamil, cimetidine, trimethoprim, or ketoconazole **Disp:** Caps 125, 250, 500 mcg **SE:** Ventricular arrhythmias, HA, CP, dizziness

Notes: Avoid w/ other drugs that prolong the QT interval; hold class I or III antiarrhythmics for at least 3 ½-lives prior to dofetilide; amiodarone level should be < 0.3 mg/L prior to dosing **Interactions:** ↑ Effects w/ amiloride, amiodarone, azole antifungals, cimetidine, diltiazem, macrolides, metformin, megestrol, nefazodone, norfloxacin, SSRIs, TCAs, triamterene, trimethoprim, verapamil, zafirlukast, quinine, grapefruit juice **NIPE:** Take w/o regard to food; monitor LFTs, BUN, creatinine

Dolasetron (Anzemet) [Antiemetic/Selective Serotonin 5-HT3 Receptor Antagonist]

Uses: *Prevent chemo-associated N/V* **Action:** 5-HT$_3$ receptor antagonist **Dose:** *Adults & Peds.* IV: 1.8 mg/kg IV as single dose 30 min prior to chemo *Adults.* PO: 100 mg PO as a single dose 1 h prior to chemo *Peds.* PO: 1.8 mg/kg PO to max 100 mg as single dose **Caution:** [B, ?] **Contra:** Component sensitivity **Disp:** Tabs 50, 100 mg; inj 20 mg/mL **SE:** Prolongs QT interval, HTN, HA, abdominal pain, urinary retention, transient ↑ LFTs **Interactions:** ↑ Effects w/ cimetidine; ↑ risk of arrhythmias w/ diuretics; ↓ effects w/ rifampin **Labs:** ↑ ALT, AST, alkaline phosphatase, PTT **NIPE:** Monitor LFTs, PTT, CBC, plts, & alkaline phosphatase w/ prolonged use

Dopamine (Intropin) [Vasopressor/Adrenergic]

Uses: *Short-term use in cardiac decompensation secondary to ↓ contractility; ↑ organ perfusion (at low dose)* **Action:** Positive inotropic agent w/ dose response: 2–10 mcg/kg/min β-effects (↑ CO & renal perfusion); 10–20 mcg/kg/min β-effects (peripheral vasoconstriction, pressor). >20 mcg/kg/min peripheral & renal vasoconstriction **Dose:** *Adults & Peds.* 5 mcg/kg/min by cont inf, ↑ increments of 5 mcg/kg/min to 50 mcg/kg/min max based on effect **Caution:** [C, ?] **Contra:** Pheochromocytom, VF, sulfite sensitivity **Disp:** Inj 40, 80, 160 mg/mL **SE:** Tachycardia, vasoconstriction, ↓ BP, HA, N/V, dyspnea **Notes:** Dosage >10 mcg/kg/min may ↓ renal perfusion; monitor urinary output; monitor ECG for ↑ in heart rate, BP, & ectopic activity; monitor PCWP & cardiac output if possible **Interactions:** ↑ Effects w/ α-blockers, diuretics, ergot alkaloids, MAOIs, BBs, anesthetics, phenytoin; ↓ effects w/ guanethidine **Labs:** False ↑ urine catecholamines, urine amino acids; false ↓ SCr **NIPE:** Maintain adequate hydration

Dornase Alfa (Pulmozyme) [Respiratory Inhalant/Enzyme]

Uses: *↓ Frequency of resp Infxns in CF* **Action:** Enzyme that selectively cleaves DNA **Dose:** Inhal 2.5 mg/d, BID dosing w/FVC > 85% w/ recommended nebulizer **Caution:** [B, ?] **Contra:** Allergy to Chinese hamster products **Disp:** Soln for inhal 1 mg/mL **SE:** Pharyngitis, voice alteration, CP, rash **Interactions:** None noted **NIPE:** ⊘ Mix or dilute w/ other meds

Dorzolamide (Trusopt) [Carbonic Anhydrase Inhibitor, Sulfonamide/Glaucoma Agent]

Uses: *Glaucoma* **Action:** Carbonic anhydrase inhibitor **Dose:** 1 gtt in eye(s) tid **Caution:** [C, ?] **Contra:** Component sensitivity **Disp:** 2% soln **SE:** Irritation, bitter taste, punctate keratitis, ocular allergic Rxn **Interactions:** ↑ Effects w/ oral carbonic anhydrase inhibitors, salicylates **NIPE:** ⊘ Wear soft contact lenses

Dorzolamide & Timolol (Cosopt) [Carbonic Anhydrase Inhibitor/Beta Adrenergic Blocker] Uses: *Glaucoma* Action: Carbonic anhydrase inhibitor w/ β-adrenergic blocker Dose: 1 gtt in eye(s) bid Caution: [C, ?] Contra: Component sensitivity Disp: Soln dorzolamide 2% & timolol 0.5% SE: Local irritation, bitter taste, superficial punctate keratitis, ocular allergic Rxn

Doxazosin (Cardura) [Antihypertensive/Alpha Blocker] Uses: *HTN & symptomatic BPH* Action: α$_1$-Adrenergic blocker; relaxes bladder neck smooth muscle Dose: *HTN:* Initial 1 mg/d PO, may be ↑ to 16 mg/d PO. *BPH:* Initial 1 mg/d PO, may be ↑ to 8 mg/d PO; XL 2–8 mg Q AM Caution: [B, ?] Contra: Component sensitivity Disp: Tabs 1, 2, 4, 8 mg; XL 4, 8 mg SE: Dizziness, HA, drowsiness, sexual dysfunction, doses >4 mg ↑ likelihood of postural ↓ BP Notes: First dose hs; syncope may occur w/in 90 mins of initial dose Interactions: ↑ effects w/ nitrates, antihypertensives, EtOH; ↓ effects w/ NSAIDs, butcher's broom; ↓ effects OF clonidine NIPE: May be taken w/ food

Doxepin (Sinequan, Adapin) [Antidepressant/TCA] WARNING: Closely monitor for worsening depression or emergence of suicidality Uses: *Depression, anxiety, chronic pain* Action: TCA; ↑ synaptic CNS conc of serotonin or norepinephrine Dose: 25–150 mg/d PO, usually hs but can be in ÷ doses; up to 300 mg/day for depression; ↓ in hepatic impair Caution: [C, ?/–] Contra: NA glaucoma Disp: Caps 10, 25, 50, 75, 100, 150 mg; PO conc 10 mg/mL SE: Anticholinergic SEs, ↓ BP, tachycardia, drowsiness, photosensitivity Interactions: ↑ Effects w/ fluoxetine, MAOIs, albuterol, CNS depressants, anticholinergics, cimetidine, oral contraceptives, propoxyphene, quinidine, EtOH, grapefruit juice; ↑ effects OF carbamazepine, anticoagulants, amphetamines, thyroid drugs, sympathomimetics; ↓ effects w/ ascorbic acid, cholestyramine, tobacco; ↓ effects OF bretylium, guanethidine, levodopa Labs: ↑ Serum bilirubin, alkaline phosphatase, glucose NIPE: Risk of photosensitivity—use sunscreen, urine may turn blue-green, may take 4–6 wk for full effect

Doxepin, Topical (Zonalon) [Antipruritic] Uses: *Short-term Rx pruritus (atopic dermatitis or lichen simplex chronicus)* Action: Antipruritic; H$_1$- & H$_2$-receptor antagonism Dose: Apply thin coating qid, 8 d max Caution: [C, ?/–] Contra: Component sensitivity Disp: 5% cream SE: ↓ BP, tachycardia, drowsiness, photosensitivity Notes: Limit application area to avoid systemic tox

Doxorubicin (Adriamycin, Rubex) [Antineoplastic/Antthracycline Antibiotic] Uses: *Acute leukemias; Hodgkin Dz & NHLs; soft tissue & osteosarcomas; Ewing sarcoma; Wilms tumor; neuroblastoma; bladder, breast, ovarian, gastric, thyroid, & lung CAs* Action: Intercalates DNA; ↓ DNA topoisomerases I & II Dose: 60–75 mg/m^2 q3wk; ↓ cardiotox w/ weekly (20 mg/m^2/wk) or cont inf (60–90 mg/m^2 over 96 h); (Per protocols) Caution: [D, ?] Contra: Severe CHF, cardiomyopathy, preexisting myelosuppression, previous Rx w/ complete cumulative doses of doxorubicin, idarubicin, daunorubicin Disp: Inj

10, 20, 50, 75, 200 mg **SE:** Myelosuppression, venous streaking & phlebitis, N/V/D, mucositis, radiation recall phenomenon, cardiomyopathy rare but dose-related; limit of 550 mg/m² cumulative dose (400 mg/m² w/ prior mediastinal irradiation) **Notes:** Dexrazoxane may limit cardiac tox; extravasation leads to tissue damage; discolors urine red/orange **Interactions:** ↑ Effects w/ streptozocin, verapamil, green tea; ↑ bone-marrow depression w/ antineoplastic drugs and radiation; ↓ effects w/ phenobarbital; ↓ effects OF digoxin, phenytoin, live virus vaccines **Labs:** ↑ Urine and plasma uric acid levels **NIPE:** ⊘ PRG, use contraception at least 4 mo after drug Rx

Doxycycline (Vibramycin) [Antibiotic/Tetracycline] Uses: *Broad-spectrum antibiotic activity, acne vulgaris, uncomplicated GC, chlamydia, PID, Lyme disease, skin infections, anthrax, malaria prophylaxis* **Action:** Tetracycline; bacteriostatic; interferes w/ protein synthesis. *Spectrum: Rickettsia* sp, *Chlamydia,* & *M. pneumoniae, B. Anthraxus* **Dose:** *Adults.* 100 mg PO q12h on 1st day, then 100 mg PO daily–bid or 100 mg IV q12h; acne QD dosing, Chlamydia 7d, Lyme disease 14-21 d, PID 14 d; *Peds >8y.* 5 mg/kg/24 h PO, to a max of 200 mg/d ÷ daily–bid **Disp:** Tabs 50, 75, 100, 150 mg; caps 50, 100 mg; syrup 50 mg/5 mL; susp 25 mg/5 mL; inj 100, 200 mg/vial **Caution:** [D, +] **Contra:** Children <8 y, severe hepatic dysfunction **SE:** D, GI disturbance, photosensitivity **Notes:** ↓ effect w/ antacids, tetracycline of choice in renal impair; for inhalational anthrax use w/ 1–2 additional antibiotics, not for CNS anthrax; **Interactions:** ↑ Effects OF digoxin, warfarin; ↓ effects w/ antacids, Fe, barbiturates, carbamazepine, phenytoins, food; ↓ effects OF penicillins **Labs:** False – urine glucose, false ↑ urine catecholamines; false ↓ urine urobilinogen **NIPE:** ↑ Risk of superinfection, ⊘ PRG, use barrier contraception

Dronabinol (Marinol) [C-II] [Antiemetic, Appetite Stimulant/Antivertigo] Uses: *N/V associated w/ CA chemo; appetite stimulation* **Action:** Antiemetic; ↓ vomiting center in the medulla **Dose:** *Adults & Peds.* Antiemetic: 5–15 mg/m²/dose q4–6h PRN. *Adults.* Appetite stimulant: 2.5 mg PO before lunch & dinner; max 20 mg/day **Caution:** [C, ?] **Contra:** Hx schizophrenia **Disp:** Caps 2.5, 5, 10 mg **SE:** Drowsiness, dizziness, anxiety, mood change, hallucinations, depersonalization, orthostatic ↓ BP, tachycardia **Notes:** Principal psychoactive substance present in marijuana **Interactions:** ↑ Effects w/ anticholinergics, CNS depressants, EtOH; ↓ effects OF theophylline **Labs:** ↓ FSH, LH, growth hormone, testosterone

Droperidol (Inapsine) [General Anesthetic] Uses: *N/V;* anesthetic premedication* **Action:** Tranquilizer, sedation, & antiemetic **Dose:** *Adults.* Nausea: initial max 2.5 mg IV/IM, may repeat 1.25 mg based on response; *Premed:* 2.5–10 mg IV, 30–60 min preop. *Peds.* Premed: 0.1–0.15 mg/kg/dose **Caution:** [C, ?] **Contra:** Component sensitivity **Disp:** Inj 2.5 mg/mL **SE:** Drowsiness, ↓ BP, occasional tachycardia & extrapyramidal Rxns, QT interval prolongation, arrhythmias **Notes:** Give IVP slowly over 2–5 min **Interactions:** ↑ Effects w/ CNS depressants, fentanyl, EtOH; ↑ hypotension w/ antihypertensives, nitrates

Drospirenone/Estradiol (Angelia) [Estrogen & Progestin Supl] Uses: Women w/uterus for moderate to severe vasomotor symp of menopause; symptoms of vulvar & vaginal atrophy d/t menopause Action: Estrogen & progestin supl Dose: 1 tab PO OD Caution: [X, –] Contra: Genital bleeding of unknown cause, breast CA, estrogen-dependent tumors, thromboembolic disorders, thrombophlebitis, recent MI, hepatic impair, adrenal insuff, renal insuff Disp: Tabs drospirenone 0.5 mg/estradiol 1 mg SE: HA, breast pain, irreg vaginal bleeding/spotting, abd cramps/bloating, N, V, hair loss, HTN, edema, yeast infection, fibroid enlargement Interactions: ↑ risk of hyperkalemia w/ ACEIs, ARBs, aldosterone antagonists, heparin, NSAIDs, spirolactone, K^+ sparing diuretics, K^+ supplements Labs: ↑ Uptake OF T_3, ↓ T_4 sex hormone-binding globulin levels; ↑ lipids; ↑ Prothrombin & factors VII, VIII, IX, X, plt aggregability NIPE: Antialdosterone activity ↑ risk of hyperkalemia in high-risk pts; in pts taking meds that ↑ K^+ monitor serum K^+ during first treatment cycle; not effected by food intake

Drospirenone/Ethinyl Estradiol (YAZ) [Estrogen & Progestin Supl] WARNING: Cigarette smoking & use of estrogen-based oral contraceptives have ↑ risk of serious cardiovascular side effects; risk ↑ w/age (esp.> 35 yrs) and smoking > 15 cig/d) Uses: Oral contraception; premenstrual dysphoric disorder Action: Suppresses ovulation by imitating the feedback inhibition of endogenous estrogen and progesterone on the pituitary and hypothalamus Dose: 1 tab PO OD x 28 d, repeat. Caution: [X,-], has antimineralocorticoid activity w/ potential hyperkalemia in renal insuff, adrenal insuff, hepatic insuff Contra: Pts w/ renal insuff, hepatic impair, adrenal insuff, DVT, PE, CVD, CAD, estrogen-dependent neoplasms, abnormal uterine bleeding, pregnancy, heavy smokers > 35 yr Disp: Drospirenone (3 mg)/ Ethinyl estradiol (20 mcg), 28-day pack has 24 active tabs & 4 inert tabs SE: Hyperkalemia, HTN, V, HA, breakthrough bleeding, amenorrhea, mastodynia, ↑ risk of gallbladder disease & thromboembolic disorders Interactions: ↑ Risk of hyperkalemia w/ ACEIs, ARBs, aldosterone antagonists, heparin, NSAIDs, spirolactone, K sparing diuretics, K^+ supplements, ↑ Effects OF cyclosporine, prednisolone, theophylline; ↓ effects w/ barbiturates, carbamazepine, griseofulvin, modafinil, phenobarbital, phenylbutazone, phenytoin, pioglitazone, rifabutin, rifampin, ritonavir, topiramate, St John's wort Labs: ↑ uptake OF T_3, ↓ T_4 sex hormone-binding globulin levels; triglycerides NIPE: Antimineralocorticoid activity comparable to spirolactone 25 mg; in pts taking meds that ↑ K^+ monitor serum K^+ during first treatment cycle; Sunday start regimen or postpartum use requires additional contraceptive methods during first cycle; use barrier contraception if taking anticonvulsants; may cause vision changes or ↓ contact lens tolerability; ⊘ protection against HIV or STDs; ⊘ smoke cigarettes

Drotrecogin Alfa (Xigris) [Antithrombotic] Uses:* Mortality in adults w/ severe sepsis (associated w/ acute organ dysfunction) at high risk of death (eg, as determined by APACHE II, WWW.NCEMI.ORG)* Action:

Recombinant human activated protein C; mechanism unknown **Dose:** 24 mcg/kg/h, total of 96 h **Caution:** [C, ?] **Contra:** Active bleeding, recent stroke or CNS surgery, head trauma, epidural catheter, CNS lesion w/ herniation risk **Disp:** 5-, 20-mg vials **SE:** Bleeding **Notes:** W/ single organ dysfunction & recent surgery may not be at high risk of death irrespective of APACHE II score & therefore not indicated. *Percutaneous procedures:* Stop inf 2 h before the procedure & resume 1 h after; major surgery: stop inf 2 h before surgery & resume 12 h after surgery in absence of bleeding **Interactions:** ↑ Risk of bleeding w/ plt inhibitors, anticoagulants **Labs:** ↑ PTT **NIPE:** DC drug 2 h before invasive procedures

Duloxetine (Cymbalta) [Antidepressant/SSNRI] WARNING:
Antidepressants may ↑ risk of suicidality; consider risks/benefits of use. Closely monitor for clinical worsening, suicidality, or behavior changes **Uses:** *Depression. DM peripheral neuropathic pain* **Action:** Selective serotonin & norepinephrine reuptake inhibitor (SSNRI) **Dose:** *Depression:* 40–60 mg/d PO ÷ bid *DM neuropathy:* 60 mg/d PO; **Caution:** [C, ?/–]; use in 3rd tri; avoid if CrCl < 30 mL/min; NA glaucoma; w/fluvoxamine, inhibitors of CYP2D6 (Table 13), TCAs, phenothiazines, type 1C antiarrhythmics **Contra:** MAOI use w/in 14 d, w/ thioridazine, NA glaucoma, hepatic insuff **Disp:** Caps delayed-release 20, 30, 60 mg **SE:** N, dizziness, somnolence, fatigue, sweating, xerostomia, constipation, decreased appetite, sexual dysfunction, urinary hesitancy, ↑ LFTs, HTN **Notes:** Swallow whole; monitor BP, avoid abrupt D/C **Interactions:** ↑ effects OF flecainide, propafenone, phenothiazines, TCAs; ↑ effects w/ cimetidine, fluvoxamine, quinolones ↑ risk OF hypertensive crisis w/ MAOIs within 14 days of taking duloxetine **NIPE:** ↑ Risk of liver damage w/ ETOH use; ⊘ d/c drug abruptly

Dutasteride (Avodart) [Androgen Hormone Inhibitor/BPH Agent]
Uses: *Symptomatic BPH* **Action:** 5α-Reductase inhibitor **Dose:** 0.5 mg PO daily **Caution:** [X, –] Hepatic impair; pregnant women should not handle pills **Contra:** Women & children **Disp:** Caps 0.5 mg **SE:** ↓ PSA levels, impotence, ↓ libido, gynecomastia **Notes:** Do not donate blood until 6 mo after D/C drug **Interactions:** ↑ Effects w/ cimetidine, ciprofloxacin, diltiazem, ketoconazole, ritonavir, verapamil **Labs:** ↓ PSA levels **NIPE:** ⊘ Handling by PRG women, take w/o regard to food

Echothiophate Iodine (Phospholine Ophthalmic) [Cholinesterase Inhibitor/Glaucoma Agent]
Uses: *Glaucoma* **Action:** Cholinesterase inhibitor **Dose:** 1 gtt eye(s) bid w/ one dose hs **Caution:** [C, ?] **Contra:** Active uveal inflammation or any inflammatory Dz of iris/ciliary body; glaucoma associated w/ iridocyclitis **Disp:** Powder to reconstitute 1.5 mg/0.03%; 3 mg/0.06%; 6.25 mg/0.125%; 12.5 mg/0.25% **SE:** Local irritation, myopia, blurred vision, ↓ BP, bradycardia **Interactions:** ↑ Effects w/ cholinesterase inhibitors, pilocarpine, succinylcholine, carbamate or organophosphate insecticides; ↑ effects OF cocaine; ↓ effects w/ anticholinergics, atropine, cyclopentolate, ophthalmic adrenocorticoids **NIPE:** ⊘ Drug 2 wk before surgery if succinylcholine to be administered, keep drug refrigerated, monitor for lens opacities

Econazole (Spectazole) [Topical Antifungal] Uses: *Tinea, cutaneous *Candida*, & tinea versicolor Infxns* **Action:** Topical antifungal **Dose:** Apply to areas bid (daily for tinea versicolor) for 2–4 wk **Caution:** [C, ?] **Contra:** Component sensitivity **Disp:** Topical cream 1% **SE:** Local irritation, pruritus, erythema **Notes:** Early symptom/clinical improvement; complete course of therapy to avoid recurrence **Interactions:** ↓ Effects w/ corticosteroids **NIPE:** Topical use only, ⊘ eye area

Edrophonium (Tensilon) [Cholinergic Muscle Stimulant/Anticholinesterase] Uses: *Diagnosis of MyG; acute MyG crisis; curare antagonist* **Action:** Anticholinesterase **Dose:** *Adults.* Test for MyG: 2 mg IV in 1 min; if tolerated, give 8 mg IV; (+) test is brief ↑ in strength. *Peds.* Test for MyG: Total dose 0.2 mg/kg; 0.04 mg/kg test dose; if no Rxn, give remainder in 1-mg increments to 10 mg max; ↓ in renal impair **Caution:** [C, ?] **Contra:** GI or GU obstruction; allergy to sulfite **Disp:** Inj 10 mg/mL **SE:** N/V/D, excessive salivation, stomach cramps, ↑ aminotransferases **Notes:** Can cause severe cholinergic effects; keep atropine available **Interactions:** ↑ Effects w/ tacrine; ↑ cardiac effects w/ digoxin; ↑ effects OF neostigmine, pyridostigmine, succinylcholine, jaborandi tree, pill-bearing spurge; ↓ effects w/ corticosteroids, procainamide, quinidine **Labs:** ↑ AST, ALT, serum amylase **NIPE:** ↑ Risk uterine irritability & premature labor in PRG pts near term

Efalizumab (Raptiva) [Antipsoriatic/Immunosuppressant] **WARNING:** Associated w/serious Infxns, malignancy, thrombocytopenia Uses: *Chronic moderate–severe plaque psoriasis* **Action:** MoAb **Dose:** *Adults.* 0.7 mg/kg SQ conditioning dose, followed by 1 mg/kg/wk; single doses should not exceed 200 mg **Caution:** [C, +/−] **Contra:** Admin of most vaccines **Disp:** 125-mg vial **SE:** First-dose Rxn, HA, worsening psoriasis, ↑ LFT, immunosuppressive-related Rxns (see warning) **Notes:** Minimize 1st-dose Rxn by administering conditioning dose; monitor plts monthly, then every 3 mo & dose ↑; pts may be trained in self-admin **Interactions:** ↑ Risk of infection & malignancy w/ immunosuppressive agents; ↓ immune response w/ live virus vaccines **Labs:** ↑ Lymphocytes **NIPE:** Reconstituted soln may be stored for 8 h; monitor for bleeding gums & bruising

Efavirenz (Sustiva) [Antiretroviral/NNRTI] Uses: *HIV Infxns* **Action:** Antiretroviral; nonnucleoside RTI **Dose:** *Adults.* 600 mg/d PO q hs. *Peds.* See insert; avoid high-fat meals **Caution:** [D, ?] CDC recommends HIV-infected mothers not breast-feed due to risk of HIV transmission **Contra:** Component sensitivity **Disp:** Caps 50, 100, 200 mg **SE:** Somnolence, vivid dreams, dizziness, rash, N/V/D **Notes:** Monitor LFT, cholesterol **Interactions:** ↑ Effects w/ ritonavir; ↑ effects OF CNS depressants, ergot derivatives, midazolam, ritonavir, simvastatin, triazolam, warfarin; ↓ effects w/ carbamazepine, phenobarbital, rifabutin, rifampin, saquinavir, St. John's wort; ↓ effects OF amprenavir, carbamazepine, clarithromycin, indinavir, phenobarbital, saquinavir, warfarin; may alter effectiveness of oral contraceptive **Labs:** ↑ AST, ALT, amylase, total cholesterol, triglycerides;

false + urine cannabinoid test **NIPE:** ⊘ High-fat foods, take w/o regard to food, use barrier contraception

Efavirenz, emtricitabine, tenofovir (Atripla) [Antiretroviral]

WARNING: Lactic acidosis and severe hepatomegaly with steatosis, including fatal cases, have been reported with the use of nucleoside analogs alone or in combination with other antiretrovirals **Uses:** *HIV Infxns* **Action:** Triple fixed-dose combination antiretroviral **Dose:** *Adults.* 1 tab QD on empty stomach; HS dose may ↓ CNS effects **Caution:** [D, ?] CDC recommends HIV-infected mothers not breast-feed (risk of HIV transmission) **Contra:** w/ astemizole, cisapride, midazolam, triazolam or ergot derivatives (competition for CYP3A4 by efavirenz could result in serious and/or life-threatening; <18 yrs, component sensitivity **Disp:** Tab containing efavirenz 600 mg/emtricitabine 200 mg/tenofovir/300 mg **SE:** Somnolence, vivid dreams, HA, dizziness, rash, N/V/D **Interactions:** ↑ Effects of ritonavir, tenofovir, ethinyl estradiol levels ↓ w/ phenobarbital, rifampin, rifabutin, saquinavir, ↓ effects of indinavir, amprenavir, clarithromycin, methadone, rifabutin, sertraine, statins, saquinavir; monitor warfarin levels **Labs:** Monitor LFT, cholesterol **NIPE:** ⊘ ETOH; ⊘ PRG & breast-feeding; register pregnant patients exposed to this drug (800) 258-4263; see individual agents for additional info

Eletriptan (Relpax) [Analgesic/Antimigraine Agent] Uses:

Acute Rx of migraine **Action:** Selective serotonin receptor (5-HT$_1$B/D) agonist **Dose:** 20–40 mg PO, may repeat in 2 h; 80 mg/24h max **Caution:** [C, +] **Contra:** Hx ischemic heart Dz, coronary artery spasm, stroke or TIA, peripheral vascular Dz, IBD, uncontrolled HTN, hemiplegic or basilar migraine, severe hepatic impair, w/in 24 h of another 5-HT$_1$ agonist or ergot, w/in 72 h of CYP3A4 inhibitors **Disp:** Tabs 20, 40 mg **SE:** Dizziness, somnolence, N, asthenia, xerostomia, paresthesias; pain, pressure, or tightness in chest, jaw or neck; serious cardiac events **Interactions:** ↑ Risk of serotonin syndrome w/ SSRIs; ↑ risk of prolonged vasospasms w/ ergot-containing medications **abs:** None known **NIPE:** Not for migraine prevention; ⊘ ETOH; ⊘ use for more than 3 migraine attacks/month

Emedastine (Emadine) [Antihistamine] Uses: *Allergic conjunctivitis*

Action: Antihistamine; selective H$_1$-antagonist **Dose:** 1 gtt in eye(s) up to qid **Caution:** [B, ?] **Contra:** Allergy to ingredients (preservatives benzalkonium, tromethamine) **Disp:** 0.05% soln **SE:** HA, blurred vision, burning/stinging, corneal infiltrates/staining, dry eyes, foreign body sensation, hyperemia, keratitis, tearing, pruritus, rhinitis, sinusitis, asthenia, bad taste, dermatitis, discomfort **Notes:** Do not use contact lenses if eyes are red **NIPE:** ⊘ Wear soft contact lens for 15 min after use

Emtricitabine (Emtriva) [Antiretroviral/NRTI] WARNING: Class

warning for lipodystrophy, lactic acidosis, & severe hepatomegaly **Uses:** HIV-1 Infxn **Action:** Nucleoside RT inhibitor (NRTI) **Dose:** 200 mg PO daily or 240 mg sol po daily; ↓ dose for renal impair **Caution:** [B, –] risk of liver dz **Contra:** Component sensitivity **Disp:** Solution: 10 mg/mL, 200 mg caps **SE:** HA, D, nausea, rash, rare hyperpigmentation of feet & hands, Posttreatment exacerbation of hepatitis **Notes:** First NRTI with once-daily dosing; caps/sol not equivalent; not rec as monotherapy; screen for HepB. **Interactions:** None noted w/ additional NRTIs **NIPE:** Take w/o regard to food, causes redistribution and accumulation of body fat; take w/ other antiretrovirals; not a cure for HIV or prevention of opportunistic infections

Enalapril (Vasotec) [Antihypertensive/ACEI] Uses: *HTN, CHF, LVD,* DN Action: ACE inhibitor Dose: *Adults.* 2.5–40 mg/d PO; 1.25 mg IV q6h. **Peds.** 0.05–0.08 mg/kg/dose PO q12–24h; ↓ in renal impair **Caution** [C (1st tri; D 2nd & 3rd tri), +] Use with NSAIDs, K⁺ suppls **Contra:** Bilateral renal artery stenosis, angioedema **Disp:** Tabs 2.5, 5, 10, 20 mg; IV 1.25 mg/mL (1, 2 mL) **SE:** Symptomatic ↓ BP with initial dose (especially with concomitant diuretics), ↑ K⁺, nonproductive cough, angioedema **Notes:** Monitor Cr; D/C diuretic for 2–3 d prior to initiation **Interactions:** ↑ Effects w/ loop diuretics; ↑ risk of cough w/ capsaicin; ↑ effects OF α-blockers, insulin, Li; ↑ risk of hyperkalemia w/ K suppl, K-sparing diuretics, salt substitutes, trimethoprim; ↓ effects w/ ASA, NSAIDs, rifampin **Labs:** May cause ↑ serum K⁺, direct Coombs' test, false + urine acetone **NIPE:** Several weeks needed for full hypotensive effect

Enfuvirtide (Fuzeon) [Antiretroviral/Fusion Inhibitor] WARNING: Rarely causes allergy; never rechallenge Uses: *W/ antiretroviral agents for HIV-1 Infxn in treatment-experienced pts with evidence of viral replication despite ongoing antiretroviral therapy* Action: Fusion inhibitor Dose: 90 mg (1 mL) SQ bid in upper arm, anterior thigh, or abdomen; rotate site Caution: [B, –] Contra: Previous allergy to drug Disp: 90 mg/mL on reconstitution; dispensed as pt convenience kit with monthly supplies SE: Inj site reactions (in nearly all pts); pneumonia, D, nausea, fatigue, insomnia, peripheral neuropathy Notes: Rotate inj site; available only via restricted drug distribution system; immediately administer on reconstitution or refrigerate for up to 24 h max. Interactions: None noted w/ other antiretrovirals NIPE: Does not cure HIV; does not ↓ risk of transmission or prevent opportunistic infections; take w/o regard to food

Enoxaparin (Lovenox) [Anticoagulant/Low Molecular Wt Heparin Derivative] WARNING: Recent or anticipated epidural/spinal anesthesia ↑ risk of spinal/epidural hematoma w/subsequent paralysis Uses: *Prevention & Rx of DVT; Rx PE; unstable angina & non-Q-wave MI* Action: LMW heparin Dose: *Adults.* Prevention: 30 mg SQ bid or 40 mg SQ q24h. *DVT/PE Rx:* 1 mg/kg SQ q12h or 1.5 mg/kg SQ q24h. *Angina:* 1 mg/kg SQ q12h. **Peds.** Prevention: 0.5 mg/kg SQ q12h. *DVT/PE Rx:* 1 mg/kg SQ q12h; ↓ dose w CrCl <30 mL/min **Caution** [B, ?] Not for prophylaxis in prosthetic heart valves **Contra:** Active bleeding, HIT Ab(+) **Disp:** Inj 10 mg/0.1 mL (30-, 40-, 60-, 80-, 100-, 120-, & 150-mg syringes) **SE:** Bleeding, hemorrhage, bruising, thrombocytopenia, pain/hematoma at site, ↑ AST/ALT **Notes:** No effect on bleeding time, plt Fxn, PT, or aPTT; monitor plt (HIT), clinical bleeding; may monitor anti-factor Xa

Interactions: ↑ Bleeding effects w/ ASA, anticoagulants, cephalosporins, NSAIDs, penicillin, chamomile, garlic, ginger, ginkgo biloba, feverfew, horse chestnut **Labs:** ↑ AST, ALT **NIPE:** No need to monitor aPTT, admin deep SQ ⊘ IM

Entacapone (Comtan) [Antiparkinsonian Agent/COMT Inhibitor] **Uses:** *Parkinson Dz* **Action:** Selective & reversible carboxymethyl transferase inhibitor **Dose:** 200 mg with each levodopa/carbidopa dose; max 1600 mg/d; ↓ levodopa/carbidopa dose by 25% if levodopa dose >800 mg **Caution:** [C, ?] Hepatic impair **Contra:** use w/ MAOI **Disp:** Tabs 200 mg **SE:** Dyskinesia, hyperkinesia, nausea, dizziness, hallucinations, orthostatic ↓ BP, brown-orange urine, D; **Interactions:** ↑ Effects w/ ampicillin, chloramphenicol, cholestyramine, erythromycin, MAOIs, probenecid, rifampin; ↑ risk of arrhythmias & HTN w/ bitolterol, dopamine, dobutamine, epinephrine, isoetharine, methyldopa, norepinephrine **Labs:** Monitor LFTs **NIPE:** ⊘ DC abruptly, breast-feed

Ephedrine [Vasopressor/Decongestant/Bronchodilator] **Uses:** *Acute bronchospasm, bronchial asthma, nasal congestion,* ↓ BP, narcolepsy, enuresis, & MyG **Action:** Sympathomimetic; stimulates α- & β-receptors; bronchodilator **Dose:** *Adults. Congestion:* 25–50 mg PO q6h; ↓ BP: 25–50 mg IV q 5–10 min to a max of 150 mg/d *Peds.* 0.2–0.3 mg/kg/dose IV q4–6h PRN **Caution:** [C, ?/–] **Contra:** Cardiac arrhythmias; angle-closure glaucoma **Disp:** Nasal solution 0.48%, 0.5%, oral capsule: 25, 37.5, 50 mg; Inj 50 mg/mL; nasal spray 0.25% **SE:** CNS stimulation (nervousness, anxiety, trembling), tachycardia, arrhythmia, HTN, xerostomia, painful urination **Notes:** Protect from light; monitor BP, HR, urinary output; can cause false (+) amphetamine EMIT; take last dose 4–6h before hs; abuse potential, OTC sales banned/restricted in most states. **Interactions:** ↑ Effects w/ acetazolamide, antacids, MAOIs, TCAs, urinary alkalinizers; ↑ effects OF sympathomimetics; ↓ response w/ diuretics, methyldopa, reserpine, urinary acidifiers; ↓ effects OF antihypertensives, BBs, dexamethasone, guanethidine **Labs:** False ↑ urine amino acids **NIPE:** ⊘ EtOH, store away from light/heat

Epinephrine (Adrenalin, Sus-Phrine, EpiPen, EpiPen Jr, others) [Vasopressor/Bronchodilator/Cardiac Stimulant, Local Anesthetic] **Uses:** *Cardiac arrest, anaphylaxis Rxn, bronchospasm, openangle glaucoma* **Action:** β-adrenergic agonist, some α-effects **Dose:** *Adults.* ACLS: 0.5–1 mg (5–10 mL of 1:10,000) IV q 5 min to response. *Anaphylaxis:* 0.3–0.5 mL SQ of 1:1000 dilution, may repeat q5–15min to a max of 1 mg/dose & 5 mg/d. *Asthma:* 0.1–0.5 mL SQ of 1:1000 dilution, repeated at 20-min to 4-h intervals or 1 inhal (met-dose) repeat in 1–2 min or susp 0.1–0.3 mL SQ for extended effect. *Peds.* ACLS: 1st dose 0.1 mL/kg IV of 1:10,000 dilution, then 0.1 mL/kg IV of 1:1000 dilution q3–5min to response. *Anaphylaxis:* 0.15—0.3 mg IM depending on weight < 30 kg 0.01 mg/kg . *Asthma:* 0.01 mL/kg SQ of 1:1000 dilution q8–12h. **Caution:** [C, ?] ↓ bronchodilation with β-blockers **Contra:** Cardiac arrhythmias, angle-closure glaucoma **Disp:** Inj 1:1000, 1:2000, 1:10,000, 1:100,000; susp for inj 1:200; aerosol 220 mcg/spray; 1% inhal soln ; EpiPen Autoinjector one dose 0.30

mg; EpiPen Jr 0.15 mg **SE:** CV (tachycardia, HTN, vasoconstriction), CNS stimulation (nervousness, anxiety, trembling), ↓ renal blood flow **Notes:** Can give via ET tube if no central line (use 2–2.5 × IV dose); EpiPen for pt self-use (www.EpiPen.com) **Interactions:** ↑ HTN effects w/ α-blockers, BBs, ergot alkaloids, furazolidone, MAOIs; ↑ cardiac effects w/ antihistamines, cardiac glycosides, levodopa, thyroid hormones, TCAs; ↑ effects OF sympathomimetics; ↓ effects OF diuretics, guanethidine, hypoglycemics, methyldopa **Labs:** ↑ Serum bilirubin, glucose, & uric acid, urine catecholamines **NIPE:** ⊘ OTC inhalation drugs

Epinastine (Elestat) [Antihistamine]
Uses: Itching w/ allergic conjunctivitis **Action:** Antihistamine **Dose: 1 gtt bid** **Caution:** [C, ?/–] **Disp:** Soln 0.05% **SE:** Burning, folliculosis, hyperemia, pruritus, URI, HA, rhinitis, sinusitis, cough, pharyngitis **NIPE:** Remove contacts before, reinsert in 10 min if eye not red; caution in pregnancy & lactation

Epirubicin (Ellence) [Antineoplastic/Anthracycline]
Uses: *Adjuvant therapy with evidence of axillary nodal involvement following resection of primary breast CA* **Actions:** Anthracycline cytotoxic agent **Dose:** Per protocols; ↓ dose with hepatic impair. **Caution:** [D, –] **Contra:** Baseline neutrophil count < 1500 cells/mm³, severe myocardial insuff, recent MI, severe arrhythmias, severe hepatic dysfunction, previous Rx with anthracyclines up to max cumulative dose **Disp :** Inj 50 mg/25 mL, 200 mg/100 mL **SE:** Mucositis, N/V/D, alopecia, myelosuppression, cardiotox, secondary AML, tissue necrosis w/ extravasation **Interactions:** ↑ Effects w/ cimetidine; ↑ effects OF cytotoxic drugs, radiation therapy; ↑ risk of HF w/ CCBs, trastuzumab; incompatible chemically w/ fluorouracil, heparin **Labs:** Monitor before & after treatment AST, total bilirubin, creatinine, CBC, LVEF **NIPE:** ⊘ Handle if PRG breast-feeding; urine reddish up to 2 d after treatment, use contraception during treatment, burning at inj site indicates infiltration, menstruation may cease permanently

Eplerenone (Inspra) [Antihypertensive/Selective Aldosterone Receptor Antagonist]
Uses: *HTN* **Action:** Selective aldosterone antagonist **Dose: Adults:** 50 mg PO daily–bid, doses >100 mg/d no benefit w/ ↑ K⁺; ↓ to 25 mg PO daily if giving w/ CYP3A4 inhibitors **Caution:** [B, +/–] Use of CYP3A4 inhibitors (Table 13); monitor K⁺ with ACE inhibitor, ARBs, NSAIDs, K⁺-sparing diuretics; grapefruit juice, St. John's wort **Contra:** K⁺ >5.5 mEq/L; NIDDM w/ microalbuminuria; SCr >2 mg/dL (males), >1.8 mg/dL (females); CrCl <50 mL/min; concurrent K⁺ suppls/K⁺-sparing diuretics **Disp:** Tabs 25, 50, 100 mg **SE:** Hypertriglyceridemia, ↑ K⁺, HA, dizziness, gynecomastia, hypercholesterolemia, orthostatic ↓ BP **Notes:** May take 4 wk to see full effect **Interactions:** ↑ Risk hyperkalemia w/ ACEis; ↑ risk of toxic effects w/ azole antifungals, erythromycin, saquinavir, verapamil, ↑ effects OF Li; ↓ effects w/ NSAIDs **NIPE:** ⊘ High-K foods, may cause reversible breast pain or enlargement w/ use

Epoetin Alfa [Erythropoietin, EPO] (Epogen, Procrit) [Recombinant Human Erythropoietin]
Uses: * CRF associated anemia*

zidovudine Rx in HIV-infected pts, CA chemo; ↓ transfusions associated with surgery **Action:** Induces erythropoiesis **Dose:** *Adults & Peds.* 50–150 units/kg IV/SQ 3×/wk; adjust dose q4–6wk PRN. *Surgery:* 300 units/kg/d × 10 d prior to surgery to 4 d after; ↓ dose if Hct approaches 36% or Hgb, ↑ >4 points in 2-wk period **Caution:** [C, +] **Contra:** Uncontrolled HTN **Disp:** Inj 2000, 3000, 4000, 10,000, 20,000, 40,000 units/mL **SE:** HTN, HA, fatigue, fever, tachycardia, N/V **Notes:** Store in refrigerator; monitor baseline & posttreatment Hct/Hgb, BP, ferritin **Interactions:** None noted **Labs:** ↑ WBCs, plts **NIPE:** Monitor for access line clotting, ⊘ shake vial

Epoprostenol (Flolan) [Antihypertensive]
Uses: *Pulmonary HTN* **Action:** Dilates pulmonary/systemic arterial vascular beds; ↓ plt aggregation **Dose:** Initial 2 ng/kg/min; ↑ by 2 ng/kg/min q15min until dose-limiting SE (CP, dizziness, N/V, HA, ↓ BP, flushing); IV cont inf 4 ng/kg/min < maximum-tolerated rate; adjust based on response; see package insert guidelines **Caution:** [B, ?] ↑ tox w/diuretics, vasodilators, acetate in dialysis fluids, anticoagulants **Contra:** Chronic use in CHF 2nd-deg severe LVSD **Disp:** Inj 0.5, 1.5 mg **SE:** Flushing, tachycardia, CHF, fever, chills, nervousness, HA, N/V/D, jaw pain, flu-like Sxs **Notes:** Abrupt D/C can cause rebound pulmonary HTN; monitor bleeding if using other antiplatelet/anticoagulants; watch ↓ BP effects with other vasodilators/diuretics **Interactions:** ↑ Risk of bleeding w/anticoagulants, antiplts; ↑ effects OF digoxin; ↓ BP w/ antihypertensives, diuretics, vasodilators **NIPE:** ⊘ Mix or administer w/ other drugs

Eprosartan (Teveten) [Antihypertensive/ARB]
Uses: *HTN,* DN, CHF **Action:** ARB **Dose:** 400–800 mg/d single dose or bid **Caution:** [C (1st tri); D (2nd & 3rd tri), –] Lithium; ↑ K+ with K+-sparing diuretics/suppls/high-dose trimethoprim **Contra:** Bilateral renal artery stenosis, 1st-deg aldosteronism **Disp:** Tabs 400, 600 mg **SE:** Fatigue, depression, hypertriglyceridemia, URI, UTI, abdominal pain, rhinitis/pharyngitis/cough **Interactions:** ↑ Risk of hyperkalemia w/ K-sparing diuretics, K suppls, trimethoprim; ↑ effects OF Li **Labs:** ↑ ALT, AST, alkaline phosphatase, BUN, creatinine; ↓ Hmg **NIPE:** Monitor LFTs, CBC & differential, renal Fxn; ⊘ PRG, breast-feeding

Eptifibatide (Integrilin) [Antiplatelet Agent]
Uses: *ACS, PCI* **Action:** Glycoprotein IIb/IIIa inhibitor **Dose:** 180 mcg/kg IV bolus, then 2 mcg/kg/min cont inf; ↓ in renal impair (SCr >2 mg/dL, <4 mg/dL: 135 mcg/kg bolus & 0.5 mcg/kg/min inf) **Caution:** [B, ?] Monitor bleeding with other anticoagulants **Contra:** Other GPIIb/IIIa inhibitors, Hx abnormal bleeding, hemorrhagic stroke (within 30 d), severe HTN, major surgery (within 6 wk), plt count <100,000 cells/mm³, renal dialysis **Disp:** Inj 0.75, 2 mg/mL **SE:** Bleeding, ↓ BP, inj site Rxn, thrombocytopenia **Notes:** Monitor bleeding, coags, plts, SCr, activated coagulation time (ACT) with prothrombin consumption index (maintain ACT between 200–300 s) **Interactions:** ↑ Bleeding w/ ASA, cephalosporins, clopidogrel, heparin, NSAIDs, thrombolytics, ticlopidine, warfarin, evening primrose oil, feverfew, garlic, ginger, ginkgo biloba, ginseng, grapeseed extract

associated with menopause*; female hypogonadism **Ac-**
se: *Menopause:* 0.3–1.25 mg/d, cyclically 3 wk on, 1 wk
–7.5 mg/d PO × 20 d, off × 10 d **Caution:** [X, –] **Contra:**
own cause, breast CA, estrogen-dependent tumors, throm-
rombophlebitis, recent MI, PRG, severe hepatic Dz **Disp**
5 mg **SE:** Nausea, HA, bloating, breast enlargement/ten
thromboembolism, hypertriglyceridemia, gallbladder Dz
for shortest time; (see Women's Health Initiatives (WHI
eractions: ↑ Effects OF corticosteroids, cyclosporine
feine, tobacco; ↓ effects w/ barbiturates, phenytoin, ri
nticoagulants, hypoglycemics, insulin, tamoxifen **Labs**
VII, VIII, IX, X, plt aggregability, thyroid-binding globu
tithrombin III, folate **NIPE:** ⊘ PRG, breast-feeding

s + Methyltestosterone (Estratest, Estrat
& Androgen Supl] Uses: *Vasomotor Sxs*; post
nt **Action:** Estrogen & androgen supl **Dose:** 1 tab/d ×
X, –] **Contra:** Genital bleeding of unknown cause, breas
umors, thromboembolic disorders, thrombophlebitis, re
s (estrogen/methyltestosterone) 0.625 mg/1.25 mg (hs
ea, HA, bloating, breast enlargement/tenderness, edema
rromboembolism, gallbladder Dz **Notes:** Use lowest dos
en's Health Initiatives (WHI) data www.whi.org) **Addi**
ects OF insulin; ↓ effects OF oral anticoagulants

[Estrogen Supl] Uses: *Atrophic vaginitis, vasc
nenopause, osteoporosis* **Action:** Estrogen supl **Dose**
to control Sxs. *Vaginal cream:* 2–4 g/d × 2 wk, then 1
Contra: Genital bleeding of unknown cause, breast CA
s, thromboembolic disorders, thrombophlebitis; **Disp**
Tabs 0.5, 1, 2 mg; vaginal cream 0.1 mg/g **SE:** Nause
rgement/tenderness, edema, ↑ triglycerides, venou
dder Dz **Interactions:** ↑ Effects w/grapefruit juic
s, cyclosporine, TCAs, theophylline, caffeine, tobacco
rbamazepine, phenytoin, primidone, rifampin; ↓ effec
ics, insulin, tamoxifen, warfarin **Labs:** ↑ Prothromb
plt aggregability, thyroid-binding globulin, T₄, trigly
blate **NIPE:** ⊘ PRG, breast-feeding

e & Medroxyprogesterone Aceta
Progestin Supl] **WARNING:** Cigarette sm
e effects from contraceptives containing estrogen. T
vy smoking (> 15 cigarettes/d) & is quite marked
use Lunelle should be strongly advised not to sm
on: Estrogen & progestin **Dose:** 0.5 mL IM (delt

Erlotinib (Tarceva) [Antineoplastic] Uses: *NSCLC after failure of 1 chemo agent* **Action:** HER1/EGFR tyrosine kinase inhibitor **Dose:** 150 mg/d PO 1 h ac or 2 h pc; ↓ (in 50-mg decrements) w/severe Rxn or w/ CYP3A4 inhibitors (Table 13); Per protocols **Caution:** [D, ?/–]; use w/ CYP3A4 (Table 13) inhibitors **Disp:** Tabs 25, 100, 150 mg **SE:** Rash, N/V/D, anorexia, abdominal pain, fatigue, cough, dyspnea, stomatitis, conjunctivitis, pruritus, dry skin, Infxn, ↑ LFT, interstitial lung disease **Notes:** May ↑ INR w/warfarin, monitor INR **Interactions:** ↑ drug plasma levels w/ CYP3A4 inhibitors (clarithromycin, ritonavir, ketoconazole); ↓ drug plasma levels w/ CYP3A4 inducers (carbamazepine, rifampicin, phenytoin, phenobarbital, St John's wort); ↑ risk of bleeding w/ anticoagulants, NSAIDs **Labs:** Monitor LFTs, PT, INR **NIPE:** ⊘ Pregnancy or lactation; use adequate contraception; ↑ drug metabolism in smokers

Ertapenem (Invanz) [Anti-infective/Carbapenem] Uses: *Complicated intraabdominal, acute pelvic, & skin Infxns, pyelonephritis, community-acquired pneumonia* **Action:** A carbapenem; β-lactam antibiotic, ↓ cell wall synthesis. *Spectrum:* Good gram(+/–) & anaerobic coverage, but not *Pseudomonas,* PCN-resistant pneumococci, MRSA, *Enterococcus,* β-lactamase(+) *H. influenza, Mycoplasma, Chlamydia* **Dose:** *Adults.* 1 g IM/IV qd; 500 mg/d in CrCl <30 mL/min **Caution:** [C, ?/–] Probenecid ↓ renal clearance **Contra:** <18 y, PCN allergy **Disp:** Inj 1 g/vial **SE:** HA, N/V/D, inj site Rxns, thrombocytosis, ↑ LFTs **Notes:** Can give IM × 7 d, IV × 14 d; 137 mg Na⁺(6 mEg)/g ertapenem **Interactions:** ↑ Effects w/ probenecid; **Labs:** ↑ AST, ALT, serum alkaline phosphatase, bilirubin, glucose, creatinine, PT, RBCs, urine WBCs **NIPE:** Monitor for superinfection

Erythromycin (E-Mycin, E.E.S., Ery-Tab, EryPed, Ilotycin) [Antibiotic/Macrolide] Uses: *Bacterial Infxns; bowel prep;* GI motility; *acne vulgaris* **Action:** Bacteriostatic; interferes with protein synthesis. *Spectrum:* Group A streptococci (*S. pyogenes*), *S. pneumoniae, N. meningitides, N. gonorrhea* (in PCN-allergic pts), *Legionella, M. pneumoniae* **Dose:** *Adults.* Base 250–500 mg PO q6–12h or ethylsuccinate 400–800 mg q6–12h; 500 mg–1 g IV q6h. *Prokinetic:* 250 mg PO tid 30 mins ac. *Peds.* 30–50 mg/kg/d PO ÷ q6–8h or 20–40 mg/kg/d IV ÷ q6h, max 2 g/d ↑ tox of carbamazepine, cyclosporine, digoxin, methylprednisolone, theophylline, felodipine, warfarin, simvastatin/lovastatin; ↓ sildenafil dose w/ use **Caution:** [B, +] ↑ tox of carbamazepine, cyclosporine, digoxin, methylprednisolone, theophylline, felodipine, warfarin, simvastatin/lovastatin; ↓ sildenafil dose w/ use **Contra:** Hepatic impair, preexisting liver Dz (estolate), use with pimozide **Disp:** *lactobionate (Ilotycin):* Powder for inj 500 mg, 1 g. *Base:* Tabs 250, 333, 500 mg; caps 250 mg. *Estolate (Ilosone):* Susp 125, 250 mg/5 mL. *Stearate (Erythrocin):* Tabs 250, 500 mg. *Ethylsuccinate (EES, EryPed):* Chew tabs 200 mg; tabs 400 mg; susp 200, 400 mg/5 mL **SE:** HA, abdominal pain, N/V/D; [QT prolongation, torsades de pointes, ventricular arrhythmias/tachycardias (rarely)]; cholestatic jaundice (estolate) **Notes:** 400 mg ethylsuccinate = 250 mg base/estolate; w/ food to minimize GI upset; lactobionate salt contains benzyl alcohol (caution in neonates) **Interactions:** ↑ Effects w/

amprenavir, indinavir, ritonavir, saquinavir, grapefruit juice; ↑ effects OF alprazolam, benzodiazepines, buspirone, carbamazepine, clozapine, colchicines, cyclosporine, digoxin, felodipine, lovastatin, midazolam, quinidine, sildenafil, simvastatin, tacrolimus, theophylline, triazolam, valproic acid; ↑ QT w/ astemizole, cisapride; ↓ effects OF penicillin, zafirlukast **Labs:** False ↑ AST, ALT, serum bilirubin, urine amino acids, false ↓ folate assay **NIPE:** Take w/ food if GI upset, monitor for superinfection & ototoxicity

Erythromycin & Benzoyl Peroxide (Benzamycin) [Anti-infective, Macrolide/Keratolytic] Uses: Topical Rx of *acne vulgaris* Action: Macrolide antibiotic with keratolytic **Dose:** Apply bid (AM & PM) **Caution:** [C, ?] **Contra:** Component sensitivity **Disp:** Gel erythromycin 30 mg/benzoyl peroxide 50 mg/g **SE:** Local irritation, dryness

Erythromycin & Sulfisoxazole (Eryzole, Pediazole) [Anti-infective, Macrolide/Sulfonamide] Uses: *Upper & lower resp tract; bacterial Infxns; otitis media in children due to *H. influenzae*; Infxns in PCN-allergic pts **Action:** Macrolide antibiotic w sulfonamide **Dose:** Based on erythromycin content. *Adults.* 400 mg erythromycin/1200 mg sulfisoxazole PO q6h. *Peds >2 mo.* 40–50 mg/kg/d erythromycin & 150 mg/kg/d sulfisoxazole PO ÷ q6h; max 2 g/d erythromycin or 6 g/d sulfisoxazole × 10 d; ↓ in renal impair **Caution:** [C (D if given near term), +] PO anticoagulants, MRX, hypoglycemics, phenytoin, cyclosporine **Contra:** Infants <2 mo **Disp:** Susp erythromycin ethylsuccinate 200 mg/sulfisoxazole 600 mg/5 mL (100, 150, 200 mL) **SE:** GI disturbance **Additional Interactions:** ↑ Effects of sulfonamides w/ ASA, diuretics, NSAIDs, probenecid **Labs:** False ↑ urine protein **NIPE:** ↑ Risk of photosensitivity—use sunscreen, ↑ fluid intake

Erythromycin, Ophthalmic (Ilotycin Ophthalmic) [Anti-infective, Macroloid, Opht agent] Uses: *Conjunctival/corneal Infxns* Action: Macrolide antibiotic **Dose:** ½ in. 2–6 ×/d **Caution:** [B, +] **Contra:** Erythromycin hypersensitivity **Disp:** 0.5% oint **SE:** Local irritation **NIPE:** May cause burning, stinging, blurred vision

Erythromycin, Topical (A/T/S, Eryderm, Erycette, T-Stat) [Topical Anti-infective, Macroloid] Uses: *Acne vulgaris* Action: Macrolide antibiotic **Dose:** Wash & dry area, apply 2% product over area bid **Caution:** [B, +] **Contra:** Component sensitivity **Disp:** Soln 1.5%, 2%; gel 2%; impregnated pads & swabs 2% **SE:** Local irritation

Escitalopram (Lexapro) [Antidepressant/SSRI] WARNING: Closely monitor for worsening depression or emergence of suicidality, particularly in ped pts Uses: Depression, anxiety Action: SSRI **Dose:** *Adults.* 10–20 mg PO qd; 10 mg in elderly & hepatic impair **Caution:** [C, +/–] ↑ Risk of serotonin syndrome (Table 14) **Contra:** With or w/in 14 d of MAOI **Disp:** Tabs 5, 10, 20 mg; soln 1 mg/mL **SE:** N/V/D, sweating, insomnia, dizziness, xerostomia, sexual dysfunction, anger, aggression, delusions, nightmares, photosensitivity **Interactions:**

↑ Risk of serotonin syndrome ASA, NSAIDs; may ↑ CNS may take up to 2–4 wk for fu petite & weight gain

Esmolol (Brevibloc) [A pensatory sinus tachycardia, antiarrhythmic **Dose:** *Adults* then 50 mcg/kg/min × 4 mi maint inf of 100 mcg/kg/mi ↑ in the maint dose of 50 mc ↓ BP; average dose 100 m **Contra:** Sinus bradycardia ↓ BP **Disp:** Inj 10, 20, 250 diaphoresis, dizziness, pai w/in 30 mins after D/C i digoxin, antihypertensives, epinephrine, MAOIs, nore OF glucagons, insulin, hyp hormones **Labs:** ↑ Glucos

Esomeprazole (N Pump Inhibitor] GERD; *H. pylori* Infxn i ↓ gastric acid **Dose:** *Ad* 20–40 mg IV 10—30 min *H. pylori* Infxn: 40 mg/c 1000 mg/bid for 10 d; Caps 20, 40 mg **SE:** HA sule & sprinkle on a ithromycin; ↑ effects ketoconazole, iron salt platelets, K+, thyroxine

Estazolam (Pro Uses: *Short-term ma mg PO qhs PRN; ↓ in w/ CNS depressants U ness, palpitations **Not** abrupt D/C after pro ithromycin; ↑ effects fects OF azole antifun ↓ Hgb, WBC, plts, K

Esterified Estro WARNING: Do not

---

vulvar/vaginal atrophy **tion:** Estrogen supl **Do** off. *Hypogonadism:* 2.5 Genital bleeding of unkr boembolic disorders, th Tabs 0.3, 0.625, 1.25, 2 derness, edema, venous **Notes:** Use lowest dose data www.whi.org) **Int** TCAs, theophylline, caf fampin; ↓ effects OF a ↑ Prothrombin & factors lin, T$_4$, triglycerides; ↓ an

Esterified Estrogen est HS) [Estrogen partum breast engorgeme wk, 1 wk off **Caution:** CA, estrogen-dependent I cent MI, PRG **Disp:** Tab 1.25 mg/2.5 mg **SE:** Naus ↑ triglycerides, venous th for shortest time (see Wor **tional Interactions:** ↑ Eff

Estradiol (Estrace) motor Sxs associated w/ PO: 1–2 mg/d, adjust PRN 1–3×/wk **Caution:** [X, –] estrogen-dependent tumor MI; hepatic impair **Disp:** HA, bloating, breast enl thromboembolism, gallbla ↑ effects OF corticosteroid ↓ effects w/ barbiturates, ca OF clofibrate, hypoglyceme & factors VII, VIII, IX, X, erides; ↓ antithrombin III,

Estradiol Cypionat (Lunelle) [Estrogen & ing ↑ risk of serious CV si risk ↑ with age & with hea women > 35 y. Women who Uses: *Contraceptive* Acti

ant thigh, buttock) monthly, do not exceed 33 d **Caution:** [X, M] HTN, gallbladder Dz, ↑ lipids, migraines, sudden HA, valvular heart Dz with complications **Contra:** PRG, heavy smokers >35 y, DVT, PE, cerebro/CV Dz, estrogen-dependent neoplasm, undiagnosed abnormal uterine bleeding, hepatic tumors, cholestatic jaundice **Disp:** Estradiol cipionate (5 mg), medroxyprogesterone acetate (25 mg) single-dose vial or prefilled syringe (0.5 mL) **SE:** Arterial thromboembolism, HTN, cerebral hemorrhage, MI, amenorrhea, acne, breast tenderness **Notes:** Start w/in 5 d of menstruation See Estradiol. **Additional Interactions:** ↓ Effects w/ aminoglutethimide

Estradiol, Transdermal (Estraderm, Climara, Vivelle) [Estrogen Supl]
Uses: *Severe menopausal vasomotor Sxs; female hypogonadism* **Action:** Estrogen supl **Dose:** 0.1 mg/d patch 1–2×/wk depending on product; adjust PRN to control Sxs **Caution:** [X, –] (See estradiol) **Contra:** PRG, undiagnosed genital bleeding, carcinoma of breast, estrogen-dependent tumors, Hx thrombophlebitis, thrombosis, **Disp:** TD patches (deliver mg/24 h) 0.025, 0.0375, 0.05, 0.075, 0.1 **SE:** Nausea, bloating, breast enlargement/tenderness, edema, HA, hypertriglyceridemia, gallbladder Dz **Notes:** Do not apply to breasts, place on trunk of body & rotate sites See Estradiol. **Additional NIPE:** Rotate application sites

Estramustine Phosphate (Estracyt, Emcyt) [Antimicrotubule Agent]
Uses: *Advanced CAP* **Action:** Antimicrotubule agent; weak estrogenic & antiandrogenic activity **Dose:** 14 mg/kg/d in 3–4 ÷ doses; take on empty stomach, do not take with milk/milk products **Caution:** [NA, not used in females] **Contra:** Active thrombophlebitis or thromboembolic disorders **Disp:** Caps 140 mg **SE:** N/V, exacerbation of preexisting CHF, thrombophlebitis, MI, PE, gynecomastia in 20–100% **Interactions:** ↓ Effects w/ antacids, Ca suppls, Ca-containing foods; ↓ effects OF anticoagulants **NIPE:** Take on empty stomach, several wk may be needed for full effects, store in refrigerator

Estrogen, Conjugated (Premarin) [Estrogen/Hormone]
WARNING: Should not be used for the prevention of CV Dz. The WHI reported ↑ risk of MI, stroke, breast CA, PE, & DVT when combined with methoxyprogesterone over 5 y of Rx; ↑ risk of endometrial CA **Uses:** *Moderate–severe menopausal vasomotor Sxs; atrophic vaginitis; palliative for advanced prostatic carcinoma; prevention & Rx of estrogen deficiency osteoporosis* **Action:** Hormonal replacement **Dose:** 0.3–1.25 mg/d PO cyclically; prostatic carcinoma requires 1.25–2.5 mg PO tid; **Caution:** [X, –] **Contra:** Severe hepatic impair, genital bleeding of unknown cause, breast CA, estrogen-dependent tumors, thromboembolic disorders, thrombosis, thrombophlebitis, recent MI **Disp:** Tabs 0.3, 0.625, 0.9, 1.25, 2.5 mg; inj 25 mg/mL; vag cream 0.625 mg/gm **SE:** ↑ Risk of endometrial carcinoma, gallbladder Dz, thromboembolism, HA, & possibly breast CA; generic products not equivalent **Interactions:** ↑ Effects OF corticosteroids, cyclosporine, TCAs, theophylline, tobacco; ↓ effects OF anticoagulants, clofibrate; ↓ effects w/ barbiturates, carbamazepine, phenytoin, rifampin **Labs:** ↑ Prothrom-

bin & factors VII, VIII, IX, X, plt aggregability, thyroid-binding globulin, T_4, triglycerides; ↓ antithrombin III, folate **NIPE:** ⊘ PRG, breast-feeding

Estrogen, Conjugated-Synthetic (Cenestin) [Estrogen/Hormone] Uses: *Rx of moderate–severe vasomotor Sxs associated with menopause* **Action:** Hormonal replacement **Dose:** 0.45–1.25 mg PO daily **Caution:** [X, –] **Contra:** See estrogen, conjugated **Disp:** Tabs 0.3, 0.45, 0.625, 0.9, 1.25 mg **SE:** Associated with an ↑ risk of endometrial CA, gallbladder Dz, thromboembolism, & possibly breast CA See Estrogen, Conjugated

Estrogen, Conjugated + Medroxyprogesterone (Prempro, Premphase) [Estrogen/Progestin Hormones] WARNING: Should not be used for the prevention of CV Dz; the WHI study reported ↑ risk of MI, stroke, breast CA, PE, & DVT over 5 y of Rx **Uses:** *Moderate–severe menopausal vasomotor Sxs; atrophic vaginitis; prevent postmenopausal osteoporosis* **Action:** Hormonal replacement **Dose:** Prempro 1 tab PO daily; Premphase 1 tab PO daily **Caution:** [X, –] **Contra:** Severe hepatic impair, genital bleeding of unknown cause, breast CA, estrogen-dependent tumors, thromboembolic disorders, thrombosis, thrombophlebitis **Disp:** (expressed as estrogen/medroxyprogesterone) *Prempro:* Tabs 0.625/2.5, 0.625/5 mg *Premphase:* Tabs 0.625/0 (days 1–14) & 0.625/5 mg (days 15–28) **SE:** Gallbladder Dz, thromboembolism, HA, breast tenderness **Notes:** See www.whi.org; See Estrogen, Conjugated **Additional Interactions:** ↓ Effects w/ aminoglutethimide

Estrogen, Conjugated + Methylprogesterone (Premarin + Methylprogesterone) [Estrogen & Androgen Hormones] Uses: *Menopausal vasomotor Sxs; osteoporosis* **Action:** Estrogen & androgen combo **Dose:** 1 tab/d **Caution:** [X, –] **Contra:** Severe hepatic impair, genital bleeding of unknown cause, breast CA, estrogen-dependent tumors, thromboembolic disorders, thrombosis, thrombophlebitis **Disp:** Tabs 0.625 mg estrogen, conjugated, & 2.5 or 5 mg of methylprogesterone **SE:** Nausea, bloating, breast enlargement/tenderness, edema, HA, hypertriglyceridemia, gallbladder Dz; See Estrogen, Conjugated

Estrogen, Conjugated + Methyltestosterone (Premarin + Methyltestosterone) [Estrogen & Androgen Hormones] Uses: *Moderate–severe menopausal vasomotor Sxs*; postpartum breast engorgement **Action:** Estrogen & androgen combo **Dose:** 1 tab/d × 3 wk, then 1 wk off **Caution:** [X, –] **Contra:** Severe hepatic impair, genital bleeding of unknown cause, breast CA, estrogen-dependent tumors, thromboembolic disorders, thrombosis, thrombophlebitis **Disp:** Tabs (estrogen/methyltestosterone) 0.625 mg/5 mg, 1.25 mg/10 mg **SE:** Nausea, bloating, breast enlargement/tenderness, edema, HA, hypertriglyceridemia, gallbladder Dz; See Estrogen, Conjugated **Additional Interactions:** ↑ Effects of insulin

Eszopiclone (Lunesta) [C-IV] [Hypnotic/nonbenzodiazepine] Uses: *Insomnia* **Action:** Nonbenzodiazepine hypnotic **Dose:** 2–3 mg/d hs *El-*

derly: 1–2 mg/d hs; hepatic impair/use w/ CYP3A4 inhibitor (Table 13): 1 mg/d hs **Caution:** [C, ?/–] **Contra:** None known **Disp:** Tabs 1-, 2-, 3-mg **SE:** HA, xerostomia, dizziness, somnolence, hallucinations, rash, Infxn, unpleasant taste **Notes:** High-fat meals slows absorption

Etanercept (Enbrel) [Antirheumatic/TNF blocker] **Uses:** *Reduces Sxs of RA in pts who fail other DMARD,* Crohn Dz **Action:** Binds TNF **Dose:** *Adults.* RA 50 mg sc weekly or 25 mg sc 2 times/wk (separated by at least 72–96 h). *Peds 4–17 y.* 0.8 mg/kg SQ 2×/wk (max 50 mg/week) 72–96 h apart **Caution:** [B, ?] conditions that predispose to Infxn (ie, DM) **Contra:** Active Infxn; **Disp:** Inj 25 mg/vial **SE:** HA, rhinitis, inj site Rxn, URI, rhinitis **Interactions:** ↓ Response to live virus vaccine **NIPE:** Rotate inj sites, ⊘ live vaccines

Ethambutol (Myambutol) [Antitubercular Agent] **Uses:** *Pulmonary TB* & other mycobacterial Infxns, MAC **Action:** ↓ RNA synthesis **Dose:** *Adults & Peds >12 y.* 15–25 mg/kg/d PO as a single dose; ↓ in renal impair, take w/ food, avoid antacids **Caution:** [B, +] **Contra:** Optic neuritis **Disp:** Tabs 100, 400 mg **SE:** HA, hyperuricemia, acute gout, abdominal pain, ↑ LFTs, optic neuritis, GI upset **Interactions:** ↑ Neurotoxicity w/ neurotoxic drugs; ↓ effects w/ Al salts **NIPE:** Monitor visual acuity

Ethinyl Estradiol (Estinyl, Feminone) [Estrogen Supl] **Uses:** *Menopausal vasomotor Sxs; female hypogonadism* **Action:** Estrogen supl **Dose:** 0.02–1.5 mg/d ÷ daily–tid **Caution:** [X, –] **Contra:** Severe hepatic impair; genital bleeding of unknown cause, breast CA, estrogen-dependent tumors, thromboembolic disorders, thrombosis, thrombophlebitis **Disp:** Tabs 0.02, 0.05, 0.5 mg **SE:** Nausea, bloating, breast enlargement/tenderness, edema, HA, hypertriglyceridemia, gallbladder Dz **Interactions:** ↑ Effects OF corticosteroids; ↓ effects w/ barbiturates, carbamazepine, hypoglycemics, insulin, phenytoin, primidone, rifampin, ↓ effects OF anticoagulants, tamoxifen; **Labs:** ↑ Prothrombin & factors VII, VIII, IX, X, plt aggregability, thyroid-binding globulin, T$_4$, triglycerides; ↓ antithrombin III, folate **NIPE:** ⊘ PRG, breast-feeding

Ethinyl Estradiol & Drospirenone (YAZ) [Estrogen & Progestin Supl] **WARNING:** Cigarette smoking & use of estrogen-based oral contraceptives have ↑ risk of serious cardiovascular side effects; risk ↑ w/age (esp. > 35 yrs) and smoking > 15 cig/d **Uses:** *Oral contraception; premenstrual dysphoric disorder* **Action:** Suppresses ovulation by imitating the feedback inhibition of endogenous estrogen and progesterone on the pituitary and hypothalamus **Dose:** 1 tab PO OD × 28 days, repeat. Caution: [X,–], has antimineralocorticoid activity w/ potential hyperkalemia in renal insuff, adrenal insuff, hepatic insuff **Contra:** Pts w/ renal insuff, hepatic impair, adrenal insuff, DVT, PE, CVD, CAD, estrogen dependent neoplasms, abnormal uterine bleeding, pregnancy, heavy smokers > 35 yr **Disp:** Ethinyl estradiol (20 mcg), drospirenone (3 mg) 28-day pack has 24 active tabs & 4 inert tabs **SE:** Hyperkalemia, HTN, N, V, HA, breakthrough bleeding, amenorrhea, mastodynia, ↑ risk of gallbladder disease & thromboembolic disorders **Interactions:** ↑ risk of hyperkalemia w/ ACEIs, ARBs, aldosterone antagonists, heparin, NSAIDs, spironolactone, K⁺ sparing diuretics, K⁺ supplements, ↑ effects OF cyclosporine, prednisolone, theophylline; ↓ effects w/ barbiturates, carbamazepine, griseofulvin, modafinil, phenobarbital, phenylbutazone, phenytoin, pioglitazone, rifabutin, rifampin, ritonavir, topiramate, St John's wort **Labs:** ↑ Uptake OF T₃, ↓ T₄ sex hormone-binding globulin levels; triglycerides **NIPE:** Antimineralocorticoid activity comparable to spironolactone 25 mg; in pts taking meds that ↑ K⁺ monitor serum K⁺ during first treatment cycle; Sunday start regimen or postpartum use requires additional contraceptive methods during first cycle; use barrier contraception if taking anticonvulsants; may cause vision changes or ↓ contact lens tolerability; ⊘ protection against HIV or STDs; ⊘ smoke cigarettes

Ethinyl Estradiol & Levonorgestrel (Preven) [Estrogen & Progestin Supl] **Uses:** *Emergency contraceptive* ("morning-after pill"); prevent PRG after contraceptive failure or unprotected intercourse **Actions:** Estrogen & progestin; interferes with implantation **Dose:** 4 tabs, take 2 tabs q12h × 2 (w/in 72 h of intercourse) **Caution:** [X, M] **Contra:** Known/suspected PRG, abnormal uterine bleeding **Disp:** Kit: ethinyl estradiol (0.05), levonorgestrel (0.25) blister pack with 4 pills & urine PRG test **SE:** Peripheral edema, N/V/D, bloating, abdominal pain, fatigue, HA, & menstrual changes **Notes:** Will not induce abortion; may ↑ risk of ectopic PRG See Ethinyl Estradiol **Additional Interactions:** ↑ Effects OF ASA, benzodiazepines, metoprolol, TCAs **NIPE:** Monitor for vision changes or ↓ tolerance of contact lens

Ethinyl Estradiol/Levonorgestrel (Seasonale) [Estrogen & Progestin Supl] **WARNING:** Cigarette smoking & use of estrogen based oral contraceptives have ↑ risk of serious cardiovascular side effects; risk ↑ w/age (esp. > 35 yrs) and smoking > 15 cig/d; **Uses:** Oral contraceptive **Action:** Suppresses ovulation by imitating the feedback inhibition of endogenous estrogen and progesterone on the pituitary and hypothalamus **Dose:** 1 tab PO OD for 91 days; repeat. Use Sunday start for first cycle **Caution:** [X,-] **Contra:** Pts w/ DVT, PE, CVD, CAD, estrogen dependent neoplasms, abnormal uterine bleeding, pregnancy, hepatic impair **Disp:** Tabs levonorgestrel 0.15 mg and ethinyl estradiol 30 mcg; 91-day pack has 84 active tabs & 7 inert tabs **SE:** HTN, N, V, HA, breakthrough bleeding, amenorrhea, mastodynia, ↑ risk of gallbladder disease & thromboembolic disorders **Interactions:** ↓ Effects w/ barbiturates, carbamazepine, griseofulvin, modafinil, phenobarbital, phenytoin, ↑ pioglitazone, rifabutin, rifampin, ritonavir, topiramate, St John's wort **Labs:** ↑ Uptake OF T₃, ↓ T₄ sex hormone-binding globulin levels **NIPE:** Sunday start regimen requires additional contraceptive methods during first cycle; use barrier contraception if taking anticonvulsants; may cause vision changes or ↓ contact lens tolerability; ⊘ protection against HIV or STDs; ⊘ smoke cigarettes

Ethinyl Estradiol & Norelgestromin (Ortho Evra) [Estrogen & Progestin Hormones] **Uses:** *Contraceptive patch* **Action:** Estrogen

& progestin **Dose:** Apply patch to abdomen, buttocks, upper torso (not breasts), or upper outer arm at the beginning of the menstrual cycle; new patch is applied weekly for 3 wk; week 4 is patch-free **Caution:** [X, M] **Contra:** Thrombophlebitis, undiagnosed vaginal bleeding, PRG, carcinoma of breast, estrogen-dependent tumor **Disp:** 20 cm^2 patch (6 mg norelgestromin (active metabolite norgestimate) & 0.75 mg of ethinyl estradiol) **SE:** Breast discomfort, HA, site Rxns, nausea, menstrual cramps; thrombosis risks similar to OCP **Notes:** Less effective in women >90 kg; See Ethinyl Estradiol **Additional Labs:** ↑ Serum amylase, Na, Ca, protein; **NIPE:** instruct patient that drug does not protect against STD/HIV

Ethosuximide (Zarontin) [Anticonvulsant] Uses: *Absence (petit mal) Szs* **Action:** Anticonvulsant; ↑ Sz threshold **Dose:** *Adults.* Initial, 250 mg PO ÷ bid; ↑ by 250 mg/d q4–7d PRN (max 1500 mg/d), usual maint 20–30 mg/kg. *Peds 3–6 y.* Initial: 15 mg/kg/d PO ÷ bid. *Maint:* 15–40 mg/kg/d ÷ bid, max 1500 mg/d **Caution:** [C, +] in renal/hepatic impair **Contra:** Component sensitivity **Disp:** Caps 250 mg; syrup 250 mg/5 mL **SE:** Blood dyscrasias, GI upset, drowsiness, dizziness, irritability **Interactions:** ↑ Effects w/ INH, phenobarbital, EtOH; ↑ effects OF CNS depressants, phenytoin; ↓ effects w/ carbamazepine, valproic acid, ginkgo biloba; ↓ effects OF phenobarbital **NIPE:** Take w/ food

Etidronate Disodium (Didronel) [Hormone/Biphosphonates] Uses: *↑ Ca^{2+} of malignancy, Paget Dz, & heterotopic ossification* **Action:** ↓ Nl & abnormal bone resorption **Dose:** *Paget Dz:* 5–10 mg/kg/d PO ÷ doses (for 3–6 mo). *↑ Ca^{2+}:* 7.5 mg/kg/d IV inf over 2 h × 3 d, then 20 mg/kg/d PO on last day of inf × 1–3 mo **Caution:** [B PO (C parenteral), ?] **Contra:** SCr >5 mg/dL **Disp:** Tabs 200, 400 mg; inj 50 mg/mL **SE:** GI intolerance (↓ by ÷ daily doses); hypophosphatemia, hypomagnesemia, bone pain, abnormal taste, fever, convulsions, nephrotox **Notes:** Take PO on empty stomach 2 h before any meal **Interactions:** ↓ Effects w/ antacids, foods that contain Ca **NIPE:** ⊘ Take w/ food, improvement may take 3 mo

Etodolac (Lodine) [Antiarthritic/NSAID] WARNING: May ↑ risk of cardiovascular events & GI bleeding **Uses:** *Osteoarthritis & pain,* RA **Action:** NSAID **Dose:** 200–400 mg PO bid–qid (max 1200 mg/d) **Caution:** [C (D 3rd tri), ?] ↑ bleeding risk with aspirin, warfarin; ↑ nephrotox w/ cyclosporine; Hx CHF, HTN, renal/hepatic impair, PUD **Contra:** Active GI ulcer **Disp:** Tabs 400, 500 mg; ER tabs 400, 500, 600 mg; caps 200, 300 mg **SE:** N/V/D, gastritis, abdominal cramps, dizziness, HA, depression, edema, renal impair **Notes:** Do not crush tabs **Interactions:** ↑ Risk of bleeding w/ anticoagulants, antiplts; ↑ effects OF Li, MTX, digoxin, cyclosporine; ↓ effects w/ ASA; ↓ effects OF antihypertensives **Labs:** False + of urine ketones & bilirubin **NIPE:** Take w/ food

Etonogestrel/Ethinyl Estradiol (NuvaRing) [Estrogen & Progestin hormones] Uses: *Contraceptive* **Action:** Estrogen & progestin combo **Dose:** Rule out PRG first; insert ring vaginally for 3 wk, remove for

1 wk; insert new ring 7 d after last removed (even if still bleeding) at same time of day ring removed. First day of menses is day 1, insert prior to day 5 even if still bleeding. Use other contraception for first 7 d of starting therapy. See insert if converting from other contraceptive; after delivery or 2nd tri abortion, insert 4 wk postpartum (if not breast-feeding) **Caution:** [X, ?/–] HTN, gallbladder Dz, ↑ lipids, migraines, sudden HA **Contra:** PRG, heavy smokers >35 y, DVT, PE, cerebro-/CV Dz, estrogen-dependent neoplasm, undiagnosed abnormal genital bleeding, hepatic tumors, cholestatic jaundice **Disp:** Intravaginal ring: ethinyl estradiol 0.015 mg/d & etonogestrel 0.12 mg/d **Notes:** If ring removed, rinse with cool/lukewarm H_2O (not hot) & reinsert ASAP; if not reinserted w/in 3 h, effectiveness ↓; do not use with diaphragm; See Ethinyl Estradiol

Etoposide [VP-16] (VePesid, Toposar) [Antineoplastic]
Uses: *Testicular CA, non-small-cell lung CA, Hodgkin Dz & NHLs, ped ALL, & allogeneic/autologous BMT in high doses* **Action:** Topoisomerase II inhibitor **Dose:** 50 mg/m^2/d IV for 3–5 d; 50 mg/m^2/d PO for 21 d (PO bioavailability = 50% of the IV form); 2–6 g/m^2 or 25–70 mg/kg used in BMT (Per protocols); ↓ in renal/hepatic impair **Caution:** [D, –] **Contra:** IT administration **Disp:** Caps 50 mg; inj 20 mg/mL **SE:** Myelosuppression, N/V, alopecia, ↓ BP if infused rapidly, anorexia, anemia, leukopenia, potential for secondary leukemias **Notes:** Emesis in low (10–30%) **Interactions:** ↑ Bleeding w/ ASA, NSAIDs, warfarin; ↑ bone marrow suppression w/ antineoplastics & radiation; ↑ effects OF cisplatin; ↓ effects OF live vaccines **Labs:** ↑ Uric acid **NIPE:** ⊘ EtOH, immunizations, PRG, breast-feeding; use contraception, 2–3 L/d fluids

Exemestane (Aromasin) [Antineoplastic]
Uses: *Advanced breast CA in postmenopausal women whose Dz has progressed following tamoxifen therapy* **Action:** An irreversible, steroidal aromatase inhibitor; ↓ circulating estrogens **Dose:** 25 mg PO daily after a meal **Caution:** [D, ?/–] **Contra:** Component sensitivity **Disp:** Tabs 25 mg **SE:** Hot flashes, nausea, fatigue **Interactions:** ↓ Effects w/ erythromycin, ketoconazole, phenobarbital, rifampin, other drugs that inhibit P4503A4, St John's wort, black cohosh, dong quai **Labs:** ↑ Alkaline phosphatase, AST, ALT **NIPE:** ⊘ PRG, breast-feeding; take pc and same time each day; monitor BP

Exenatide (Byetta) [Hypoglycemic/Incretin]
Uses: Type 2 DM combined w/ metformin &/or sulfonylurea **Action:** An incretin mimetic: ↑ insulin release, ↓ glucagon secretion, ↓ gastric emptying, promotes satiety **Dose:** 5 mcg SQ bid w/in 60 min before AM & PM meals; ↑ to 10 mcg SQ bid after 1 mo PRN; do not give w/ meal **Caution:** [C, ?/–] may ↓ absorption of other oral drugs (take antibiotics/contraceptives 1 h before) **Contra:** CrCl < 30 mL/min **Disp:** Soln 5, 10 mcg/dose (prefilled pen) **SE:** Hypoglycemia, N/V/D, dizziness, HA, dyspepsia, ↓ appetite, jittery **NIPE:** Consider ↓ sulfonylurea to ↓ risk of hypoglycemia; discard pen 30 d after 1st use

Ezetimibe (Zetia) [Antilipemic/Selective Cholesterol Absorption Inhibitor]
Uses: *Primary hypercholesterolemia alone or in combo with

an HMG-CoA reductase inhibitor* **Action:** ↓ intestinal absorption of cholesterol & phytosterols **Dose:** *Adults & Peds >10 y.* 10 mg/d PO **Caution:** [C, +/–] Bile acid sequestrants ↓ bioavailability **Contra:** Hepatic impair **Disp:** Tabs 10 mg **SE:** HA, D, abdominal pain, ↑ transaminases in combo with an HMG-CoA reductase inhibitor **Interactions:** ↑ Effects w/ cyclosporine; ↓ effects w/ cholestyramine, fenofibrate, gemfibrozil **NIPE:** If used w/ fibrates ↑ risk of cholethiasis

Ezetimibe/Simvastatin (Vytorin) [Antilipemic/HMG-CoA Reductase Inhibitor] **Uses:** *Hypercholesterolemia* **Action:** ↓ Absorption of cholesterol & phytosterols w/HMG-CoA-reductase inhibitor **Dose:** 10/10–10/80 mg/d PO; w/cyclosporine or danazol:10/10 mg/d max; w/ amiodarone or verapamil: 10/20 mg/d max; ↓ in severe renal insuff **Caution:** [X, –]; w/ CYP3A4 inhibitors (Table 13), gemfibrozil, niacin > 1 g/d, danazol, amiodarone, verapamil **Contra:** PRG/lactation; liver disease or ↑ LFTs **Disp:** Tabs (ezetimibe/simvastatin) 10/10, 10/20, 10/40, 10/80 mg **SE:** HA, GI upset, myalgia, myopathy manifested as muscle pain, weakness or tenderness w/ creatine kinase 10 × ULN, rhabdomyolysis, hepatitis, Infxn **Interactions:** ↑ Risk of myopathy w/ clarithromycin, erythromycin, itraconazole, ketoconazole **Labs:** Monitor LFTs **NIPE:** ⊘ In pregnancy or lactation; use adequate contraception; ⊘ ETOH

Famciclovir (Famvir) [Antiviral] **Uses:** *Acute herpes zoster (shingles) & genital herpes* **Action:** ↓ viral DNA synthesis **Dose:** *Zoster:* 500 mg PO q8h × 7 d. *Simplex:* 125–250 mg PO bid; ↓ in renal impair **Caution:** [B, –] **Contra:** Component sensitivity **Disp:** Tabs 125, 250, 500 mg **SE:** Fatigue, dizziness, HA, pruritus, N/D **Interactions:** ↑ Effects w/ cimetidine, probenecid, theophylline; ↑ effects OF digoxin **NIPE:** Not affected by food, therapy most effective if taken w/in 72 h of rash

Famotidine (Pepcid) [Antisecretory/H₂-receptor Antagonist] **Uses:** *Short-term Tx of duodenal ulcer & benign gastric ulcer; maint for duodenal ulcer, hypersecretory conditions, GERD, & heartburn* **Action:** H₂-antagonist; ↓ gastric acid secretion **Dose:** *Adults.* Ulcer: 20 mg IV q12h or 20–40 mg PO qhs × 4–8 wk. *Hypersecretion:* 20–160 mg PO q6h. *GERD:* 20 mg PO bid ×6 wk; maint: 20 mg PO hs. *Heartburn:* 10 mg PO PRN q12h. *Peds.* 0.5–1 mg/kg/d; ↓ in severe renal insuff **Caution:** [B, M] **Contra:** Component sensitivity **Disp:** Tabs 10, 20, 40 mg; chew tabs 10 mg; susp 40 mg/5 mL; gelatin cap 10 mg; inj 10 mg/2 mL **SE:** Dizziness, HA, constipation, D, thrombocytopenia **Notes:** Chewable tabs contain phenylalanine **Interactions:** ↑ Effects OF glipizide, glyburide, nifedipine, nitrendipine, nisoldipine, tolbutamide; ↓ effects w/ antacids; ↓ effects OF azole antifungals, cefuroxime, enoxacin, diazepam **NIPE:** ⊘ ASA, EtOH, tobacco, caffeine; take hs

Felodipine (Plendil) [Antihypertensive/CCB] **Uses:** *HTN & CHF* **Action:** CCB **Dose:** 2.5–10 mg PO daily; swallow whole; ↓ in hepatic impair **Caution:** [C, ?] ↑ effect with azole antifungals, erythromycin, grapefruit juice **Contra:** Component sensitivity **Disp.:** ER tabs 2.5, 5, 10 mg **SE:** Peripheral edema, flushing, tachycardia, HA, gingival hyperplasia **Notes:** Follow BP in elderly & in impaired hepatic Fxn; **Interactions:** ↑ Effects w/ azole antifungals, cimetidine, cyclosporine, ranitidine, propranolol, EtOH, grapefruit juice; ↑ effects OF digoxin, erythromycin; ↓ effects w/ barbiturates, carbamazepine, nafcillin, oxcarbazepine, phenytoin; rifampin; ↓ effects OF theophylline **NIPE:** ⊘ DC abruptly

Fenofibrate (TriCor) [Antilipemic/Fibric Acid Derivative]
Uses: *Hypertriglyceridemia* **Action:** ↓ Triglyceride synthesis **Dose:** 48–145 mg daily; ↓ in renal impair, take w/ meals **Caution:** [C, ?] **Contra:** Hepatic/severe renal insuff, 1st-deg biliary cirrhosis, unexplained persistent ↑ LFTs, gallbladder Dz **Disp:** Tabs 48, 145 mg **SE:** GI disturbances, cholecystitis, arthralgia, myalgia, dizziness **Notes:** Monitor LFTs **Interactions:** ↑ Effects OF anticoagulants; ↓ effects w/ BBs, cholestyramine, colestipol, estrogens, resins, rifampin, thiazide diuretics **Labs:** ↑ LFTs, BUN, creatinine; ↓ Hgb, Hct, WBCs, uric acid

Fenoldopam (Corlopam) [Antihypertensive/Vasodilator]
Uses: *Hypertensive emergency* **Action:** Rapid vasodilator **Dose:** Initial 0.03–0.1 mcg/kg/min IV inf, titrate q 15 min in 0.05–0.1 mcg/kg/min increments **Caution:** [B, ?] ↓ BP w/ β-blockers **Contra:** Allergy to sulfites **Disp:** Inj 10 mg/mL **SE:** ↓ BP, edema, facial flushing, N/V/D, atrial flutter/fibrillation, ↑ intraocular pressure **Notes:** Avoid concurrent β-blockers **Interactions:** ↑ Effects w/ acetaminophen ↑ hypotension w/ BBs **Labs:** ↑ Serum urea nitrogen, creatinine, LFTs, LDH; ↑ K⁺

Fenoprofen (Nalfon) [Analgesic/NSAID]   WARNING: May ↑ risk of cardiovascular events & GI bleeding
Uses: *Arthritis & pain* **Action:** NSAID **Dose:** 200–600 mg q4–8h, to 3200 mg/d max; take with food **Caution:** [B (D 3rd tri), +/–] CHF, HTN, renal/hepatic impair, Hx PUD **Contra:** NSAID sensitivity **Disp.:** Caps 200, 300 mg **SE:** GI disturbance, dizziness, HA, rash, edema, renal impair, hepatitis **Notes:** Swallow whole **Interactions:** ↑ Effects w/ ASA, anticoagulants; ↑ hyperkalemia w/ K-sparing diuretics; ↑ effects OF aminoglycoside, anticoagulants, Li, MTX, phenytoin, sulfonamides, sulfonylureas; ↓ effects w/ phenobarbital; ↓ effects OF antihypertensives **Labs:** False ↑ free and total T₃ levels, false + urine barbiturates & benzodiazepines; ↑ serum Na & Cl **NIPE:** ⊘ ASA, EtOH, OTC drugs

Fentanyl (Sublimaze) [Opioid Analgesic] [C-II]
Uses: *Short-acting analgesic* in anesthesia & PCA **Action:** Narcotic analgesic **Dose:** *Adults.* 25–100 mcg/kg/dose IV/IM titrated to effect. *Peds.* 1–2 mcg/kg IV/IM q1–4h titrated to effect; ↓ in renal impair **Caution:** [B, +] **Contra:** ↑ ICP, resp depression, severe renal/hepatic impair **Disp.:** Inj 0.05 mg/mL **SE:** Sedation, ↓ BP, bradycardia, constipation, nausea, resp depression, miosis **Notes:** 0.1 mg of fentanyl = 10 mg of morphine IM **Interactions:** ↑ Effects w/ CNS depressants, cimetidine, phenothiazines, ritonavir, TCAs, EtOH, grapefruit juice; ↑ risks OF HTN crisis w/ MAOIs; ↓ effects w/ buprenorphine, dezocine, nalbuphine, pentazocine **Labs:** False ↑ serum amylase, lipase

Fentanyl Buccal (Fentora) [C-II] [Opioid Analgesic] WARNING: ⊘ Substitute Fentora on a mcg to mcg basis w/ other oral fentanyl products;

NOT for opioid naive **Uses:** *Persistent moderate-severe chronic pain in patients already tolerant to opioids **Dose:** 100 mcg tab in buccal cavity above rear molar, may repeat > 30 min; reevaluate maintenance dose if > 4 doses/24 hrs **Caution:** [C, –] **Contra:** ⊘ To manage acute or postoperative pain; ⊘ children < 18 y **Disp:** Buccal tabs 100, 200, 400, 600, 800 mcg **SE:** Sedation, resp depression, hypotension, N, V, fatigue, anemia, dizziness, constipation, edema, HA **Interactions:** ↑ Effects w/ CNS depressants, cimetidine, phenothiazines, ritonavir, TCAs, EtOH, grapefruit juice; ↑ risks of HTN crisis w/ MAOIs; ↓ effects w/ buprenorphine, dezocine, nalbuphine, pentazocine **Labs:** Effect has not been eval. **NIPE:** ⊘ Use within 14 d of MAOI; use w/ other CNS depressants causes profound sedation, hypoventilation, hypotension

Fentanyl, Transdermal (Duragesic) [C-II] [Opioid Analgesic]
WARNING: Potential for abuse and fatal overdose. **Uses:** *Persistent moderate-severe chronic pain in patients already tolerant to opioids* **Action:** Narcotic **Dose:** Apply patch to upper torso q72h; dose based on narcotic requirements in previous 24 h; start 25 mcg/h patch q72h; ↓ in renal impair **Caution:** [B, +] CYP3A4 inhibitors (Table 13) may ↑ fentanyl effect, in pts w/Hx substance abuse **Contra:** Not opioid tolerant, short-term ↑ pain management; postop pain in outpatient surgery, mild pain, PRN use ↑ ICP, resp depression, severe renal/hepatic impair; peds < 2 yr **Disp:** TD patches 12.5, 25, 50, 75, 100 mcg/h **SE:** Resp depression (fatal), sedation, ↓ BP, bradycardia, constipation, nausea, miosis **Notes:** 0.1 mg of fentanyl = 10 mg of morphine IM; peak level 24–72 h; See Fentanyl Patch; ⊘ Cut patch; ↑ risk of ↑ absorption w/ elevated temperature; cleanse skin only w/ water, ⊘ soap, lotions, or EtOH because they may ↑ absorption; ⊘ use in children < 110 lb

Fentanyl, Transmucosal System (Actiq) [C-II] [Opioid Analgesic] **Uses:** *Induction of anesthesia; breakthrough CA pain* **Action:** Narcotic analgesic **Dose:** *Adults.* Anesthesia: 5–15 mcg/kg. *Pain:* 200 mcg over 15 min, titrate to effect; ↓ in renal impair **Caution:** [B, +] **Contra:** ↑ ICP, resp depression, severe renal/hepatic impair **Disp:** Lozenges on stick 200, 400, 600, 800, 1200, 1600 mcg **SE:** Sedation, ↓ BP, bradycardia, constipation, nausea, resp depression, miosis **Notes:** 0.1 mg of fentanyl = 10 mg of morphine IM; **Additional NIPE:** ⊘ Use for children < 33 lb and < 2 y old

Ferrous Gluconate (Fergon) [Oral Iron Supl] **Uses:** *Iron deficiency anemia* & Fe supl **Action:** Dietary supl **Dose:** *Adults.* 100–200 mg of elemental Fe/d ÷ doses. *Peds.* 4–6 mg/kg/d ÷ doses; take on empty stomach (OK w/ meals if GI upset occurs); avoid antacids **Caution:** [A, ?] **Contra:** Hemochromatosis, hemolytic anemia **Disp:** Tabs 300 (34 mg Fe), 325 mg (36 mg Fe) **SE:** GI upset, constipation, dark stools, discoloration of urine, may stain teeth **Notes:** 12% elemental Fe; **Interactions:** ↑ Effects w/ chloramphenicol, citrus fruits or juices, vitamin C; ↓ effects w/ antacids, cimetidine, fluoroquinolones, proton pump inhibitors, tetracycline, black cohosh, chamomile, feverfew, gossypol, hawthorn, nettle, plantain, St. John's wort, whole-grain breads, cheese, eggs, milk, coffee, tea, yogurt; ↓ effects OF fluoroquinolones, levodopa **Labs:** False + stool guaiac test **NIPE:** ⊘ Antacids, tetracyclines, take liq form in liquids and through a straw to prevent teeth staining

Ferrous Gluconate Complex (Ferrlecit) [Iron Supl] **Uses:** *Iron deficiency anemia or supl to erythropoietin therapy* **Action:** Fe Supl **Dose:** Test dose: 2 mL (25 mg Fe) IV over 1 h. If no reaction, 125 mg (10 mL) IV over 1 h. Usual cumulative dose 1 g Fe over 8 sessions (until favorable Hct) **Caution:** [B, ?] **Contra:** Anemia not due to Fe deficiency; CHF; Fe overload **Disp:** Inj 12.5 mg/mL Fe **SE:** ↓ BP, serious allergic Rxns, GI disturbance, inj site Rxn **Notes:** Dose expressed as mg Fe; may infuse during dialysis; See Ferrous Gluconate

Ferrous Sulfate [Iron Supl] **Uses:** *Fe deficiency anemia & Fe supl* **Action:** Dietary supl **Dose:** *Adults.* 100–200 mg elemental Fe/d in ÷ doses. *Peds.* 1–6 mg/kg/d ÷ daily–tid; on empty stomach (OK w/ meals if GI upset occurs); avoid antacids **Caution:** [A, ?] ↑ absorption w/ vitamin C; ↓ absorption w/ tetracycline, fluoroquinolones, antacids, H₂-blockers, proton pump inhibitors **Contra:** Hemochromatosis, hemolytic anemia **Disp.:** Tabs 187 (60 mg Fe), 200 (65 mg Fe), 324 (65 mg Fe), 325 (65 mg Fe); SR caplets & tabs 160 mg (50 mg Fe), 200 mg (65 mg Fe); gtt 75 mg/0.6 mL (15 mg Fe/0.6 mL); elixir 220 mg/5 mL (44 mg Fe/5 mL); syrup 90 mg/5 mL (18 mg Fe/5 mL) **SE:** GI upset, constipation, dark stools, discolored urine; See Ferrous Gluconate

Fexofenadine (Allegra, Allegra-D) [Antihistamine] **Uses:** *Allergic rhinitis* **Action:** Antihistamine **Dose:** *Adults & Peds >12 y.* 60 mg PO bid or 180 mg/d; ↓ in renal impair **Caution:** [C, ?] **Contra:** Component sensitivity **Disp:** Caps 60 mg; tabs 30, 60, 180 mg; Allegra-D (60 mg fexofenadine/120 mg pseudoephedrine) **SE:** Drowsiness (rare) **Interactions:** ↑ Effects w/ erythromycin, ketoconazole; ↓ effects w/ antacids **NIPE:** ⊘ EtOH or CNS depressants

Filgrastim [G-CSF] (Neupogen) [Colony-Stimulating Factor] **Uses:** *↓ Incidence of Infxn in febrile neutropenic pts; Rx chronic neutropenia* **Action:** Recombinant G-CSF **Dose:** *Adults & Peds.* 5 mcg/kg/d SQ or IV single daily dose; D/C therapy when ANC >10,000 **Caution:** [C, ?] Interactions w/ drugs that potentiate release of neutrophils (eg, lithium) **Contra:** Allergy to *E. coli*-derived proteins or G-CSF **Disp:** Inj 300 mcg/mL **SE:** Fever, alopecia, N/V/D, splenomegaly, bone pain, HA, rash **Notes:** monitor for cardiac events; no benefit w/ ANC >10,000/mm³ **Interactions:** ↑ Interference w/ cytotoxic drugs; ↑ release of neutrophils w/ Li **NIPE:** Monitor CBC & plts

Finasteride (Proscar, Propecia) [Androgen Hormone Inhibitor/Steroid] **Uses:** *BPH & androgenetic alopecia* **Action:** ↓ 5α-Reductase **Dose:** *BPH:* 5 mg/d PO. *Alopecia:* 1 mg/d PO; food may ↓ absorption **Caution:** [X, –] Hepatic impair **Contra:** Pregnant women should avoid handling pills **Disp:** Tabs 1 mg (Propecia), 5 mg (Proscar) **SE:** ↓ PSA level (↓ by ≈50%) **Notes:** Reestablish PSA baseline at 6 mo; 3–6 mo for effect on urinary Sxs; continue therapy to maintain new hair **Interactions:** ↑ Effects w/ saw palmetto; ↓ effects w/ anticholinergics, adrenergic bronchodilators, theophylline; **NIPE:** ↓ libido, impotence (rare)

Flavoxate (Urispas) [Antispasmotic] **Uses:** *Relief of Sx of dysuria, urgency, nocturia, suprapubic pain, urinary frequency, incontinence* **Action:** Antispasmotic **Dose:** 100–200 mg PO tid–qid **Caution:** [B, ?] **Contra:** Pyloric or duodenal obstruction, GI hemorrhage, GI obstruction, ileus, achalasia, BPH **Disp:** Tabs 100 mg **SE:** Drowsiness, blurred vision, xerostomia **Interactions:** ↑ Effects OF CNS depressants **NIPE:** ↑ Risk of heat stroke w/ exercise and in hot weather

Flecainide (Tambocor) [Antiarrhythmic] **Uses:** Prevent AF/flutter & PSVT, *prevent/suppress life-threatening ventricular arrhythmias* **Action:** Class 1C antiarrhythmic **Dose:** *Adults.* 100 mg PO q12h; ↑ by 50 mg q12h q4d to max 400 mg/d. *Peds.* 3–6 mg/kg/d in 3 ÷ doses; ↓ in renal impair, **Caution:** [C, +] monitor in hepatic impair ↑ conc with amiodarone, digoxin, quinidine, ritonavir/amprenavir, BB, verapamil **Contra:** 2nd-/3rd-degree AV block, RBBB w/ bifascicular or trifascicular block, cardiogenic shock, CAD, ritonavir/amprenavir, alkalinizing agents **Disp:** Tabs 50, 100, 150 mg **SE:** Dizziness, visual disturbances, dyspnea, palpitations, edema, tachycardia, CHF, HA, fatigue, rash, nausea **Notes:** May cause new/worsened arrhythmias; initiate Rx in hospital; dose q8h if pt is intolerant/condition is uncontrolled at 12-h intervals **Interactions:** ↑ Effects w/ alkalinizing drugs, amiodarone, cimetidine, propranolol, quinidine; ↑ effects OF digoxin; ↑ risk of arrhythmias w/ CCBs, antiarrhythmics, disopyramide; ↓ effects w/ acidifying drugs, tobacco **Labs:** ↑ Alkaline phosphatase **NIPE:** Full effects may take 3–5 d

Floxuridine (FUDR) [Pyrimidine Antimetabolite] **Uses:** *GI adenoma, liver, ↓ renal cancers*; colon & pancreatic CAs **Action:** Inhibits thymidylate synthase; ↓ DNA synthesis (S-phase specific) **Dose:** 0.1–0.6 mg/kg/d for 1–6 wk (Per protocols) **Caution:** [D, –] Drug interaction w/ live & rotavirus vaccine **Contra:** BM suppression, poor nutritional status, potentially serious Infxn **Disp:** Inj 500 mg **SE:** Myelosuppression, anorexia, abdominal cramps, N/V/D, mucositis, alopecia, skin rash, & hyperpigmentation; rare neurotox (blurred vision, depression, nystagmus, vertigo, & lethargy); intra-arterial catheter-related problems (ischemia, thrombosis, bleeding, & Infxn) **Notes:** Palliative Rx for inoperable/incurable pts **Interactions:** ↑ Effects w/ metronidazole **Labs:** ↑ LFTs, 5-HIAA urine excretion; ↓ plasma albumin **NIPE:** Need effective birth control; ↑ risk of photosensitivity—use sunscreen

Fluconazole (Diflucan) [Antifungal] **Uses:** *Candidiasis (esophageal, oropharyngeal, urinary tract, vaginal, prophylaxis); cryptococcal meningitis* **Action:** Antifungal, ↓ fungal cytochrome P-450 sterol demethylation. *Spectrum:* All *Candida* sp except *C. krusei* **Dose:** *Adults.* 100–400 mg/d PO or IV. *Vaginitis:* 150 mg PO qd. *Crypto:* 400 mg day 1, then 200 mg × 10–12wk after CSF (–). *Peds.* 3–6 mg/kg/d PO or IV; 12 mg/kg/d/systemic Infxn; ↓ in renal impair **Caution:** [C, –] **Contra:** w/ terfenadine **Disp:** Tabs 50, 100, 150, 200 mg; susp 10,

40 mg/mL; inj 2 mg/mL **SE:** HA, rash, GI upset, ↓ K⁺ **Notes:** PO use produces the same levels as IV; PO preferred **Interactions:** ↑ Effects w/ HCTZ, benzodiazepines, anticoagulants; ↑ effects OF amitriptyline, carbamazepine, cyclosporine, hypoglycemics, losartan, methadone, phenytoin, quinidine, tacrolimus, TCAs, theophylline, caffeine, zidovudine; ↓ effects w/ cimetidine, rifampin **Labs:** ↑ LFTs

Fludarabine Phosphate (Flamp, Fludara) [Antineoplastic]
Uses: *Autoimmune hemolytic anemia, CLL, cold agglutinin hemolysis,* low-grade lymphoma, mycosis fungoides **Action:** ↓ Ribonucleotide reductase; blocks DNA polymerase-induced DNA repair **Dose:** 18–30 mg/m²/d for 5 d, as a 30-min inf (Per protocols) **Caution:** [D, –] Give cytarabine before fludarabine (↓ its metabolism) **Contra:** Severe Infxns; CrCl < 30 mL/min **Disp:** Inj 50 mg **SE:** Myelosuppression, N/V/D, ↑ LFT, edema, CHF, fever, chills, fatigue, dyspnea, nonproductive cough, pneumonitis, severe CNS tox rare in leukemia **Interactions:** ↑ Effects w/ other myelosuppressive drugs; ↑ risk of pulmonary effects w/ pentostatin **NIPE:** May take several weeks for full effect, use barrier contraception

Fludrocortisone Acetate (Florinef) [Hormone/Mineralocorticoid] **Uses:** *Adrenocortical insuff, Addison Dz, salt-wasting syndrome* **Action:** Mineralocorticoid replacement **Dose:** *Adults.* 0.1–0.2 mg/d PO. *Peds.* 0.05–0.1 mg/d PO **Caution:** [C, ?] **Contra:** Systemic fungal Infxns; known allergy **Disp:** Tabs 0.1 mg **SE:** HTN, edema, CHF, HA, dizziness, convulsions, acne, rash, bruising, hyperglycemia, HPA suppression, cataracts **Notes:** For adrenal insuff, use w/ glucocorticoid; dosage changes based on plasma renin activity **Interactions:** ↑ Risk of hypokalemia w/ amphotericin B, thiazide diuretics, loop diuretics; ↓ effects w/ rifampin, barbiturates, hydantoins; ↓ effects OF ASA, INH **Labs:** ↓ Serum K⁺ **NIPE:** Eval for fluid retention

Flumazenil (Romazicon) [Antidote/Benzodiazepine] Uses: *Reverse sedative effects of benzodiazepines & general anesthesia* **Action:** Benzodiazepine receptor antagonist **Dose:** *Adults.* 0.2 mg IV over 15 s; repeat PRN, to 1 mg max (3 mg max in benzodiazepine OD). *Peds.* 0.01 mg/kg (0.2 mg/dose max) IV over 15 s; repeat 0.005 mg/kg at 1-min intervals to max 1 mg total; ↓ in hepatic impair **Caution:** [C, ?] **Contra:** In TCA OD; if pts given benzodiazepines to control life-threatening conditions (ICP/status epilepticus) **Disp:** Inj 0.1 mg/mL **SE:** N/V, palpitations, HA, anxiety, nervousness, hot flashes, tremor, blurred vision, dyspnea, hyperventilation, withdrawal syndrome **Notes:** Does not reverse narcotic Sx or amnesia **Interactions:** ↑ Risk of Szs and arrhythmias when benzodiazepine action is reduced **NIPE:** Food given during IV administration will reduce drug serum level

Flunisolide (AeroBid, Nasalide) [Corticosteroid] Uses: *Asthma in pts requiring chronic steroid therapy; relieve seasonal/perennial allergic rhinitis* **Action:** Topical steroid **Dose:** *Adults.* Met-dose inhal: 2 inhal bid (max 8/d). *Nasal:* 2 sprays/nostril bid (max 8/d). *Peds >6 y.* Met-dose inhal: 2 inhal bid (max 4/d). *Nasal:* 1–2 sprays/nostril bid (max 4/d) **Caution:** [C, ?] **Contra:** Status asthmaticus **Disp:** Aerobid-0.25mg/inh; Nasarel 29 mcg/spray **SE:** Tachycardia, bitter taste, local effects, oral candidiasis **Notes:** Not for acute asthma **NIPE:** Shake well before use

Fluorouracil [5-FU] (Adrucil) [Antineoplastic/Antimetabolite]

Uses: *Colorectal, gastric, pancreatic, breast, basal cell,* head, neck, bladder, CAs **Action:** Inhibitor of thymidylate synthetase (interferes with DNA synthesis, S-phase specific) **Dose:** 370–1000 mg/m²/d for 1–5 d IV push to 24-h cont inf; protracted venous inf of 200–300 mg/m²/d (Per protocol); 800 mg/d max **Caution:** [D, ?] ↑ tox w/ allopurinol; do not give MRX before 5-FU **Contra:** Poor nutritional status, depressed BM Fxn, thrombocytopenia, major surgery w/in past mo, G6PD enzyme deficiency, PRG, serious Infxn, bilirubin >5 mg/dL **Disp:** Inj 50 mg/mL **SE:** Stomatitis, esophagopharyngitis, N/V/D, anorexia, myelosuppression (leukocytopenia, thrombocytopenia, & anemia), rash/dry skin/photosensitivity, tingling in hands/feet w/pain (palmar–plantar erythrodysesthesia), phlebitis/discoloration at inj sites **Notes:** ↑ Thiamine intake; **Interactions:** ↑ Effects w/ leucovorin, Ca **Labs:** ↑ LFTs **NIPE:** ⊘ EtOH, ↑ risk of photosensitivity—use sunscreen, ↑ fluids 2–3 L/d, use barrier contraception

Fluorouracil, Topical [5-FU] (Efudex) [Antineoplastic/Antimetabolite]

Uses: *Basal cell carcinoma; actinic/solar keratosis* **Action:** Inhibitor of thymidylate synthetase (↓ DNA synthesis, S-phase specific) **Dose:** Apply 5% cream bid × 3–6 wk **Caution:** [D, ?] Irritant chemo **Contra:** Component sensitivity **Disp:** Cream 0.5, 1, 5%; soln 1, 2, 5% **SE:** Rash, dry skin, photosensitivity **Notes:** Healing may not be evident for 1–2 mo; do not overuse; See Fluorouracil **Additional NIPE:** ⊘ Use occlusive dressing; wash hands immediately after application

Fluoxetine (Prozac, Sarafem) [Antidepressant/SSRI]

WARNING: Closely monitor for worsening depression or emergence of suicidality, particularly in ped pts **Uses:** *Depression, OCD, panic disorder, bulimia, PMDD* (Sarafem) **Action:** SSRI **Dose:** 20 mg/d PO (max 80 mg/d ÷); weekly regimen 90 mg/wk after 1–2 wk of standard dose. *Bulimia:* 60 mg q AM. *Panic disorder:* 20 mg/d. *OCD:* 20–80 mg/d. *PMDD:* 20 mg/d or 20 mg intermittently, start 14 d prior to menses, repeat with each cycle; ↓ in hepatic failure **Caution:** [B, ?/–] Serotonin syndrome with MAOI, SSRI, serotonin agonists, linezolid; risk of QT prolongation w/ phenothiazines **Contra:** MAOI/thioridazine (wait 5 wk after D/C before starting MAOI) **Disp:** *Prozac:* Caps 10, 20, 40 mg; scored tabs 10 mg; SR cap 90 mg; soln 20 mg/5mL. *Sarafem:* Caps 10, 20 mg **SE:** Nausea, nervousness, weight loss, HA, insomnia **Interactions:** ↑ Effects w/ CNS depressants, MAOIs, EtOH, St. John's wort; ↑ effects OF alprazolam, BBs, carbamazepine, clozapine, cardiac glycosides, diazepam, dextromethorphan, loop diuretics, haloperidol, phenytoin, Li, ritonavir, thioridazine, tryptophan, warfarin, sympathomimetic drugs; ↓ effects w/ cyproheptadine; ↓ effects OF buspirone, statins **Labs:** ↑ LFTs, BUN, creatinine, urine albumin

Fluoxymesterone (Halotestin) [Hormone] Uses: Androgen-responsive metastatic *breast CA, hypogonadism* **Action:** ↓ Secretion of LH & FSH (feedback inhibition) **Dose:** *Breast CA:* 10–40 mg/d ÷ × 1–3 mo. *Hypogonadism:* 5–20 mg/d **Caution:** [X, ?/–] ↑ effect w/ anticoagulants, cyclosporine, insulin, lithium, narcotics **Contra:** Serious cardiac, liver, or kidney Dz; PRG **Disp:** Tabs 2, 5, 10 mg **SE:** Virilization, amenorrhea & menstrual irregularities, hirsutism, alopecia, acne, nausea, & cholestasis. *Hematologic tox:* Suppression of clotting factors II, V, VII, & X & polycythemia; ↑ libido, HA, & anxiety **Notes:** ↓ Total T₄ levels **Interactions:** ↑ Effects w/ narcotics, EtOH, echinacea; ↑ effects OF anticoagulants, cyclosporine, insulin, hypoglycemics, tacrolimus; ↓ effects w/ anticholinergics, barbiturates **Labs:** ↑ Creatinine, creatinine clearance; ↓ thyroxine-binding globulin, serum total T₄ **NIPE:** Radiographic studies of skeletal maturation (hand/wrist) q6mo in prepubertal children; monitor fluid retention

Fluphenazine (Prolixin, Permitil) [Antipsychotic/Phenothiazine] Uses: *Schizophrenia* **Action:** Phenothiazine antipsychotic; blocks postsynaptic mesolimbic dopaminergic brain receptors **Dose:** 0.5–10 mg/d in ÷ doses PO q6–8h, average maint 5 mg/d; or 1.25 mg IM, then 2.5–10 mg/d in ÷ doses q6–8h PRN; ↓ in elderly **Caution:** [C, ?/–] **Contra:** Severe CNS depression, coma, subcortical brain damage, blood dyscrasias, hepatic Dz, w/ caffeine, tannic acid, or pectin-containing products **Disp:** Tabs 1, 2.5, 5, 10 mg; elixir 2.5 mg/5 mL; inj 2.5 mg/mL; depot inj 25 mg/mL **SE:** Drowsiness, extrapyramidal effects **Notes:** Monitor LFTs; less sedative/hypotensive than chlorpromazine **Interactions:** ↑ Effects w/ antimalarials, BBs, CNS depressants, EtOH, kava kava; ↑ effects OF anticholinergics, BBs, nitrates; ↓ effects w/ antacids, caffeine, tobacco; ↓ effects OF anticonvulsants, guanethidine, levodopa, sympathomimetics **Labs:** False + urine PRG test; ↑ serum cholesterol, glucose, LFTs, ↓ uric acid **NIPE:** Photosensitivity—use sunscreen, urine may turn pink or red in color, ↑ risk of heatstroke in hot weather

Flurazepam (Dalmane) [C-IV] [Sedative/Hypnotic/Benzodiazepine] Uses: *Insomnia* **Action:** Benzodiazepine **Dose:** *Adults & Peds >15 y.* 15–30 mg PO qhs PRN; ↓ in elderly **Caution:** [X, ?/–] Elderly, low albumin, hepatic impair **Contra:** NA glaucoma; PRG **Disp:** Caps 15, 30 mg **SE:** "Hangover" due to accumulation of metabolites, apnea **Notes:** May cause dependency **Interactions:** ↑ CNS depression w/ antidepressants, antihistamines, opioids, EtOH; ↑ effects OF digoxin, phenytoin; ↑ effects w/ cimetidine, disulfiram, fluoxetine, isoniazid, ketoconazole, metoprolol, oral contraceptives, propranolol, SSRIs, valproic acid, chamomile, kava, passion flower, valerian; ↓ effects OF levodopa; ↓ effects w/ barbiturates, rifampin, theophylline, nicotine **Labs:** ↑ LFTs **NIPE:** ⊘ In pregnancy or lactation; use adequate contraception; ⊘ EtOH; ⊘ d/c abruptly with long-term use.

Flurbiprofen (Ansaid) [Analgesic/NSAID]   WARNING: May ↑ risk of cardiovascular events & GI bleeding Uses: *Arthritis* **Action:** NSAID **Dose:** 50–300 mg/d ÷ bid–qid, max 300 mg/d w/ food **Caution:** [B (D in 3rd tri), +]

Contra: PRG (3rd tri); aspirin allergy **Disp:** Tabs 50, 100 mg **SE:** Dizziness, GI upset, peptic ulcer Dz **Interactions:** ↑ Effects w/ amprenavir, anticonvulsants, azole antifungals, BBs, CNS depressants, cimetidine, ciprofloxin, clozapine, digoxin, disulfiram, diltiazem, INH, levodopa, macrolides, oral contraceptives, rifampin, ritonavir, SSRIs, valproic acid, verapamil, EtOH, grapefruit juice, kava kava, valerian; ↓ effects w/ aminophylline, carbamazepine, rifampin, rifabutin, theophylline; ? ↓ effects OF levodopa **Labs:** ↑ LFTs, false − urine glucose **NIPE:** ⊘ PRG, breast-feeding; take with food to ↓ GI upset

Flutamide (Eulexin) [Antineoplastic/Antiandrogen] WARN-ING: Liver failure & death reported. Measure LFT before, monthly, & periodically after; D/C immediately if ALT 2× upper limits of nl or jaundice develops **Uses:** Advanced *CAP* (in combo with LHRH agonists, eg, leuprolide or goserelin); with radiation & GnRH for localized CAP **Action:** Nonsteroidal antiandrogen **Dose:** 250 mg PO tid (750 mg total) **Caution:** [D, ?] **Contra:** Severe hepatic impair **Disp:** Caps 125 mg **SE:** Hot flashes, loss of libido, impotence, N/V/D, gynecomastia **Interactions:** ↑ Effects w/ anticoagulants **Labs:** ↑ LFTs (monitor), BUN **NIPE:** ⊘ EtOH; urine amber/yellow-green in color

Fluticasone, Nasal (Flonase) [Anti-inflammatory/Corticosteroid] Uses: *Seasonal allergic rhinitis* **Action:** Topical steroid **Dose:** *Adults & Adolescents.* Nasal: 2 sprays/nostril/d. *Peds 4–11 y.* Nasal: 1–2 sprays/nostril/d **Caution:** [C, M] **Contra:** Primary Rx of status asthmaticus **Disp:** Nasal spray 50 mcg/actuation **SE:** HA, dysphonia, oral candidiasis **Interactions:** ↑ Effects w/ ketoconazole **Labs:** ↑ Cholesterol **NIPE:** Clear nares of exudate before use

Fluticasone, Oral (Flovent, Flovent Rotadisk) [Anti-inflammatory/Corticosteroid] Uses: Chronic *asthma* **Action:** Topical steroid **Dose:** *Adults & Adolescents.* 2–4 puffs bid. *Peds 4–11 y.* 50 mcg bid **Caution:** [C, M] **Contra:** Primary Rx of status asthmaticus **Disp:** Met-dose inhal 44, 110, 220 mcg/activation; Rotadisk dry powder: 50, 100, 250 mcg/activation **SE:** HA, dysphonia, oral candidiasis **Notes:** Counsel on use of device **Interactions:** ↑ Effects w/ ketoconazole **Labs:** ↑ Cholesterol **NIPE:** Risk of thrush, rinse mouth after use; ⊘ & report exposure to measles & chickenpox

Fluticasone Propionate & Salmeterol Xinafoate (Advair Diskus) [Anti-inflammatory/Corticosteroid] Uses: *Maint therapy for asthma* **Action:** Corticosteroid w/ long-acting bronchodilator **Dose:** *Adults & Peds >12 y.* 1 inhal bid q 12 h **Caution:** [C, M] **Contra:** Not for acute attack or in conversion from PO steroids or acute asthma **Disp:** Met-dose inhal powder (fluticasone/salmeterol in mcg) 100/50, 250/50, 500/50 **SE:** Upper resp Infxn, pharyngitis, HA **Notes:** Combo of Flovent & Serevent; do not use with spacer, do not wash mouthpiece, do not exhale into device **Interactions:** ↑ Bronchospasm w/ BBs; ↑ hypokalemia W/ loop and thiazide diuretics; ↑ effects w/ ketoconazole, MAOIs, TCAs **Labs:** ↑ Cholesterol **NIPE:** ⊘ & report exposure to measles & chickenpox, rinse mouth after use

Fluvastatin (Lescol) [Antilipemic/HMG-CoA Reductase Inhibitor] Uses: *Atherosclerosis, primary hypercholesterolemia, hypertriglyceridemia* Action: HMG-CoA reductase inhibitor Dose: 20–80 mg PO qhs; ↓ w/ hepatic impair Caution: [X, –] Contra: Active liver Dz, ↑ LFTs, PRG, breast-feeding Disp: Caps 20, 40 mg; XL 80 mg SE: HA, dyspepsia, N/D, abdominal pain Interactions: ↑ Effects w/ azole antifungals, cimetidine, danazol, glyburide, macrolides, phenytoin, ritonavir, EtOH, grapefruit juice; ↑ effects OF diclofenac, glyburide, phenytoin, warfarin; ↓ effects w/ cholestyramine, colestipol, isradipine, rifampin Labs: ↑ LFTs, CPK, thyroid Fxn NIPE: Take hs, ↑ photosensitivity—use sunscreen

Fluvoxamine (Luvox) [Antidepressant/SSRI WARNING: Closely monitor for worsening depression or emergence of suicidality, particularly in ped pts Uses: *OCD* Action: SSRI Dose: Initial 50 mg single qhs dose, ↑ to 300 mg/d in ÷ doses; ↓ in elderly/hepatic impair, titrate slowly; ÷ doses > 100 mg Caution: [C, ?/–] Numerous interactions (MAOIs, phenothiazines, SSRIs, serotonin agonists) Contra: MAOI w/in 14 days Disp: Tabs 25, 50, 100 mg SE: HA, nausea, D, somnolence, insomnia Interactions: ↑ Effects w/ melatonin, MAOIs; ↑ effects OF BBs, benzodiazepines, methadone, carbamazepine, haloperidol, Li, phenytoin, TCAs, theophylline, warfarin, St. John's wort; ↑ risks of serotonin syndrome w/ buspirone, dexfenfluramine, fenfluramine, tramadol, nefazodone, sibutramine, tryptophan; ↓ effects w/ buspirone, cyproheptadine, tobacco; ↓ effects OF buspirone, HMG-CoA reductase inhibitors NIPE: ⊘ MAOIs for 14 d before start of drug; ⊘ EtOH

Folic Acid [Vitamin Supl] Uses: *Megaloblastic anemia; folate deficiency* Action: Dietary supl Dose: *Adults.* Supl 0.4 mg/d PO. *PRG:* 0.8 mg/d PO. *Folate deficiency:* 1 mg PO qd–tid. *Peds.* Supl 0.04–0.4 mg/24 h PO, IM, IV, or SQ. *Folate deficiency:* 0.5–1 mg/24 h PO, IM, IV, or SQ Caution: [A, +] Contra: Pernicious, aplastic, normocytic anemias Disp: Tabs 0.4, 0.8, 1 mg; inj 5 mg/mL SE: Well tolerated Notes: OK for all women of childbearing age; ↓ fetal neural tube defects by 50%; no effect on normocytic anemias Interactions: ↓ Effects w/ anticonvulsants, sulfasalazine, aminosalicylic acid, chloramphenicol, MTX, oral contraceptives, pyrimethamine, triamterene, trimethoprim; ↓ effects OF phenobarbital, phenytoin

Fondaparinux (Arixtra) [Anticoagulant] WARNING: When epidural/spinal anesthesia or spinal puncture is used, pts anticoagulated or scheduled to be anticoagulated with LMW heparins, heparinoids, or fondaparinux for prevention of thromboembolic complications are at risk for epidural or spinal hematoma, which can result in long-term or permanent paralysis Uses: *DVT prophylaxis* in hip fracture or replacement or knee replacement; w/DVT or PE in combo w/ warfarin Action: Synthetic, specific inhibitor of activated factor X; a LMW heparin Dose: 2.5 mg SQ qd, up to 5–9 d; start at least 6 h postop Caution: [B, ?] ↑ bleeding risk w/ anticoagulants, antiplatelets, drotrecogin alfa, NSAIDs

Contra: Wt <50 kg, CrCl <30 mL/min, active bleeding, bacterial endocarditis, thrombocytopenia associated w/ antiplatelet Ab **Disp:** Prefilled syringes 2.5/0.5, 10/0.8, 5/0.4, 7.5/0.6 mg/mL **SE:** Thrombocytopenia, anemia, fever, nausea **Notes:** D/C if plts <100,000 mm³; only give SQ; may monitor anti-factor Xa levels **Interactions:** ↑ Effects w/ anticoagulants, cephalosporins, NSAIDs, penicillins, salicylates **Labs:** ↑ LFTs

Formoterol (Foradil Aerolizer) [Bronchodilator/Beta-2 Adrenergic Agonist]

Uses: Maint Rx of *asthma & prevention of bronchospasm* with reversible obstructive airway Dz; exercise-induced bronchospasm **Action:** Long-acting β₂-adrenergic agonist, bronchodilator **Dose:** *Adults & Peds* >5 y. Asthma: Inhale one 12-mcg cap q12h w/ aerolizer, 24 mcg/d max. *Adults & Peds > 12 y.* Exercise-induced bronchospasm: 1 inhal 12-mcg cap 15 min before exercise **Caution:** [C, ?] **Contra:** Need for acute bronchodilation; use w/in 2 wk of MAOI **Disp:** 12-mcg powder for inhal (as caps) for use in Aerolizer **SE:** Paradoxical bronchospasm; URI, pharyngitis, back pain **Notes:** Do not swallow caps—for use only with inhaler; do not start with worsening or acutely deteriorating asthma **Interactions:** ↑ Effects w/ adrenergics; ↑ effects OF BBs; ↑ risk of hypokalemia w/ corticosteroids, diuretics, xanthines; ↑ risk of arrhythmias w/ MAOIs, TCAs

Fosamprenavir (Lexiva) [Antiretroviral/Protease Inhibitor]

WARNING: Do **not** use with severe liver dysfunction, reduce dose with mild–moderate liver impair (fosamprenavir 700 mg bid w/o ritonavir) **Uses:** HIV Infxn **Action:** Protease inhibitor **Dose:** 1400 mg bid w/o ritonavir; if w/ritonavir, fosamprenavir 1400 mg + ritonavir 200 mg qd or fosamprenavir 700 mg + ritonavir 100 mg bid. If w/ efavirenz & ritonavir: fosamprenavir 1400 mg + ritonavir 300 mg qd **Caution:** [C, ?/–]; **Contra:** w/ergot alkaloids, midazolam, triazolam, or pimozide; avoid if sulfa allergy **Disp:** Tabs 700 mg **SE:** N/V/D, HA, fatigue, rash **Notes:** Numerous drug interactions because of hepatic metabolism **Interactions:** ↑ Effects w/ indinavir, nelfinavir; ↑ effects OF antiarrhythmics, amitriptyline, atorvastatin, benzodiazepine, bepridil, CCBs, cyclosporine, ergotamine, ethinyl estradiol, imipramine, itraconazole, ketoconazole, midazolam, norethindrone, rapamycin, rifabutin, sildenafil, tacrolimus, TCA, vardenafil, warfarin; ↓ effects w/ antacids, carbamazepine, dexamethasone, didanosine, efavirenz, H₂-receptor antagonists, nevirapine, phenobarbital, phenytoin, proton pump inhibitors, rifampin St. John's wort; ↓ effects OF methadone **Labs:** ↑ ALT, AST, triglycerides, glucose, lipase **NIPE:** Take w/o regard to food, use barrier contraception, monitor for opportunistic infection, inform about fat redistribution/accumulation

Foscarnet (Foscavir) [Antiviral]

Uses: *CMV retinitis*; acyclovir-resistant *herpes Infxns* **Action:** ↓ Viral DNA polymerase & RT **Dose:** *CMV retinitis: Induction:* 60 mg/kg IV q8h or 100 mg/kg q12h × 14–21 d. *Maint:* 90–120 mg/kg IV q24h (Monday–Friday). *Acyclovir-resistant HSV induction:* 40 mg/kg IV q8–12h × 14–21 d; use central line; ↓ with renal impair **Caution:** [C, –] ↑ Sz potential w/ fluoroquinolones; avoid nephrotoxic Rx (cyclosporine, aminoglycosides, ampho B, protease inhibitors) **Contra:** Significant renal impair (CrCl <0.4 mL/min/kg) **Disp:** Inj 24 mg/mL **SE:** Nephrotox, electrolyte abnormalities **Notes:** Sodium loading (500 mL 0.9% NaCl) before & after helps minimize nephrotox; monitor ionized calcium; **Interactions:** ↑ Risks of Sz w/ quinolines; ↑ risks of nephrotoxicity w/ aminoglycosides, amphotericin B, didanosine, pentamidine, vancomycin **Labs:** ↑ LFTs, CPK, BUN, SCr; ↓ Hmg, Hct, Ca^{2+}, Mg^{2+}, K^+, P **NIPE:** ↑ Fluids; perioral tingling, extremity numbness & paresthesia indicates electrolyte imbalance

Fosfomycin (Monurol) [Antibiotic] **Uses:** *Uncomplicated UTI* **Action:** ↓ bacterial cell wall synthesis. *Spectrum:* Gram(+) (staph, pneumococci); gram(–) (*E. coli, Enterococcus, Salmonella, Shigella, H. influenzae, Neisseria,* indole-negative *Proteus, Providencia*); *B. fragilis* & anaerobic gram(–) cocci are resistant **Dose:** 3 g PO dissolved in 90–120 mL of H_2O single dose; ↓ in renal impair **Caution:** [B, ?] ↓ absorption w/ antacids/Ca salts **Contra:** Component sensitivity **Disp:** Granule packets 3 g **SE:** HA, GI upset **Notes:** May take 2–3 d for Sxs to improve **Interactions:** ↓ Effects w/ antacids, metoclopramide **Labs:** ↑ LFTs; ↓ Hmg, Hct **NIPE:** May take w/o regard to food

Fosinopril (Monopril) [Antihypertensive/ACEI] **Uses:** *HTN, CHF,* DN **Action:** ACE inhibitor **Dose:** 10 mg/d PO initial; max 40 mg/d PO; ↓ in elderly; ↓ in renal impair **Caution:** [D, +] ↑ K^+ w/ K^+ suppls, ARBs, K^+-sparing diuretics; ↑ renal AE w/ NSAIDs, diuretics, hypovolemia **Contra:** Hereditary/idiopathic angioedema or angioedema with ACE inhibitor, bilateral renal artery stenosis **Disp:** Tabs 10, 20, 40 mg **SE:** Cough, dizziness, angioedema, ↑ K^+ **Interactions:** ↑ Effects w/ antihypertensives, diuretics; ↑ effects OF Li; ↑ risk of hyperkalemia w/ K-sparing diuretics, salt substitutes; ↑ cough w/ capsaicin; ↓ effects w/ antacids, ASA, NSAIDs **Labs:** ↓ Hmg, Hct **NIPE:** ⊘ PRG, breast-feeding

Fosphenytoin (Cerebyx) [Anticonvulsant/Hydantoin] **Uses:** *Status epilepticus* **Action:** ↓ Sz spread in motor cortex **Dose:** Dose as phenytoin equivalents (PE). **Load:** 15–20 mg PE/kg. **Maint:** 4–6 mg PE/kg/d; ↓ dosage, monitor levels in hepatic impair **Caution:** [D, +] May ↑ phenobarbital **Contra:** Sinus bradycardia, SA block, 2nd-/3rd-degree AV block, Adams–Stokes syndrome, rash during Rx **Disp:** Inj 75 mg/mL **SE:** ↓ BP, dizziness, ataxia, pruritus, nystagmus **Notes:** 15 min to convert fosphenytoin to phenytoin; admin <150 mg PE/min to prevent ↓ BP; administer with BP monitoring **Interactions:** ↑ Effects w/ amiodarone, chloramphenicol, cimetidine, diazepam, disulfiram, estrogens, INH, omeprazole, phenothiazines, salicylates, sulfonamides, tolbutamide; ↓ effects w/ TCAs, antituberculosis drugs, carbamazepine, EtOH, nutritional suppls, ginkgo biloba; ↓ effects OF anticoagulants, corticosteroids, digitoxin, doxycycline, oral contraceptives, folic acid, Ca, vitamin D, rifampin, quinidine, theophylline **Labs:** ↑ Serum glucose, alkaline phosphatase; ↓ serum thyroxine, Ca **NIPE:** Breast-feeding, for short-term use

Frovatriptan (Frova) [Migraine Suppressant/5 HT Agonist] See Table 11

Fulvestrant (Faslodex) [Antineoplastic/Antiestrogen] Uses: Hormone receptor(+) metastatic *breast CA* in postmenopausal women with Dz progression following antiestrogen therapy **Action:** Estrogen receptor antagonist **Dose:** 250 mg IM monthly, either a single 5-mL inj or two concurrent 2.5-mL IM inj into buttocks **Caution:** [X, ?/–] ↑ effects w/ CYP3A4 inhibitors (Table 13) w/ hepatic impair **Contra:** PRG **Disp:** Prefilled syringes 50 mg/mL (single 5 mL, dual 2.5 mL) **SE:** N/V/D, constipation, abdominal pain, HA, back pain, hot flushes, pharyngitis, inj site Rxns **Notes:** Only use IM **Interactions:** ↑ Risk of bleeding w/ anticoagulants **NIPE:** ⊘ PRG, breast-feeding; use barrier contraception

Furosemide (Lasix) [Antihypertensive/Loop Diuretic] Uses: *CHF, HTN, edema,* ascites **Action:** Loop diuretic; ↓ Na & Cl reabsorption in ascending loop of Henle & distal tubule **Dose:** *Adults.* 20–80 mg PO or IV bid. *Peds.* 1 mg/kg/dose IV q6–12h; 2 mg/kg/dose PO q12–24h (max 6 mg/kg/dose) **Caution:** [C, +] ↓ K⁺, ↑ risk of digoxin tox; ↑ risk of ototox w/ aminoglycosides, cis-platinum (esp in renal dysfunction) **Contra:** Allergy to sulfonylureas; anuria; hepatic coma/severe electrolyte depletion **Disp:** Tabs 20, 40, 80 mg; soln 10 mg/mL, 40 mg/5 mL; inj 10 mg/mL **SE:** ↓ BP, hyperglycemia, ↓ K⁺ **Notes:** Monitor electrolytes, renal Fxn; high doses IV may cause ototox **Interactions:** ↑ Nephrotoxic effects w/ cephalosporins; ↑ ototoxicity w/ aminoglycosides, cis-platin; ↑ risk of hypokalemia w/ antihypertensives, carbenoxolone, corticosteroids, digitalis glycosides, terbutaline; ↓ effects w/ barbiturates, cholestyramine, colestipol, NSAIDs, phenytoin, dandelion, ginseng; ↓ effects OF hypoglycemics **Labs:** ↑ BUN, serum amylase, cholesterol, glucose, triglycerides, uric acid, ↓ serum K⁺, Na⁺, Ca²⁺, Mg²⁺ **NIPE:** Risk of photosensitivity—use sunscreen

Gabapentin (Neurontin) [Anticonvulsant] Uses: Adjunct therapy in the Rx of *partial Szs*; postherpetic neuralgia (PHN)*; chronic pain syndromes **Action:** Anticonvulsant **Dose:** *Anticonvulsant:* 300–1200 mg PO tid (max 3600 mg/d). *PHN:* 300 mg day 1, 300 mg bid day 2, 300 mg tid day 3, titrate (1800–3600 mg/d); ↓ in renal impair **Caution:** [C, ?] **Contra:** Component sensitivity **Disp:** Caps 100, 300, 400, 800 mg; soln 250 mg/5mL; tab 600, 800 mg **SE:** Somnolence, dizziness, ataxia, fatigue **Notes:** Not necessary to monitor levels **Interactions:** ↑ Effects w/ cimetidine, CNS depressants; ↑ effects OF phenytoin; ↓ effects w/ antacids, ginkgo biloba **Labs:** False + urinary protein **NIPE:** Take w/o regard to food

Galantamine (Reminyl) [Cholinesterase Inhibitor] Uses: *Alzheimer Dz* **Action:** Acetylcholinesterase inhibitor **Dose:** 4 mg PO bid, ↑ to 8 mg PO bid after 4 wk; may ↑ to 12 mg bid in 4 wk **Caution:** [B, ?] ↑ effect w/ succinylcholine, amiodarone, diltiazem, verapamil, NSAIDs, digoxin; ↓ effect w/ anticholinergics **Contra:** Severe renal/hepatic impair **Disp:** Tabs 4, 8, 12 mg; soln 4 mg/mL **SE:** GI disturbances, weight loss, sleep disturbances, dizziness, HA **Notes:** Caution w/ urinary outflow obstruction, Parkinson Dz, severe asthma/COPD, severe heart Dz or ↓ BP **Interactions:** ↑ Effects w/ amitriptyline, cimetidine, erythromycin, fluoxetine, fluvoxamine, ketoconazole, paroxetine, quinidine **Labs:** ↑ Alkaline phosphatase **NIPE:** ↑ Dosage q4wk, if DC several days then restart at lowest dose; take w/ food and maintain adequate fluid intake

Gallium Nitrate (Ganite) [Hormone] Uses: *↑ Ca^{2+} of malignancy*; bladder CA **Action:** ↓ bone resorption of Ca^{2+} **Dose:** ↑ Ca^{2+}: 200 mg/m² × 5 d. *CA:* 350 mg/m² cont inf × 5 d to 700 mg/m² rapid IV inf q2wk in antineoplastic settings (Per protocols) **Caution:** [C, ?] Do not give with live vaccines or rotavirus vaccine **Contra:** SCr >2.5 mg/dL **Disp:** Inj 25 mg/mL **SE:** Renal insuff, ↓ Ca^{2+}, hypophosphatemia, ↓ bicarbonate, <1% acute optic neuritis **Notes:** Bladder CA: use in combo with vinblastine & ifosamide **Interactions:** ↑ Risks of nephrotoxicity w/ amphotericin B, aminoglycosides, vancomycin **NIPE:** Monitor SCr, adequate fluids

Ganciclovir (Cytovene, Vitrasert) [Antiviral] Uses: *Rx & prevent CMV retinitis, prevent CMV Dz* in transplant recipients **Action:** ↓ viral DNA synthesis **Dose:** *Adults & Peds.* IV: 5 mg/kg IV q12h for 14–21 d, then maint 5 mg/kg/d IV × 7 d/wk or 6 mg/kg/d IV × 5 d/wk. *Ocular implant:* One implant q5–8mo. *Adults.* PO: following induction, 1000 mg PO tid. *Prevention:* 1000 mg PO tid; with food; ↓ in renal impair **Caution:** [C, –] ↑ effect w/ immunosuppressives, imipenem/cilastatin, zidovudine, didanosine, other nephrotoxic Rx **Contra:** ANC <500, plt <25,000), intravitreal implant **Disp:** Caps 250, 500 mg; inj 500 mg; ocular implant 4.5 mg **SE:** Granulocytopenia & thrombocytopenia, fever, rash, GI upset **Notes:** Not a cure for CMV; handle inj w/ cytotox cautions; implant confers no systemic benefit **Interactions:** ↑ Effects w/ cytotoxic drugs, immunosuppressive drugs, probenecid; ↑ risks of nephrotoxicity w/ amphotericin B, cyclosporine; ↑ effects w/ didanosine **Labs:** ↑ LFTs; ↓ blood glucose **NIPE:** Take w/ food, ⊘ PRG, breast-feeding, EtOH, NSAIDs; photosensitivity—use sunscreen

Gatifloxacin (Tequin, Zymar Ophthalmic) [Antibiotic/Fluoroquinolone] Uses: *Bronchitis, sinusitis, community-acquired pneumonia, UTI, uncomplicated skin/soft tissue Infxn* **Action:** Quinolone antibiotic, ↓ DNA-gyrase. *Spectrum:* Gram(+) (except MRSA, *Listeria*), gram(–) (not *Pseudomonas*), atypicals, some anaerobes (*Clostridium*, not *C. difficile*) **Dose:** 400 mg/d PO or IV; *Ophth:* Day 1 & 2 one gt q2h in eye while awake (8 ×/day max) day 3–7, one gt 4×d while awake; (↓ in renal impair) **Caution:** [C, M] **Contra:** Prolonged QT interval, w/ other Rx that prolong QT interval (Class Ia & III antiarrhythmics, erythromycin, antipsychotics, TCA); uncorrected ↓ K⁺; children < 18 y or in PRG/lactating women **Disp:** Oral susp 200 mg/5 mL; tabs 200, 400 mg; inj 10 mg/mL; premixed infuse D₅W 200 mg, 400 mg; ophth soln 0.3% **SE:** Prolonged QT interval, HA, N/D, tendon rupture, photosensitivity **Notes:** Reliable activity against *S. pneumoniae;* **Interactions:** ↑ Effects w/ antiarrhythmics, antipsychotics, cimetidine, erythromycin, loop diuretics, probenecid, TCAs; ↑ CNS effects and Szs w/ NSAIDs; ↑ effects OF digoxin, warfarin; ↓ effects w/ antacids, didanosine, H₂ antagonists, proton pump inhibitors, Fe **NIPE:** Take 4 h after antacids containing Mg, Al, Fe, or Zn; drink plenty of fluids, avoid direct sunlight

Gefitinib (Iressa) [Antineoplastic] Uses: *Rx locally advanced or metastatic non-small-cell lung CA after failure of both platinum-based & docetaxel chemotherapies* Action: ↓ intracellular phosphorylation of tyrosine kinases Dose: 250 mg/d PO Caution: [D, –] Disp: Tabs 250 mg SE: D, rash, acne, dry skin, N/V, interstitial lung Dz, ↑ liver transaminases Notes: Follow LFTs Interactions: ↑ effects w/ ketoconazole, itraconazole, and other CYP3A4 inhibitors; ↑ risk of bleeding w/ warfarin; ↓ effects w/ cimetidine, ranitidine and other H2 receptor antagonists; ↓ effects w/ phenytoin, rifampin, and other CYP3A4 inducers Labs: ↑ ALT, AST, PT NIPE: ⊘ PRG or breast-feeding; take w/o regard to food; ↑ risk of corneal erosion/ulcer

Gemcitabine (Gemzar) [Antineoplastic/Nucleoside Analog] Uses: *Pancreatic CA, brain mets, NSCLC,* gastric CA Action: Antimetabolite; ↓ ribonucleotide reductase; produces false nucleotide base-inhibiting DNA synthesis Dose: 1000 mg/m² over 30 min–1 h IV inf/wk × 3–4 wk or 6–8 wk; dose modifications based on hematologic Fxn (Per protocol) Caution: [D, ?/–] Contra: PRG Disp: Inj 200 mg, 1 g SE: Myelosuppression, N/V/D, drug fever, skin rash Notes: Reconstituted soln concn 38 mg/mL (not 40 mg/mL as earlier labeling); monitor hepatic/renal Fxn prior & during Rx Interactions: ↑ Bone marrow depression w/ radiation therapy, antineoplastic drugs; ↓ live virus vaccines Labs: ↑ LFTs, BUN, SCr NIPE: ⊘ EtOH, NSAIDs, immunizations, PRG?

Gemfibrozil (Lopid) [Antilipemic/Fibric Acid Derivative] Uses: *Hypertriglyceridemia, coronary heart Dz* Action: Fibric acid Dose: 1200 mg/d PO ÷ bid 30 min ac AM & PM Caution: [C, ?] Enhances the effect of warfarin, sulfonylureas; ↑ risk of rhabdomyopathy w/ HMG-CoA reductase inhibitors; ↓ effects w/ cyclosporine Contra: Renal/hepatic impair (SCr >2.0 mg/dL), gallbladder Dz, primary biliary cirrhosis Disp: Tabs 600 mg SE: Cholelithiasis, GI upset Notes: Avoid concurrent use with the HMG-CoA reductase inhibitors; monitor LFTs & serum lipids Interactions: ↑ Effects OF anticoagulants, sulfonylureas; ↓ effects w/ rifampin; ↓ effects OF cyclosporine Labs: ↑ LFTs, + ANA, ↓ Hmg, Hct, WBCs

Gemifloxacin (Factive) [Antibiotic/Fluoroquinolone] Uses: Community-acquired pneumonia, acute exacerbation of chronic bronchitis Action: ↓ DNA gyrase & topoisomerase IV; *Spectrum:* S. *pneumoniae* (including MDR strains), *H. influenzae, H. parainfluenzae, M. catarrhalis, M. pneumoniae, Chlamydia pneumoniae, K. pneumoniae* Dose: 320 mg PO qd; CrCl < 40 mL/min: 160 mg PO qd Caution: [C, ?/–]; children < 18 y; Hx of ↑ QTc interval, electrolyte disorders, w/ Class IA/III antiarrhythmics, erythromycin, TCAs, antipsychotics Contra: Fluoroquinolone allergy Disp: Tab 320 mg SE: Rash, N/V/D, abdominal pain, dizziness, xerostomia, arthralgia, allergy/anaphylactic reactions, peripheral neuropathy, tendon rupture Notes: Take 3 h before or 2 h after Al/Mg-containing antacids, Fe, Z or other metal cations Interactions: ↑ risk of prolonged QT interval w/ amiodarone, antipsychotics, erythromycin, procainamide, quinidine, sotalol, TCAs; ↑ effect OF warfarin; ↑ effects w/ probenecid; ↓ effects w/ antacids, didanosine, iron, sucralfate **Labs:** ↑ BUN, creatinine, CPK, K+ LFTs; ↓ albumin, protein, sodium **NIPE:** ↑ fluid intake; d/c if c/o tenderness/pain in muscles/tendons; ⊘ excessive sunlight exposure—use sunscreen

Gemtuzumab Ozogamicin (Mylotarg) [Chemotherapeutic Agent]

WARNING: Can cause severe allergic Rxns & other infusion related reactions including severe pulmonary events; hepatotox, including severe hepatic venoocclusive Dz (VOD) reported **Uses:** *Relapsed CD33+ AML in pts > 60 who are poor candidates for chemo* **Action:** MoAb linked to calicheamicin; selective for myeloid cells **Dose:** Per protocol **Caution:** [D,?/–] **Contra:** Component sensitivity **Disp:** 5 mg/20 mL vial **SE:** Myelosuppression, allergy (including anaphylaxis), inf Rxns (chills, fever, N/V, HA), pulmonary events, hepatotox **Notes:** Only use as single agent, not in combo w/ other agents; premedicate (diphenhydramine & acetaminophen) **Interactions:** ↑ Risk for allergic or hypersensitive reaction and thrombocytopenia w/ abciximab; ↓ effects w/ abciximab **Labs:** Monitor before & after therapy CBC, ALT, AST, electrolytes **NIPE:** Monitor for bleeding, myelosuppression, BP; ⊘ ASA, PRG, breast-feeding

Gentamicin (Garamycin, G-Mycitin, others) [Antibiotic/Aminoglycoside]

Uses: *Serious Infxns* caused by *Pseudomonas, Proteus, E. coli, Klebsiella, Enterobacter,* & *Serratia* & initial Rx of gram(–) sepsis **Action:** Bactericidal; ↓ protein synthesis. *Spectrum:* Synergy w/ PCNs; gram(–) (not *Neisseria, Legionella, Acinetobacter*) **Dose:** *Adults.* 3–7 mg/kg/24h IV ÷ q8–24h. *Synergy:* 1 mg/kg q8h. *Peds.* Infants <7 d <1200 g: 2.5 mg/kg/dose q18–24h. *Infants >1200 g:* 2.5 mg/kg/dose q12–18h. *Infants >7 d:* 2.5 mg/kg/dose IV q8–12h. *Children:* 2.5 mg/kg/d IV q8h; ↓ with renal insuff **Caution:** [C, +/–] Avoid other nephrotoxic Rxs **Contra:** Aminoglycoside sensitivity **Disp:** Premixed infus 40, 60, 70, 80, 90, 100, 120 mg; ADD-Vantage inj vials 10 mg/mL; inj 40 mg/mL; IT preservative-free 2 mg/mL **SE:** Nephrotox/ototox/neurotox **Notes:** Follow CrCl, SCr & serum conc for dose adjustments (Table 2); once daily dosing popular; follow; use IBW to dose (use adjusted if obese >30% IBW) **Interactions:** ↑ Ototoxicity, neurotoxicity, nephrotoxicity w/ aminoglycosides, amphotericin B, cephalosporins, loop diuretics, penicillins; ↑ effects w/ NSAIDs; ↓ effects w/ carbenicillin; **Labs:** False ↑ AST, urine protein; ↑ urine amino acids **NIPE:** Photosensitivity—use sunscreen

Gentamicin & Prednisolone, Ophthalmic (Pred-G Ophthalmic) [Antibiotic/Anti-inflammatory]

Uses: *Steroid-responsive ocular & conjunctival Infxns* sensitive to gentamicin **Action:** Bactericidal; ↓ protein synthesis plus anti-inflammatory. *Spectrum: Staphylococcus, E. coli, H. influenzae, Klebsiella, Neisseria, Pseudomonas, Proteus,* & *Serratia* sp **Dose:** Oint. ½ in. in conjunctival sac daily-tid. *Susp:* 1 gt bid–qid, up to 1 gt/h for severe Infxns **Contra:** Aminoglycoside sensitivity **Caution:** [C, ?] **Disp:** Oint, ophth: Prednisolone acetate 0.6% & gentamicin sulfate 0.3% (3.5 g). Susp, ophth: Prednisolone acetate 1% & gentamicin sulfate 0.3% (2, 5, 10 mL) **SE:** Local irritation; See Gentamicin **Additional NIPE:** Systemic effects w/ long-term use

Gentamicin, Ophthalmic (Garamycin, Genoptic, Gentacidin, Gentak, others) [Antibiotic] **Uses:** *Conjunctival Infxns* **Action:** Bactericidal; ↓ protein synthesis **Dose:** *Oint:* Apply ½ in. bid–tid. *Soln:* 1–2 gtt q2–4h, up to 2 gtt/h for severe Infxn **Caution:** [C, ?] **Contra:** Aminoglycoside sensitivity **Disp:** Soln & oint 0.3% **SE:** Local irritation **Notes:** Do not use other eye drops w/in 5–10 mins; do not touch dropper to eye; **NIPE:** ⊘ Other eye drops for 10 min after administering this drug

Gentamicin, Topical (Garamycin, G-Mycitin) [Antibiotic] **Uses:** *Skin Infxns* caused by susceptible organisms **Action:** Bactericidal; ↓ protein synthesis **Dose:** *Adults & Peds >1 y.* Apply tid–qid **Caution:** [C, ?] **Contra:** Aminoglycoside sensitivity **Disp:** Cream & oint 0.1% **SE:** Irritation **NIPE:** ⊘ Apply to large denuded areas

Glimepiride (Amaryl) [Hypoglycemic/Sulfonylurea] **Uses:** *Type 2 DM* **Action:** Sulfonylurea; ↑ pancreatic insulin release; ↑ peripheral insulin sensitivity; ↓ hepatic glucose output & production **Dose:** 1–4 mg/d, max 8 mg **Caution:** [C, –] **Contra:** DKA **Disp:** Tabs 1, 2, 4 mg **SE:** HA, nausea, hypoglycemia **Notes:** Give w/ 1st meal of day **Interactions:** ↑ Effects w/ ACEIs, adrenergic antagonists, BBs, chloramphenicol, MAOIs, NSAIDs, probenecid, salicylates, sulfonamides, warfarin, ginseng, garlic; ↓ effects w/ corticosteroids, estrogens, INH, oral contraceptives, nicotinic acid, phenytoin, sympathomimetics, thiazide diuretics, thyroid hormones **NIPE:** Antabuse-like effect w/ EtOH

Glipizide (Glucotrol, Glucotrol XL) [Hypoglycemic/Sulfonylurea] **Uses:** *Type 2 DM* **Action:** Sulfonylurea; ↑ pancreatic insulin release; ↑ peripheral insulin sensitivity; ↓ hepatic glucose output & production; ↓ intestinal absorption of glucose **Dose:** 5 mg initial, ↑ by 2.5–5 mg/d, max 40 mg/d; XL max 20 mg; 30 min ac; hold if pt NPO **Caution:** [C, ?/–] Severe liver Dz **Contra:** DKA, Type 1 DM, sensitivity to sulfonamides **Disp:** Tabs 5, 10 mg; XL tabs 2.5, 5, 10 mg **SE:** HA, anorexia, N/V/D, constipation, fullness, rash, urticaria, photosensitivity **Notes:** Counsel pt about diabetes management; wait several days before adjusting dose; monitor glucose **Interactions:** ↑ Effects w/ azole antifungals, anabolic steroids, chloramphenicol, cimetidine, clofibrate, MAOIs, NSAIDs, probenecid, salicylates, sulfonamides, TCAs, warfarin, celery, coriander, dandelion root, fenugreek, ginseng, garlic, juniper berries; ↓ effects w/ amphetamines, corticosteroids, epinephrine, estrogens, glucocorticoids, oral contraceptives, phenytoin, rifampin, sympathomimetics, thiazide diuretics, thyroid hormones, tobacco **LABS:** ↑ BUN, Cr, AST, lipids; ↓ glucose, hmg, wbc, platelets **NIPE:** Antabuse-like effect w/ EtOH; give 30 min before meal; hold dose if pt NPO

Glucagon [Antihypoglycemic/Hormone] **Uses:** Severe *hypoglycemic* Rxns in DM with sufficient liver glycogen stores or β-blocker OD **Action:** Accelerates liver gluconeogenesis **Dose:** *Adults.* 0.5–1 mg SQ, IM, or IV;

repeat in 20 min PRN. *β-Blocker OD:* 3–10 mg IV; repeat in 10 min PRN; ma[y] give cont infus 1–5 mg/h. **Peds.** Neonates: 0.3 mg/kg/dose SQ, IM, or IV q4h PRN *Children:* 0.025–0.1 mg/kg/dose SQ, IM, or IV; repeat in 20 min PRN **Caution** [B, M] **Contra:** Known pheochromocytoma **Disp:** Inj 1 mg **SE:** N/V, ↓ BP **Notes** Administration of glucose IV necessary; ineffective in starvation, adrenal insuff, o[r] chronic hypoglycemia **Interactions:** ↑ Effect w/ epinephrine, phenytoin; ↑ effect OF anticoagulants **Labs:** ↓ Serum K⁺; **NIPE:** Response w/in 20 min after inj

Glyburide (DiaBeta, Micronase, Glynase) [Hypoglycemic, Sulfonylurea] Uses: *Type 2 DM* Action: Sulfonylurea; ↑ pancreatic in[-] sulin release; ↑ peripheral insulin sensitivity; ↓ hepatic glucose output & produc[-] tion; ↓ intestinal absorption of glucose **Dose:** 1.25–10 mg qd–bid, max 20 mg/[d] *Micronized:* 0.75–6 mg qd–bid, max 12 mg/d **Caution:** [C, ?] Renal impair **Con**[-] **tra:** DKA, Type I DM **Disp:** Tabs 1.25, 2.5, 5 mg; micronized tabs 1.5, 3, 6 m[g] **SE:** HA, hypoglycemia **Notes:** Not OK for CrCl <50 mL/min; hold dose if pt NP[O] **Interactions:** ↑ Effects w/ anticoagulants, anabolic steroids, BBs, chlorampheni[-] col, cimetidine, clofibrate, MAOIs, NSAIDs, probenecid, salicylates, sulfon[-] amides, TCAs, EtOH, celery, coriander, dandelion root, fenugreek, ginseng, garli[c] juniper berries; ↓ effects w/ amphetamines, corticosteroids, baclofen, epinephrin[e] glucocorticoids, oral contraceptives, phenytoin, rifampin, sympathomimetics, thi[-] azide diuretics, thyroid hormones, tobacco **Labs:** False ↑ urine protein **NIPE**[:] Antabuse-like effect w/ EtOH

Glyburide/Metformin (Glucovance) [Hypoglycemic/Sul[-] fonylurea & Biguanide] Uses: *Type 2 DM* Action: Sulfonylurea: ↑ Pancreatic insulin release. *Metformin:* ↑ Peripheral insulin sensitivity; ↓ hepati[c] glucose output & production; ↓ intestinal absorption of glucose **Dose:** 1st lin[e] (naive pts), 1.25/250 mg PO daily–bid; 2nd line, 2.5/500 mg or 5/500 mg bid (ma[x] 20/2000 mg); take w/ meals, ↑ dose gradually hold prior to & 48 h after ionic con[-] trast media **Caution:** [C, –] **Contra:** SCr >1.4 in females or >1.5 in males; hypox[-] emic conditions (CHF, sepsis, recent MI); alcoholism; metabolic acidosis; liver D[z] **Disp:** Tabs 1.25/250 mg, 2.5/500 mg, 5/500 mg **SE:** HA, hypoglycemia, lactic aci[-] dosis, anorexia, N/V, rash **Notes:** Avoid EtOH; hold dose if NPO; monitor folat[e] levels for megaloblastic anemia; See Glyburide **Additional Interactions:** ↑ Ef[-] fects w/ amiloride, ciprofloxacin cimetidine, digoxin, miconazole, morphine nifedipine, procainamide, quinidine, quinine, ranitidine, triamterene, trimethoprim vancomycin; ↓ effects w/ CCBs, INH, phenothiazines

Glycerin Suppository [Laxative] Uses: *Constipation* Action: Hyper osmolar laxative **Dose:** *Adults.* 1 adult supp PR PRN. **Peds.** 1 infant supp P[R] daily–bid PRN **Caution:** [C, ?] **Disp:** Supp (adult, infant); liq 4 mL/applicatorful **SE**[:] Can cause D **Interactions:** ↑ Effects w/ diuretics **Labs:** ↑ Serum triglycerides, phos[-] phatidylglycerol in amniotic fluid; ↓ serum Ca **NIPE:** Insert and retain for 15 min

Gonadorelin (Lutrepulse) [Gonadotropin-releasing Hor[-] mone] Uses: *Primary hypothalamic amenorrhea* Action: Stimulates pitu[-] itary release of LH & FSH **Dose:** 5 mcg IV q 90 min × 21 d using Lutrepulse pump kit **Caution:** [B, M] ↑ levels w/ androgens, estrogens, progestins, glucocorticoids, spironolactone, levodopa; ↓ levels with OCP, digoxin, dopamine antagonists **Contra:** Any condition exacerbated by PRG or reproductive hormones, ovarian cysts, causes of anovulation other than hypothalamic, hormonally dependent tumor **Disp:** Inj 100 mcg **SE:** Risk of multiple pregnancies; inj site pain **Notes:** Monitor LH, FSH **Interactions:** ↑ Effects w/ androgens, estrogens, glucocorticoids, levodopa, progestins, spironolactone; ↓ effects w/ digoxin, dopamine antagonists, oral contraceptives, phenothiazines

Goserelin (Zoladex) [Antineoplastic/Gonadotropin-releasing Hormone]

Uses: Advanced *CAP* & w/ radiation for localized high-risk CAP, *endometriosis, breast CA* **Action:** LHRH agonist, transient ↑ then ↓ in LH, resulting in ↓ testosterone **Dose:** 3.6 mg SQ (implant) q 28d or 10.8 mg SQ q3mo; usually into lower abdominal wall **Caution:** [X, –] **Contra:** PRG, breast-feeding, 10.8-mg implant not for women **Disp:** SQ implant 3.6 (1 mo), 10.8 (3 mo) **SE:** Hot flashes, ↓ libido, gynecomastia, & transient exacerbation of CA-related bone pain ("flare reaction") 7–10 d after 1st dose) **Notes:** Inject SQ into fat in abdominal wall; do not aspirate; females must use contraception **Interactions:** None noted **Labs:** ↑ Alkaline phosphatase, estradiol, HDL, LDL, triglycerides; initial ↑ then ↓ after 1–2 wk FSH, LH, testosterone

Granisetron (Kytril) [Antiemetic/5 HT3 antagonist]

Uses: *Prevention of N/V* **Action:** Serotonin receptor antagonist **Dose:** *Adults & Peds.* 10 mcg/kg/dose IV 30 min prior to chemo *Adults.* Inj 0.1, 1 mg/mL, 2 mg PO 1 h prior to chemo, then 12 h later. *Postop N/V:* 1 mg IV before end of OR case **Caution:** [B, +/–] St. John's wort ↓ levels **Contra:** Liver Dz, children <2 y **Disp:** Tabs 1 mg; inj 0.1, 1 mg/mL; soln 2 mg/10 mL **SE:** HA, constipation **Interactions:** ↑ Serotonergic effects w/ horehound; ↑ extrapyramidal Rxns w/ drugs causing these effects **Labs:** ↑ ALT, AST **NIPE:** May cause anaphylactic Rxn

Guaifenesin (Robitussin, others) [Expectorant]

Uses: *Relief of dry, nonproductive cough* **Action:** Expectorant **Dose:** *Adults.* 200–400 mg (10–20 mL) PO q4h (max 2.4 g/d). *Peds.* <2 y: 12 mg/kg/d in 6 ÷ doses. *2–5 y:* 50–100 mg (2.5–5 mL) PO q4h (max 600 mg/d). *6–11 y:* 100–200 mg (5–10 mL) PO q4h (max 1.2 g/d) **Caution:** [C, ?] **Disp:** Tabs 100, 200; SR tabs 600, 1200 mg; caps 200 mg; SR caps 300 mg; liq 100 mg/5 mL **SE:** GI upset **Notes:** Give w/ large amount of H_2O; some dosage forms contain EtOH **Interactions:** ↑ Bleeding w/ heparin **Labs:** False results of urine 5-HIAA, VMA **NIPE:** ↑ Fluid intake

Guaifenesin & Codeine (Robitussin AC, Brontex, others) [C-V] [Expectorant/Analgesic/Antitussive]

Uses: *Relief of dry, nonproductive cough* **Action:** Antitussive w/ expectorant **Dose:** *Adults.* 5–10 mL or 1 tab PO q6–8h (max 60 mL/24 h). *Peds.* 2–6 y: 1–1.5 mg/kg codeine/d ÷ dose q4–6h (max 30 mg/24 h). *6–12 y:* 5 mL q4h (max 30 mL/24 h) **Caution:** [C, +] **Disp:** Brontex tab 10 mg codeine/300 mg guaifenesin; liq 2.5 mg codeine/75 mg guaifenesin/5 mL; others 10 mg codeine/100 mg guaifenesin/5 mL **SE:** Somnolence **Interactions:** ↑ CNS depression w/ barbiturates, antihistamines, glutethimide, methocarbamol, cimetidine, EtOH; ↓ effects w/ quinidine **Labs:** ↑ Urine morphine; false ↑ amylase, lipase **NIPE:** Take w/ food

Guaifenesin & Dextromethorphan (many OTC brands) [Expectorant/Antitussive]

Uses: *Cough* due to upper resp tract irritation **Action:** Antitussive w/ expectorant **Dose:** *Adults & Peds >12 y.* 10 mL PO q6–8h (max 40 mL/24 h). *Peds. 2–6 y:* Dextromethorphan 1–2 mg/kg/24 h ÷ 3–4 × d (max 10 mL/d). *6–12 y:* 5 mL q6–8h (max 20 mL/d) **Caution:** [C, +] **Contra:** Administration w/ MAOI **Disp:** Many OTC formulations **SE:** Somnolence **Notes:** Give with plenty of fluids **Interactions:** ↑ Effects w/ quinidine, terbinafine; ↑ effects OF isocarboxazid, MAOIs, phenelzine; ↑ risk of serotonin syndrome w/ sibutramine

Haemophilus B Conjugate Vaccine (ActHIB, HibTITER, PedvaxHIB, Prohibit, others) [Vaccine/Inactivated]

Uses: Routine *immunization* of children against *H. influenzae* type B Dzs **Action:** Active immunization against *Haemophilus* B **Dose:** *Peds.* 0.5 mL (25 mg) IM in deltoid or vastus lateralis **Caution:** [C, +] **Contra:** Febrile illness, immunosuppression, allergy to thimerosal **Disp:** Inj 7.5, 10, 15, 25 mcg/0.5 mL **SE:** Observe for anaphylaxis; edema, ↑ risk of *Haemophilus* B Infxn the week after vaccination **Notes:** Booster not required; report all serious adverse Rxn to VAERS: 1-800-822-7967 **Interactions:** ↓ Effects w/ immunosuppressives, steroids

Haloperidol (Haldol) [Antipsychotic/Butyrophenone]

Uses: *Psychotic disorders, agitation, Tourette disorders, & hyperactivity in children* **Action:** Antipsychotic, neuroleptic **Dose:** *Adults.* Moderate Sxs: 0.5–2 mg PO bid–tid. *Severe Sxs/agitation:* 3–5 mg PO bid–tid or 1–5 mg IM q4h PRN (max 100 mg/d). *Peds.* 3–6 y: 0.01–0.03 mg/kg/24 h PO qd. *6–12 y:* Initial, 0.5–1.5 mg/24 h PO; ↑ by 0.5 mg/24 h to maintenance of 2–4 mg/24 h (0.05–0.1 mg/kg/24 h) or 1–3 mg/dose IM q4–8h to 0.1 mg/kg/24 h max; Tourette Dz may require up to 15 mg/24 h PO; ↓ in elderly **Caution:** [C, ?] ↑ effects w/ SSRIs, CNS depressants, TCA, indomethacin, metoclopramide; avoid levodopa (↓ antiparkinsonian effects) **Contra:** NA glaucoma, severe CNS depression, coma, Parkinson Dz, BM suppression, severe cardiac/hepatic Dz **Disp:** Tabs 0.5, 1, 2, 5, 10, 20 mg; conc liq 2 mg/mL; inj 5 mg/mL; decanoate inj 50, 100 mg/mL **SE:** Extrapyramidal Sxs (EPS), ↓ BP, anxiety, dystonias **Notes:** Do not give decanoate IV; dilute PO conc liq w/ H₂O/juice; monitor for EPS **Interactions:** ↑ Effects w/ CNS depressants, quinidine, EtOH; ↑ hypotension w/ antihypertensives, nitrates; ↑ anticholinergic effects w/ antihistamines, antidepressants, atropine, phenothiazines, quinidine, disopyramide; ↓ effects w/ antacids, carbamazepine, Li, nutmeg, tobacco; ↓ effects OF anticoagulants, levodopa, guanethidine **Labs:** False + PRG test, ↓ serum cholesterol **NIPE:** ↑ Risk of photosensitivity—use sunscreen

Haloprogin (Halotex) [Antifungal]

Uses: *Topical Rx of tinea pedis, tinea cruris, tinea corporis, tinea manus* **Action:** Topical antifungal **Dose:** *Adults.*

Apply bid for ≤ 2 wk; intertriginous may require **Caution:** [B, ?] **Contra:** Component sensitivity **Disp:** 1% cream; soln **SE:** Local irritation **Notes:** Avoid contact w/ eyes; improvement should occur w/in 4 wk

Heparin [Anticoagulant] Uses: *Rx & prevention of DVT & PE,* unstable angina, AF w/ emboli formation, & acute arterial occlusion **Action:** Acts w/ antithrombin III to inactivate thrombin & ↓ thromboplastin formation **Dose:** *Adults.* Prophylaxis: 3000–5000 units SQ q8–12h. *Thrombosis Rx:* Load 50–80 units/kg IV, then 10–20 units/kg IV qh (adjust based on PTT). *Peds.* Infants: Load 50 units/kg IV bolus, then 20 units/kg/h IV by cont inf. *Children:* Load 50 units/kg IV, then 15–25 units/kg cont inf or 100 units/kg/dose q4h IV intermittent bolus (adjust based on PTT) **Caution:** [B, +] ↑ risk of hemorrhage w/ anticoagulants, aspirin, antiplatelets, cephalosporins w/ MTT side chain **Contra:** Uncontrolled bleeding, severe thrombocytopenia, suspected ICH **Disp:** Inj 10, 100, 1000, 2000, 2500, 5000, 7500, 10,000, 20,000, 40,000 units/mL **SE:** Bruising, bleeding, thrombocytopenia **Notes:** Follow PTT, thrombin time, or activated clotting time to monitor; little PT effect; therapeutic PTT 1.5–2 × control for most conditions; monitor for HIT; follow plt counts **Interactions:** ↑ Effects w/ anticoagulants, antihistamines, ASA, clopidogrel, cardiac glycosides, cephalosporins, Pyridamole, NSAIDs, quinine, tetracycline, ticlopidine, feverfew, ginkgo biloba, ginger, valerian; ↓ effects w/ nitroglycerine, ginseng, goldenseal, ↓ effects OF insulin **Labs:** ↑ LFTs, TFTs

Hepatitis A Vaccine (Havrix, Vaqta) [Vaccine/Inactivated] Uses: *Prevent hepatitis A* in high-risk individuals (eg, travelers, certain professions, or high-risk behaviors) **Action:** Provides active immunity **Dose:** (Expressed as ELISA units [EL.U.]) *Havrix:* *Adults.* 1440 EL.U. single IM dose. *Peds >2 y.* 720 EL.U. single IM dose. *Vaqta:* *Adults.* 50 units single IM dose. *Peds.* 25 units single IM dose **Caution:** [C, +] **Contra:** Allergy to any component of formulation **Disp:** Inj 720 EL.U./0.5 mL, 1440 EL.U./1 mL; 50 units/mL **SE:** Fever, fatigue, pain at inj site, HA **Notes:** Booster OK 6–12 mo after primary; report serious adverse effects to VAERS: 1-800-822-7967 **Interactions:** None noted **NIPE:** ⊘ If pt febrile

Hepatitis A (Inactivated) & Hepatitis B (Recombinant) Vaccine (Twinrix) [Vaccine/Inactivated] Uses: *Active immunization against hepatitis A/B* **Action:** Active immunity **Dose:** 1 mL IM at 0, 1, & 6 mo **Caution:** [C, +] **Contra:** Component sensitivity **Disp:** Single-dose vials, syringes **SE:** Fever, fatigue, pain at site, HA **Notes:** Booster OK 6–12 mo after vaccination; report all serious adverse effects to VAERS: 1-800-822-7967 **Interactions:** ↓ Immune response w/ corticosteroids, immunosuppressants **NIPE:** ↑ Response if inj in deltoid vs gluteus

Hepatitis B Immune Globulin (HyperHep, H-BIG) [Immunoglobulin] Uses: *Exposure to HBsAg(+) materials,* eg, blood, plasma, or serum (accidental needle-stick, mucous membrane contact, or PO

146   Hepatitis B Vaccine

ingestion) **Action:** Passive immunization **Dose:** *Adults & Peds.* 0.06 mL/kg IM to a max of 5 mL; w/in 24 h of exposure; w/in 14 d of sexual contact; repeat 1 & 6 mo after exposure **Caution:** [C, ?] **Contra:** Allergies to γ-globulin or antiimmunoglobulin Ab; allergies to thimerosal; IgA deficiency **Disp:** Inj **SE:** Inj site pain, dizziness **Notes:** Administered IM in gluteal or deltoid; if exposure continues, pt should also receive hepatitis B vaccine **Interactions:** ↓ Immune response if given w/ live virus vaccines

Hepatitis B Vaccine (Engerix-B, Recombivax HB) [Vaccine/Inactivated]

Uses: *Prevention of hepatitis B* **Action:** Active immunization; recombinant DNA **Dose:** *Adults.* 3 IM doses of 1 mL each; 1st 2 doses 1 mo apart; the 3rd 6 mo after the 1st. *Peds.* 0.5 mL IM given on adult schedule **Caution:** [C, +] ↓ effect w/ immunosuppressives **Contra:** Yeast allergy **Disp:** *Engerix-B:* Inj 20 mcg/mL; peds inj 10 mcg/0.5 mL. *Recombivax HB:* Inj 10 & 40 mcg/mL; peds inj 5 mcg/0.5 mL **SE:** Fever, inj site pain **Notes:** IM inj for adults & older peds in the deltoid; in other peds, administer in the anterolateral thigh **Interactions:** ↓ Immune response w/ corticosteroids, immunosuppressants **NIPE:** ↑ Response inj in deltoid vs gluteus

Hetastarch (Hespan) [Plasma Volume Expander]

Uses: *Plasma volume expansion* as adjunct in shock & leukapheresis **Action:** Synthetic colloid; action similar to albumin **Dose:** *Volume expansion:* 500–1000 mL (1500 mL/d max) IV (20 mL/kg/h max rate). *Leukapheresis:* 250–700 mL; ↓ in renal failure **Caution:** [C, +] **Contra:** Severe bleeding disorders, CHF, or oliguric/anuric renal failure **Disp:** Inj 6 g/100 mL **SE:** Bleeding (prolongs PT, PTT, bleed time, etc) **Notes:** Not blood or plasma substitute **NIPE:** Monitor CBC, PT, PTT; observe for anaphylactic Rxns

Human Papillomavirus (Types 6, 11, 16, 18) Recombinant Vaccine (Gardasil) [Vaccine]

Uses: *Prevent cervical CA, precancerous genital lesions, and genital warts due to HPV types 6, 11, 16, 18 in females 9–26 yrs* **Action:** Recombinant vaccine, passive humoral immunity **Dose:** 0.5 mL IM initial, then 2 and 6 mo **Caution:** [B, ?/–] **Disp:** Single-dose vial and prefilled syringe: 0.5 mL **SE:** Site Rxn (pain, erythema, swelling, pruritus), fever **Interactions:** w/ immunosuppressants, may get decreased response **NIPE:** Give IM in deltoid or upper thigh; first approved cancer vaccine; report adverse events to VAERS 1-800-822-7967; register pregnant patients exposed to drug (800) 986-8999

Hydralazine (Apresoline, others) [Antihypertensive/Vasodilator]

Uses: *Moderate–severe HTN; CHF* (w/ Isordil) **Action:** Peripheral vasodilator **Dose:** *Adults.* Initial 10 mg PO qid, ↑ to 25 mg qid 300 mg/d max. *Peds.* 0.75–3 mg/kg/24 h PO ÷ q6–12h; ↓ in renal impair; check CBC & ANA before starting **Caution:** [C, +] ↓ hepatic Fxn & CAD; ↑ tox w/ MAOI, indomethacin, β-blockers **Contra:** Dissecting aortic aneurysm, mitral valve rheumatic heart Dz **Disp:** Tabs 10, 25, 50, 100 mg; inj 20 mg/mL **SE:** SLE-like syndrome w/ chronic high doses; SVT following IM route, peripheral neuropathy **Notes:** Compensatory sinus tachycardia eliminated w/ β-blocker **Interactions:** ↑ Effects w/ antihypertensives, diazoxide, diuretics, MAOIs, nitrates, EtOH; ↓ pressor response w/ epinephrine; ↓ effects w/ NSAIDs; **NIPE:** Take w/ food

Hydrochlorothiazide (HydroDIURIL, Esidrix, others) [Antihypertensive/Thiazide Diuretic]

Uses: *Edema, HTN* **Action:** Thiazide diuretic; ↓ Na reabsorption in the distal tubule **Dose:** *Adults.* 25–100 mg/d PO single or ÷ doses. *Peds.* <6 mo: 2–3 mg/kg/d in 2 ÷ doses. >6 mo: 2 mg/kg/d in 2 ÷ doses **Caution:** [D, +] **Contra:** Anuria, sulfonamide allergy, renal insuff **Disp:** Tabs 25, 50, 100 mg; caps 12.5 mg; PO soln 50 mg/5 mL **SE:** ↓ K⁺, hyperglycemia, hyperuricemia, ↓ Na⁺ **Interactions:** ↑ Hypotension w/ ACEIs, antihypertensives, carbenoxolone, ↑ hypokalemia w/ carbenoxolone, corticosteroids; ↑ hyperglycemia w/ BBs, diazoxide, hypoglycemic drugs; ↑ effects OF Li, MRX; ↓ effects w/ amphetamines, cholestyramine, colestipol, NSAIDs, quinidine, dandelion **Labs:** False ↓ urine estriol **NIPE:** Monitor uric acid, take w/ food, ↑ risk of photosensitivity—use sunscreen

Hydrochlorothiazide & Amiloride (Moduretic) [Antihypertensive/Thiazide & K+ Sparing Diuretic]

Uses: *HTN* **Action:** Combined thiazide & a K⁺-sparing diuretic **Dose:** 1–2 tabs/d PO **Caution:** [D, ?] **Contra:** w/renal failure, sulfonamide allergy **Disp:** Tabs (amiloride/HCTZ) 5 mg/50 mg **SE:** ↓ BP, photosensitivity, ↑ K⁺/↓ K⁺, hyperglycemia, ↓ Na⁺, hyperlipidemia, hyperuricemia **Interactions:** ↑ Hypotension w/ACEIs, antihypertensives, carbenoxolone, ↑ hypokalemia w/ amphotericin B, carbenoxolone, corticosteroids, licorice; ↑ risk OF hyperkalemia w/ ACE-I, K-sparing diuretics, NSAIDs, K salt substitutes; ↑ hyperglycemia w/ BBs, diazoxide, hypoglycemic drugs; ↑ effects OF amantadine, antihypertensives, digoxin, Li, MTX; ↑ effects w/ CNS depressants; ↓ effects w/ amphetamines, cholestyramine, colestipol, NSAIDs, quinidine, dandelion **Labs:** False ↓ urine estriol; interferes w/ glucose tolerance test; monitor electrolytes, LFTs, uric acid; **NIPE:** take w/ food, I&O, daily weights, ⊘ salt substitutes, bananas, & oranges; ↑ risk of photosensitivity—use sunscreen

Hydrochlorothiazide & Spironolactone (Aldactazide) [Antihypertensive/Thiazide & K+ sparing Diuretic]

Uses: *Edema, HTN* **Action:** Combined thiazide & K⁺-sparing diuretic **Dose:** 25–200 mg each component/d, ÷ doses **Caution:** [D, +] **Contra:** Sulfonamide allergy **Disp:** Tabs (HCTZ/spironolactone) 25 mg/25 mg, 50 mg/50 mg **SE:** Photosensitivity, ↓ BP, ↑ or ↓ K⁺, ↓ Na⁺, hyperglycemia, hyperlipidemia, hyperuricemia **Additional Interactions** ↑ Risk OF hyperkalemia w/ ACEIs, K-sparing diuretics, K suppls, salt substitutes; ↓ effects of digoxin **NIPE:** DC drug 3 d before glucose tolerance test

Hydrochlorothiazide & Triamterene (Dyazide, Maxzide) [Antihypertensive/Thiazide & K⁺ sparing Diuretic]

Uses: *Edema & HTN* **Action:** Combined thiazide & K⁺-sparing diuretic **Dose:** *Dyazide:* 1–2 caps PO qd–bid. *Maxzide:* 1 tab/d PO **Caution:** [D, +/–] **Contra:**

Sulfonamide allergy **Disp:** (Triamterene/HCTZ) 37.5 mg/25 mg, 75 mg/50 mg **SE:** Photosensitivity, ↓ BP, ↑ or ↓ K⁺, ↓ Na⁺, hyperglycemia, hyperlipidemia, hyperuricemia **Notes:** HCTZ component in Maxzide more bioavailable than in Dyazide; See Hydrochlorothiazide **Additional Interactions:** ↑ Risk OF hyperkalemia w/ ACEIs, K-sparing diuretics, K suppls, salt substitutes; ↑ effects w/ cimetidine, licorice root, ↓ effects OF digoxin **Labs:** ↑ Serum glucose, BUN, creatinine K⁺, Mg²⁺, uric acid, urinary Ca²⁺; interference w/ assay of quinidine & lactic dehydrogenase **NIPE:** Urine may turn blue

Hydrocodone & Acetaminophen (Lorcet, Vicodin, others) [C-III] [Narcotic Analgesic/Antitussive]
Uses: *Moderate–severe pain*; **Action:** Narcotic analgesic w/ nonnarcotic analgesic; hydrocodone is antitussive **Dose:** 1–2 caps or tabs PO q4–6h PRN **Caution:** [C, M] **Contra:** CNS depression, severe resp depression **Disp:** Many formulations; specify hydrocodone/APAP dose; caps 5/500; tabs 2.5/500, 5/400, 5/500, 7.5/400, 10/400, 7.5/500, 7.5/650, 7.5/750, 10/325, 10/400, 10/500, 10/650; elixir & soln (fruit punch) 2.5 mg hydrocodone/167 mg APAP/5 mL **SE:** GI upset, sedation, fatigue **Notes:** Do not exceed >4 g acetaminophen/d **Interactions:** ↑ Effects w/ antihistamines, cimetidine, CNS depressants, dextroamphetamines, glutethimide, MAOIs, protease inhibitors, TCAs, EtOH, St. John's wort; ↑ effects OF warfarin; ↓ effects w/ phenothiazines **Labs:** False ↑ amylase, lipase **NIPE:** Take w/ food, ↑ fluid intake

Hydrocodone & Aspirin (Lortab ASA, others) [C-III] [Narcotic Analgesic]
Uses: *Moderate–severe pain* **Action:** Narcotic analgesic with NSAID **Dose:** 1–2 PO q4–6h PRN, w/ food/milk **Caution:** [C, M] ↓ renal Fxn, gastritis/PUD. **Contra:** Component sensitivity; children w/chickenpox (Reye's syndrome) **Disp:** 5 mg hydrocodone/500 mg ASA/tab **SE:** GI upset, sedation, fatigue **Notes:** Monitor for GI bleed; See Hydrocodone and Acetaminophen

Hydrocodone & Guaifenesin (Hycotuss Expectorant, others) [C-III]
Uses: *Nonproductive cough* associated with resp Infxn **Action:** Expectorant w/ cough suppressant **Dose:** *Adults & Peds >12 y.* 5 mL q4h & hs. *Peds.* < 2 y: 0.3 mg/kg/d ÷ qid. *2–12 y:* 2.5 mL q4h pc & hs **Caution:** [C, M] **Contra:** Component sensitivity **Disp:** Hydrocodone 5 mg/guaifenesin 100 mg/5 mL **SE:** GI upset, sedation, fatigue; See Hydrocodone and Acetaminophen **Additional Interactions:** ↑ Bleeding w/ heparin **Labs:** False results of urine 5-HIAA, VMA

Hydrocodone & Homatropine (Hycodan, Hydromet, others) [C-III] [Narcotic Analgesic/Antitussive]
Uses: *Relief of cough* **Action:** Combo antitussive **Dose:** (Based on hydrocodone) *Adults.* 5–10 mg q4–6h. *Peds.* 0.6 mg/kg/d ÷ tid–qid **Caution:** [C, M] **Contra:** NA glaucoma, ↑ ICP, depressed ventilation **Disp:** Syrup 5 mg hydrocodone/5 mL; tabs 5 mg hydrocodone **SE:** Sedation, fatigue, GI upset **Notes:** Do not give >q4h; see individual drugs; See Hydrocodone and Acetaminophen **Additional Labs:** ↑ ALT, AST

Hydrocodone & Ibuprofen (Vicoprofen) [C-III] [Narcotic Analgesic/NSAID]
Uses: *Moderate–severe pain (<10 d)* **Action:** Nar-

cotic w/ NSAID **Dose:** 1–2 tabs q4–6h PRN **Caution:** [C, M] Renal insuff; ↓ effect w/ ACE inhibitors & diuretics; ↑ effect w/ CNS depressants, EtOH, MAOI, aspirin, TCA, anticoagulants **Contra:** Component sensitivity **Disp:** Tabs 7.5 mg hydrocodone/200 mg ibuprofen **SE:** Sedation, fatigue, GI upset; See Hydrocodone and Acetaminophen **Additional Interactions:** ↓ Effects OF ACEIs, diuretics

Hydrocodone & Pseudoephedrine (Detussin, Histussin-D, others) [C-III] [Antitussive/Decongestant] Uses: *Cough & nasal congestion* **Action:** Narcotic cough suppressant with decongestant **Dose:** 5 mL qid, PRN **Caution:** [C, M] **Contra:** MAOIs **Disp:** 5 mg hydrocodone/60 mg pseudoephedrine/5 mL **SE:** ↑ BP, GI upset, sedation, fatigue; See Hydrocodone and Acetaminophen **Additional Interactions:** ↑ Effects w/ sympathomimetics

Hydrocodone, Chlorpheniramine, Phenylephrine, Acetaminophen, & Caffeine (Hycomine Compound) [C-III] [Narcotic Analgesic/Antitussive/Antihistamine] Uses: *Cough & Sxs of URI* **Action:** Narcotic cough suppressant w/ decongestants & analgesic **Dose:** 1 tab PO q4h PRN **Caution:** [C, M] **Contra:** NA glaucoma **Disp:** Hydrocodone 5 mg/chlorpheniramine 2 mg/phenylephrine 10 mg/APAP 250 mg/caffeine 30 mg/tab **SE:** ↑BP, GI upset, sedation, fatigue; See Hydrocodone and Acetaminophen

Hydrocortisone, Rectal (Anusol-HC Suppository, Cortifoam Rectal, Proctocort, others) [Corticosteroid] Uses: *Painful anorectal conditions,* radiation proctitis, management of ulcerative colitis **Action:** Antiinflammatory steroid **Dose:** *Adults.* Ulcerative colitis: 10–100 mg PR qd–bid for 2–3 wk **Caution:** [B, ?/–] **Contra:** Component sensitivity **Disp:** *Hydrocortisone acetate:* Rectal aerosol 90 mg/applicator; supp 25 mg. *Hydrocortisone base:* Rectal 1%; rectal susp 100 mg/60 mL **SE:** Minimal systemic effect **NIPE:** Administer after BM, insert supp blunt end first, admin enema w/ pt lying on side and retain for 1 h

Hydrocortisone, Topical & Systemic (Cortef, Solu-Cortef) [Corticosteroid] See Steroids, Tables 4 & 5 **Caution:** [B, –] **Contra:** Viral, fungal, or tubercular skin lesions; serious Infxns (except septic shock or tuberculous meningitis) **SE:** Systemic forms: ↑ appetite, insomnia, hyperglycemia, bruising **Notes:** May cause HPA axis suppression **Interactions:** ↑ Effects w/ cyclosporine, estrogens; ↑ effects OF cardiac glycosides, cyclosporine; ↑ risk OF GI bleed w/ NSAIDs; ↓ effects w/ aminoglutethimide, antacids, barbiturates, cholestyramine, colestipol, ephedrine, phenobarbital, phenytoin, rifampin; ↓ effects OF anticoagulants, hypoglycemics, insulin, INH, salicylates **Labs:** False − in skin allergy tests **NIPE:** ⊘ EtOH, live virus vaccines, abrupt DC of drug; take w/ food; may mask S/Sxs infection

Hydromorphone (Dilaudid) [C–II] [Narcotic Analgesic] Uses: *Moderate/severe pain* **Action:** Narcotic analgesic **Dose:** tabs: 1–4 mg PO q 4–6 hr PRN; parental:1–2 mg SC or IM q 4–6 hr PRN; rectal suppositories: 1 rectally q 6–8 hr PRN; oral liquid: 2.5–20 mg q 3–6 hr PRN; ↓ w/ hepatic failure **Caution:** [B (D if prolonged use or high doses near term), ?] ↑ effects w/ CNS depressants, phenothiazines, TCA **Contra:** Component sensitivity **Disp:** Tabs 2, 4, 8 mg; liq 5 mg/mL or 1 mg/mL; inj 1, 2, 4, 10 mg/mL; supp 3 mg **SE:** Sedation, dizziness, GI upset **Notes:** Morphine 10 mg IM = hydromorphone 1.5 mg IM **Interactions:** ↑ Effects w/ CNS depressants, phenothiazines, TCAs, EtOH, St. John's wort; ↓ effects w/ nalbuphine, pentazocine **Labs:** ↑ Serum amylase, lipase **NIPE:** Take w/ food, ↑ fluids & fiber to prevent constipation

Hydroxyurea (Hydrea, Droxia) [Antineoplastic/Antimetabolite]
Uses: *CML, head & neck, ovarian & colon CA, melanoma, acute leukemia, sickle cell anemia, polycythemia vera, HIV* **Action:** ↓ ribonucleotide reductase system **Dose:** (per protocol) 50–75 mg/kg for WBC >100,000 cells/mL; 20–30 mg/kg in refractory CML. *HIV:* 1000–1500 mg/d in single or ÷ doses; ↓ in renal insuff **Caution:** [D, –] ↑ effects w/ zidovudine, zalcitabine, didanosine, stavudine, fluorouracil **Contra:** Severe anemia, BM suppression, WBC <2500 or plt <100,000, PRG **Disp:** Caps 200, 300, 400, 500 mg, tabs 1000 mg **SE:** Myelosuppression (primarily leukopenia), N/V, rashes, facial erythema, radiation recall Rxns, & renal dysfunction **Notes:** Capsules can be opened & emptied into H₂O **Interactions:** ↑ Risk of pancreatitis w/ didanosine, indinavir, stavudine; ↑ bone marrow depression w/ antineoplastic drugs or radiation therapy **Labs:** ↑ Serum uric acid, BUN, creatinine **NIPE:** ↑ Fluids 10–12 glasses/d, use barrier contraception, ↑ risk OF infertility

Hydroxyzine (Atarax, Vistaril) [Antipsychotic, Sedative/Hypnotic/Antihistamine]
Uses: *Anxiety, sedation, itching* **Action:** Antihistamine, antianxiety **Dose:** *Adults.* Anxiety or sedation: 50–100 mg PO or IM qid or PRN (max 600 mg/d). *Itching:* 25–50 mg PO or IM tid–qid. *Peds.* 0.5–1.0 mg/kg/24 h PO or IM q6h; ↓ in hepatic failure **Caution:** [C, +/–] ↑ effects w/ CNS depressants, anticholinergics, EtOH **Contra:** Component sensitivity **Disp:** Tabs 10, 25, 50, 100 mg; caps 25, 50, 100 mg; syrup 10 mg/5 mL; susp 25 mg/5 mL; inj 25, 50 mg/mL **SE:** Drowsiness & anticholinergic effects **Notes:** Useful to potentiate narcotics effects; not for IV/SQ (thrombosis & digital gangrene) **Interactions:** ↑ Effects w/ antihistamines, anticholinergics, CNS depressants, EtOH **Labs:** False – skin allergy tests; false ↑ in urinary 17-hydroxycorticosteroid levels

Hyoscyamine (Anaspaz, Cystospaz, Levsin, others) [Antispasmodic/Anticholinergic]
Uses: *Spasm associated w/ GI & bladder disorders* **Action:** Anticholinergic **Dose:** *Adults.* 0.125–0.25 mg (1–2 tabs) SL/PO tid–qid, ac & hs; 1 SR cap q12h **Caution:** [C, +] ↑ effects w/ anamantadine, antihistamines, antimuscarinics, haloperidol, phenothiazines, TCA, MAOI **Contra:** BOO, GI obstruction, glaucoma, MyG, paralytic ileus, severe ulcerative colitis, MI **Disp:** (Cystospaz-M, Levsinex): timed release caps 0.375 mg; elixir (EtOH); soln 0.125 mg/5 mL; inj 0.5 mg/mL; tab 0.125 mg; tab (Cystospaz) 0.15 mg; XR tab (Levbid): 0.375 mg; SL (Levsin SL) 0.125 mg **SE:** Dry skin, xerosto-

mia, constipation, anticholinergic SE, heat prostration may occur in hot weather **Notes:** Administer tabs before meals/food **Interactions:** ↑ Effects w/ amantadine, antimuscarinics, haloperidol, phenothiazines, quinidine, TCAs, MAOIs; ↓ effects w/ antacids, antidiarrheals; ↓ effects OF levodopa **NIPE:** ↑ Risk of heat intolerance, photophobia

Hyoscyamine, Atropine, Scopolamine, & Phenobarbital (Donnatal, others) [Antispasmotic/Anticholinergic]

Uses: *Irritable bowel, spastic colitis, peptic ulcer, spastic bladder* **Action:** Anticholinergic, antispasmodic **Dose:** 0.125–0.25 mg (1–2 tabs) tid–qid, 1 cap q12h (SR), 5–10 mL elixir tid–qid or q8h **Caution:** [D, M] **Contra:** NA glaucoma **Disp:** Many combos/manufacturers; *Cap* (Donnatal, others): Hyosc. 0.1037 mg/atropine 0.0194 mg/scop. 0.0065 mg/phenobarbital 16.2 mg. *Tabs* (Donnatal, others): Hyosc. 0.1037 mg/atropine 0.0194 mg/scop. 0.0065 mg/phenobarbital 16.2 mg. *Long-acting* (Donnatal): Hyosc. 0.311 mg/atropine 0.0582 mg/scop. 0.0195 mg/phenobarbital 48.6 mg. *Elixirs* (Donnatal, others): Hyosc. 0.1037 mg/atropine 0.0194 mg/scop. 0.0065 mg/phenobarbital 16.2 mg/5 mL **SE:** Sedation, xerostomia, constipation

Ibandronate (Boniva) [Bone Resorption Inhibitor/Bisphosphonate]

Uses: Rx & prevent osteoporosis in postmenopausal women **Action:** Bisphosphonate, ↓ osteoclast-mediated bone-resorption **Dose:** 2.5 mg PO qd or 150 mg once each month on the same day (do not lie down for 60 min after); 3 mg IV over 15–30 sec q 3 mo **Caution:** [C, ?/–] avoid w/ CrCl < 30 mL/min **Contra:** Uncorrected ↓ Ca^{2+}; inability to stand/sit upright for 60 min **Disp:** Tabs 2.5, 150 mg, inj IV 3 mg/3 mL **SE:** N/D, HA, dizziness, asthenia, HTN, Infxn, dysphagia, esophagitis, esophageal/gastric ulcer, musculoskeletal pain, jaw osteonecrosis (avoid extensive dental procedures) **Notes:** Take 1st thing in AM w/ H_2O (6–8 oz) > 60 min before 1st food/beverage & any meds containing multivalent cations; adequate Ca^{2+} & vit D supls necessary **Interactions:** ↑ Effects w/ anticoagulants, amantadine, antihistamines, antidiarrheals, anticonvulsants, CNS depressants, corticosteroids, digitalis, griseofulvin, MAOIs, phenothiazides, tetracyclines, TCAs **NIPE:** ↑ Risk OF photophobia, constipation, urinary hesitancy

Ibuprofen (Motrin, Rufen, Advil, others) [OTC] [Anti-inflammatory, Anti-pyretic, Analgesic/NSAID]

WARNING: May ↑ risk of cardiovascular events & GI bleeding **Uses:** *Arthritis, pain, fever* **Action:** NSAID **Dose:** *Adults.* 200–800 mg PO bid–qid (max 2.4 g/d). *Peds.* 30–40 mg/kg/d in 3–4 ÷ doses (max 40 mg/kg/d); w/ food **Caution:** [B, +] **Contra:** 3rd tri PRG severe hepatic impair, allergy & use w/ other NSAIDs, UGI bleed, ulcers, **Disp:** Tabs 100, 200, 400, 600, 800 mg; chew tabs 50, 100 mg; caps 200 mg; susp 100 mg/2.5 mL, 100 mg/5 mL, 40 mg/mL (200 mg is OTC preparation) **SE:** Dizziness, peptic ulcer, plt inhibition, worsening of renal insuff **Interactions:** ↑ Effects w/ ASA, corticosteroids, probenecid, EtOH; ↑ effects of aminoglycosides, anticoagulants, digoxin, hypoglycemics, Li, MTX; ↑ risks of bleeding w/ abciximab, cefotetan, valproic acid, thrombolytic drugs, warfarin, ticlopidine, garlic, ginger, ginkgo biloba; ↓ effects w/ feverfew; ↓ effects OF antihypertensives **Labs:** ↑ BUN, creatinine; ↓ Hmg, Hct, BS, plts **NIPE:** Take w/ food

Ibutilide (Corvert) [Antiarrhythmic] Uses: *Rapid conversion of AF/flutter* **Action:** Class III antiarrhythmic **Dose:** 0.01 mg/kg (max 1 mg) IV inf over 10 min; may repeat once; w/ECG monitoring **Caution:** [C, –] Do not use w/ class I or III antiarrhythmics or w/in 4 h of ibutilide **Contra:** QTc > 440 ms **Disp:** Inj 0.1 mg/mL **SE:** Arrhythmias, HA **Interactions:** ↑ Refractory effects w/ amiodarone, disopyramide, procainamide, quinidine, sotalol; ↑ QT interval w/ antihistamines, antidepressants, erythromycin, phenothiazines, TCAs

Idarubicin (Idamycin) [Antineoplastic/Anthracycline] Uses: *Acute leukemias* (AML, ALL, ANLL), *CML in blast crisis, breast CA* **Action:** DNA intercalating agent; ↓ DNA topoisomerases I & II **Dose:** (per protocol) 10–12 mg/m²/d for 3–4 d; ↓ in renal/hepatic impairment **Caution:** [D, –] **Contra:** Bilirubin >5 mg/dL, PRG **Disp:** Inj 1 mg/mL (5-, 10-, 20-mg vials) **SE:** Myelosuppression, cardiotox, N/V, mucositis, alopecia, & IV site Rxns, rare changes in renal/hepatic Fxn **Notes:** Avoid extravasation—potent vesicant; only given IV **Interactions:** ↑ Myelosuppression w/ antineoplastic drugs and radiation therapy; ↓ effects OF live virus vaccines **NIPE:** ↑ Fluids to 2–3 L/d

Ifosfamide (Ifex, Holoxan) [Antineoplastic/Alkylating Agent] Uses: Lung, breast, pancreatic & gastric CA, HL/NHL, soft tissue sarcoma **Action:** Alkylating agent **Dose:** (per protocol) 1.2 g/m²/d for 5 d by bolus or cont inf; 2.4 g/m²/d for 3 d; w/ mesna uroprotection; ↓ in renal/hepatic impair **Caution:** [D, M] ↑ effect w/ phenobarbital, carbamazepine, phenytoin; St. John's wort may ↓ levels **Contra:** ↓ BM Fxn, PRG **Disp:** Inj 1, 3 g **SE:** Hemorrhagic cystitis, nephrotox, N/V, mild–moderate leukopenia, lethargy & confusion, alopecia, & ↑ hepatic enzyme **Notes:** Administer w/ mesna to prevent hemorrhagic cystitis **Interactions:** ↑ Effects w/ allopurinol, chloral hydrate, phenobarbital, phenytoin, grapefruit juice; ↑ myelosuppression w/ antineoplastic drugs and radiation therapy; ↓ effects OF live virus vaccines **NIPE:** ↑ Fluids to 2–3 L/d

Iloprost (Ventavis) [Prostaglandin Analog] WARNING: Associated with syncope; may require dosage adjustment Uses: NYHA Class III/IV pulmonary arterial HTN * **Action:** Prostaglandin analog **Dose:** If initial 2.5 mcg tolerated, ↑ to 5 mcg inh 6–9 ×/d (at least 2 h apart) while awake **Caution:** [C, ?/–] Antiplatelet effects, ↑ bleeding risk w/anticoagulants; may have additive hypotensive effects **Contra:** SBP <85 mm Hg **Disp:** Inh soln 10 mcg/mL **SE:** Syncope, ↓ BP, vasodilation, cough, HA, trismus **Notes:** Requires Pro-Dose AAD nebulizer **Interactions:** ↑ effects OF anticoagulants, antihypertensives, antiplatelets **NIPE:** instruct pt of syncope risk; monitor BP

Imatinib (Gleevec) [Antineoplastic/Tyrosin Kinase Inhibitor] Uses: *Rx of CML, blast crisis, gastrointestinal stromal tumors (GIST)* **Action:** ↓ BCL-ABL tyrosine kinase (signal transduction) **Dose:** *Chronic phase CML:*

400–600 mg PO qd. *Accelerated/blast crisis:* 600–800 mg PO qd. *GIST:* 400–600 mg PO qd **Caution:** [D, ?/–] w/CYP3A4 meds (Table 13), warfarin, **Contra:** Component sensitivity **Disp:** Caps 100, 400 mg **SE:** GI upset, fluid retention, muscle cramps, musculoskeletal pain, arthralgia, rash, HA, neutropenia, thrombocytopenia **Notes:** Follow CBCs & LFTs baseline & monthly **Additional Interactions:** ↓ Effects w/ St. John's wort **NIPE:** Take w/ food & ↑ fluids to decrease GI irritation, use barrier contraception

Imipenem–Cilastatin (Primaxin) [Antibiotic/Carbapenem]

Uses: *Serious Infxns* caused by a wide variety of susceptible bacteria **Action:** Bactericidal; interferes with cell wall synthesis. *Spectrum:* Gram(+) (inactive against *S. aureus*, group A & B streptococci), gram(–) (not *Legionella*), anaerobes **Dose:** *Adults.* 250–1000 mg (imipenem) IV q6–8h. *Peds.* 60–100 mg/kg/24 h IV ÷ q6h; ↓ in renal Dz if CrCl is <70 mL/min **Caution:** [C, +/–] Probenecid may ↑ tox **Contra:** Ped pts w/ CNS Infxn (↑ Sz risk) & <30 kg w/ renal impair **Disp:** Inj (imipenem/cilastatin) 250/250 mg, 500/500 mg, 750/750 mg **SE:** Szs may occur w/ drug accumulates, GI upset, thrombocytopenia **Interactions:** ↑ Risks OF Szs w/ ganciclovir, theophylline; ↓ effects w/ aztreonam, cephalosporins, chloramphenicol, penicillins, probenicid **Labs:** ↑ LFTs, BUN, creatinine; ↓ Hmg, Hct **NIPE:** Eval for superinfection

Imipramine (Tofranil) [Antidepressant/TCA]

Uses: *Depression, enuresis,* panic attack, chronic pain **Action:** TCA; ↑ synaptic conc of serotonin or norepinephrine in the CNS **Dose:** *Adults.* Hospitalized: Initial 100 mg/24 h PO in ÷ doses; can ↑ over several wks to max 300 mg/d. *Outpatient:* Maint 50–150 mg PO hs, 300 mg/24 h max. *Peds.* Antidepressant: 1.5–5 mg/kg/24 h ÷ qd–qid. *Enuresis:* >6 y: 10–25 mg PO qhs; ↑ by 10–25 mg at 1–2-wk intervals (max 50 mg for 6–12 y, 75 mg for >12 y); treat for 2–3 mo, then taper **Caution:** [D, ?/–] **Contra:** Use with MAOIs, NA glaucoma, acute recovery phase of MI, PRG, CHF, angina, CVD, arrhythmias **Disp:** Tabs 10, 25, 50 mg; caps 75, 100, 125, 150 mg **SE:** CV Sxs, dizziness, xerostomia, discolored urine **Notes:** Less sedation than with amitriptyline **Interactions:** ↑ Effects w/ amiodarone, anticholinergics, BBs, cimetidine, diltiazem, Li, oral contraceptives, quinidine, phenothiazines, ritonavir, verapamil, EtOH, evening primrose oil; ↑ effects OF CNS depressants, hypoglycemics, warfarin; ↑ risk OF serotonin syndrome w/ MAOIs; ↓ effects w/ carbamazepine, phenobarbital, rifampin, tobacco; ↓ effects OF clonidine, guanethidine, methyldopa, reserpine **Labs:** ↑ Serum glucose, bilirubin, alkaline phosphatase **NIPE:** D/C 48 h before surgery, D/C MAOIs 2 wk before admin this drug, 4–6 wk for full effects, take w/ food

Imiquimod Cream, 5% (Aldara) [Topical Immunomodulator]

Uses: *Anogenital warts, HPV, condylomata acuminata* **Action:** Unknown; may induce cytokines **Dose:** Applied 3×/wk, leave on skin for 6–10 h & wash off with soap & water, continue therapy 16 wk max **Caution:** [B, ?] **Contra:** Component sensitivity **Disp:** Single-dose packets 5% (250 mg cream) **SE:** Local skin reactions common **Notes:** Not a cure; wash hands before & after application **NIPE:** Condoms & diaphragms may be weakened—⊘ contact

Immune Globulin, IV (Gamimune N, Sandoglobulin, Gammar IV) [Immune Serum]
Uses: *IgG Ab deficiency Dz states, (eg, congenital agammaglobulinemia, CVH, & BMT), HIV, hepatitis A prophylaxis, ITP* **Action:** IgG supl **Dose:** *Adults & Peds.* Immunodeficiency: 100–200 mg/kg/mo IV at a rate of 0.01–0.04 mL/kg/min to a max of 400 mg/kg/dose. *ITP:* 400 mg/kg/dose IV qd × 5 d. *BMT:* 500 mg/kg/wk; ↓ in renal insuff **Caution:** [C, ?] Separate administration of live vaccines by 3 mo **Contra:** Isolated immunoglobulin A deficiency w/ Abs to IgA, severe thrombocytopenia or coagulation disorders **Disp:** Inj **SE:** Adverse effects associated mostly w/ rate of inf, GI upset **Interactions:** ↓ Effects OF live virus vaccines **NIPE:** Give live virus vaccines 3 mo after this drug; rapid inf can cause anaphylactoid Rxn

Inamrinone [Amrinone] (Inocor) [Inotropic]
Uses: *Acute CHF, ischemic cardiomyopathy* **Action:** Positive inotrope w/ vasodilator **Dose:** IV bolus 0.75 mg/kg over 2–3 min. Maint 5–10 mcg/kg/min; 10 mg/d max; ↓ if ClCr <10 mL/min **Caution:** [C, ?] **Contra:** Allergy to bisulfites **Disp:** Inj 5 mg/mL **SE:** Monitor for fluid, electrolyte, & renal changes **Notes:** Incompatible w/ dextrose solns **Interactions:** Precipitates form if contact made with furosemide; diuretics cause significant hypovolemia; ↑ effects OF digitalis **Labs:** Monitor ALT, AST, BUN, creatinine, electrolytes, plts **NIPE:** Monitor I&O, daily weights, BP, pulse

Indapamide (Lozol) [Antihypertensive/Thiazide Diuretic]
Uses: *HTN, edema, CHF* **Action:** Thiazide diuretic; ↑ Na, Cl, & H$_2$O excretion in the proximal segment of the distal tubule **Dose:** 1.25–5 mg/d PO **Caution:** [D, ?] ↑ effect w/ loop diuretics, ACE inhibitors, cyclosporine, digoxin, Li **Contra:** Anuria, thiazide/sulfonamide allergy, renal insuff, PRG **Disp:** Tabs 1.25, 2.5 mg **SE:** ↓ BP, dizziness, photosensitivity **Notes:** No additional effects on BP w/ doses >5 mg, take early to avoid nocturia **Interactions:** ↑ Effects w/ antihypertensives, diazoxide, nitrates, EtOH; ↑ effects OF ACEIs, Li; ↑ risk of gout w/ cyclosporine, thiazides; ↑ risk OF hypokalemia w/ amphotericin B, corticosteroids, mezlocillin, piperacillin, ticarcillin; ↓ effects w/ cholestyramine, colestipol, NSAIDs; ↓ effects OF hypoglycemics **Labs:** ↑ Serum glucose, uric acid, ↓ K$^+$, Na, Cl **NIPE:** ↑ Risk photosensitivity—use sunscreen, take w/ food

Indinavir (Crixivan) [Antiretroviral/Protease Inhibitor]
Uses: *HIV Infxn* **Action:** Protease inhibitor; ↓ maturation of immature noninfectious virions to mature infectious virus **Dose:** 800 mg PO q8h; in combo w/ other antiretrovirals; on empty stomach; ↓ in hepatic impair **Caution:** [C, ?] Numerous drug interactions **Contra:** Concomitant use w/ triazolam, midazolam, pimozide, ergot alkaloids, simvastatin, lovastatin, sildenafil, St. John's wort **Disp:** Caps 100, 200, 333, 400 mg **SE:** Nephrolithiasis, dyslipidemia, lipodystrophy, GI effects **Interactions:** ↑ Effects w/ aldesleukin, azole antifungals, clarithromycin,

delavirdine, interleukins, quinidine, zidovudine; ↑ effects OF amiodarone, cisapride, clarithromycin, ergot alkaloids, fentanyl, HMG-CoA reductase inhibitors, INH, oral contraceptives, phenytoin, rifabutin, ritonavir, sildenafil, stavudine, zidovudine; ↓ effects w/ efavirenz, fluconazole, phenytoin, rifampin, St. John's wort, high-fat/protein foods, grapefruit juice; ↓ effects OF midazolam, triazolam **Labs:** ↑ Serum glucose, LFTs, ↓ Hmg, plts, neutrophils **NIPE:** ↑ Fluids 1–2 L/d, capsules moisture sensitive—keep desiccant in container

Indomethacin (Indocin) [Analgesic, anti-inflammatory, antipyretic/NSAID]

WARNING: May ↑ risk of cardiovascular events & GI bleeding **Uses:** *Arthritis; close ductus arteriosus; ankylosing spondylitis* **Action:** ↓ prostaglandins **Dose:** *Adults.* 25–50 mg PO bid–tid, max 200 mg/d. *Infants:* 0.2–0.25 mg/kg/dose IV; may repeat in 12–24 h up to 3 doses; w/ food **Caution:** [B, +] **Contra:** ASA/NSAID sensitivity, peptic ulcer Dz/active GI bleed, precipitation of asthma/urticaria/rhinitis by NSAIDs/aspirin, premature neonates w/ NEC, ↓ renal Fxn, active bleeding, thrombocytopenia, 3rd tri PRG **Disp:** Inj 1 mg/vial; caps 25, 50 mg; SR caps 75 mg; susp 25 mg/5 mL **SE:** GI bleeding or upset, dizziness, edema **Notes:** Monitor renal Fxn **Interactions:** ↑ Effects w/ acetaminophen, anti-inflammatories, gold compounds, diflunisal, probenicid; ↑ effects of aminoglycosides, anticoagulants, digoxin, hypoglycemics, Li, MTX, nifedipine, phenytoin, penicillamine, verapamil; ↓ effects w/ ASA; ↓ effects OF antihypertensives **Labs:** ↑ Serum K+, BUN, creatinine, AST, ALT, urine glucose, protein, PT; ↓ Hmg, Hct, leukocytes, plts **NIPE:** Take w/ food

Infliximab (Remicade) [Anti-inflammatory/Monoclonal Antibody]

WARNING: TB, invasive fungal Infxns, & other opportunistic Infxns reported, some fatal: perform TB skin testing prior to therapy **Uses:** *Moderate–severe Crohn Dz; fistulizing Crohn Dz; RA (w/ MTX), ulcerative colitis* **Action:** IgG1K neutralizes TNFα (human & murine regions) **Dose:** *Crohn Dz: Induction:* 5 mg/kg IV inf, w/doses 2 & 6 wk after. *Maint:* 5 mg/kg IV inf q8wk. *RA:* 3 mg/kg IV inf at 0, 2, 6 wk, then q8wk **Caution:** [B, ?/–] Active Infxn; moderate–severe CHF, hepatic impairment **Contra:** Murine allergy, moderate–severe CHF **Disp:** 100 mg inj **SE:** Allergic Rxns; pts predisposed to Infxn (especially TB); HA, fatigue, GI upset, infusion Rxns; hepatotoxicity or reactivation, hepatitis B, pneumonia, BM suppression, systemic vasculitis, pericardial effusion **Interactions:** May ↓ effects OF live virus vaccines; **Labs:** May ↑ + ANA; Monitor LFTs **NIPE:** ↑ Susceptibility to infection

Influenza Vaccine (Fluzone, FluShield, Fluvirin) [Antiviral/Vaccine]

Uses: *Prevent influenza*; all adults >50 y, children 6–23 mo, pregnant women (2nd/3rd tri during flu season), nursing home residents, chronic Dzs, health care workers & household contacts of high-risk pts, children < 9 y receiving vaccine for the first time **Action:** Active immunization **Dose:** *Adults.* 0.5 mL/dose IM. *Peds.* ≥ 3 y: 0.5 mL IM; 6–35 mo 0.25 mL IM; *6 mo to < 9 y* (first-time vaccination): 2 doses > 4 wk apart, 2nd dose before Dec if possible **Caution:** [C, +]

Contra: Egg, gentamicin, or thimerosal allergy, Infxn at site; high risk of influenza complications, Hx of Guillain–Barré, asthma, children 5–17 y on aspirin **Disp:** Based on specific manufacturer, 0.25- & 0.5-mL prefilled syringes **SE:** Soreness at inj site, fever, myalgia, malaise, Guillain–Barré syndrome (controversial) **Notes:** Optimal in U.S.: Oct–Nov, protection begins 1–2 wk after, lasts up to 6 mo; each yr, vaccines based on predictions of flu active in flu season (December–Spring in U.S.); whole or split virus for adults; Peds <13 y split virus or purified surface antigen to ↓ febrile Rxns **Interactions:** ↑ Effects OF theophylline, warfarin; ↓ effects w/ corticosteroids, immunosuppressants; ↓ effects OF aminopyrine, phenytoin

Influenza Virus Vaccine Live, Intranasal (FluMist) [Antiviral/Vaccine] Uses: *Prevent influenza* **Action:** Live-attenuated vaccine **Dose:** *Adults 9–49 y.* 1 dose (0.5 mL)/season **Caution:** [C,?/–] **Contra:** Egg allergy, PRG, Hx Guillain–Barré syndrome, known/suspected immune deficiency, asthma or reactive airway Dz **Disp:** Prefilled, single-use, intranasal sprayer **SE:** Runny nose, nasal congestion, HA, cough **Notes:** 0.25 mL into each nostril; do not administer concurrently w/ other vaccines; avoid contact w/ immunocompromised individuals for 21 days **NIPE:** ⊘ Take w/ antivirals, ASA, NSAIDs, immunosuppressants, corticosteroids, radiation therapy

Insulin [Hypoglycemic/Hormone] Uses: *Type 1 or type 2 DM refractory to diet or PO hypoglycemic agents; acute life-threatening ↑ K^+* **Action:** Insulin supl **Dose:** Based on serum glucose; usually SQ; can give IV (only regular)/IM; type I typical start dose 0.5–1 units/kg/d; type 2 0.3–0.4 Units/kg/d; renal failure may ↓ insulin needs **Caution:** [B, +] **Contra:** Hypoglycemia **Disp:** Table 6 **SE:** Highly purified insulins ↑ free insulin; monitor for several wks when changing doses/agents **Interactions:** ↑ Hypoglycemic effects w/ α-blockers, anabolic steroids, BBs, clofibrate, fenfluramine, guanethidine, MAOIs, NSAIDs, pentamidine, phenylbutazone, salicylates, sulfinpyrazone, tetracyclines, EtOH, celery, coriander, dandelion root, fenugreek, ginseng, garlic, juniper berries; ↓ hypoglycemic effects w/ corticosteroids, dextrothyroxine, diltiazem, dobutamine, epinephrine, niacin, oral contraceptives, protease inhibitor antiretrovirals, rifampin, thiazide diuretics, thyroid preps, marijuana, tobacco **NIPE:** If mixing insulins, draw up short-acting preps first in syringe

Insulin Human Inhalation Powder (Exubera) [Hypoglycemic/Hormone] Uses: *Type-1 DM in adults combo w/long-acting insulin; Type-2 DM monotherapy or w/other agents* **Action:** Regulates glucose metabolism **Dose:** Premeal (mg) = BW(kg) (times) 0.05 mg/kg; round down to nearest whole mg; give w/in 10 min prior to meal; titrate based on glucose; 1 mg blister = 3 IU of SC regular human insulin; 3 mg blister = 8 IU of SC regular human insulin **Caution:** [C, M] **Contra:** Smoker or if D/C smoking < 6 months before start; D/C if smoking resumes; unstable or poorly controlled lung disease **Disp:** Unit dose blisters: 1, 3 mg; Exubera Inhaler **SE:** Hypoglycemia, dry mouth, chest pain, otitis media, cough, dyspnea, pharyngitis, rhinitis, sinusitis, epistaxis,

↑ sputum **Interactions:** ↑ effects w/albuterol within 30 min; salicylates, MAOIs, sulfonamides, ACEIs, active cigarette smoke; ↓ absorption with bronchodilators and other inhaled agents; ↓ effects w/ corticosteroids, thiazides, phenothiazines, sympathomimetics, and passive cigarette smoke **NIPE:** Assess pulmonary fxn before Tx and 6–12 months; store blisters at room temperature

Interferon Alfa (Roferon-A, Intron A) [Antineoplastic/Immunomodulator]

WARNING: Can cause or aggravate fatal or life-threatening neuropsychiatric, autoimmune, ischemic, and infectious disorders. Monitor patients closely. **Uses:** *Hairy cell leukemia, Kaposi sarcoma, melanoma, CML, chronic hepatitis C, chronic hep B, follicular NHL, condylomata acuminata **Action:** Antiproliferative against tumor cells; modulates host immune response; inhibits viral replication in infected cells **Dose:** Per protocols. *Adults.* Hairy cell leukemia: Alfa-2a (Roferon-A): 3 M units/d for 16–24 wk SQ/IM then 3 M units 3 times/wk for up to 6–24 mo; Alfa-2b (Intron A): 2 M units/m² IM/ SQ 3×/wk for 2–6 mo; *Chronic hepatitis B:* Alfa-2b (Intron A): 3 M units/m² SQ 3×/wk × 1 wk, then 6 M units/m² 3×/wk (Max 10M units 3×/wk, total duration 16–24 wks). *Follicular NHL* (Intron A) 5 M units SQ 3×/wk for 18 mo; *Melanoma* (Intron A) 20 M units m² IV × 5 days/wk for 4 wks, then 10 M units/m² SQ 3×/wk for 48 wks; *Kaposi sarcoma* (Intron A) 30 M units/m IM/SQ 3×/wk for 10–12 wks, then 36 M units IM/SQ 3×/wk; *Chronic hep C* (Intron A) 3m units 3×/wk for 16 wks (continue 18–24 mo if response) Roferon A: 3 M units 3×/wk for 12 mo SQ/IM; *Condyloma acuminata* (Intron A) 1 M units/lesion (max 5 lesions) 3×/wk for 3 wks. *Peds.* CML: Alfa-2a (Roferon-A): 2.5–5 M units/m² IM qd. **Contra:** Benzyl alcohol sensitivity, decompensated liver Dz, autoimmune Dz, immunosuppressed transplant recipients, neonates, infants **Disp:** Injectable forms (see also peg interferon) **SE:** Flu-like Sxs; fatigue; anorexia in 20–30%; neurotox at high doses; neutralizing Ab in up to 40% of pts receiving prolonged systemic therapy **Interactions:** ↑ Effects of antineoplastics, CNS depressants, doxorubicin, theophylline; ↓ effects of live virus vaccine **Labs:** ↑ LFTs, BUN, SCr, glucose, phosphorus, ↓ Hmg, Hct, Ca **NIPE:** ASA & EtOH use may cause GI bleed, ↑ fluids to 2–3 L/d

Interferon Alfa-2b & Ribavirin Combo (Rebetron) [Antineoplastic/Immunomodulator]

WARNING: Can cause or aggravate fatal or life-threatening neuropsychiatric, autoimmune, ischemic, and infectious disorders. Monitor patients closely. Contraindicated in pregnant females & their male partners **Uses:** *Chronic hepatitis C in pts w/ compensated liver Dz who have relapsed following α-interferon therapy* **Action:** Combo antiviral agents (see individual agents) **Dose:** 3 M units Intron A SQ 3×/wk w/ 1000–1200 mg of Rebetron PO ÷ bid dose for 24 wk. *Pts <75 kg:* 1000 mg of Rebetrol/d **Caution:** [X, ?] **Contra:** PRG, males w/ PRG female partner, autoimmune hepatitis, creatinine clearance < 50 mL/min **Disp:** *Pts <75 kg:* Combo packs: 6 vials Intron A (3 M Units/0.5 mL) w/ 6 syringes & EtOH swabs, 70 Rebetron caps; one 18 M units multidose vial of

Intron A inj (22.8 M units/3.8 mL; 3 M units/0.5 mL) & 6 syringes & swabs, 70 Rebetron caps; one 18 M units Intron A inj multidose pen (22.5 M units/1.5 mL; 3 M units/0.2 mL) w/ 6 needles & swabs, 70 Rebetron caps. *Pts >75 kg:* Identical except 84 Rebetron caps/pack **SE:** See warning, flu-like syndrome, HA, anemia **Notes:** Negative PRG test required monthly; instruct pts in self-administration of SQ Intron A; See Interferon Alfa **Additional Labs:** ↑ Uric acid

Interferon Alfacon-1 (Infergen) [Immunomodulator] WARNING: Can cause or aggravate fatal or life-threatening neuropsychiatric, autoimmune, ischemic, and infectious disorders. Monitor patients closely. **Uses:** *Chronic hepatitis C* **Action:** Biologic response modifier **Dose:** 9 mcg SQ 3×/wk × 24 wk **Caution:** [C, M] **Contra:** Allergy to *E. coli*–derived products **Disp:** Inj 9, 15 mcg **SE:** Flu-like syndrome, depression, blood dyscrasias **Notes:** Allow > 48 h between inj **Interactions:** ↑ Effects OF theophylline **Labs:** ↑ Triglycerides, TSH; ↓ Hmg, Hct **NIPE:** Refrigerate, ⊘ shake, use barrier contraception

Interferon beta 1a (Rebif) [Immunomodulator] **Uses:** *MS, relapsing* **Action:** Biologic response modifier **Dose:** 44 mcg SC 3×/wk; start 8.8 mcg SC 3 ×/wk for 2 wk, then 22 mcg SC 3 ×/wk for 2 wk then to 44 mcg SC 3 × wk **Caution:** [C, ?] w/ hepatic impair, depression, Sz disorder, thyroid Dz **Contra:** Human albumin allergy **Disp:** Inj **SE:** Inj site rxn, HA, flu like Sx, malaise, fatigue, rigors, myalgia, depression w/suicidal ideation, hepatotoxicity, myelosuppression **Interactions:** Caution with other hepatotoxic drugs **Labs:** Monitor CBC 1, 3, and 6 mo; TFTs q 6mo w/hx thyroid dz **NIPE:** Dose > 48 h apart; D/C if jaundice occurs; may have abortifacient effects

Interferon β-1b (Betaseron) [Immunomodulator] **Uses:** *MS, relapsing-remitting & secondary progressive* **Action:** Biologic response modifier **Dose:** 0.25 mg SQ qod **Caution:** [C, ?] **Contra:** Allergy to human albumin products **Disp:** Powder for inj 0.3 mg **SE:** Flu-like syndrome, depression, blood dyscrasias; **Interactions:** ↑ Effects OF theophylline, zidovudine **Labs:** ↑ LFTs, BUN, urine protein **NIPE:** ↑ Risk of photosensitivity—use sunscreen, abortion; ↑ fluid intake, use barrier contraception

Interferon γ-1b (Actimmune) [Immunomodulator] **Uses:** *↓ Incidence of serious Infxns in chronic granulomatous Dz (CGD), osteopetrosis* **Action:** Biologic response modifier **Dose:** *Adults.* CGD: 50 mcg/m² SQ (1.5 million units/m²) BSA >0.5 m²; if BSA <0.5 m², give 1.5 mcg/kg/dose; given 3×/wk. *Peds.* BSA ≤ 0.5 m²; 1.5 mcg/kg/ SQ tid; BSA > 0.5 m2: 50 mcg/m2 SQ tid **Caution:** [C, ?] **Contra:** Allergy to *E. coli*–derived products **Disp:** Inj 100 mcg (2 million units) **SE:** Flu-like syndrome, depression, blood dyscrasias

Ipecac Syrup [OTC] [Antidote] **Uses:** *Drug OD, certain cases of poisoning* **NOTE:** Usage is falling out of favor & is no longer recommended by some groups **Action:** Irritation of the GI mucosa; stimulation of the chemoreceptor trigger zone **Dose:** *Adults.* 15–30 mL PO, followed by 200–300 mL of H₂O; if no emesis in 20 min, repeat once. *Peds.* 6–12 y: 5–10 mL PO, followed by 10–20 mL/kg of H_2O; if no emesis in 20 min, repeat once. *1–12 y:* 15 mL PO followed by 10–20 mL/kg of H_2O; if no emesis in 20 min, repeat once **Caution:** [C, ?] **Contra:** Ingestion of petroleum distillates, strong acid, base, or other caustic agents; comatose/unconscious **Disp:** Syrup 15, 30 mL (OTC) **SE:** Lethargy, D, cardiotox, protracted vomiting (www.clintox.org/Pos_Statements/Ipecac.html) **Interactions:** ↑ Effects OF myelosuppressives, theophylline, zidovudine **NIPE:** ↑ Fluids to 2–3 L/d, ⊘ EtOH, CNS depressants; activated charcoal more effective

Ipratropium (Atrovent) [Bronchodilator/Anticholinergic] Uses: *Bronchospasm w/ COPD, rhinitis, rhinorrhea* **Action:** Synthetic anticholinergic similar to atropine **Dose:** *Adults & Peds >12 y.* 2–4 puffs qid. *Nasal:* 2 sprays/nostril bid–tid **Caution:** [B, +/–] **Contra:** Allergy to soya lecithin/related foods **Disp:** Metdose inhaler 18 mcg/dose; inhal soln 0.02%; nasal spray 0.03%, 0.06%; nasal inhaler 20 mcg/dose **SE:** Nervousness, dizziness, HA, cough, bitter taste, nasal dryness **Notes:** Not for acute bronchospasm **Interactions:** ↑ Effects w/ albuterol; ↑ effects OF anticholinergics, antimuscarinics; ↓ effects w/ jaborandi tree, pill-bearing spurge **NIPE:** Adequate fluids, separate inhalation of other drugs by 5 min

Irbesartan (Avapro) [Antihypertensive/ARB] Uses: *HTN*, DN, CHF **Action:** Angiotensin II receptor antagonist **Dose:** 150 mg/d PO, may ↑ to 300 mg/d **Caution:** [C (1st tri; D 2nd/3rd), ?/–] **Disp:** Tabs 75, 150, 300 mg **SE:** Fatigue, ↓ BP **Interactions:** ↑ Risk OF hyperkalemia w/ K-sparing diuretics, trimethoprim, K supls; ↑ effects OF Li **Labs:** ↑ BUN, SCr; ↓ Hmg **NIPE:** ⊘ PRG, breast-feeding

Irinotecan (Camptosar) [Antineoplastic] Uses: *Colorectal* & lung CA **Action:** Topoisomerase I inhibitor; ↓DNA synthesis **Dose:** Per protocol; 125–350 mg/m² qwk–q3wk (↓ hepatic dysfunction, as tolerated per tox) **Caution:** [D, –] **Contra:** Allergy to component **Disp:** Inj 20 mg/mL **SE:** Myelosuppression, N/V/D, abdominal cramping, alopecia; D is dose-limiting; Rx acute D w/ atropine; Rx subacute D w/ loperamide **Notes:** D correlated to levels of metabolite SN-38 **Interactions:** ↑ Effects OF antineoplastics; ↑ risk OF akathisia w/ prochlorperazine **Labs:** ↑ LFTs **NIPE:** Use barrier contraception, ⊘ exposure to infection

Iron Dextran (Dexferrum, INFeD) [Iron Supl] Uses: *Fe deficiency when cannot supplement PO* **Action:** Fe supl **Dose:** Estimate Fe deficiency, give IM/IV. Do a 0.5-mL test dose; total replacement dose (mL) = 0.0476 × weight (kg) × [desired Hgb (g/dL) – measured Hgb (g/dL)] + 1 mL/5 kg weight (max 14 mL). *Adults.* Max daily dose: 100 mg Fe. *Peds.* Max daily dose: *<5 kg:* 25 mg Fe. *5–10 kg:* 50 mg Fe. *10–50 kg:* 100 mg Fe **Caution:** [C, M] **Contra:** Anemia w/o Fe deficiency. **Disp:** Inj 50 mg (Fe)/mL **SE:** Anaphylaxis, flushing, dizziness, inj site & inf Rxns, metallic taste **Notes:** Give deep IM using "Z-track" technique; IV preferred **Interactions:** ↓ Effects w/ chloramphenicol, ↓ absorption OF oral Fe **Labs:** False ↓ serum Ca; false + guaiac test **NIPE:** ⊘ Take oral Fe

Iron Sucrose (Venofer) [Iron Supl] Uses: *Fe deficiency anemia w/chronic HD in those receiving erythropoietin* **Actions:** Fe replacement. **Dose:**

5 mL (100 mg) IV during dialysis, 1 mL (20 mg)/min max. **Caution:** [C, M] **Contra:** Anemia w/o Fe deficiency **Disp:** 20 mg elemental Fe per mL, 5-mL vials. **SE:** Anaphylaxis, ↓ BP, cramps, N/V/D, HA **Notes:** Most pts require cumulative doses of 1000 mg; administer at slow rate **Interactions:** ↓ Absorption OF oral iron supplements **Labs:** Monitor ferritin, hmg, hct, transferrin saturation; obtain iron levels 48 h > IV dose; ↑ LFTs **NIPE:** ⊘ Use oral & IV supplements together

Isoniazid (INH) [Antitubercular]

Uses: *Rx & prophylaxis of TB* **Action:** Bactericidal; interferes w/ mycolic acid synthesis, disrupts cell wall **Dose:** **Adults.** Active TB: 5 mg/kg/24 h PO or IM (usually 300 mg/d) or DOT: 15 mg/kg (max 900 mg) 3 ×/wk. *Prophylaxis:* 300 mg/d PO for 6–12 mo. Or 900 mg 2 ×/wk. **Peds.** Active TB: 10–15 mg/kg/d PO or IM 300 mg/d max. *Prophylaxis:* 10 mg/kg/24 h PO; ↓ in hepatic/renal dysfunction **Caution:** [C, +] Liver Dz, dialysis; avoid EtOH **Contra:** Acute liver Dz, Hx INH hepatitis **Disp:** Tabs 100, 300 mg; syrup 50 mg/5 mL; inj 100 mg/mL **SE:** Hepatitis, peripheral neuropathy, GI upset, anorexia, dizziness, skin Rxn **Notes:** Give w/ 2–3 other drugs for active TB, based on INH resistance patterns when TB acquired & sensitivity results; prophylaxis usually w/ INH alone. IM rarely used. ↓ Peripheral neuropathy w/ pyridoxine 50–100 mg/d. Check CDC guidelines (in MMWR) for current recommendations **Interactions:** ↑ Effects OF acetaminophen, anticoagulants, carbamazepine, cycloserine, diazepam, meperidine, hydantoins, theophylline, valproic acid, EtOH; ↑ effects w/ rifampin; ↓ effects w/ Al salts; ↓ effects OF anticoagulants, ketoconazole **Labs:** False + urine glucose, false ↑ AST, uric acid, false ↓ serum glucose **NIPE:** Only take w/ food if GI upset

Isoproterenol (Isuprel) [Bronchodilator/Sympathomimetic]

Uses: *Shock, bronchospasm, cardiac arrest, AV nodal block* **Action:** β₁- & β₂-receptor stimulant **Dose:** **Adults.** 2–10 mcg/min IV inf; titrate to effect. *Inhal:* 1–2 inhal 4–6×/d. **Peds.** 0.2–2 mcg/kg/min IV inf; titrate to effect. *Inhal:* 1–2 inhal 4–6×/d **Caution:** [C, ?] **Contra:** Angina, tachyarrhythmias (digitalis-induced or others) **Disp:** Met-inhaler; soln for neb 0.5%, 1%; inj 0.02 mg/mL, 0.2 mg/mL **SE:** Insomnia, arrhythmias, HA, trembling, dizziness **Notes:** Pulse > 130 bpm may induce arrhythmias **Interactions:** ↑ Effects w/ albuterol, guanethidine, oxytocic drugs, sympathomimetics, TCAs; ↑ risk of arrhythmias w/ amitriptyline, bretylium, cardiac glycosides, K-depleting drugs, theophylline; ↓ effects w/ BBs **Labs:** False ↑ serum AST, bilirubin, glucose **NIPE:** Saliva may turn pink in color, ↑ fluids to 2–3 L/d; more specific β 2 agonists preferred d/t excessive β 1 cardiac stimulation of drug; drug induces ischemia & dysrhythmias

Isosorbide Dinitrate (Isordil, Sorbitrate, Dilatrate-SR) [Antianginal/Nitrate]

Uses: *Rx & prevent angina,* CHF (w/ hydralazine) **Action:** Relaxes vascular smooth muscle **Dose:** *Acute angina:* 5–10 mg PO (chew tabs) q2–3h or 2.5–10 mg SL PRN q5–10min; do not give >3 doses in a 15–30-min period. *Angina prophylaxis:* 5–40 mg PO q6h; do not give nitrates on a chronic q6h or qid basis >7–10 d; tolerance may develop; provide 10–12-h drug-free intervals

Caution: [C, ?] **Contra:** Severe anemia, closed-angle glaucoma, postural ↓ BP, cerebral hemorrhage, head trauma (can ↑ ICP), w/ sildenafil, tadalafil, vardenafil **Disp:** Tabs 5, 10, 20, 30 mg; SR tabs 40 mg; SL tabs 2.5, 5, 10 mg; chew tabs 5, 10 mg; SR caps 40 mg **SE:** HA, ↓ BP, flushing, tachycardia, dizziness **Notes:** Higher PO dose usually needed to achieve same results as SL forms **Interactions:** ↑ Hypotension w/ antihypertensives, ASA, CCBs, phenothiazides, sildenafil, EtOH **Labs:** False ↓ serum cholesterol **NIPE:** ⊘ Nitrates for a 8–12-h period/d to avoid tolerance

Isosorbide Dinitrate & Hydralazine HCL (BiDil) [Antianginal, Antihypertensive/Vasodilator, Nitrate]

Uses: HF in AA pts; improve survival & functional status, prolong time between hospitalizations for HF **Action:** Relaxes vascular smooth muscle; peripheral vasodilator **Dose:** Initially: 1 tab TID PO (if not tolerated reduce to ½ tab TID) , titrate > 3–5 d as tolerated; Max: 2 tabs TID **Caution:** [C, ?/–] recent MI, syncope, hypovolemia, hypotension, hep impair **Contra:** ⊘ for children, concomitant use w/ PDE5 inhibitor (sildenafil) **Disp:** isosorbide dinitrate 20 mg/ hydralazine HCL 37.5 mg tabs **SE:** HA, dizziness, orthostatic hypotension, sinusitis, GI distress, tachycardia, paresthesia, amblyopia **Interactions:** ↑ risk of severe hypotension w/ antihypertensives, ASA, CCBs, MAOIs, phenothiazides, sildenafil, tadalafil, vardenafil, ETOH; ↓ pressor response w/ epinephrine; ↓ effects w/ NSAIDs; **Labs:** False ↓ serum cholesterol **NIPE:** ⊘ Nitrates for a 8–12-h period/d to avoid tolerance; take w/ food.

Isosorbide Mononitrate (Ismo, Imdur) [Antianginal/Nitrate]

Uses: *Prevention/Rx of angina pectoris* **Action:** Relaxes vascular smooth muscle **Dose:** 5-10 mg PO bid, w/ the 2 doses 7 h apart or XR (Imdur) 30–60 mg/d PO, max 240 mg **Caution:** [C, ?] **Contra:** Head trauma/cerebral hemorrhage (can ↑ ICP), w/ sildenafil, tadalafil, vardenafil **Disp:** Tabs 10, 20 mg; XR 30, 60, 120 mg **SE:** HA, dizziness, ↓ BP **Interactions:** ↑ Hypotension w/ ASA, CCB, nitrates, sildenafil, EtOH **Labs:** False ↓ serum cholesterol

Isotretinoin [13-*cis* Retinoic Acid] (Accutane, Amnesteem, Claravis, Sotret) [Anti-acne Agent]

WARNING: Must not be used by PRG females; can induce severe birth defects; pt must be capable of complying w/ mandatory contraceptive measures; prescribed according to product-specific risk management system. Because of teratogenicity, Accutane is approved for marketing only under a special restricted distribution FDA program called iPLEDGE **Uses:** *Refractory severe acne* **Action:** Retinoic acid derivative **Dose:** 0.5–2 mg/kg/d PO ÷ bid (↓ in hepatic Dz, take w/ food) **Caution:** [X, –] Avoid tetracyclines **Contra:** Retinoid sensitivity, PRG **Disp:** Caps 10, 20, 30, 40 mg **SE:** Rare: Depression, psychosis, suicidal thoughts; dermatologic sensitivity, xerostomia, photosensitivity, ↑ LFTs, ↑ triglycerides **Notes:** Risk management program requires 2 (–) PRG tests before Rx & use of 2 forms of contraception 1 mo before, during, & 1 mo after therapy; to prescribe isotretinoin, the Prescriber must access the iPLEDGE system via the Internet (www.ipledgeprogram.com); monitor LFTs

& lipids **Interactions:** ↑ Effects w/ corticosteroids, phenytoin, vitamin A; ↑ risk of pseudotumor cerebri w/ tetracyclines; ↑ triglyceride levels w/ EtOH; ↓ effects OF carbamazepine **NIPE:** ↑ Risk of photosensitivity—use sunscreen, take w/ food, ⊘ PRG; low-dose progesterone only hormonal contraceptives may not be adequate birth control alone.

Isradipine (DynaCirc) [Antihypertensive/CCB]
Uses: *HTN* Action: CCB Dose: *Adults.* 2.5–10 mg PO bid. Caution: [C, ?] Contra: Severe heart block, sinus bradycardia, CHF, dosing w/in several hours of IV β-blockers Disp: Caps 2.5, 5 mg; tabs CR 5, 10 mg SE: HA, edema, flushing, fatigue, dizziness, palpitations Interactions: ↑Effects w/ azole antifungals, BBs, cimetidine; ↑ effects OF carbamazepine, cyclosporine, digitalis glycosides, prazosin, quinidine; ↓ effects w/ Ca, rifampin; ↓ effects OF lovastatin **Labs:** ↑ LFTs **NIPE:** ⊘ D/C abruptly

Itraconazole (Sporanox) [Antifungal]
WARNING: Potential for negative inotropic effects on the heart; if signs or Sxs of CHF occur during administration, continued use should be assessed Uses: *Fungal Infxns (aspergillosis, blastomycosis, histoplasmosis, candidiasis)* Action: ↓ Ergosterol synthesis Dose: 200 mg PO or IV qd–bid (capsule w/ meals or cola/grapefruit juice); PO soln on empty stomach; avoid antacids Caution: [C, ?] Numerous drug interactions Contra: Inj. If CrCl <30 mL/min, Hx of CHF or ventricular dysfunction, or w/ H₂-antagonist, omeprazole Disp: Caps 100 mg; soln 10 mg/mL; inj 10 mg/mL SE: Nausea, rash, hepatitis, ↓ K⁺, CHF (mostly w/ IV use) Notes: PO soln & caps not interchangeable; useful in pts who cannot take amphotericin B; Interactions: ↑ Effects w/ clarithromycin, erythromycin; ↑ effects OF alprazolam, anticoagulants, atevirdine, atorvastatin, buspirone, cerivastatin, chlordiazepoxide, cyclosporine, diazepam, digoxin, felodipine, fluvastatin, indinavir, lovastatin, methadone, methylprednisolone, midazolam, nelfinavir, pravastatin, ritonavir, saquinavir, simvastatin, tacrolimus, tolbutamide, triazolam, warfarin; ↑ QT prolongation w/ astemizole, cisapride, pimozide, quinidine, terfenadine; ↓ effects w/ antacids, Ca, cimetidine, didanosine, famotidine, lansoprazole, Mg, nizatidine, omeprazole, phenytoin, rifampin, sucralfate, grapefruit juice **Labs:** ↑ LFTs, BUN, SCr **NIPE:** Take capsule w/ food & soln w/o food, ⊘ PRG or breast-feeding, ↑ risk of disulfiram-like response w/ EtOH

Kaolin-Pectin (Kaodene, Kao-Spen, Kapectolin) [OTC] [Antidiarrheal/Absorbent]
Uses: *Diarrhea* Action: Absorbent demulcent Dose: *Adults.* 60–120 mL PO after each loose stool or q3–4h PRN. *Peds.* 3–6 y: 15–30 mL/dose PO PRN. *6–12 y:* 30–60 mL/dose PO PRN Caution: [C, +] Contra: D secondary to pseudomembranous colitis Disp: Multiple OTC forms; also available w/ opium (Parepectolin CII) SE: Constipation, dehydration Interaction: ↓ Effects OF ciprofloxacin, clindamycin, digoxin, lincomycin, lovastatin, penicillamine, quinidine, tetracycline **NIPE:** Take other meds 2–3 h before or after this drug

Ketoconazole (Nizoral, Xolegel gel, Nizoral AD Shampoo) [Shampoo–OTC] [Antifungal]
Uses: *Systemic fungal Infxns; topical

for local fungal Infxns due to dermatophytes & yeast; shampoo for dandruff,* short term in CAP when rapid ↓ testosterone needed (ie, cord compression) **Action:** ↓ fungal cell wall synthesis **Dose:** *Adults.* PO: 200 mg PO qd; ↑ to 400 mg PO qd for serious Infxn; CAP 400 mg PO tid (short-term). *Topical:* Apply qd (cream/shampoo) **Peds >2 y.** 5–10 mg/kg/24 h PO ÷ q12–24h (↓ in hepatic Dz) **Caution:** [C, +/–] Any agent ↑ gastric pH prevents absorption; may enhance anticoagulants; w/ EtOH (disulfiram-like Rxn) numerous drug interactions **Contra:** CNS fungal Infxns (poor CNS penetration); concurrent astemizole, cisapride, PO triazolam **Disp:** Tabs 200 mg; topical cream 2%; shampoo 10% **SE:** N **Notes:** Monitor LFTs w/ systemic use **Interactions:** ↑ Effects OF alprazolam, anticoagulants, atevirdine, atorvastatin, buspirone, chlordiazepoxide, cyclosporine, diazepam, felodipine, fluvastatin, indinavir, lovastatin, methadone, methylprednisolone, midazolam, nelfinavir, pravastatin, ritonavir, saquinavir, simvastatin, tacrolimus, tolbutamide, triazolam, warfarin; ↑ QT prolongation w/ astemizole, cisapride, quinidine, terfenadine; ↓ effects w/ antacids, Ca, cimetidine, didanosine, famotidine, lansoprazole, Mg, nizatidine, omeprazole, phenytoin, rifampin, sucralfate **Labs:** ↑ LFTs **NIPE:** Take tabs w/ citrus juice, take w/ food; shampoo wet hair 1 min, rinse, repeat for 3 min; ⊘ PRG or breast-feeding

Ketoprofen (Orudis, Oruvail) [Analgesic/NSAID] WARNING:

May ↑ risk of cardiovascular events & GI bleeding **Uses:** *Arthritis, pain* **Action:** NSAID; ↓ prostaglandins **Dose:** 25–75 mg PO tid–qid, 300 mg/d/max; w/ food **Caution** [B (D 3rd tri), ?] **Contra:** NSAID/ASA sensitivity **Disp:** Tabs 12.5 mg; caps 25, 50, 75 mg; caps, SR 100, 150, 200 mg **SE:** GI upset, peptic ulcers, dizziness, edema, rash **Interactions:** ↑ Effects w/ ASA, corticosteroids, NSAIDs, probenicid, EtOH; ↑ effects OF antineoplastics, hypoglycemics, insulin, Li, MTX; ↑ risk of nephrotoxicity w/ aminoglycosides, cyclosporines; ↑ risk of bleeding w/ anticoagulants, cefamandole, cefotetan, cefoperazone, clopidogrel, eptifibatide, plicamycin, thrombolytics, tirofiban, valproic acid, dong quai, feverfew, garlic, ginkgo biloba, ginger, horse chestnut, red clover; ↓ effects OF antihypertensives, diuretics **Labs:** ↑ LFTs, BUN, serum Na^+, creatinine, Cl^-, K^+, PT; ↑ or ↓ glucose; ↓ Hmg, Hct, plts, leukocytes **NIPE:** ↑ Risk of photosensitivity—use sunscreen, take w/ food

Ketorolac (Toradol) [Analgesic/NSAID] WARNING: Indicated for

short term (≥ 5 d) Rx of moderate–severe acute pain that requires opioid analgesia levels **Uses:** *Pain* **Action:** NSAID; ↓ prostaglandins **Dose:** 15–30 mg IV/IM q6h or 10 mg PO qid; max IV/IM 120 mg/d, max PO 40 mg/d; do not use for > 5 d; ↓ for age & renal dysfunction **Caution:** [B (D 3rd tri), –] **Contra:** Peptic ulcer Dz, NSAID sensitivity, advanced renal Dz, CNS bleeding, anticipated major surgery, labor & delivery, nursing mothers **Disp:** Tabs 10 mg; inj 15 mg/mL, 30 mg/mL **SE:** Bleeding, peptic ulcer Dz, renal failure, edema, dizziness, allergy **Notes:** PO only as continuation of IM/IV therapy **Interactions:** ↑ Effects w/ ASA, corticosteroids, NSAIDs, probenicid, EtOH; ↑ effects OF antineoplastics, hypoglycemics, insulin,

Li, MTX; ↑ risk of nephrotoxicity w/ aminoglycosides, cyclosporines; ↑ risk of bleeding w/ anticoagulants, cefamandole, cefotetan, cefoperazone, clopidogrel, eptifibatide, plicamycin, thrombolytics, tirofiban, valproic acid, dong quai, feverfew, garlic, ginkgo biloba, ginger, horse chestnut, red clover; ↓ effects OF antihypertensives, diuretics **Labs:** ↑ LFTs, PT, BUN, SCr, Na⁺, Cl⁻, K⁺ **NIPE:** 30-mg dose equals comparative analgesia of meperidine 100 mg or morphine 12 mg

Ketorolac Ophthalmic (Acular, Acular LS, Acular PF) [Analgesic, Anti-inflammatory/NSAID] Uses: *Ocular itching w/ seasonal allergies; inflammation w/ cataract extraction; pain/photophobia w/ incisional refractive surgery (Acular PF); Pain w/ corneal refractive surgery (Acular LS)* **Action:** NSAID **Dose:** 1 gt qid **Caution:** [C, +] **Disp:** Acular LS: 0.4%; Acular, Acular PF Soln 0.5% **SE:** Local irritation

Ketotifen (Zaditor) [Opht Antihistamine] Uses: *Allergic conjunctivitis* **Action:** H₁-receptor antagonist, mast cell stabilizer **Dose:** *Adults & Peds.* 1 gt in eye(s) q8–12h **Caution:** [C,?/–] **Disp:** Soln 0.025%/5 mL **SE:** Local irritation, HA, rhinitis **NIPE:** Insert soft contact lenses 10 min after drug use

Labetalol (Trandate, Normodyne) [Antihypertensive/Alpha & Beta Blocker] Uses: *HTN* & hypertensive emergencies (IV) **Action:** α- & β-Adrenergic blocking agent **Dose:** *Adults.* HTN: Initial, 100 mg PO bid, then 200–400 mg PO bid. Increase by 100-mg increments OD q 2–3 days until BP controlled *Hypertensive emergency:* 20–80 mg IV bolus, then 2 mg/min IV inf, titrate up to 300 mg. *Peds.* PO: 3–20 mg/kg/d in ÷ doses. *Hypertensive emergency:* 0.4–1.5 mg/kg/h IV cont inf **Caution:** [C (D in 2nd or 3rd tri), +] **Contra:** Asthma/COPD, cardiogenic shock, uncompensated CHF, heart block **Disp:** Tabs 100, 200, 300 mg; inj 5 mg/mL **SE:** Dizziness, nausea, ↓ BP, fatigue, CV effects; **Notes:** When BP controlled w/ IV Labetalol, convert to 200 mg PO for 1 dose, then 200–400 mg PO q 6–12 h **Interactions:** ↑ Effects w/ cimetidine, diltiazem, nitroglycerine, quinidine, paroxetine, verapamil; ↑ tremors w/ TCAs; ↓ effects w/ glutethimide, NSAIDs, salicylates; ↓ effects of antihypertensives, β-adrenergic bronchodilators, sulfonylureas **Labs:** False + urine catecholamines **NIPE:** May have transient tingling of scalp

Lactic Acid & Ammonium Hydroxide [Ammonium Lactate] (Lac-Hydrin) [Emollient] Uses: *Severe xerosis & ichthyosis* **Action:** Emollient moisturizer **Dose:** Apply bid **Caution:** [B, ?] **Disp:** Cream, lotion, lactic acid 12% w/ ammonium hydroxide **SE:** Local irritation **NIPE:** ⊘ children < 2 years; ↓ sun exposure—use sunscreen; risk of hyperpigmentation

Lactobacillus (Lactinex Granules) [Antidiarrheal] [OTC] Uses: Control of D, especially after antibiotic therapy **Action:** Replaces nl intestinal flora **Dose:** *Adults & Peds >3 y.* 1 packet, 1–2 caps, or 4 tabs PO qd–qid (w/ meals or liq) **Caution:** [A, +] **Contra:** Milk/lactose allergy **Disp:** Tabs; caps; EC caps; powder in packets (all OTC) **SE:** Flatulence

Lactulose (Chronulac, Cephulac, Enulose) [Laxative] Uses: *Hepatic encephalopathy; constipation* **Action:** Acidifies the colon, allows ammonia to diffuse into colon **Dose:** *Acute hepatic encephalopathy:* 30–45 mL PO q1h until soft stools, then tid–qid. *Chronic laxative therapy:* 30–45 mL PO tid–qid; adjust q1–2d to produce 2–3 soft stools/d. *Rectally:* 200 g in 700 mL of H₂O PR. *Peds.* Infants: 2.5–10 mL/24 h ÷ tid–qid. *Peds:* 40–90 mL/24 h ÷ tid–qid **Caution:** [B, ?] **Contra:** Galactosemia **Disp:** Syrup 10 g/15 mL, soln 10 g/15 mL, 10, 20 g/packet **SE:** Severe D, flatulence; life-threatening electrolyte disturbances **Interactions:** ↓ Effects w/ antacids, neomycin **Labs:** ↓ Serum ammonia **NIPE:** May take 24–48 h for results

Lamivudine (Epivir, Epivir-HBV) [Antiretroviral/NRTI] **WARNING:** Lactic acidosis & severe hepatomegaly w/ steatosis reported w/ nucleoside analogs **Uses:** *HIV Infxn, chronic hepatitis B* **Action:** ↓ HIV RT & hepatitis B viral polymerase, resulting in viral DNA chain termination **Dose:** *HIV: Adults & Peds >16 y.* 150 mg PO bid or 300 mg PO qd. *Peds <16 y.* 4 mg/kg PO bid. *HBV: Adults.* 100 mg/d PO. *Peds 2–17 y.* 3 mg/kg/d PO, 100 mg max; ↓ in renal impair **Caution:** [C, ?] **Contra:** Component hypersensitivity **Disp:** Tabs 100 mg (HBV) 150 mg, 300 mg; soln 5 mg/mL (HBV), 10 mg/mL **SE:** HA, pancreatitis, GI upset, lactic acidosis, peripheral neuropathy **Interactions:** ↑ Effects w/ co-trimoxazole, trimethoprim/sulfamethoxazole; ↑ risk OF lactic acidosis w/ antiretrovirals, reverse transcriptase inhibitors **Labs:** ↑ LFTs

Lamotrigine (Lamictal) [Anticonvulsant] **WARNING:** Serious rashes requiring hospitalization & D/C of Rx reported; rash less frequent in adults **Uses:** *Partial Szs, bipolar disorder, Lennox–Gastaut syndrome* **Action:** Phenyltriazine antiepileptic, Ø[CN1] glutamate, stabilize neuronal membrane **Dose:** *Adults.* Szs: Initial 50 mg PO, then 50 mg PO bid for 2 wk, then maint 300–500 mg/d in ÷ doses. *Bipolar:* Initial 25 mg/d PO, then 50 mg PO qd for 2 wk, then 100 mg PO qd for 1 wk; Maint 200 mg/d. *Peds.* 0.6 mg/kg in ÷ doses for wk 1 & 2, then 1.2 mg/kg for wk 3 & 4, then Maint 15 mg/kg/d (max 400 mg/d) in 1–2 ÷; ↓ in hepatic Dz or if w/ enzyme inducers or valproic acid) **Caution:** [C, –] **Interactions w/** other antiepileptics **Disp:** Tabs 25, 100, 150, 200 mg; chew tabs 2, 5, 25 mg **SE:** Photosensitivity; HA, GI upset, dizziness, ataxia, rash (potentially life-threatening in children > adults) **Notes:** Value of therapeutic monitoring not established **Interactions:** ↑ Effects of valproic acid; ↑ effects OF carbamazepine; ↓ effects w/ phenobarbital, phenytoin, primidone **NIPE:** ↑ Risk of photosensitivity—use sunscreen

Lansoprazole (Prevacid, Prevacid IV) [Antisecretory/Proton-Pump Inhibitor] **Uses:** *Duodenal ulcers, prevent & Rx NSAID gastric ulcers, IV alternative for ≤ 7 d /w erosive esophagitis.* H. pylori Infxn, erosive esophagitis, & hypersecretory conditions, GERD **Action:** Proton pump inhibitor **Dose:** 15–30 mg/d PO; NSAID ulcer prevention 15 mg/d PO ≤ 12 wk, NSAID ulcers 30 mg/d PO, ×8 wk; 30 mg IV qd ≤ 7 d change to PO for 6–8 wk; ↓ in severe hepatic impair **Caution:** [B, ?/–] **Disp:** Caps 15, 30 mg; granules for suspension 15, 30 mg OD tabs 15, 30 mg; inj set w/ filter **SE:** HA, fatigue **Notes:** For IV provided in-line filter must be used **Interactions:** ↑ Effects OF hypoglycemics, nifedipine; ↓ effects w/ sucralfate; ↓ effects OF ampicillin, cefpodoxime, cefuroxime, digoxin, enoxacin ketoconazole, theophylline **Labs:** ↑ LFTs, SCr, LDH, gastrin, lipids **NIPE:** Take ac

Lanthanum Carbonate (Fosrenol) [Phosphate Binder] Uses: Hyperphosphatemia in renal disease* **Action:** Phosphate binder **Dose:** 750–150 mg PO qd ÷ doses, w/ or immed after meal; titrate every 2–3 wk based on PO_4 levels **Caution:** [C, ?/–], no data in GI disease **Disp:** Chew tabs 250, 500, 750 1000 mg **SE:** N/V, graft occlusion, HA, ↓ BP **Notes:** Chew tabs before swallow ing; separate from meds that interact with antacids by 2 h **Labs:** ↑ serum calciun level; monitor serum phosphate levels **NIPE:** use cautiously w/ GI disease; moni tor for bone pain or deformity

Latanoprost (Xalatan) [Glaucoma Agent] Uses: *open angle glaucoma, ocular HTN* **Action:** Prostaglandin, ↑ outflow of aqueous humor **Dose:** 1 gtt eye(s) hs **Caution:** [C, ?] **Disp:** 0.005% soln **SE:** May darken light irides blurred vision, ocular stinging, & itching **Interactions:** ↑ Risk OF precipitation i mixed w/ eye drops w/ thimerosal

Leflunomide (Arava) [Anti-rheumatic DMARDs/Immuno-modulator] WARNING: PRG must be excluded prior to start of Rx Uses *Active RA* **Action:** ↓ Pyrimidine synthesis **Dose:** Initial 100 mg/d PO for 3 d then 10–20 mg/d **Caution:** [X, –] **Contra:** PRG **Disp:** Tabs 10, 20, 100 mg **SE** D, Infxn, HTN, alopecia, rash, nausea, joint pain, hepatitis **Interactions:** ↑ Effects w/ rifampin; ↑ risk OF hepatotoxicity w/ hepatotoxic drugs, MRX; ↑ effects OF NSAIDs; ↓ effects w/ activated charcoal, cholestyramine **Labs:** ↑ LFTs; Monitor LFTs during initial therapy **NIPE:** ⊘ PRG, breast-feeding, live virus vaccines

Lenalidomide (Revlimid) [Immunomodulator] WARNING: Sig nificant teratogen; patient must be enrolled in RevAssist risk reduction program Uses: *MDS* multiple myeloma **Action:** Thalidomide analog, immune modula tor **Dose:** *Adults.* 10 mg PO daily; swallow whole w/water **Caution:** [X,–] w renal impair **Disp:** Caps 5, 10 mg **SE:** D, pruritus, rash, fatigue, myelosuppres sion, thromboembolism, **Labs:** ↑ LFTs, monitor for myelosuppression, throm boembolism, hepatotoxicity **NIPE:** Routine PRG tests required; Rx only in 1-mo increments; limited distribution network; males must use condom and not donate sperm; use contraception at least 4 wks beyond D/C

Lepirudin (Refludan) [Anticoagulant] Uses: *HIT* **Action:** Direc thrombin inhibitor **Dose:** Bolus 0.4 mg/kg IV, then 0.15 mg/kg/h inf (↓ dose & in rate if CrCl <60 mL/min) **Caution:** [B, ?/–] Hemorrhagic event or severe HTN **Contra:** Active bleeding **Disp:** Inj 50 mg **SE:** Bleeding, anemia, hematoma **Notes** Adjust dose based on aPTT ratio, maintain aPTT ratio of 1.5–2.0 **Interactions** ↑ Risk OF bleeding w/ antiplt drugs, cephalosporins, NSAIDs, thrombolytics, sali cylates, feverfew, ginkgo biloba, ginger, valerian

Letrozole (Femara) [Antineoplastic]   Uses: *Advanced breast CA in postmenopausal* **Action:** Nonsteroidal aromatase inhibitor **Dose:** 2.5 mg/d PO **Caution:** [D, ?] **Contra:** PRG **Disp:** Tabs 2.5 mg **SE:** Anemia, nausea, hot flashes, arthralgia **Notes:** Requires periodic CBC, thyroid Fxn, electrolyte, LFT, & renal monitoring; **Interactions:** ↑ Risk OF interference w/ action of drug w/ estrogens and oral contraceptives **Labs:** ↑ LFTs, cholesterol, Ca, ↓ lymphocytes, monitor blood work as above

Leucovorin (Wellcovorin) [Folic Acid Derivative]   Uses: *OD of folic acid antagonist; megaloblastic anemia, augmentation of 5-FU impaired MTX elimination* **Action:** Reduced folate source; circumvents action of folate reductase inhibitors (eg, MTX) **Dose:** *Adults & Peds.* Per protocol. **Caution:** [C, ?/–] **Contra:** Pernicious anemia **Disp:** Tabs 5, 10, 15, 25 mg; inj 50, 100, 200, 350, 500 **SE:** Allergic Rxn, N/V/D, fatigue **Notes:** Many dosing schedules for leucovorin rescue following MTX therapy; do not use intrathecally/intraventrically **Interactions:** ↑ Effects OF fluorouracil; ↓ effects OF MTX, phenobarbital, phenytoin, primidone, trimethoprim/sulfamethoxazole **NIPE:** ↑ Fluids to 3 L/d

Leuprolide (Lupron, Lupron DEPOT, Lupron DEPOT-Ped, Viadur, Eligard) [Antineoplastic]   Uses: *Advanced CAP (all products except Depot-Ped), endometriosis (Lupron), uterine fibroids (Lupron), & CPP (Lupron-Ped)* **Action:** LHRH agonist; paradoxically ↑ release of gonadotropin, resulting in ↓ pituitary gonadotropins (↓ LH); in men ↓ testosterone **Dose:** *Adults. CAP: Lupron Depot:* 7.5 mg IM q28d or 22.5 mg IM q3mo or 30 mg IM q4mo; Eligard: 45 mg SQ 6 mo; Viadur implant (CAP only); insert in inner upper arm using local anesthesia, replace q12mo. *Endometriosis (Lupron DEPOT):* 3.75 mg IM qmo ×6. *Fibroids:* 3.75 mg IM qmo ×3. *Peds.* CPP (Lupron-Ped): 50 mcg/kg/d SQ inj; ↑ by 10 mcg/kg/d until total down-regulation achieved. *DEPOT: <25 kg:* 7.5 mg IM q4wk. *>25–37.5 kg:* 11.25 mg IM q4wk. *>37.5 kg:* 15 mg IM q4wk **Caution:** [X, ?] w/ impending cord compression in CAP **Contra:** Undiagnosed vaginal bleeding, implant dosage form in women & peds; PRG **Disp:** Inj 5 mg/mL; Lupron DEPOT 3.75 (1 mo for fibroids, endometriosis); Lupron DEPOT for CAP: 7.5 mg (1 mo), 11.25 mg (3 mo), 22.5 (3 mo), 30 mg (4 mo); Eligard depot for CAP: 7.5 mg (1 mo); 22.5 mg (3 mo), 30 mg (4 mo), 45 mg (6 mo); Viadur 65 mg 12-mo SQ implant, Lupron-Ped 7.5, 11.25, 15 mg **SE:** Hot flashes, gynecomastia, N/V, alopecia, anorexia, dizziness, HA, insomnia, paresthesias, depression exacerbation, peripheral edema, & bone pain (transient "flare Rxn" at 7–14 d after the 1st dose [LH/testosterone surge before suppression]) may block flare **Interactions:** ↓ Effects w/ androgens, estrogens **Labs:** ↑ LFTs, BUN, serum Ca, uric acid, glucose, lipids, WBC, PT; ↓ serum K⁺, plts **NIPE:** Nonsteroidal antiandrogen (eg bicalutamide)

Levalbuterol (Xopenex) [Bronchodilator/Beta 2 Agonist]   Uses: *Asthma (Rx & prevention of bronchospasm)* **Action:** Sympathomimetic bronchodilator **Dose:** *Adult > 12 yrs.* 0.63–1.25 mg neb q6–8h; *Peds > 4 yrs.* 1–2 puffs q4-6h **Caution:** [C, ?] **Disp.:** Multidose inhaler 45 mcg/puff (15 gm); Soln for inhal 0.31, 0.63, 1.25 mg/3 mL, 1.25 mg/0.5 mL **SE:** Tachycardia, nervousness, trembling, flu syndrome **Notes:** *R*-isomer of albuterol; may ↓ CV side effects compared with albuterol **Interactions:** ↑ Effects w/ MAOIs, TCAs; ↑ risk OF hypokalemia w/ loop & thiazide diuretics; ↓ effects w/ BBs; ↓ effects OF digoxin **Labs:** ↑ Serum glucose, ↓ serum K⁺ **NIPE:** Use other inhalants 5 min after this drug

Levetiracetam (Keppra) [Anticonvulsant] Uses: *Partial onset Szs* **Action:** Unknown **Dose:** *Adults.* 500 mg PO bid, may ↑ 3000 mg/d max; *Peds.* 4–16 y: 10–20 mg/kg/d ÷ in 2 doses, 60 mg/kg/d max (↓ in renal insuff) **Caution:** [C, ?/–] **Contra:** Component allergy **Disp:** Tabs 250, 500, 750, 1000 mg; Sol 100 mg/mL **SE:** Dizziness & somnolence; impaired coordination **Interactions:** ↑ Effects w/ antihistamines, TCAs, benzodiazepines, narcotics, EtOH **NIPE:** May take w/ food

Levobunolol (A-K Beta, Betagan) [Glaucoma Agent/Beta Adrenergic Blocker] Uses: *Glaucoma* **Action:** β-Adrenergic blocker **Dose:** 1 gt qd–bid **Caution:** [C, ?] **Disp:** Soln 0.25, 0.5% **SE:** Ocular stinging or burning **Notes:** Possible systemic effects if absorbed **Interactions:** ↑ Effects w/ BBs; ↑ risk OF hypotension & bradycardia w/ quinidine, verapamil; ↓ intraocular pressure w/ carbonic anhydrase inhibitors, epinephrine, pilocarpine **NIPE:** Night vision and acuity may be decreased

Levocabastine (Livostin) [Antihistamine] Uses: *Allergic seasonal conjunctivitis* **Action:** Antihistamine **Dose:** 1 gt in eye(s) qid = 2 wk **Caution:** [C, +/–] **Disp:** 0.05% gtt **SE:** Ocular discomfort **NIPE:** ⊘ Insert soft contact lenses

Levofloxacin (Levaquin, Quixin & Iquix Ophthalmic) [Antibiotic/Fluoroquinolone] Uses: *Lower resp tract Infxns, sinusitis, UTI; topical for bacterial conjunctivitis, skin Infxns* **Action:** Quinolone antibiotic, ↓ DNA gyrase. *Spectrum:* Excellent gram(+) except MRSA & *E. faecium*; excellent gram(–) except *S. maltophilia* & *Acinetobacter* sp; poor anaerobic **Dose:** 250–500 mg/d PO or IV; community acquired pneumonia 750 mg/day for 5 d; ophth 1–2 gtt in eye(s) q2h while awake for 2 d, then q4h while awake for 5 d; ↓ in renal insuff, avoid antacids if PO **Caution:** [C, –] **Interactions** w/ cation-containing products (eg, antacids) **Contra:** Quinolone sensitivity **Disp:** Tabs 250, 500, 750 mg; premixed IV 250, 500, 750 mg, inj 25 mg/mL; Leva-Pak 750 mg × 5 d; Sol: 25 mg/mL ophth soln 0.5% (Quixin), 1.5% (Iquix) **SE:** N/D, dizziness, rash, GI upset, photosensitivity **Interactions:** ↑ Effects OF cyclosporine, digoxin, theophylline, warfarin, caffeine; ↑ risk OF Szs w/ foscarnet, NSAIDs; ↑ risk OF hyperor hypoglycemia w/ hypoglycemic drugs; ↓ effects w/ antacids, antineoplastics, Ca, cimetidine, didanosine, famotidine, Fe, lansoprazole, Mg, nizatidine, omeprazole, phenytoin, ranitidine, NaHCO₃, sucralfate, Zn **NIPE:** Risk of tendon rupture & tendonitis—DC if pain or inflammation; ↑ fluids, use sunscreen, antacids 2 h before or after this drug

Levonorgestrel (Plan B) [Progestin/Hormone] Uses: *Emergency contraceptive ("morning-after pill")*; prevents PRG if taken < 72 h after unprotected sex/contraceptive fails **Action:** Progestin **Dose:** 0.75 mg q12h × 2 **Caution:** [X, M] **Contra:** Known/suspected PRG, abnormal uterine bleeding **Disp:** Tab, 0.75 mg, 2 blister pack **SE:** N/V, abdominal pain, fatigue, HA, menstrual changes. **Notes:** Will not induce abortion; ↑ risk of ectopic PRG **Interactions:** ↓ Effects w/ barbiturates, carbamazepine, modafinil, phenobarbital, phenytoin, pioglitazone, rifabutin, rifampin, ritonavir, topiramate

Levonorgestrel Implant (Norplant II, Jadelle) [Progestin/ Hormone] Uses: *Contraceptive* **Action:** Progestin **Dose:** Implant 150 mg in midforearm **Caution:** [X, +/–] **Contra:** Undiagnosed abnormal uterine bleeding, Hepatic Dz, thromboembolism, Hx of intracranial HTN, breast CA, renal impair **Disp:** 75 mg implant times 5 **SE:** Uterine bleeding, HA, acne, nausea **Notes:** Prevents PRG for up to 5 y; remove if PRG desired **Interactions:** ↓ Effects w/ barbiturates, carbamazepine, modafinil, phenobarbital, phenytoin, pioglitazone, rifabutin, rifampin, ritonavir, topiramate **Labs:** ↑ uptake OF T_3, ↓ T_4 sex hormone-binding globulin levels **NIPE:** Menstrual irregularities 1st y after implant, use barrier contraception if taking anticonvulsants, may cause vision changes or contact lens tolerability

Levonorgestrel/Ethinyl Estradiol (Seasonale) Levorphanol (Levo-Dromoran) [C-II] [Narcotic Analgesic] Uses: *Moderate– severe pain; chronic pain* **Action:** Narcotic analgesic **Dose:** 2–4 mg PO PRN q6–8h; 1–2 mg IM/SQ PRN q6–8h (↓ in hepatic failure) **Caution:** [B/D (prolonged use or high doses at term), ?] **Contra:** Component allergy **Disp:** Tabs 2 mg; inj 2 mg/mL **SE:** Tachycardia, ↓ BP, drowsiness, GI upset, constipation, resp depression, pruritus **Interactions:** ↑ CNS effects w/ antihistamines, cimetidine, CNS depressants, glutethimide, methocarbamol, EtOH, St. John's wort **Labs:** False ↑ amylase, lipase **NIPE:** ↑ Fluids & fiber, take w/ food

Levothyroxine (Synthroid, Levoxyl, others) [Thyroid Hormone] Uses: *Hypothyroidism, myxedema coma* **Action:** Supplement L-thyroxine **Dose:** *Adults.* Hypothyroid Initial, 12/5-50 mcg/d PO; ↑ by 25–50 mcg/d every mo; usual 100–200 mcg/d. Myxedema: 200-500 mcg IV, then 100-300 mct/d **Peds.** Hypothyroid: *0–3 mo:* 10–15 mcg/kg/24 h PO. *3–6 mo:* 8–10 mcg/kg/d PO; *6–12 mo:* 6–8 mcg/kg/d PO; *1–5 yr:* 5–6 mcg/kg/d PO; *6–12 yr:* 4–5 mcg/kd/d PO; *> 12 yr:* 2–3 mcg/kd/d PO; Reduce dose by 50% if IV; titrate based on response & thyroid tests; dose can ↑ rapidly in young/middle-aged **Caution:** [A, +] **Contra:** Recent MI, uncorrected adrenal insuff **Disp:** Tabs 25, 50, 75, 88, 100, 112, 125, 137, 150, 175, 200, 300 mcg; inj 200, 500 mcg **SE:** Insomnia, weight loss, alopecia, arrhythmia **Notes:** Take w/ full glass of water (prevents choking) **Interactions:** ↑ Effects OF anticoagulants, sympathomimetics, TCAs, warfarin; ↓ effects w/ antacids, BBs, carbamazepine, cholestyramine, estrogens, Fe salts, phenytoin, phenobarbital, rifampin, simethicone, sucralfate; ↓ effects OF digoxin, hypoglycemics, theophylline **Labs:** False ↑ serum T_3; drug alters thyroid uptake of radioactive I—DC drug 4 wk before studies **NIPE:** ⊘ Switch brands due to different bioavailabilities

Lidocaine (Anestacon Topical, Xylocaine, others) [Antiarrhythmic/Local Anesthetic] **Uses:** Local anesthetic; Rx cardiac arrhythmias **Action:** Anesthetic; class IB antiarrhythmic **Dose:** *Adults.* Antiarrhythmic, ET: 5 mg/kg; follow w/ 0.5 mg/kg in 10 min if effective. *IV load:* 1 mg/kg/dose bolus over 2–3 min; repeat in 5–10 min; 200–300 mg/h max; cont inf 20–50 mcg/kg/min or 1–4 mg/min. *Peds.* Antiarrhythmic, ET, load: 1 mg/kg; repeat in 10–15 min 5 mg/kg max total, then IV inf 20–50 mcg/kg/min. *Topical:* Apply max 3 mg/kg/dose. *Local inj anesthetic:* Max 4.5 mg/kg (Table 3) **Caution:** [C, +] **Contra:** Do not use lidocaine w/ epi on digits, ears, or nose (risk of vasoconstriction & necrosis) heart block **Disp:** *Inj local:* 0.5, 1, 1.5, 2, 4, 10, 20%. *Inj IV:* 1% (10 mg/mL), 2% (20 mg/mL); admixture 4, 10, 20%. *IV inf:* 0.2%, 0.4%; cream 2%; gel 2, 2.5%; oint 2.5, 5%; liq 2.5%; soln 2, 4%; viscous 2% **SE:** Dizziness, paresthesias, & convulsions associated w/ tox **Notes:** 2nd line to amiodarone in ECC; dilute ET dose 1–2 mL w/ NS; epi may be added for local anesthesia to ↑ effect & ↓ bleeding; for IV forms, ↓ w/ liver Dz or CHF; see Table 2 for systemic levels **Interactions:** ↑ Effects w/ amprenavir, BBs, cimetidine; ↑ neuromuscular blockade w/ aminoglycosides, tubocurarine, pareira; ↑ cardiac depression w/ procainamide, tocainide; ↑ effects OF succinylcholine **Labs:** False ↑ SCr, ↑ CPK for 48 h after IM inj **NIPE:** Oral spray/soln may impair swallowing

Lidocaine/Prilocaine (EMLA, LMX) [Topical Anesthetic] **Uses:** *Topical anesthetic*; adjunct to phlebotomy or dermal procedures **Action:** Topical anesthetic **Dose:** *Adults.* EMLA cream, anesthetic disc (1 g/10 cm^2): Thick layer 2–2.5 g to intact skin, cover w/ occlusive dressing (eg, Tegaderm) for at least 1 h. *Anesthetic disc:* 1 g/10 cm^2 for at least 1 h. *Peds.* Max dose: <3 mo or <5 kg: 1 g/10 cm^2 for 1 h. *3–12 mo & >5 kg:* 2 g/20 cm^2 for 4 h. *1–6 y & >10 kg:* 10 g/100 cm^2 for 4 h. *7–12 y & >20 kg:* 20 g/200 cm^2 for 4 h **Caution:** [B, +] Methemoglobinemia **Contra:** Use on mucous membranes, broken skin, eyes; allergy to amide-type anesthetics **Disp:** Cream 2.5% lidocaine/2.5% prilocaine; anesthetic disc (1 g) **SE:** Burning, stinging, methemoglobinemia **Notes:** Longer contact time ↑ effect; See Lidocaine **NIPE:** Low risk of systemic adverse effects

Lidocaine/Tetracaine Transdermal (Synera) **Uses:** Topical anesthetic; adjunct to phlebotomy or dermal procedures **Action:** Topical anesthetic **Dose:** *Adults & Children > 3 yrs.* Phlebotomy: Apply to intact skin 20–30 min prior to venipuncture; *Dermal procedures:* Apply to intact skin 30 min prior to procedure **Caution:** (B, ±) **Contra:** Pts w/allergy to lidocaine/tetracaine/amide & ester type anesthetics; use on mucous membranes, broken skin, eyes; pts w/ para-aminobenzoic acid (PABA) hypersensitivity **Supplied:** TD patch lidocaine 70 mg/tetracaine 70 mg SE: Erythema, blanching, edema, rash, burning, dizziness, HA, paresthesias **Notes:** ⊘ Use multiple patches simultaneously or sequentially **Interactions:** ↑ Systemic effects of Class I antiarrhythmic drugs (tocainide, mexiletine); ↑ systemic effects with other local anesthetics **NIPI:** ⊘ Cut patch/remove top cover—may cause thermal injury; low risk of systemic adverse effects

Lindane [OTC] (Kwell) [Scabicide/Pediculicide] Uses: *Head lice, crab lice, scabies* **Action:** Ectoparasiticide & ovicide **Dose:** *Adults & Peds.* Cream or lotion: Thin layer after bathing, leave for 8–12 h, pour on laundry. *Shampoo:* Apply 30 mL, develop a lather w/ warm water for 4 min, comb out nits **Caution:** [C, +/–] **Contra:** Open wounds, Sz disorder **Disp:** Lotion 1%; shampoo 1% **SE:** Arrhythmias, Szs, local irritation, GI upset **Notes:** Caution w/ overuse (may be absorbed); may repeat Rx in 7 days **Interactions:** Oil-based hair creams ↑ drug absorption **NIPE:** Apply to dry hair/dry, cool skin

Linezolid (Zyvox) [Antibiotic/Oxazolidinones] Uses: *Infxns caused by gram(+) bacteria (including vancomycin-resistant enterococcus, VRE), pneumonia, skin Infxns* **Action:** Unique, binds ribosomal bacterial RNA; bactericidal for strep, bacteriostatic for enterococci & staph. *Spectrum:* Excellent gram(+) activity including VRE & MRSA **Dose:** *Adults.* 400–600 mg IV or PO q12h. *Peds.* 10 mg/kg IV or PO q8h (q12h in preterm neonates) **Caution:** [C, ?/–] w/ reversible MAOI, avoid foods w/ tyramine & cough/cold products w/ pseudoephedrine; w/ myelosuppression **Disp:** Inj 2 mg/mL; tabs 400, 600 mg; susp 100 mg/5 mL **SE:** HTN, N/D, HA, insomnia, GI upset, myelosuppression, tongue discoloration **Interactions:** ↑ Risk OF serotonin syndrome w/ SSRIs, sibutramine, trazodone, venlafaxine; ↑ HTN w/ amphetamines, dextromethorphan, dopamine, epinephrine, levodopa, MAOIs, meperidine, metaraminol, phenylephrine, phenylpropanolamine, pseudoephedrine, tyramine, ginseng, ephedra, ma huang, tyramine containing foods; ↑ risk OF bleeding w/ antiplts **Labs:** Follow weekly CBC **NIPE:** Take w/o regard to food, ⊘ tyramine-containing foods

Liothyronine (Cytomel) [Thyroid Hormone] Uses: *Hypothyroidism, goiter, myxedema coma, thyroid suppression therapy* **Action:** T_3 replacement **Dose:** *Adults.* Initial 25 mcg/24 h, titrate q1–2wk to response & TFT; initial of 25–100 mcg/24 h PO. *Myxedema coma:* 25–50 mcg IV. *Peds.* Initial 5 mcg/24 h, titrate by 5-mcg/24 h increments at 1–2-wk intervals; Maint 20–75 mcg/24 h PO qd; ↓ in elderly **Caution:** [A, +] **Contra:** Recent MI, uncorrected adrenal insuff, uncontrolled HTN **Disp:** Tabs 5, 25, 50 mcg; inj 10 mcg/mL **SE:** Alopecia, arrhythmias, CP, HA, sweating **Interactions:** ↑ Effects OF anticoagulants; ↓ effects w/ bile acid sequestrants, carbamazepine, estrogens, phenytoin, rifampin; ↓ effects OF hypoglycemics, theophylline; **Labs:** Monitor TFT; **NIPE:** Monitor cardiac status, take in AM

Lisinopril (Prinivil, Zestril) [Antihypertensive/ACEI] Uses: *HTN, CHF, prevent DN & AMI* **Action:** ACE inhibitor **Dose:** 5–40 mg/24 h PO qd–bid. *AMI:* 5 mg w/in 24 h of MI, then 5 mg after 24 h, 10 mg after 48 h, then 10 mg/d; ↓ in renal insuff **Caution:** [D, –] **Contra:** ACE inhibitor sensitivity **Disp:** Tabs 2.5, 5, 10, 20, 30, 40 mg **SE:** Dizziness, HA, cough, ↓ BP, angioedema, ↑ K^+ **Notes:** To prevent DN, start when urinary microalbuminemia begins **Interactions:** ↑ Effects w/ α-blockers, diuretics ↑ risk OF hyperkalemia w/ K-sparing diuretics, trimethoprim, salt substitutes; ↑ risk OF cough w/ capsaicin; ↑ effects OF insulin,

Li; ↓ effects w/ ASA, indomethacin, NSAIDs **Labs:** ↑ Serum K⁺, creatinine, BUN **NIPE:** Maximum effect may take several weeks

Lithium Carbonate (Eskalith, Lithobid, others) [Antimanic]

Uses: *Manic episodes of bipolar Dz* **Action:** Effects shift toward intraneuronal metabolism of catecholamines **Dose:** *Adults.* Acute mania: 600- 1200 mg/d PO tid–qid ÷ doses (max 2.4 g/d) or 900 mg SR bid *Peds 2–12 y.* 15–60 mg/kg/d in 3–4 ÷ doses; must titrate; follow serum levels; ↓ in renal insuff, elderly **Caution:** [D, –] Many drug interactions **Contra:** Severe renal impair or CV Dz, lactation **Disp:** Caps 150, 300, 600 mg; tabs 300 mg; SR tabs 300, CR tabs 450 mg; syrup 300 mg/5 mL **SE:** Polyuria, polydipsia, nephrogenic DI, tremor; Na retention or diuretic use may ↑tox; arrhythmias, dizziness **Notes:** See Table 2 for drug levels **Interactions:** ↑ Effects OF TCA; ↑ effects w/ ACEIs, bumetanide, carbamazepine, ethacrynic acid, fluoxetine, furosemide, methyldopa, NSAIDs, phenytoin, phenothiazines, probenecid, tetracyclines, thiazide diuretics, dandelion, juniper; ↓ effects w/ acetazolamide, antacids, mannitol, theophyllines, urea, verapamil, caffeine **Labs:** False + urine glucose, ↑ serum glucose, creatinine kinase, TSH, I-131 uptake; ↓ uric acid, T₃, T₄ **NIPE:** Several weeks before full effects of med, ↑ fluid intake to 2–3 L/d

Lodoxamide (Alomide) [Antihistamine]

Uses: *Seasonal allergic conjunctivitis; keratitis* **Action:** Stabilizes mast cells **Dose:** *Adults & Peds >2 y.* 1–2 gtt in eye(s) qid ≤ 3 mon **Caution:** [B, ?] **Disp:** Soln 0.1% **SE:** Ocular burning, stinging, HA **NIPE:** Not recommended for children < 2 years; ⊘ wear contact lens w/ drug

Lomefloxacin (Maxaquin) [Antibiotic/Fluoroquinolone]

Uses: *UTI, acute exacerbation of chronic bronchitis; prophylaxis in transurethral procedures* **Action:** Quinolone antibiotic; ↓ DNA gyrase. *Spectrum:* Good gram(–) activity including *H. influenzae* except *Stenotrophomonas maltophilia, Acinetobacter* sp, & some *P. aeruginosa* **Dose:** 400 mg PO; ↓ in renal insuff, avoid antacids **Caution:** [C, –] Interactions w/ cation-containing products **Contra:** Allergy to other quinolones, children < 18 y **Disp:** Tabs 400 mg **SE:** Photosensitivity, Szs, HA, dizziness **Interactions:** ↑ Effects w/ cimetidine, probenecid; ↑ effects OF cyclosporine, warfarin, caffeine; ↓ effects w/ antacids **Labs:** ↑ LFTs, ↓ K⁺ **NIPE:** ↑ Risk of photosensitivity—use sunscreen, ↑ fluids to 2 L/d

Loperamide (Imodium) [OTC] [Antidiarrheal]

Uses: *Diarrhea* **Action:** Slows intestinal motility **Dose:** *Adults.* Initial 4 mg PO, then 2 mg after each loose stool, up to 16 mg/d. *Peds.* 2–5 y, 13–20 kg: 1 mg PO tid. *6–8 y, 20–30 kg.* 2 mg PO bid. *8–12 y, >30 kg:* 2 mg PO tid **Caution:** [B, +] Not for acute diarrhea caused by *Salmonella, Shigella,* or *C. difficile* **Contra:** Pseudomembranous colitis, bloody diarrhea **Disp:** Caps 2 mg; tabs 2 mg; liq 1 mg/5 mL (OTC) **SE:** Constipation, sedation, dizziness **Interactions:** ↑ Effects w/ antihistamines, CNS depressants, phenothiazines, TCAs, EtOH

Lopinavir/Ritonavir (Kaletra) [Antiretroviral/Protease Inhibitor]

Uses: *HIV Infxn* **Action:** Protease inhibitor **Dose:** *Adults.* Tx naïve:

2 tab PO qd or 1 tab PO bid; Tx experienced pt: 1 tab PO bid (↑ dose if taken w/ amprenavir, efavirenz, fosamprenavir, nelfinavir, nevirapine) **Peds.** 7–15 kg: 12/3 mg/kg PO bid. *15–40 kg:* 10/2.5 mg/kg PO bid. *>40 kg:* Adult dose (w/ food) **Caution:** [C, ?/–] Numerous drug interactions **Contra:** Concomitant drugs dependent on CYP3A or CYP2D6 **Disp:** Tab 200 mg/50 mg, soln 400 mg/100 mg/5 mL **SE:** Soln has EtOH, avoid disulfiram, metronidazole; GI upset, asthenia, ↑ cholesterol/triglycerides, pancreatitis; protease metabolic syndrome **Interactions:** ↑ Effects w/ clarithromycin, erythromycin; ↑ effects OF amiodarone, amprenavir, azole antifungals, bepridil, cisapride, cyclosporine, CCBs, ergot alkaloids, flecainide, flurazepam, HMG-CoA reductase inhibitors, indinavir, lidocaine, meperidine, midazolam, pimozide, propafenone, propoxyphene, quinidine, rifabutin, saquinavir, sildenafil, tacrolimus, terfenadine, triazolam, zolpidem; ↓ effects w/ barbiturates, carbamazepine, dexamethasone, didanosine, efavirenz, nevirapine, phenytoin, rifabutin, rifampin, St. John's wort; ↓ effects OF oral contraceptives, warfarin **NIPE:** Take w/ food, use barrier contraception

Loracarbef (Lorabid) [Antibiotic/Cephalosporin-2nd gen]

Uses: *Upper & lower resp tract, skin, urinary tract* **Action:** 2nd-gen cephalosporin; ↓ cell wall synthesis. *Spectrum:* Weaker than 1st-gen against gram(+), enhanced gram(–) **Dose:** *Adults.* 200–400 mg PO qd-bid. **Peds.** 7.5–15 mg/kg/d PO ÷ bid; on empty stomach; ↓ in severe renal insuff **Caution:** [B, +] **Disp:** Caps 200, 400 mg; susp 100, 200 mg/5 mL **SE:** D **Interactions:** ↑ Effects w/ probenecid; ↑ effects OF warfarin; ↑ nephrotoxicity w/ aminoglycosides, furosemide **NIPE:** Take w/o food

Loratadine (Claritin, Alavert) [Antihistamine]

Uses: *Allergic rhinitis, chronic idiopathic urticaria* **Action:** Nonsedating antihistamine **Dose:** *Adults.* 10 mg/d PO **Peds.** 2–5 y: 5 mg/day qd. *>6 y:* Adult dose; on empty stomach; ↓ in hepatic insuff **Caution:** [B, +/–] **Contra:** Component allergy **Disp:** Tabs 10 mg (OTC); rapidly disintegrating Reditabs 10 mg; syrup 1 mg/mL **SE:** HA, somnolence, xerostomia **Interactions:** ↑ Effects w/ CNS depressants, erythromycin, ketoconazole, MAOIs, protease inhibitors, procarbazine, EtOH **NIPE:** Take w/o food

Lorazepam (Ativan, others) [C-IV] [Anxiolytic, Sedative, Hypnotic/Benzodiazepine]

Uses: *Anxiety & anxiety w/ depression; preop sedation; control status epilepticus*; EtOH withdrawal; antiemetic **Action:** Benzodiazepine; antianxiety agent **Dose:** *Adults.* Anxiety: 1–10 mg/d PO in 2–3 ÷ doses. *Preop:* 0.05 mg/kg to 4 mg max IM 2 h before surgery. *Insomnia:* 2–4 mg PO hs. *Status epilepticus:* 4 mg/dose IV PRN q10–15 min; usual total dose 8 mg. *Antiemetic:* 0.5–2 mg IV or PO q4–6h PRN. *EtOH withdrawal:* 2–5 mg IV or 1–2 mg PO initial depending on severity; titrate based on response **Peds.** Status epilepticus: 0.05 mg/kg/dose IV, repeat in 1–20 min intervals × 2 PRN. *Antiemetic, 2–15 y:* 0.05 mg/kg (to 2 mg/dose) pre chemo; ↓ in elderly; do not administer IV >2 mg/min or 0.05 mg/kg/min **Caution:** [D, ?/–] **Contra:** Severe pain, severe

↓ BP, sleep apnea, NA glaucoma, allergy to propylene glycol or benzyl alcohol **Disp:** Tabs 0.5, 1, 2 mg; soln, PO conc 2 mg/mL; inj 2, 4 mg/mL **SE:** Sedation, ataxia, tachycardia, constipation, resp depression **Notes:** ≤10 min for effect if IV **Interactions:** ↑ Effects w/ cimetidine, disulfiram, probenecid, calendula, catnip, hops, lady's slipper, passionflower, kava kava, valerian; ↑ effects OF phenytoin; ↑ CNS depression w/ anticonvulsants, antihistamines, CNS depressants, MAOIs, scopolamine, EtOH; ↓ effects w/ caffeine, tobacco; ↓ effects OF levodopa **Labs:** ↑ LFTs **NIPE:** {NR} D/C abruptly

Losartan (Cozaar) [Antihypertensive/ARB] **Uses:** *HTN,* CHF, DN **Action:** Angiotensin II antagonist **Dose:** 25–50 mg PO qd-bid, max 100 mg; ↓ in elderly/hepatic impair **Caution:** [C (1st tri, D 2nd & 3rd tri), ?/–] **Disp:** Tabs 25, 50, 100 mg **SE:** ↓ BP in pts on diuretics; GI upset, angioedema **Interactions:** ↑ Risk OF hyperkalemia w/ K-sparing diuretics, K supls, trimethoprim; ↑ effects OF Li; ↓ effects w/ diltiazem, fluconazole, phenobarbital, rifampin **NIPE:** ⊘ PRG, breast-feeding

Lovastatin (Mevacor, Altocor) [Antilipemic/HMG-CoA Reductase Inhibitor] **Uses:** *Hypercholesterolemia* **Action:** HMG-CoA reductase inhibitor **Dose:** 20 mg/d PO w/ PM meal; may ↑ at 4-wk intervals to 80 mg/d max or 60 mg ER tab; take w/ meals **Caution:** [X, –] Avoid w/ grapefruit juice, gemfibrozil **Contra:** Active liver Dz **Disp:** Tabs 10, 20, 40 mg; ER tabs 10, 20, 40, 60 mg **SE:** HA & GI intolerance common; promptly report any unexplained muscle pain, tenderness, or weakness (myopathy) **Notes:** Maintain cholesterol-lowering diet; monitor LFT q12wk × 1 y, then q6mo **Interactions:** ↑ Effects w/ grapefruit juice; ↑ risk of severe myopathy w/ azole antifungals, cyclosporine, erythromycin, gemfibrozil, HMG-CoA inhibitors, niacin; ↑ effects OF warfarin; ↓ effects w/ isradipine, pectin **Labs:** ↑ LFTs **NIPE:** ⊘ PRG, take drug in evening, periodic eye exams

Lubiprostone (Amitiza) [Laxative] **Uses:** *Chronic idiopathic constipation in adults* **Action:** Selective Cl channel activator **Dose:** *Adults.* 24 mcg PO bid w/ food **Contra:** Mechanical GI obstruction **Caution:** [C,?/–] Severe D, severe renal or moderate–severe hepatic impair **Disp:** Gelcaps 24 mcg **SE:** N, HA, D, GI distention, abd pain **Labs:** Monitor LFTs and BUN/Crea **NIPE:** Requires (–) pregnancy test before Tx; utilize contraception; ⊘ breast-feed; periodically reassess drug need; not for chronic use; suspend drug if diarrhea occurs

Lutropin Alfa (Luveris) [Hormone] **Uses:** *Infertility* **Action:** Recombinant LH **Dose:** 75 units SC w/ 75–150 units FSH, 2 separate injs max 14 d **Caution:** [X, ?/M] **Contra:** Primary ovarian failure, uncontrolled thyroid/adrenal dysfunction, intracranial lesion, abnormal uterine bleeding, hormone-dependent GU tumor, ovarian cyst, PRG **Disp:** Inj 75 units **SE:** HA, N, ovarian hyperstimulation syndrome, breast pain, ovarian cysts;↑ risk of multiple births **NIPE:** Rotate inj sites; do not exceed 14 d duration unless signs of imminent follicular development

Lymphocyte Immune Globulin [Antithymocyte Globulin, ATG] (Atgam) [Immunosuppressant] **Uses:** *Allograft rejection in transplant pts; aplastic anemia if not candidates for BMT* **Action:** ↓ circulating T lymphocytes **Dose:** *Adults.* Prevent rejection: 15 mg/kg/day IV ×14 d, then qod ×7; initial w/in 24 h before/after transplant. *Rx rejection:* Same except use 10–15 mg/kg/d; max 28 doses in 21 d. *Peds.* 5–25 mg/kg/d IV. **Caution:** [C, ?] **Contra:** Hx Rxn to other equine γ-globulin preparation, leukopenia, thrombocytopenia **Disp:** Inj 50 mg/mL **SE:** D/C w/ severe thrombocytopenia/leukopenia; rash, fever, chills, ↓ BP, HA, ↑ K+ **Notes:** *Test dose:* 0.1 mL 1:1000 dilution in NS **Interactions:** ↑ Immunosuppression w/ azathioprine, corticosteroids, immunosuppressants **Labs:** ↑ LFTs **NIPE:** Risk of febrile Rxn

Magaldrate (Riopan, Lowsium) [OTC] [Antacid/Aluminum & Magnesium Salt]
Uses: *Hyperacidity associated w/ peptic ulcer, gastritis, & hiatal hernia* **Action:** Low-Na antacid **Dose:** 5–10 mL PO between meals & hs **Caution:** [B, ?] **Contra:** Ulcerative colitis, diverticulitis, ileostomy/colostomy, renal insuff (Mg content) **Disp:** Susp (OTC) **SE:** GI upset **Notes:** <0.3 mg Na/tab or tsp **Interactions:** ↑ Effects OF levodopa, quinidine; ↓ effects OF allopurinol, anticoagulants, cefpodoxime, ciprofloxacin, clindamycin, digoxin, indomethacin, INH, ketoconazole, lincomycin, phenothiazines, quinolones, tetracyclines **NIPE:** ⊘ Other meds w/in 1–2 h

Magnesium Citrate (various) [OTC] [Laxative/Magnesium Salt]
Uses: *Vigorous bowel preparation*; constipation **Action:** Cathartic laxative **Dose:** *Adults.* 120–300 mL PO PRN. *Peds.* 0.5 mL/kg/dose, to 200 mL PO max; w/ a beverage **Caution:** [B, +] **Contra:** Severe renal Dz, heart block, N/V, rectal bleeding **Disp:** Effervescent soln (OTC) **SE:** Abdominal cramps, gas **Interactions:** ↓ Effects OF anticoagulants, digoxin, fluoroquinolones, ketoconazole, nitrofurantoin, phenothiazines, tetracyclines **Labs:** ↑ Mg2+, ↓ protein, Ca2+, K+ **NIPE:** ⊘ Other meds w/in 1–2 h

Magnesium Hydroxide (Milk of Magnesia) [OTC] [Laxative/Magnesium Salt]
Uses: *Constipation; hyperacidity, Mg replacement* **Action:** NS laxative **Dose:** *Adults.* Antacid 5—15 mL PO PRN qid, 2–4 tab PO PRN QID; laxative 30–60 mL PO qd or in ÷ doses *Peds.* <2 yrs 0.5 mL/kg/dose PO PRN (follow dose w/ 8 oz of H2O) **Caution:** [B, +] **Contra:** Renal insuff or intestinal obstruction, ileostomy/colostomy **Disp:** Tabs 311 mg; liq 400, 800 mg/5 mL (OTC) **SE:** D, abdominal cramps **Interactions:** ↓ Effects OF chlordiazepoxide, dicumarol, digoxin, indomethacin, INH, quinolones, tetracyclines **Labs:** ↑ Mg2+, ↓ protein, Ca2+, K+ **NIPE:** ⊘ Other meds w/in 1–2 h

Magnesium Oxide (Mag-Ox 400, others) [OTC] [Antacid, Mg Supl/Magnesium Salt]
Uses: *Replacement for low Mg levels* **Action:** Mg supl **Dose:** 400–800 mg/d ÷ qd–qid w/ full glass of H2O **Caution:** [B, +] **Contra:** Ulcerative colitis, diverticulitis, ileostomy/colostomy, heart block, renal insuff **Disp:** Caps 140 mg; tabs 400 mg (OTC) **SE:** D, N **Interactions:** ↓ Effects OF chlordiazepoxide, dicumarol, digoxin, indomethacin, INH, quinolones, tetracyclines **Labs:** ↑ Mg2+, ↓ protein, Ca2+, K+ **NIPE:** ⊘ Other meds w/in 1–2 h

Magnesium Sulfate (various) [Mg Supl/Magnesium Salt]
Uses: *Replacement for low Mg levels; preeclampsia & premature labor*; refractory ↓ K+ & ↓ Ca2+ **Action:** Mg supl **Dose:** *Adults.* 3 gm PO q6h times 4 PRN; *Supl:* 1–2 g IM or IV; repeat PRN. *Preeclampsia/premature labor:* 4 g load then 1–4 g/h IV inf. *Peds.* 25–50 mg/kg/dose IM or IV q4–6h for 3–4 doses; repeat PRN; ↓ dose w/ low urine output or renal insuff **Caution:** [B, +] **Contra:** Heart block, renal failure **Disp:** Inj 10, 20, 40, 80, 125, 500 mg/mL; bulk powder; **SE:** CNS depression, D, flushing, heart block **Interactions:** ↑ CNS depression w/ antidepressants, antipsychotics, anxiolytics, barbiturates, hypnotics, narcotics; EtOH; ↑ neuromuscular blockade w/ aminoglycosides, atracurium, gallamine, pancuronium, tubocurarine, vecuronium **Labs:** ↑ Mg2+; ↓ protein, Ca2+, K+ **NIPE:** Check for absent patellar reflexes

Mannitol (various) [Osmotic Diuretic]   Uses: *Cerebral edema, ↑ intraocular pressure, renal impair, poisonings* **Action:** Osmotic diuretic **Dose:** *Diuresis: Adults.* Test dose: 0.2 g/kg/dose IV over 3–5 min; if no diuresis w/in 2 h, D/C; *Oliguria:* 50 g–100 g IV over 90 min; ↑ IOP: 0.5–2 gm/kg IV over 30 min; *Cerebral edema:* 0.25–1.5 g/kg/dose IV >30 min **Caution:** [C, ?] w/ CHF or volume overload **Contra:** Anuria, dehydration, heart failure, PE **Disp:** Inj 5, 10, 15, 20, 25% **SE:** Initial volume ↑ may exacerbate CHF; N/V/D; **Notes:** monitor for volume depletion **Interactions:** ↑ Effects OF cardiac glycosides; ↓ effects OF barbiturates, imipramine, Li, salicylates **Labs:** ↑/↓ Serum phosphate

Measles, Mumps, Rubella and Varicella Virus Vaccine Live (Proquad) [Vaccine/Live Attenuated]   Uses: *Simultaneous vaccination against measles, mumps, rubella, & varicella in peds 12 mo–12 y or for second dose of MMR* **Action:** Active immunization, live attenuated virus **Dose:** 1 vial SQ inj **Caution:** [N/A] Hx of cerebral injury or Szs (febrile reaction) **Contra:** Hx anaphylaxis to neomycin, blood dyscrasia, lymphoma, leukemia, immunosuppressive steroids, febrile illness, untreated TB **Disp:** Inj **SE:** Fever, inj site Rxn, rash **Notes:** Allow 1 mo between inj & any other measles vaccine

Mecasermin (Increlex) [Human IGF-1]   Uses: *Growth failure in IGF-1 deficiency or HGH antibodies* **Action:** Human IGF-1 **Dose:** *Peds.* 0.04–0.09 mg/kg SQ BID; may ? by 0.04 mg/kg to 0.12 mg/kg; take w/in 20 min of meal **Caution:** [C,+/–] **Disp:** Vial 40 mg **SE:** HA, inj site rxn, V, hypoglycemia **Labs:** Monitor BS with rapid dose, may cause hypoglycemia **NIPE:** Limited distribution network

Mechlorethamine (Mustargen) [Antineoplastic/Alkylating Agent]   WARNING: Highly toxic, handle w/ care   Uses: *Hodgkin Dz & NHL, cutaneous T-cell lymphoma (mycosis fungoides), lung CA, CML, malignant pleural effusions,* & CLL **Action:** Alkylating agent (bifunctional) **Dose:** Per protocol: 0.4 mg/kg single dose or 0.1 mg/kg/d for 4 d; 6 mg/m2 1–2 ×/mo **Caution:** [D, ?] **Contra:** Known infectious Dz **Disp:** Inj 10 mg **SE:** Myelosuppression, thrombosis, or thrombophlebitis at site; tissue damage w/ extravasation (Na thiosulfate used topically to treat); N/V, skin rash, amenorrhea, sterility (especially in men), secondary leukemia if treated for Hodgkin Dz **Notes:** Highly volatile; administer w/in 30–60 min of prep **Interactions:** ↑ Risk OF blood dyscrasias w/ amphotericin B; ↑ risk OF bleeding w/ anticoagulants, NSAIDs, plt inhibitors, salicylates; ↑ myelosuppression w/ antineoplastic drugs, radiation therapy; ↓ effects OF live virus vaccines **Labs:** ↑ Serum uric acid **NIPE:** ↑ Fluids to 2–3 L/d; ⊘ PRG, breast-feeding, vaccines, exposure to infection; ↑ risk of tinnitus

Meclizine (Antivert) [Antiemetic/Antivertigo/Anticholinergic] Uses: *Motion sickness; vertigo* **Action:** Antiemetic, anticholinergic, & antihistaminic properties **Dose:** *Adults & Peds >12 y.* 12.5–100 mg PO tid–qid PRN **Disp:** [B, ?] **Disp:** Tabs 12.5, 25, 50 mg; chew tabs 25 mg; caps 25, 30 mg (OTC) **SE:** Drowsiness, xerostomia, & blurred vision common **Interactions:** ↑ Sedation w/ antihistamines, CNS depressants, neuroleptics, EtOH; ↑ anticholinergic effects w/ anticholinergics, atropine, disopyramide, haloperidol, phenothiazines, quinidine **NIPE:** Use prophylactically

Medroxyprogesterone (Provera, Depo-Provera) [Antineoplastic/Progestin] **WARNING:** May cause loss of bone density; associated w/ duration of use Uses: * Contraception; secondary amenorrhea, abnormal uterine bleeding (AUB) caused by hormonal imbalance; endometrial CA* **Action:** Progestin supl **Dose:** *Contraception:* 150 mg IM q3mo depo or 104 mg SQ q3 mo (depo SQ). *Secondary amenorrhea:* 5–10 mg/d PO for 5–10 d. *AUB:* 5–10 mg/d PO for 5–10 d beginning on the 16th or 21st d of menstrual cycle. *Endometrial CA:* 400–1000 mg/wk IM; ↓ in hepatic insuff **Caution:** [X, +] **Contra:** Hx of thromboembolic disorders, hepatic Dz, PRG **Disp:** Tabs 2.5, 5, 10 mg; depot inj 150, 400 mg/mL; depo SQ inj 104 mg/10.65 mL **SE:** Breakthrough bleeding, spotting, altered menstrual flow, anorexia, edema, thromboembolic complications, depression, weight gain **Notes:** Perform breast exam & Pap smear before contraceptive therapy; obtain PRG test if last inj > 3 mo **Interactions:** ↓ Effects w/ aminoglutethimide, phenytoin, carbamazepine, phenobarbital, rifampin, rifabutin **NIPE:** Sunlight exposure may cause melasma, if GI upset take w/ food

Megestrol Acetate (Megace) [Antineoplastic/Progestin] Uses: *Breast/endometrial CAs; appetite stimulant in cachexia (CA & HIV)* **Action:** Hormone; progesterone analog **Dose:** *CA:* 40–320 mg/d PO in ÷ doses. *Appetite:* 800 mg/d PO ÷ **Caution:** [X, –] Thromboembolism **Contra:** PRG **Disp:** Tabs 20, 40 mg; soln 40 mg/mL **SE:** May induce DVT; edema, menstrual bleeding; insomnia, rash, myelosuppression **Interactions:** ↑ Effects OF warfarin **Labs:** ↑ LDH **NIPE:** ↑ Risk of photosensitivity—use sunscreen; do not D/C abruptly

Meloxicam (Mobic) [Analgesic/Anti-inflammatory/NSAIDs] **WARNING:** May ↑ risk of cardiovascular events & GI bleeding Uses: *Osteoarthritis, RA, JRA* **Action:** NSAID w/ ↑ COX-2 activity **Dose:** *Adults.* 7.5–15 mg/d PO; *Peds.* (> 2 yr): 0.125 mg/kg/d, max 7.5 mg; ↓ in renal insuff; take w/food **Caution:** [C,D (3rd trimester) ?/–] Peptic ulcer, NSAID, or ASA sensitivity **Disp:** Tabs 7.5 mg; susp. 7.5 mg/5 mL **SE:** HA, dizziness, GI upset, GI bleeding, edema **Interactions:** ↑ Effects OF ASA, anticoagulants, corticosteroids, Li, EtOH, tobacco; ↓ effects w/ cholestyramine; ↓ effects OF antihypertensives **Labs:** False + guaiac test, ↑ LFTs **NIPE:** Take w/ food, may take several days for full effect

Melphalan [L-PAM] (Alkeran) [Antineoplastic/Alkylating Agent] WARNING: Severe BM depression, leukemogenic, & mutagenic
Uses: *Multiple myeloma, ovarian CAs,* breast, testicular CAs, melanoma; allogenic & ABMT (high dose) **Action:** Alkylating agent (bifunctional) **Dose:** (Per protocol) 6 mg/d or 0.15–0.25 mg/kg/d for 4–7 d, repeat 4–6-wk intervals, or 1-mg/kg ×1 q4–6wk; 0.15 mg/kg/d for 5 d q6wk. *High-dose high-risk multiple myeloma:* Single dose 140 mg/m². *ABMT:* 140–240 mg/m² IV; ↓ in renal insuff **Caution:** [D, ?] **Contra:** Allergy or resistance **Disp:** Tabs 2 mg; inj 50 mg **SE:** ↓ BM, secondary leukemia, alopecia, dermatitis, stomatitis, & pulmonary fibrosis; rare allergic Rxns **Interactions:** ↑ Risk of nephrotoxicity w/ cisplatin, cyclosporine; ↓ effects w/ cimetidine, interferon alfa **Labs:** ↑ Uric acid, urine 5-HIAA **NIPE:** ↑ Fluids, ⊘ PRG, breast-feeding; take PO on empty stomach.

Memantine (Namenda) [Anti-Alzheimer's Agent/NMDA Receptor Antagonist]
Uses: *Moderate/severe Alzheimer Dz* **Action:** *N*-methyl-D-aspartate receptor antagonist **Dose:** Target 20 mg/d, start 5 mg/d, ↑ 5 mg/d to 20 mg/d, wait > 1 wk before ↑ dose; use ÷ doses >5 mg/d **Caution:** [B, ?/–] Hepatic/mild–moderate renal impair **Disp:** Tabs 5, 10 mg, combo pak: 5 mg × 28 + 10 mg × 21; sol 2 mg/mL **SE:** Dizziness **Notes:** Renal clearance ↓ by alkaline urine (↓ 80% pH 8) **Interactions:** ↑ Effects w/ amantadine, carbonic anhydrase inhibitors, dextromethorphan, ketamine, sodium bicarbonate; ↑ effects w/ any drug, herb, food that alkalinizes urine **Labs:** Monitor BUN, SCr **NIPE:** Take w/o regard to food, EtOH ↓ adverse effects & ↓ effectiveness

Meningococcal Polysaccharide Vaccine (Menomune) [Vaccine/Live]
Uses: *Immunize against N. meningitidis* (meningococcus)* OK in some complement deficiency, asplenia, lab workers w/ exposure; college students by some professional groups **Action:** Live vaccine, active immunization **Dose:** *Adults & Peds >2 y.* 0.5 mL SQ (not IM, intradermally or IV); **Caution:** [C, ?/–] **Contra:** Thimerosal sensitivity **Disp:** Inj **SE:** Local inj site Rxns, HA **Notes:** Active against meningococcal serotypes A, C, Y, & W-135; not group B **Interactions:** ↓ Effects w/ immunoglobulin if admin. w/in 1 mo **NIPE:** Pain & inflammation at inj site; keep epi (1:1000) available for anaphylactic/allergic Rxns

Meperidine (Demerol) [C–II] [Opioid Analgesic]
Uses: *Moderate–severe pain* **Action:** Narcotic analgesic **Dose:** *Adults.* 50–150 mg PO or IM q3–4h PRN. *Peds.* 1–1.5 mg/kg/dose PO or IM/SQ q3–4h PRN, up to 100 mg/dose; ↓ in elderly/renal impair **Caution:** [C/D (prolonged use or high dose at term), +] ↓ Sz threshold **Contra:** Recent/concomitant MAOIs, renal failure **Disp:** Tabs 50, 100 mg; syrup 50 mg/mL; inj 10, 25, 50, 75, 100 mg/mL **SE:** Resp depression, Szs,

sedation, constipation **Notes:** Analgesic effects potentiated w/ use of hydroxyzine; 75 mg IM = 10 mg morphine IM **Interactions:** ↑ Effects w/ antihistamines, barbiturates, cimetidine, MAOIs, neuroleptics, selegiline, TCAs, St. John's wort, EtOH; ↑ effects OF INH; ↓ effects w/ phenytoin **Labs:** ↑ Serum amylase, lipase

Meprobamate (Equinil, Miltown) [C-IV] [Antianxiety]

Uses: *Short-term relief of anxiety* **Action:** Mild tranquilizer; antianxiety **Dose:** *Adults.* 400 mg PO tid-qid, max 2400 mg/d; *Peds 6–12 y.* 100–200 mg bid-tid; ↓ in renal/liver impair **Caution:** [D, +/–] **Contra:** NA glaucoma, porphyria, PRG **Disp:** Tabs 200, 400 mg **SE:** May cause drowsiness, syncope, tachycardia, edema **Interactions:** ↑ Effects w/ antihistamines, barbiturates, CNS depressants, narcotics, EtOH

Mercaptopurine [6-MP] (Purinethol) [Antineoplastic/Antimetabolite]

Uses: *Acute leukemias,* 2nd-line Rx of CML & NHL, maint ALL in children, immunosuppressant w/ autoimmune Dzs (Crohn Dz) **Action:** Antimetabolite, mimics hypoxanthine **Dose:** 80–100 mg/m²/d or 2.5–5 mg/kg/d; maint 1.5–2.5 mg/kg/d; w/ allopurinol requires a 67–75% ↓ dose of 6-MP (interference w/ xanthine oxidase metabolism); ↓ in renal/hepatic insuff; take on empty stomach **Caution:** [D, ?] **Contra:** Severe hepatic Dz, BM suppression, PRG **Disp:** Tabs 50 mg **SE:** Mild hematotox; mucositis, stomatitis, & D; rash, fever, eosinophilia, jaundice, hepatitis **Notes:** Handle properly; ensure adequate hydration **Interactions:** ↑ Effects w/ allopurinol; ↑ risk OF bone marrow suppression w/ trimethoprim-sulfamethoxazole; ↓ effects OF warfarin **Labs:** False ↑ serum glucose, uric acid **NIPE:** ↑ Fluid intake to 2–3 L/d, may take 4+ wk for improvement

Meropenem (Merrem) [Antibiotic/Carbapenem]

Uses: *Intraabdominal Infxns, bacterial meningitis* **Action:** Carbapenem; ↓ cell wall synthesis, a β-lactam. *Spectrum:* Excellent gram(+) (except MRSA & E. faecium); excellent gram(–) including extended-spectrum β-lactamase producers; good anaerobic **Dose:** *Adults.* 1 to 2 g IV q8h. *Peds.* > 3 mo, < 50 kg, 10–40 mg/kg IV q 8h; ↓ in renal insuff **Caution:** [B, ?] **Contra:** β-Lactam sensitivity **Disp:** Inj 1 g, 500 mg **SE:** Less Sz potential than imipenem; D, thrombocytopenia **Notes:** Overuse can ↑ bacterial resistance **Interactions:** ↑ Effects w/ probenecid **Labs:** ↑ LFTs, BUN, creatinine, eosinophils ↓ Hmg, Hct, WBCs **NIPE:** Monitor for superinfection

Mesalamine (Rowasa, Asacol, Pentasa) [Anti-inflammatory]

Uses: *Mild–moderate distal ulcerative colitis, proctosigmoiditis, proctitis* **Action:** Unknown; may inhibit prostaglandins **Dose:** *Rectal:* 60 mL QHS, retain 8 h (enema), 500 mg bid–tid or 1000 mg qhs (supp) *PO:* Cap: 1 gm PO qid, Tab: 1.6–2.4 g/d in ÷ doses (tid-qid); ↓ initial dose in elderly **Caution:** [B, M] **Contra:** Salicylate sensitivity **Disp:** Tabs 400 mg; caps 250, 500 mg; supp 500, 1000 mg; rectal susp 4 g/60 mL **SE:** HA, malaise, abdominal pain, flatulence, rash, pancreatitis, pericarditis **Interactions:** ↓ Effect OF digoxin **Labs:** ↑ LFTs, amylase, lipase **NIPE:** May discolor urine yellow-brown

Mesna (Mesnex) [Uroprotectant/Antidote] Uses: *Prevent hemorrhagic cystitis due to ifosfamide or cyclophosphamide* Action: Antidote, reacts with acrolein and other metabolites to form stable compounds Dose: Per protocol; dose as a % of ifosfamide or cyclophosphamide dose IV bolus: 20% (er, 10–12 mg/kg) IV at 0, 4, and 8 h, then 40% at 0, 1, 4, and 7 h; *IV inf:* 20% prechemo, 50–100% w/chemo, then 25–50% for 12 h following chemo; *Oral:* 20% IV dose at hour 0, 4, and 8 h (mix with juice) Caution: [B; ?/–] Contra: Thiol sensitivity Disp: Inj 100 mg/mL; tablets 400 mg SE: ↓ BP, allergic Rxns, HA, GI upset, taste perversion Notes: Hydration helps ↓ hemorrhagic cystitis Interactions: ↓ Effects OF warfarin Labs: False + urine ketones

Mesoridazine (Serentil) [Antipsychotic/Phenothiazine]
WARNING: Can prolong QT interval in dose-related fashion; torsades de pointes reported Uses: *Schizophrenia,* acute & chronic alcoholism, chronic brain syndrome Action: Phenothiazine antipsychotic Dose: Initial, 25–50 mg PO or IV tid; ↑ to 300–400 mg/d max Caution: [C, ?/–] Contra: Phenothiazine sensitivity, coadministration w/ drugs that cause QT_c prolongation, CNS depression Disp: Tabs 10, 25, 50, 100 mg; PO conc 25 mg/mL; inj 25 mg/mL SE: Low incidence of EPS; ↓ BP, xerostomia, constipation, skin discoloration, tachycardia, lowered Sz threshold, blood dyscrasias, pigmentary retinopathy at high doses Interactions: ↑ Effects w/ antimalarials, BBs, chloroquine, TCAs, EtOH; ↑ effects OF antidepressants, nitrates, antihypertensives; ↑ QT interval w/ amiodarone, azole antifungals, disopyramide, fluoxetine, macrolides, paroxetine, procainamide, quinidine, quinolones, TCAs, verapamil; ↓ effects w/ attapulgite, barbiturates, caffeine, tobacco; ↓ effects of barbiturates, guanethidine, guanadrel, levodopa, Li, sympathomimetics Labs: False + PRG test; ↑ serum glucose, cholesterol; ↓ uric acid NIPE: Photosensitivity—use sunscreen

Metaproterenol (Alupent, Metaprel) [Bronchodilator/Beta Adrenergic Agonist] Uses: *Asthma & reversible bronchospasm* Action: Sympathomimetic bronchodilator Dose: *Adults.* Inhal: 1–3 inhal q3–4h, 12 inhal max/24 h; wait 2 min between inhal. *PO:* 20 mg q6–8h. *Peds.* Inhal: 0.5 mg/kg/dose, 15 mg 2ose max inhaled q4–6h by neb or 1–2 puffs q4-6h. *PO:* 0.3–0.5 mg/kg/dose q6–8h Caution: [C, ?/–] Contra: Tachycardia, other arrhythmias Disp: Aerosol 0.65 mg/inhal; soln for inhal 0.4, 0.6, 5%; tabs 10, 20 mg; syrup 10 mg/5 mL SE: nervousness, tremor, tachycardia, HTN Notes: Fewer β₁ effects than isoproterenol & longer acting Interactions: ↑ Effects w/ sympathomimetic drugs, xanthines; ↑ risk OF arrhythmias w/ cardiac glycosides, halothane, levodopa, theophylline, thyroid hormones; ↑ HTN w/ MAOIs; ↓ effects w/ BBs Labs: ↑ Serum K⁺ NIPE: Separate additional aerosol use by 5 min

Metaxalone (Skelaxin) [Skeletal Muscle Relaxant] Uses: *Painful musculoskeletal conditions* Action: Centrally acting skeletal muscle relaxant Dose: 800 mg PO tid–qid Caution: [C, ?/–] anemia Contra: Severe hepatic/renal impair Disp: Tabs 400, 800 mg SE: N/V, HA, drowsiness, hepatitis

Interactions: ↑ Sedating effects w/ CNS depressants, EtOH **Labs:** False + urine glucose using Benedict's test

Metformin (Glucophage, Glucophage XR, Glumetza (extended release) [Hypoglycemic/Biguanide]

WARNING: Associated w/ lactic acidosis **Uses:** *Type 2 DM; use as monotherapy or w/ sulfonylurea or insulin* **Action:** ↓ Hepatic glucose production & intestinal absorption of glucose; ↑ insulin sensitivity **Dose:** *Adults.* Initial: 500 mg PO bid; or 850 mg qd, may ↑ to 2550 mg in ÷ doses; take w/ AM & PM meals; can convert total daily dose to qd dose of XR form; Glumetza 500 mg PO OD at evening meal, initial: 1g PO OD, increase by 500 mg OD q week to max of 2 g/d OD. *Peds 10–16 y.* 500 mg PO bid, ↑ 500 mg/wk to 2000 mg/d max in ÷ doses; do not use XR formulation in peds; Glumetza ◌ < 18 y.o. **Caution:** [B, +/–]; avoid EtOH; hold dose before & 48 h after ionic contrast **Contra:** SCr >1.4 in females or >1.5 in males; contra in hypoxemic conditions (eg acute CHF/sepsis) **Disp:** Tabs 500, 850, 1000 mg; XR tabs 500, 750, 1000 mg; Glumetza 500-mg extended release **SE:** Anorexia, N/V, rash, lactic acidosis (rare, but serious) **Interactions:** ↑ Effects w/ amiloride, cimetidine, digoxin, furosemide, MAOIs, morphine, procainamide, quinidine, quinine, ranitidine, triamterene, trimethoprim, vancomycin; ↓ effects w/ corticosteroids, CCBs, diuretics, estrogens, INH, oral contraceptives, phenothiazines, phenytoin, sympathomimetics, thyroid drugs, tobacco **Labs:** monitor LFTs, BUN/Crea, serum Vit B$_{12}$ **NIPE:** Take w/ food; ◌ dehydration, EtOH, before surgery

Methadone (Dolophine) [C-II] [Opioid Analgesic]

Uses: *Severe pain; detox, maint of narcotic addiction* **Action:** Narcotic analgesic **Dose:** *Adults.* 2.5–10 mg IM q3–8h or 5–15 mg PO q8h; titrate as needed *Peds.* 0.7 mg/kg/24 h PO or IM ÷ q8h; ↑ slowly to avoid resp depression; ↓ in renal impair **Caution:** [B/D (prolonged use or high doses at term), + (w/ doses ≥ 20 mg/24 h)], severe liver Dz **Disp:** Tabs 5, 10, 40 mg; PO soln 5, 10 mg/5 mL; PO conc 10 mg/mL; inj 10 mg/mL **SE:** Resp depression, sedation, constipation, urinary retention, ventricular arrhythmias **Notes:** Equianalgesic w/ parenteral morphine; longer half-life; prolongs QT interval **Interactions:** ↑ Effects w/ cimetidine, CNS depressants, EtOH; ↑ effects OF anticoagulants, EtOH, antihistamines, barbiturates, glutethimide, methocarbamol; ↓ effects w/ carbamazepine, nelfinavir, phenobarbital, phenytoin, primidone, rifampin, ritonavir **Labs:** ↑ Serum amylase, lipase

Methenamine (Hiprex, Urex, others) [Urinary Anti-infective]

Uses: *Suppress/eliminate bacteriuria associated w/ chronic/ recurrent UTI* **Action:** Converted to formaldehyde & ammonia in acidic urine; nonspecific bactericidal action **Dose:** *Adults.* Hippurate: 0.5–1 g bid. *Mandelate:* 1 g qid PO pc & hs *Peds 6–12 y.* Hippurate: 25–50 mg/kg/d PO ÷ bid. *Mandelate:* 50–75 mg/kg/d PO ÷ qid (take w/ food, ascorbic acid w/ adequate hydration) **Caution:** [C, +] **Contra:** Renal insuff, severe hepatic Dz, & severe dehydration; sulfonamide allergy **Disp:** *Methenamine hippurate* (Hiprex, Urex): Tabs 1g. *Methenamine mandelate:* 500mg, 1g EC tabs **SE:** Rash, GI upset, dysuria, **Interactions:** ↓ Effects w/

acetazolamide, antacids **Labs:** ↑ Serum catecholamines, urine glucose, urobilinogen, LFTs; ↓ urine estriol, estrogens **NIPE:** ↑ Fluids to 2–3 L/d; take w/ food

Methimazole (Tapazole) [Anti-Thyroid Agent] Uses: *Hyperthyroidism, thyrotoxicosis,* prep for thyroid surgery or radiation **Action:** Blocks T_3 & T_4 formation **Dose:** *Adults.* Initial: 15–60 mg/d PO ÷ tid. *Maint:* 5–15 mg PO qd. *Peds.* Initial: 0.4–0.7 mg/kg/24 h PO ÷ tid. *Maint:* ⅓–{2/3} of initial dose PO qd; w/ food **Caution:** [D, +/–] **Contra:** Breast-feeding **Disp:** Tabs 5, 10, 20 mg **SE:** GI upset, dizziness, blood dyscrasias **Notes:** Follow clinically & w/ TFT **Interactions:** ↑ Effects OF digitalis glycosides, metoprolol, propranolol; ↓ effects OF anticoagulants, theophylline; ↓ effects w/ amiodarone **Labs:** ↑ LFTs, PT **NIPE:** Take w/ food

Methocarbamol (Robaxin) [Skeletal Muscle Relaxant/Centrally Acting] Uses: *Relief of discomfort associated w/ painful musculoskeletal conditions* **Action:** Centrally acting skeletal muscle relaxant **Dose:** *Adults.* 1.5 g PO qid for 2–3 d, then 1-g PO qid maint therapy; IV form rarely indicated. *Peds.* 15 mg/kg/dose IV, may repeat PRN (OK for tetanus only), max 1.8 g/m2/d for 3 d **Caution:** Sz disorders [C, +] **Contra:** MyG, renal impair **Disp:** Tabs 500, 750 mg; inj 100 mg/mL **SE:** Can discolor urine; drowsiness, GI upset **Interactions:** ↑ Effects w/ CNS depressant, EtOH **Labs:** ↑ Urine 5-HIAA, urine vanillylmandelic acid **NIPE:** Monitor for blurred vision, nystagmus, diplopia

Methotrexate (Folex, Rheumatrex) [Antineoplastic, Antirheumatic (DMARDs), Immunosuppressant/Antimetabolite] Uses: *ALL & AML including leukemic meningitis, trophoblastic tumors (chorioepithelioma, choriocarcinoma, hydatidiform mole), breast, lung, head, & neck CAs, Burkitt's lymphoma, mycosis fungoides, osteosarcoma, Hodgkin Dz & NHL, psoriasis; RA* **Action:** ↓ Dihydrofolate reductase-mediated production of tetrahydrofolate **Dose:** *CA:* Per protocol. *RA:* 7.5 mg/wk PO ×1 or 2.5 mg q12h PO for 3 doses/wk; ↓ in renal/hepatic impair **Caution:** [D, –] **Contra:** Severe renal/hepatic impair, PRG/lactation **Disp:** Tabs 2.5, 5, 7.5, 10, 15 mg; inj 2.5, 10, 25 mg/mL; powder 20 mg **SE:** Myelosuppression, N/V/D, anorexia, mucositis, hepatotox (transient & reversible; may progress to atrophy, necrosis, fibrosis, cirrhosis), rashes, dizziness, malaise, blurred vision, alopecia, photosensitivity, renal failure, pneumonitis; rarely, pulmonary fibrosis; chemical arachnoiditis & HA w/ IT delivery **Notes:** Monitor CBC, LFTs, Cr, MTX levels & CXR; "high dose" > 500 mg/m2 requires leucovorin rescue to (↓ tox; w/intrathecal, use preservative-free/alcohol-free solution. **Interactions:** ↑ Effects w/ chloramphenicol, cyclosporine, etretinate, NSAIDs, phenylbutazone, phenytoin, penicillin, probenecid, salicylates, sulfonamides, sulfonylureas, EtOH; ↑ effects OF cyclosporine, tetracycline, theophylline; ↓ effects w/ antimalarials, aminoglycosides, binding resins, cholestyramine, folic acid; ↓ effects OF digoxin **Labs:** ↑ AST, ALT, alkaline phosphatase, bilirubin, cholesterol **NIPE:** ↑ Risk of photosensitivity—use sunscreen, ↑ fluids 2–3 L/d

Methyldopa (Aldomet) [Antihypertensive/Centrally Acting Antiadrenergic] Uses: *HTN* **Action:** Centrally acting antihypertensive **Dose:** *Adults.* 250–500 mg PO bid–tid (max 2–3 g/d) or 250 mg–1 g IV q6–8h. *Peds.* 10 mg/kg/24 h PO in 2–3 ÷ doses (max 40 mg/kg/24 h ÷ q6–12h) or 5–10 mg/kg/dose IV q6–8h to total dose of 20–40 mg/kg/24 h; ↓ in renal insuff/elderly **Caution:** [B (PO), C (IV), +] **Contra:** Liver Dz; MAOIs **Disp:** Tabs 125, 250, 500 mg; inj 50 mg/mL **SE:** Discolors urine; initial transient sedation or drowsiness frequent; edema, hemolytic anemia; hepatic disorders **Interactions:** ↑ Effects w/ anesthetics, diuretics, levodopa, Li, methotrimeprazine, thioxanthenes, vasodilators, verapamil; ↑ effects OF haloperidol, Li, tolbutamide; ↓ effects w/ amphetamines, Fe, phenothiazines, TCAs; ↓ effects OF ephedrine **Labs:** Interference w/ ↓Cr, glucose, AST, catecholamines; urine catecholamines, uric acid; false ↓ serum cholesterol, triglycerides **NIPE:** After 1–2 mo tolerance may develop

Methylergonovine (Methergine) [Oxytocic/Ergot Alkaloid] Uses: *Postpartum bleeding (uterine subinvolution)* **Action:** Ergotamine derivative **Dose:** 0.2 mg IM after placental delivery, may repeat 2-4-h intervals or 0.2–0.4 mg PO q6–12h for 2–7 d **Caution:** [C, ?] **Contra:** HTN, PRG **Disp:** Injectable 0.2 mg/mL; tabs 0.2 mg **SE:** HTN, N/V **Notes:** Give IV doses over a period of >1 min w/ frequent BP monitoring **Interactions:** ↑ Vasoconstriction w/ ergot alkaloids, sympathomimetics, tobacco **NIPE:** ⊘ Smoking

Methylphenidate, Oral (Concerta, Ritalin, Ritalin SR, others) [CII] [CNS Stimulant] Uses: *ADHD, narcolepsy* depression **Action:** CNS stimulant **Dose:** *Adults.* Narcolepsy: 10 mg PO 2–3 times/day, 60 mg/day max. Depression: 2.5 mg QAM; ? slowly, 20 mg/day max; use regular release only *Peds.* Based on product; Initial total daily dose of 15–20 mg; 90 mg/max; administer once (ER/SR) to BID (regular) **Caution:** [C,+/–] Hx alcoholism or drug abuse; separate from MAOIs by 14 days **Disp:** Tabs 5, 10, 20 mg; Tabs SR (Ritalin SR) 20 mg; ER tabs (Concerta) 18, 27, 36, 54 mg **SE:** CV or CNS stimulation **Interactions:** ↑ Risk of hypertensive crisis w/MAOIs; ↑ effects of anticonvulsants, anticoagulants, TCA, SSRIs; ↓ effects of guanethidine, antihypertensives **Labs:** Monitor CBC, platelets **NIPE:** Titrate dose; take 30–45 min before meals; do not chew or crush; Concerta "ghost tablet" may appear in stool; see insert to convert to ER dose; see also transdermal methylphenidate; abuse and diversion concerns; d/c if seizures or agitation occurs

Methylphenidate, Transdermal (Daytrana) [CII] [CNS Stimulant] Uses: *ADHD in children 6–12 yrs* **Action:** CNS stimulant **Dose:** *Peds.* Apply to hip in AM (2 h before desired effect), remove 9 h later **Caution:** [C,+/–] sensitization may preclude subsequent use of oral forms; abuse and diversion concerns **Disp:** Patches 10, 15, 20, 30 mg **SE:** Local reactions, stimulation **Interactions:** ↑ effects of oral anticoagulants, Phenobarbital, phenytoin, primidone, SSRIs, TCAs; ↑ risk of hypertensive crisis w/MAOIs; caution with pressor drugs **NIPE:** Titrate dose in weekly increments; effects last several hours following removal; rotate application sites; ⊘ expose patches to direct external sources of heat

Methylprednisolone (Solu-Medrol) [Anti-inflammatory, Immunosuppressant/Corticosteroid]

[See Steroids Table 4] **Interactions** ↑ Effects w/ cyclosporine, clarithromycin, erythromycin, estrogens, ketoconazole, oral contraceptives, troleandomycin, grapefruit juice; ↑ effects OF cyclosporine; ↓ effects w/ aminoglutethimide, barbiturates, carbamazepine, cholestyramine, colestipol, INH, phenytoin, phenobarbital, rifampin; ↓ effects OF anticoagulants, hypoglycemics, INH, salicylates, vaccines **Labs:** ↓ Skin test Rxns; false ↑ serum cortisol, digoxin, theophylline, & urine glucose **NIPE:** ⊘ D/C abruptly, ⊘ infections or vaccines

Metoclopramide (Reglan, Clopra, Octamide) [Antiemetic, Dopamine Antagonist]

Uses: *Relief of diabetic gastroparesis, symptomatic GERD; chemo-induced N/V, facilitate small-bowel intubation & radiologic evaluation of the upper GI tract,* stimulate gut in prolonged postop ileus **Action:** Stimulates upper GI tract motility; blocks dopamine in chemoreceptor trigger zone **Dose:** *Adults.* Diabetic gastroparesis: 10 mg PO 30 min ac & hs for 2–8 wk PRN or same dose given IV for 10 d, then PO. *Reflux:* 10–15 mg PO 30 min ac & hs. *Antiemetic:* 1–3 mg/kg/dose IV 30 min before chemo, then q2h ×2 doses, then q3h ×3 doses. *Peds.* Reflux: 0.1 mg/kg/dose PO qid. *Antiemetic:* 1–2 mg/kg/dose IV a adults **Caution:** [B, –] Drugs w/ extrapyramidal ADRs **Contra:** Sz disorders, GI obstruction **Disp:** Tabs 5, 10 mg; syrup 5 mg/5 mL; inj 5 mg/mL **SE:** Dystonic Rxns common w/ high doses, (Rx w/ IV diphenhydramine); restlessness, drowsiness, D **Interactions:** ↑ Risk of serotonin syndrome w/ sertraline, venlafaxine; ↑ effects OF acetaminophen, ASA, CNS depressants, cyclosporine, levodopa, Li, succinylcholine, tetracyclines, EtOH; ↓ effects w/ anticholinergics, narcotics; ↓ effects OF cimetidine, digoxin **Labs:** ↑ Serum ALT, AST, amylase **NIPE:** Monitor for extrapyramidal effects

Metolazone (Mykrox, Zaroxolyn) [Antihypertensive/Thiazide Diuretic]

Uses: *Mild–moderate essential HTN & edema of renal D, or cardiac failure* **Action:** Thiazide-like diuretic; ↓ distal tubule Na reabsorption **Dose:** *HTN:* 2.5–5 mg/d PO (Zaroxolyn), 0.5–1 mg/day PO (Mykrox). *Edema:* 2.5–20 mg/d PO. *Peds.* 0.2–0.4 mg/kg/d PO ÷ q12h–qd **Caution:** [D, +] **Contra:** Thiazide/sulfonamide sensitivity, anuria **Disp:** *Tabs:* Mykrox (rapid acting) 0.5 mg, Zaroxolyn 2.5, 5, 10 mg **SE:** Monitor fluid/electrolytes; dizziness, ↓ BP, tachycardia, CP, photosensitivity **Notes:** Mykrox & Zaroxolyn not bioequivalent **Interactions:** ↑ Effects w/ antihypertensives, barbiturates, narcotics, nitrates, EtOH, food; ↑ effects OF digoxin, Li; ↑ hyperglycemia w/ BBs, diazoxide; ↑ hypokalemia w/ amphotericin B, corticosteroids, mezlocillin, piperacillin, ticarcillin; ↓ effects w/ cholestyramine, colestipol, hypoglycemics, insulin, NSAIDs, salicylates; ↓ effects OF methenamine **Labs:** ↑ Serum and urine glucose, serum cholesterol, triglycerides, uric acid **NIPE:** ↑ Risk of photosensitivity—use sunscreen; ↑ risk of gout; monitor electrolytes

Metoprolol (Lopressor, Toprol XL) [Antihypertensive/BB]
WARNING: Do not acutely stop therapy as marked worsening of angina can result **Uses:** *HTN, angina, AMI, CHF* **Action:** β-Adrenergic receptor blocker **Dose:** *Angina:* 50–200 mg PO bid max 400 mg/d. *HTN:* 50–200 mg PO BID max 450 mg/d. *AMI:* 5 mg IV q 2 min ×3 doses, then 50 mg PO q6h ×48 h, then 100 mg PO bid. *CHF:* 12–25 mg/d PO ×2 wk, ↑ at 2-wk intervals to 200 mg/max, use low dose in pts w/ greatest severity; ↓ in hepatic failure **Caution:** [C, +] Uncompensated CHF, bradycardia, heart block **Contra:** Arrhythmia w/ tachycardia **Disp:** Tabs 25, 50, 100 mg; ER tabs 25, 50, 100, 200 mg; inj 1 mg/mL **SE:** Drowsiness, insomnia, ED, bradycardia, bronchospasm **Interactions:** ↑ Effects w/ cimetidine, dihydropyridines, diltiazem, fluoxetine, hydralazine, methimazole, oral contraceptives, propylthiouracil, quinidine, quinolones; ↑ effects OF hydralazine; ↑ bradycardia w/ digoxin, dipyridamole, verapamil; ↓ effects w/ barbiturates, NSAIDs, rifampin; ↓ effects OF isoproterenol, theophylline **Labs:** ↑ BUN, SCr, LFTs, uric acid **NIPE:** Take w/ food, ⊘ D/C abruptly—withdraw over 2 wk

Metronidazole (Flagyl, MetroGel) [Antibacterial, Antiprotozoals] **Uses:** *Bone/joint, endocarditis, intraabdominal, meningitis, & skin Infxns; amebiasis; trichomoniasis; bacterial vaginosis* **Action:** Interferes w/ DNA synthesis. *Spectrum:* Excellent anaerobic coverage *C. difficile,* also *H. pylori* in combo therapy **Dose:** *Adults.* Anaerobic Infxns: 500 mg IV q6–8h. *Amebic dysentery:* 750 mg/d PO for 5–10 d. *Trichomoniasis:* 250 mg PO tid for 7 d or 2 g PO ×1. *C. difficile Infxn:* 500 mg PO or IV q8h for 7–10 d (PO preferred; IV only if pt NPO). *Vaginosis:* 1 applicatorful intravag bid or 500 mg PO bid for 7 d. *Acne rosacea/skin:* Apply bid. *Peds.* Anaerobic Infxns: 15 mg/kg/24 h PO or IV ÷ q6h. *Amebic dysentery:* 35–50 mg/kg/24 h PO in 3 ÷ doses for 5–10 d; ↓ in hepatic impair **Caution:** [B, M] Avoid EtOH **Contra:** First tri of PRG **Disp:** Tabs 250, 500 mg; XR tabs 750 mg; caps 375 mg; topical lotion & gel 0.75%; intravag gel 0.75% (5 g/applicator 37.5 mg in 70-g tube), cream 1% **SE:** Disulfiram-like Rxn; dizziness, HA, anorexia, urine discoloration **Notes:** For Trichomoniasis, Rx pt's partner; no aerobic bacteria activity; use in combo w/ serious mixed Infxns **Interactions:** ↑ Effects w/ cimetidine; ↑ effects OF carbamazepine, fluorouracil, Li, warfarin; ↓ effects w/ barbiturates, cholestyramine, colestipol, phenytoin **Labs:** May cause ↓/zero values for LFTs, triglycerides, glucose **NIPE:** Take w/ food, possible metallic taste

Mexiletine (Mexitil) [Antiarrhythmic] **Uses:** *Suppression of symptomatic ventricular arrhythmias*; diabetic neuropathy **Action:** Class IB antiarrhythmic **Dose:** *Adults.* 200–300 mg PO q8h; 1200 mg/d max. *Peds.* 2.5–5 mg/kg PO q 8h; w/ food or antacids **Caution:** [C, +] May worsen severe arrhythmias; drug interactions w/ hepatic enzyme inducers & suppressors requires dosage changes **Contra:** Cardiogenic shock or 2nd-/3rd-degree AV block w/o pacemaker **Disp:** Caps 150, 200, 250 mg **SE:** lightheadedness, dizziness, anxiety, incoordination, GI upset, ataxia, hepatic damage, blood dyscrasias **Interactions:** ↑ Effects

w/ fluvoxamine, quinidine, caffeine; ↑ effects OF theophylline; ↓ effects w/ at
ropine, hydantoins, phenytoin, phenobarbital, rifampin, tobacco **Labs:** ↑ LFTs, +
ANA; Monitor LFTs

Mezlocillin (Mezlin) [Antibiotic/Penicillin] Uses: *Infxns caused
by susceptible gram(−) bacteria (skin, bone, resp tract, urinary tract, abdomen, sep-
ticemia)* **Action:** Bactericidal; ↓ cell wall synthesis. *Spectrum:* Gram(−) *Kleb
siella, Proteus, E. coli, Enterobacter, P. aeruginosa,* & *Serratia* **Dose:** *Adults.* 3 g
IV q4–6h. *Peds.* 200–300 mg/kg/d ÷ q4–6h; ↓ in renal/hepatic insuff **Caution:**
[B, M] **Contra:** PCN sensitivity **Disp:** Inj **SE:** GI upset, agranulocytosis, thrombocytopenia **Notes:** Often used w/ aminoglycoside **Interactions:** ↑ Effects w.
probenecid; ↑ effects OF MTX **Labs:** ↑ LFTs, BUN, SCr; ↓ serum K+

Miconazole (Monistat, others) [Antifungal] Uses: *Candidal Infxns, dermatomycoses (various tinea forms)* **Action:** Fungicide; alters funga
membrane permeability **Dose:** Apply to area bid for 2–4 wk. *Intravag:* 1 applicatorful or supp hs for 3 (4% or 200 mg) or 7 d (2% or 100 mg) **Caution:** [C, ?]
Azole sensitivity **Disp:** Topical cream 2%; lotion 2%; powder 2%; spray 2%; vaginal supp 100, 200 mg; vaginal cream 2%, 4% [OTC] **SE:** Vaginal burning, may
↑ warfarin **Notes:** Antagonistic to amphotericin B in vivo **Interactions:** ↑ Effects
OF anticoagulants, cisapride, loratadine, phenytoin, quinidine; ↓ effects w/ amphotericin B; ↓ effects OF amphotericin B **Labs:** ↑ Protein

Midazolam (Versed) [C-IV] [Sedative/Benzodiazepine]
Uses: *Preop sedation, conscious sedation for short procedures & mechanically
ventilated pts, induction of general anesthesia* **Action:** Short-acting benzodiazepine **Dose:** *Adults.* 1–5 mg IV or IM; titrate to effect. *Peds.* Preop: > 6 mo
0.25–1 mg/kg PO, 20 mg max . *Conscious sedation:* 0.08 mg/kg times 1. > 6 mo
0.1–0.2 mg/kg IM x1 max 10 mg. *General anesthesia:* 0.025–0.1 mg/kg IV q2min
for 1–3 doses PRN to induce anesthesia (↓ in elderly, w/ narcotics or CNS depressants) **Caution:** [D, +/−] CYP3A4 substrate (Table 13), several drug interactions
Contra: NA glaucoma; use of amprenavir, nelfinavir, ritonavir **Disp:** Inj 1,
5 mg/mL; syrup 2 mg/mL **SE:** Monitor for resp depression; ↓ BP in conscious sedation, nausea **Notes:** Reversal w/ flumazenil **Interactions:** ↑ Effects w/ azole antifungals, antihistamines, cimetidine, CCBs, CNS depressants, erythromycin, INH,
phenytoin, protease inhibitors, grapefruit juice, EtOH; ↓ effects w/ rifampin, tobacco; ↓ effects OF levodopa NIPE: Monitor for resp depression

Mifepristone [RU 486] (Mifeprex) [Abortifacient] WARNING:
Pt counseling & information required; associated w/ fatal infections & bleeding
Uses: *Termination of intrauterine pregnancies of <49 d* **Action:** Antiprogestin;
↑ prostaglandins, results in uterine contraction **Dose:** Administered w/ 3 office vis-
its: day 1, three 200-mg tabs PO; day 3 if no abortion, two 200-mg tabs PO; on or
about day 14, verify termination of PRG **Caution:** [X, −] **Contra:** Anticoagulation
therapy, bleeding disorders **Disp:** Tabs 200 mg **SE:** Abdominal pain & 1–2 wk of
uterine bleeding **Notes:** Give under medical supervision only **Interactions:** ↑ Ef-

fects w/ azole antifungals, erythromycin, grapefruit juice; ↓ effects w/ carbamazepine, dexamethasone, phenytoin, phenobarbital, rifampin, St. John's wort

Miglitol (Glyset) [Hypoglycemic/Alpha-glucosidase Inhibitor] Uses: *Type 2 DM* Action: a-Glucosidase inhibitor; delays digestion of carbohydrates Dose: Initial 25 mg PO tid; maint 50–100 mg tid (w/ 1st bite of each meal) Caution: [B, –] Contra: DKA, obstructive/inflammatory GI disorders; SCr > 2 Disp: Tabs 25, 50, 100 mg SE: Flatulence, D, abdominal pain Interactions: ↑ Effects w/ celery, coriander, juniper berries, ginseng, garlic; ↓ effects w/ INH, niacin, intestinal absorbents, amylase, pancreatin; ↓ effects OF digoxin, propranolol, ranitidine; Labs: ⊘ use w/serum crea > 2 mg/dL NIPE: Use alone or w/ sulfonylureas

Milrinone (Primacor) [Vasodilator] Uses: *CHF* Action: Positive inotrope & vasodilator; little chronotropic activity Dose: 50 mcg/kg, then 0.375–0.75 mcg/kg/min inf; ↓ in renal impair Caution: [C, ?] Contra: Allergy to drug or amrinone Disp: Inj 200 mcg/mL, 1 mg/mL SE: Arrhythmias, ↓ BP, HA Notes: Monitor fluid/electrolyte status & BP/HR Interactions: ↑ Hypotension w/ disopyramide

Mineral Oil [OTC] [Emollient Laxative] Uses: *Constipation* Action: Emollient laxative Dose: Adults. 15–45 mL PO PRN. Peds >6 y. 5–20 mL PO q day Caution: [C, ?] N/V, difficulty swallowing, bedridden pts Contra: Colostomy/ileostomy, appendicitis, diverticulitis, ulcerative colitis Disp: Liq [OTC] SE: Lipid pneumonia, anal incontinence, ↓ vitamin absorption Interactions: ↑ Effects w/ stool softeners; ↓ effects OF cardiac glycosides, oral contraceptives, sulfonamides, warfarin

Minoxidil (Loniten, Rogaine) [Antihypertensive/Vasodilator, Topical Hair Growth] Uses: *Severe HTN; male & female pattern baldness* Action: Peripheral vasodilator; stimulates vertex hair growth Dose: Adults. PO: (HTN) 2.5–80 mg PO (divided dose) qd–bid, max 100 mg/d. Topical: (Baldness) Apply bid to affected area. Peds. 0.2–1 mg/kg/24 h ÷ PO q12–24h, max 50 mg/d; ↓ PO dose in elderly Caution: [C, +] Contra: Pheochromocytoma, allergy to components Disp: Tabs 2.5, 5, 10 mg; topical soln (Rogaine) 2%, 5% SE: Pericardial effusion & volume overload w/ PO use; hypertrichosis w/chronic use; edema, ECG changes, weight gain Interactions: ↑ Hypotension w/ guanethidine Labs: ↑ Alkaline phosphatase, BUN, creatinine; ↓ Hmg, Hct

Mirtazapine (Remeron, Remeron SolTab) [Tetracyclic Antidepressant] WARNING: Closely monitor for worsening depression or emergence of suicidality, particularly in ped pts Uses: *Depression* Action: Tetracyclic antidepressant Dose: 15 mg PO hs, up to 45 mg/d hs Caution: [C, ?] Contra: MAOIs w/in 14 d Disp: Tabs 15, 30, 45 mg; rapid dissolving tabs 15 mg, 30 mg SE: Somnolence, ↑ cholesterol, constipation, xerostomia, weight gain, agranulocytosis Notes: Do not ↑ dose at intervals of less than 1–2 wk Interactions: ↑ Effects w/ CNS depressants, fluvoxamine; ↑ risk OF HTN crisis

w/ MAOIs **Labs:** ↑ ALT, cholesterol, triglycerides **NIPE:** Handle rapid tabs with dry hands, do not cut or chew

Misoprostol (Cytotec) [Mucosal Protective Agent/Prostaglandin]

Uses: *Prevent NSAID-induced gastric ulcers*; induction of labor, incomplete & therapeutic abortion **Action:** Prostaglandin w/ both antisecretory & mucosal protective properties **Dose:** *Ulcer prevention:* 200 mcg PO qid w/ meals; in females, start on 2nd or 3rd day of next nl menstrual period; 25–50 mcg for induction of labor (term); 400 mcg on day 3 of mifepristone for PRG termination (take w/ food) **Caution:** [X, –] **Contra:** PRG, component allergy **Disp:** Tabs 100, 200 mcg **SE:** Can cause miscarriage w/ potentially dangerous bleeding; HA, GI Sxs common (D, abdominal pain, constipation) **Interactions:** ↑ HA & GI symptoms w/ phenylbutazone

Mitomycin (Mutamycin) [Antineoplastic/Alkylating Agent]

Uses: *Stomach, pancreas,* breast, colon CA; squamous cell carcinoma of the anus; non-small-cell lung, head & neck, cervical; bladder CA (intravesically) **Action:** Alkylating agent; may generate oxygen free radicals, w/ DNA strand breaks **Dose:** Per protocol; 20 mg/m² q6–8wk or 10 mg/m² in combo w/ other myelosuppressive drugs; bladder CA 20–40 mg in 40 mL NS via a urethral catheter once/wk for 8 wk, followed by monthly treatments for 1 y; ↓ in renal/hepatic impair **Caution:** [D, –] **Contra:** Thrombocytopenia, leukopenia, coagulation disorders, SCr >1.7 mg/dL **Disp:** Inj 5, 20, 40 mg **SE:** Myelosuppression (may persist up to 3–8 wk after dose, may be cumulative; minimize by a lifetime dose <50–60 mg/m²), N/V, anorexia, stomatitis, & renal tox; microangiopathic hemolytic anemia w/ progressive renal failure (similar to hemolytic–uremic syndrome); venoocclusive liver Dz, interstitial pneumonia, alopecia ; extravasation Rxns; contact dermatitis. **Interactions:** ↑ Bronchospasm w/ vinca alkaloids; ↑ bone marrow suppression w/ antineoplastics

Mitoxantrone (Novantrone) [Antineoplastic/Antibiotic]

Uses: *AML (w/ cytarabine), ALL, CML, CAP, MS,* breast CA & NHL **Action:** DNA-intercalating agent; ↓ DNA topoisomerase II **Dose:** Per protocol; ↓ in hepatic impair, leukopenia, thrombocytopenia; **Caution:** [D, –] reports of secondary AML (monitor CBC) **Contra:** PRG **Disp:** Inj 2 mg/mL **SE:** Myelosuppression, N/V, stomatitis, alopecia (infrequent), cardiotox, urine discoloration; **Interactions:** ↑ Bone marrow suppression w/ antineoplastics; ↓ effects OF live virus vaccines **Labs:** ↑ AST, ALT, uric acid **NIPE:** ↑ fluids to 2–3 L/d, maintain hydration ⊘ vaccines, infection; Cardiac monitoring prior to each dose

Modafinil (Provigil) [Analeptic/CNS Stimulant]

Uses: *Improve wakefulness in pts w/ narcolepsy & excessive daytime sleepiness* **Action:** Alters dopamine & norepinephrine release, ↓ GABA-mediated neurotransmission **Dose:** 200 mg PO q morning; ↓ dose 50% w/ elderly/hepatic impair **Caution:** [C, ?/–], CV Dz; ↑ effects of warfarin, diazepam, phenytoin; ↓ effects of oral contraceptives, cyclosporine, theophylline **Contra:** Component allergy **Disp:** Tablets 100 mg, 200 mg **SE:** HA, N, D, paresthesias, rhinitis, agitation **Interactions:** ↑ Effects OF CNS stimulants, diazepam, phenytoin, propranolol, TCAs, warfarin; ↓ effect OF cyclosporine, oral contraceptives, theophylline **NIPE:** Take w/o regard to food, monitor BP, use barrier contraception

Moexipril (Univasc) [Antihypertensive/ACEI] Uses: *HTN, post-MI.* DN **Action:** ACE inhibitor **Dose:** 7.5–30 mg in 1–2 ÷ doses 1 h ac **Caution:** [C (1st tri), D 2nd & 3rd tri), ?] **Contra:** ACE inhibitor sensitivity **Disp:** Tabs 7.5, 15 mg; ↓ in renal impair **SE:** ↓ BP, edema, angioedema, HA, dizziness, cough **Interactions:** ↑ Effects w/ diuretics, antihypertensives, EtOH, probenecid, garlic; ↑ effects OF insulin, Li; ↑ risk OF hyperkalemia with K supl, K-sparing diuretics; ↓ effects w/ antacids, ASA, NSAIDS, ephedra, yohimbe, ginseng **Labs:** ↑ BUN, creatinine, K⁺, ALT, AST, serum alkaline phosphatase; ↓ serum cholesterol; false + test for urine acetone **NIPE:** May alter sense of taste, may cause cough, ⊘ salt substitutes, ⊘ PRG, use barrier contraception

Molindone (Moban) [Antipsychotic] Uses: *Psychotic disorders* **Action:** Piperazine phenothiazine **Dose:** *Adults.* 50–75 mg/d PO, ↑ to 225 mg/d if necessary. *Peds.* 3–5 y: 1–2.5 mg/d PO in 4 ÷ doses. *5–12 y:* 0.5–1.0 mg/kg/d in 4 ÷ doses **Caution:** [C, ?] NA glaucoma **Contra:** Drug or EtOH-induced CNS depression **Disp:** Tabs 5, 10, 25, 50 mg; **SE:** BP, tachycardia, arrhythmias, EPS, Szs, constipation, xerostomia, blurred vision **Interactions:** ↑ Effects w/ antihypertensives; ↑ hyperkalemia w/ K-sparing diuretics, K supls, salt substitutes, trimethoprim; ↑ effects OF insulin, Li; ↓ effects w/ ASA, NSAIDs **Labs:** ↑ Serum K⁺, BUN, creatinine **NIPE:** Take w/o food, monitor for persistent cough

Montelukast (Singulair) [Bronchodilator/Leukotriene Receptor Antagonist] Uses: *Prophylaxis & Rx of chronic asthma, seasonal allergic rhinitis* **Action:** Leukotriene receptor antagonist **Dose:** *Asthma: Adults & Peds > 15y.* 10 mg/d PO taken in PM. *Peds.* 2–5 y: 4 mg/d PO taken in PM. *6–14 y:* 5 mg/d PO in PM. *Rhinitis: Adults & Peds > 15y.* 10 mg qd *Peds.* 2–5 y: 4 mg qd. *6-14 y:* 5 mg qd **Caution:** [B, M] **Contra:** Component allergy **Disp:** Tabs 10 mg; chew tabs 4, 5 mg **SE:** HA, dizziness, fatigue, rash, GI upset, Churg–Strauss syndrome **Notes:** Not for acute asthma attacks **Interactions:** ↑↓ Effects w/ phenobarbital, rifampin **Labs:** ↑ AST, ALT

Morphine (Avinza XR, Duramorph, Infumorph, MS Contin, Kadian SR, Oramorph SR, Roxanol) [C-II] [Narcotic Analgesic] Uses: *Relief of severe pain* **Action:** Narcotic analgesic **Dose:** *Adults.* PO: 5–30 mg q4h PRN; SR tabs 15–60 mg q8–12h (do not chew/crush). *IV/IM:* 2.5–15 mg q2–6h; supp 10–30 mg q4h. *IT:* (Duramorph, Infumorph): Per protocol *Peds.* > 6 mo 0.1–0.2 mg/kg/dose IM/IV q2–4h PRN to 15 mg/dose max; 0.2–0.5 mg/kg PO q 4–6h prn; 0.3–0.6 mg/kg SR tabs PO q12h **Caution:** [B (D if prolonged use or high doses at term), +/–] **Contra:** Severe asthma, resp depression, GI obstruction **Disp:** Immediate-release tabs 15, 30 mg; MS Contin CR tabs 15, 30, 60, 100, 200 mg; Oramorph SR CR tabs 15, 30, 60, 100 mg; Kadian SR caps 20,

30 50, 60, 100 mg; Avinza XR caps 30, 60, 90, 120 mg; soln 10, 20, 100 mg/5 mL; supp 5, 10, 20 mg; inj 2, 4, 5, 8, 10, 15, 25, 50 mg/mL; Duramorph/Infumorph inj 0.5, 1 mg/mL; supp 5, 10, 20, 30 mg **SE:** Narcotic SE (resp depression, sedation, constipation, N/V, pruritus), granulomas w/ IT **Notes:** May require scheduled dosing to relieve severe chronic pain; do not crush/chew SR/CR forms **Interactions:** ↑ Effects w/ cimetidine, CNS depressants, dextroamphetamine, TCAs, EtOH, kava kava, valerian, St. John's wort; ↑ effects OF warfarin; ↑ risk OF HTN crisis w/ MAOIs; ↓ effects w/ opioids, phenothiazines **Labs:** ↑ Serum amylase, lipase

Morphine, Liposomal (DepoDur) [Narcotic Analgesic]
Uses: *Long-lasting epidural analgesia* **Action:** ER morphine analgesia **Dose:** 10–20 mg lumbar epidural inj (c-section 10 mg after cord clamped) **Caution:** [C,+/–] elderly, biliary Dz (sphincter of Oddi spasm) **Contra:** ileus, resp depression, asthma, obstructed airway, suspected/or known head injury ↑ ICP, allergy to morphine. **Disp:** Inj 10 mg/mL **SE:** Hypoxia, resp depression, ↓ BP, retention, N/V, constipation, flatulence, pruritus, pyrexia, anemia, HA, dizziness, tachycardia, insomnia, ileus **Notes:** Effect ≤ 48 h; not for IT/IV/IM use

Moxifloxacin (Avelox, Vigamox ophthalmic) [Antibiotic/Fluoroquinolone]
Uses: *Acute sinusitis, acute bronchitis, skin/soft tissue Infxns, conjunctivitis, & community-acquired pneumonia* **Action:** 4th-gen quinolone; ↓ DNA gyrase. *Spectrum:* Excellent gram(+) coverage except MRSA & *E. faecium;* good gram(–) coverage except *P. aeruginosa, S. maltophilia,* & *Acinetobacter* sp; good anaerobic coverage **Dose:** 400 mg/d PO/IV; (avoid cation products, antacids). *Ophth:* 1 gt tid ×7d; take PO 4 h before or 8 h after antacids **Caution:** [C, ?/–] Quinolone sensitivity; interactions w/ Mg-, Ca-, Al-, & Fe-containing products & class IA & III antiarrhythmic agents **Contra:** Quinolone or component sensitivity **Disp:** Tabs 400 mg, inj, ophth 0.5% **SE:** Dizziness, nausea, QT prolongation, Szs, photosensitivity, tendon rupture **Interactions:** ↑ Effects w/ probenecid; ↑ effects OF diazepam, theophylline, caffeine, metoprolol, propranolol, phenytoin, warfarin; ↓ effects w/ antacids, didanosine, Fe salts, Mg, sucralfate, NaHCO3, zinc **Labs:** ↑ LFTs, BUN, SCr, amylase, PT, triglycerides, cholesterol; ↓ Hmg, Hct **NIPE:** ⊘ Give to children <18 y; ↑ fluids to 2–3 L/d

Multivitamins (Table 15)

Mupirocin (Bactroban) [Topical Anti-infective]
Uses: *Impetigo; eradication of MRSA in nasal carriers* **Action:** ↓ bacterial protein synthesis **Dose:** *Topical:* Apply small amount to affected area 2–5 (times)/d for 5–14 days. *Nasal:* Apply bid in nostrils × 5 d **Caution:** [B, ?] **Contra:** Do not use concurrently w/ other nasal products **Disp:** Oint 2%; cream 2% **SE:** Local irritation, rash **Interactions:** ↓ Bacterial action w/ chloramphenicol **NIPE:** ⊘ Use w/ other nasal drugs

Muromonab-CD3 (Orthoclone OKT3) [Immunosuppressant/Monoclonal Antibody]
WARNING: Can cause anaphylaxis; monitor fluid status **Uses:** *Acute rejection following organ transplantation* **Action:** Murine Ab, Blocks T-cell Fxn **Dose:** Per protocol **Adults.** 5 mg/d IV for

10–14 d. *Peds.* 0.1 mg/kg/d IV for 10–14 d **Caution:** [C, ?/–] Murine sensitivity, fluid overload **Contra:** Heart failure/fluid overload, Hx of Szs, PRG, uncontrolled HTN **Disp:** Inj 5 mg/5 mL **SE:** monitor closely for anaphylaxis or pulmonary edema, fever, & chills after the 1st dose (premedicate w/ steroid/APAP/antihistamine) **Notes:** Monitor during inf; use 0.22-micron filter for administration **Interactions:** ↑ Effects w/ immunosuppressives; ↑ effects OF live virus vaccines; ↑ risk OF CNS effects & encephalopathy w/ indomethacin **Labs:** ↑ AST, ALT **NIPE:** ⊘ Immunizations, exposure to infection

Mycophenolic Acid (Myfortic) [Immunosuppressant] WARNING: ↑ Risk of Infxns, possible development of lymphoma Uses: *Prevent rejection after renal transplant* Action: Cytostatic to lymphocytes Dose: *Adults.* 720 mg PO bid; *Peds.* BSA 400–720 mg/m²: 750 mg PO bid; ↓ in renal insuff/neutropenia; take on empty stomach Caution: [C, ?/–] Contra: Component allergy Disp: DR tabs 180, 360 mg SE: N/V/D, pain, fever, HA, Infxn, HTN, anemia, leukopenia, edema Interactions: ↓ OF phenytoin, theophylline; ↓ w/antacids, cholestyramine, iron Labs: Monitor LFTs, BUN, Creatinine, CBC NIPE: If GI distress—take with food; avoid crowds & people w/ infections

Mycophenolate Mofetil (CellCept) [Immunosuppressant] WARNING: ↑ Risk of Infxns, possible development of lymphoma Uses: *Prevent organ rejection after transplant* Action: ↓ immunologically mediated inflammatory responses Dose: *Adults.* 1 g PO bid; *Peds.* BSA 1.2–1.5 m²: 750 mg PO bid; *BSA >1.5 m²:* 1 g PO bid; may taper up to 600 mg/m² PO bid; used w/ steroids & cyclosporine; ↓ in renal insuff or neutropenia. *IV:* Infuse over at least 2 h. *PO:* Take on empty stomach, do not open capsules Caution: [C, ?/–] Contra: Component allergy, IV use in polysorbate 80 allergy Disp: Caps 250, 500 mg; susp 200 mg/mL; inj 500 mg SE: N/V/D, pain, fever, HA, Infxn, HTN, anemia, leukopenia, edema Interactions: ↑ Effects w/ acyclovir, ganciclovir, probenecid; ↑ effects OF acyclovir, ganciclovir; ↓ effects w/ antacids, cholestyramine, cyclosporine, Fe, food; ↓ effects OF oral contraceptives, phenytoin, theophylline Labs: ↑ LFTs NIPE: Use barrier contraception during and 6 wk after drug therapy, ⊘ exposure to infection; take w/o food

Nabilone (Cesamet) [CII] [Synthetic Cannabinoid] WARNING: Psychotomimetic rxns, may persist for 72 h following d/c; caregivers should be present during initial use or dosage modification; patients should not operate heavy machinery; avoid alcohol, sedatives, hypnotics, other psychoactive substances Uses: *Refractory chemo-induced emesis* Action: Synthetic cannabinoid Dose: *Adults.* 1–2 mg PO bid 1–3 h before chemo, 6 mg/d max; may continue for 48 h beyond final chemo dose Caution: [C,?/–] elderly, HTN, heart failure, underlying psychiatric illness, substance abuse; high protein binding and first-pass metabolism may lead to drug interactions Disp: Caps 1 mg SE: Drowsiness, vertigo, xerostomia, euphoria, ataxia, HA, difficulty concentrating, tachycardia, ⊘ BP Interactions: ↑ CNS depression w/ benzodiazepines, barbiturates, CNS depressants,

ETOH; ↑ effects w/ opioids; ↑ effects OF opioids; cross-tolerance w/ opioids
NIPE: May require initial dose evening before chemo; Rx only quantity for single cycle

Nabumetone (Relafen) [Analgesic, Anti-inflammatory, Antipyretic/NSAID]
WARNING: May ↑ risk of cardiovascular events & GI bleeding **Uses:** *Arthritis & pain* **Action:** NSAID; ↓ prostaglandins **Dose:** 1000–2000 mg/d ÷ qd–bid w/ food **Caution:** [C (D 3rd tri), +] **Contra:** Peptic ulcer, NSAID sensitivity, severe hepatic Dz **Disp:** Tabs 500, 750 mg **SE:** Dizziness, rash, GI upset, edema, peptic ulcer **Interactions:** ↑ Effects w/ aminoglycosides; ↑ effects OF anticoagulants, hypoglycemics, Li, MTX, thrombolytics; ↑ GI effects w/ ASA, corticosteroids, K supls, NSAIDs, EtOH; ↓ effects of antihypertensives, diuretics **Labs:** ↑ LFTs, BUN, SCr; ↓ serum glucose, Hmg, Hct, plts **NIPE:** Photosensitivity—use sunscreen

Nadolol (Corgard) [Antihypertensive, Antianginal/BB]
Uses: *HTN & angina* **Action:** Competitively blocks β-adrenergic receptors, $β_1$, $β_2$ **Dose:** 40–80 mg/d; ↑ to 240 mg/d (angina) or 320 mg/d (HTN) PRN; ↓ in renal insuff & elderly **Caution:** [C (1st tri; D if 2nd or 3rd tri), +] **Contra:** Uncompensated CHF, shock, heart block, asthma **Disp:** Tabs 20, 40, 80, 120, 160 mg **SE:** Nightmares, paresthesias, ↓ BP, bradycardia, fatigue **Interactions:** ↑ Effects w/ antihypertensives, diuretics, nitrates, EtOH; ↑ effects OF aminophylline, lidocaine; ↑ risk OF HTN w/ clonidine, ephedrine, epinephrine, MAOIs, phenylephrine, pseudoephedrine; ↑ bradycardia w/ digitalis glycosides, ephedrine, epinephrine, phenylephrine, pseudoephedrine; ↓ effects w/ ampicillin, antacids, clonidine, NSAIDs, thyroid meds; ↓ effects OF glucagon, theophylline **Labs:** ↑ K^+, cholesterol, triglycerides, BUN, uric acid **NIPE:** May ↑ cold sensitivity; ⊘ D/C abruptly

Nafcillin (Nallpen) [Antibiotic/Penicillinase-resistant Penicillin]
Uses: *Infxns caused by susceptible strains of Staphylococcus & Streptococcus* **Action:** Bactericidal β-lactamase-resistant penicillin; ↓ cell wall synthesis. *Spectrum:* Good gram(+) except MRSA and enterococcus, no gram (−), poor anaerobe **Dose:** *Adults.* 1–2 g IV q4–6h. *Peds.* 50–200 mg/kg/d ÷ q4–6h **Caution:** [B, ?] PCN allergy **Disp:** Inj powder 1, 2 gm **SE:** Interstitial nephritis, D, fever, nausea **Notes:** No adjustments for renal Fxn **Interactions:** ↑ Effects OF MTX; ↓ effects w/ chloramphenicol, macrolides, tetracyclines; ↓ effects OF cyclosporine, oral contraceptives, tacrolimus, warfarin **Labs:** ↑ Serum protein **NIPE:** Aminoglycosides not compatible, risk of drug inactivation w/ fruit juice/carbonated drinks; monitor for superinfection

Naftifine (Naftin) [Antifungal]
Uses: *Tinea pedis, cruris, & corporis* **Action:** Antifungal antibiotic; ↓ cell membrane ergosterol synthesis **Dose:** Apply bid **Caution:** [B, ?] **Contra:** Component sensitivity **Disp:** 1% cream; gel **SE:** Local irritation

Nalbuphine (Nubain) [Narcotic Agonist-Antagonist Analgesic]
Uses: *Moderate–severe pain; preop & obstetric analgesia* **Action:**

Narcotic agonist–antagonist; ↓ ascending pain pathways **Dose:** *Adults.* 10–20 mg IM or IV q4–6h PRN; max of 160 mg/d; single max dose, 20 mg. *Peds.* 0.2 mg/kg IV or IM to a max dose of 20 mg; ↓ in hepatic insuff **Caution:** [B (D if prolonged or high doses at term), ?] **Contra:** Sulfite sensitivity **Disp:** Inj 10, 20 mg/mL **SE:** CNS depression & drowsiness; caution w/ opiate use **Interactions:** ↑ CNS depression w/ cimetidine, CNS depressants; EtOH ↑ effects OF digitoxin, phenytoin, rifampin **Labs:** ↑ Serum amylase, lipase

Naloxone (Narcan) [Opioid Antagonist] **Uses:** *Opioid addiction (diagnosis) & OD* **Action:** Competitive narcotic antagonist **Dose:** *Adults.* 0.4–2.0 mg IV, IM, or SQ q5min; max total dose, 10 mg. *Peds.* 0.01–1 mg/kg/dose IV, IM, or SQ; repeat IV q3min × 3 doses PRN **Caution:** May precipitate acute withdrawal in addicts **Disp:** Inj 0.4, 1.0 mg/mL; neonatal inj 0.02 mg/mL **SE:** ↓ BP, tachycardia, irritability, GI upset, pulmonary edema **Notes:** If no response after 10 mg, suspect nonnarcotic cause **Interactions:** ↓ Effects OF opioids

Naltrexone (ReVia) [Opioid Antagonist] **Uses:** *EtOH & narcotic addiction* **Action:** Competitively binds to opioid receptors **Dose:** 50 mg/d PO; do not give until opioid-free for 7–10 d **Caution:** [C, M] **Contra:** Acute hepatitis, liver failure; opioid use **Disp:** Tabs 50 mg **SE:** May cause hepatotox; insomnia, GI upset, joint pain, HA, fatigue **Interactions:** ↑ Lethargy & somnolence w/ thioridazine; ↓ effects OF opioids

Naphazoline & Antazoline (Albalon-A Ophthalmic, others), Naphazoline & Pheniramine Acetate (Naphcon A) [Opht Antihistamine] **Uses:** *Relieve ocular redness & itching caused by allergy* **Action:** Vasoconstrictor & antihistamine **Dose:** 1–2 gtt up to qid **Caution:** [C, +] **Contra:** Glaucoma, children <6 y, & w/ contact lenses **Disp:** Soln 15 mL **SE:** CV stimulation, dizziness, local irritation **Interactions:** ↑ Risk of HTN crisis w/ MAOIs, TCAs

Naproxen (Aleve [OTC], Naprosyn, Anaprox) [Analgesic, Anti-inflammatory, Antipyretic/NSAID] **WARNING:** May ↑ risk of cardiovascular events & GI bleeding **Uses:** *Arthritis & pain* **Action:** NSAID; ↓ prostaglandins **Dose:** *Adults & Peds >12 y.* 200–500 mg bid–tid to 1500 mg/d max; ↓ in hepatic impair **Caution:** [B (D 3rd tri), +] **Contra:** NSAID sensitivity, peptic ulcer disease **Disp:** Tabs 200, 250, 375, 500 mg; delayed release: 375, 500 mg; controlled release: 375 mg, 500 mg; susp 125 mg/5 mL **SE:** Dizziness, pruritus, GI upset, peptic ulcer, edema **Interactions:** ↑ Effects w/ aminoglycosides; ↑ effects OF anticoagulants, hypoglycemics, Li, MTX, thrombolytics; ↑ GI effects w/ ASA, corticosteroids, K supls, NSAIDs, EtOH; ↓ effects OF antihypertensives, diuretics **Labs:** ↑ Urine 5-HIAA **NIPE:** Take w/ food

Naratriptan (Amerge) [Migraine Suppressant/5 HT Agonist] [OTC] **Uses:** *Acute migraine attacks* **Action:** Serotonin 5-HT₁ receptor antagonist **Dose:** 1–2.5 mg PO once; repeat PRN in 4 h; ↓ in mild renal/hepatic insuff, take w/ fluids **Caution:** [C, M] **Contra:** Severe renal/hepatic impair, avoid in angina, ischemic heart Dz, uncontrolled HTN, cerebrovascular syndromes, & ergot use **Disp:** Tabs 1, 2.5 mg **SE:** Dizziness, sedation, GI upset, paresthesias, ECG changes, coronary vasospasm, arrhythmias **Interactions:** ↑ Effects w/ MAOIs, SSRIs; ↑ effects OF ergot drugs; ↓ effects w/ nicotine

Natalizumab (Tysabri) [Immunomodulator] WARNING: Cases of progressive multifocal leukoencephalopathy (PML) reported **Uses:** *Relapsing MS to delay disability and ↓ recurrences* **Action:** Adhesion molecule inhibitor **Dose:** *Adults.* 300 mg IV q4 wk; second-line Tx only **Contra:** PML; immune compromise or w/immunosuppressant **Caution:** [C,?/–] baseline MRI to rule out PML **Disp:** Vial 300 mg **SE:** Infxn, immunosuppression; infusion rxn precluding subsequent use; HA, fatigue, arthralgia **NIPE:** Give slowly to ↓ rxns; d/c immediately w/ signs of PML (weakness, paralysis, vision loss, impaired speech, cognitive ↓); evaluate at 3 and 6 mos, then q 6 mos thereafter; limited distribution (TOUCH risk mgmt program (800) 456-2255)

Nateglinide (Starlix) [Hypoglycemic/Meglitinide] **Uses:** *Type 2 DM* **Action:** ↑ Pancreatic release of insulin **Dose:** 120 mg PO tid 1–30 min pc; ↓ to 60 mg tid if near target HbA$_{1c}$ (take 1–30 min ac) **Caution:** [C, –]. Caution w/ drugs metabolized by CYP2C9/3A4 (Table 13) **Contra:** Diabetic ketoacidosis, type 1 DM **Disp:** Tabs 60, 120 mg **SE:** Hypoglycemia, URI; salicylates, nonselective β-blockers may enhance hypoglycemia **Interactions:** ↑ Effects w/ nonselective BBs, MAOIs, NSAIDs, salicylates, ↓ effects w/ corticosteroids, niacin, sympathomimetics, thiazide diuretics, thyroid meds **Labs:** ↑ Uric acid

Nedocromil (Tilade) [Anti-inflammatory/Respiratory Inhalant] **Uses:** *Mild–moderate asthma* **Action:** Anti-inflammatory agent **Dose:** Inhal: 2 inhal qid **Caution:** [B, ?/–] **Contra:** Component allergy **Disp:** Metdose inhaler **SE:** Chest pain, dizziness, dysphonia, rash, GI upset, Infxn **Notes:** Not for acute asthma **NIPE:** May take 2–4 wk for full therapeutic effect

Nefazodone (Serzone) [Antidepressant] WARNING: Fatal hepatitis & liver failure possible, D/C if LFT >3× ULN, do not re-treat; closely monitor for worsening depression or emergence of suicidality, particularly in ped pts **Uses:** *Depression* **Action:** ↓ Neuronal uptake of serotonin & norepinephrine **Dose:** Initial 100 mg PO bid; usual 300–600 mg/d in 2 + doses **Caution:** [C, ?] **Contra:** MAOIs, pimozide, cisapride, carbamazepine **Disp:** Tabs 50, 100, 150, 200, 250, 500 mg **SE:** Postural ↓ BP & allergic Rxns; HA, drowsiness, xerostomia, constipation, GI upset, liver failure **Notes:** Monitor LFTs, HR/BP **Interactions:** ↑ Effects w/ benzodiazepines, buspirone; ↑ effects OF alprazolam, buspirone, carbamazepine, cyclosporine, digoxin, triazolam; ↑ risk OF QT prolongation w/ astemizole, cisapride, pimozide; ↑ risk OF serious and/or fatal Rxn w/ MAOIs; ↓ effects OF propranolol **Labs:** ↑ LFTs, cholesterol; ↓ Hct **NIPE:** Take w/o food; may take 2–4 wk for full therapeutic effects

Nelarabine (Arranon) [Nucleoside Analog] WARNING: Neurotoxicity possible, which may be fatal **Uses:** *T-cell ALL or T-cell LBL unresponsive > 2 other regimens* **Action:** Nucleoside analog **Dose:** *Adults.* 1500 mg/m² IV over 2 hr days 1, 3, 5 of 21-day cycle **Peds.** 650 mg/m² IV over 1 hr days 1–5 of 21-day cycle **Caution:** [D,?/–] **Disp:** Vial 250 mg **SE:** Neuropathy, ataxia, seizures, coma, hematologic toxicity, GI upset, HA, blurred vision **Notes:** Prehydration, urinary alkalinization, and allopurinol before dose **Labs:** Monitor CBC

Nelfinavir (Viracept) [Antiretroviral/Protease Inhibitor]

Uses: *HIV Infxn* **Action:** Protease inhibitor; results in formation of immature, noninfectious virion production **Dose:** *Adults.* 750 mg PO tid or 1250 mg PO bid. *Peds.* 20–30 mg/kg PO tid; take w/ food **Caution:** [B, ?] Many significant drug interactions **Contra:** Phenylketonuria, triazolam/midazolam use or any other drug highly dependent on CYP3A4 (Table 13) **Disp:** Tabs 250, 625 mg; powder 50 mg/g; **SE:** Food ↑ absorption; interacts w/ St. John's wort; dyslipidemia, lipodystrophy, D, rash **Interactions:** ↑ Effects w/ erythromycin, ketoconazole, indinavir, ritonavir; ↑ effects of barbiturates, carbamazepine, cisapride, ergot alkaloids, erythromycin, lovastatin, midazolam, phenytoin, saquinavir, simvastatin, triazolam; ↓ effects w/ barbiturates, carbamazepine, phenytoin, rifabutin, rifampin; ↓ effects OF oral contraceptives **Labs:** ↑ LFTs **NIPE:** Take w/ food; use barrier contraception

Neomycin, Bacitracin, & Polymyxin B (Neosporin Ointment) (See Bacitracin, Neomycin, & Polymyxin B Topical)

Neomycin, Colistin, & Hydrocortisone (Cortisporin-TC Otic Drops); Neomycin, Colistin, Hydrocortisone, & Thonzonium (Cortisporin-TC Otic Suspension) [Antibiotic /Anti-inflammatory]

Uses: *External otitis,* Infxns of mastoid/fenestration cavities **Action:** Antibiotic w/anti-inflammatory **Dose:** *Adults.* 4–5 gtt in ear(s) tid–qid. *Peds.* 3–4 gtt in ear(s) tid–qid **Caution:** [C, ?] **Disp:** Otic gtt & susp **SE:** Local irritation

Neomycin & Dexamethasone (AK-Neo-Dex Ophthalmic, NeoDecadron Ophthalmic) [Antibiotic/Corticosteroid]

Uses: *Steroid-responsive inflammatory conditions of the cornea, conjunctiva, lid, & anterior segment* **Action:** Antibiotic w/ anti-inflammatory corticosteroid **Dose:** 1–2 gtt in eye(s) q3–4h or thin coat tid–qid until response, then ↓ to qd **Caution:** [C, ?] **Disp:** Cream neomycin 0.5%/dexamethasone 0.1%; oint neomycin 0.35%/dexamethasone 0.05%; soln neomycin 0.35%/dexamethasone 0.1% **SE:** local irritation **Notes:** Use under ophthalmologist's supervision

Neomycin & Polymyxin B (Neosporin Cream) [OTC] [Antibiotic]

Uses: *Infxn in minor cuts, scrapes, & burns* **Action:** Bactericidal **Dose:** Apply bid–qid **Caution:** [C, ?] **Contra:** Component allergy **Disp:** Cream neomycin 3.5 mg/polymyxin B 10,000 Units/g **SE:** Local irritation **Notes:** Different from Neosporin oint

Neomycin, Polymyxin B, & Dexamethasone (Maxitrol) [Antibiotic/Corticosteroid]

Uses: *Steroid-responsive ocular conditions w/ bacterial Infxn* **Action:** Antibiotic w/ anti-inflammatory corticosteroid **Dose:** 1–2

gtt in eye(s) q4–6h; apply oint in eye(s) tid–qid **Caution:** [C, ?] **Disp:** Oint neomycin sulfate 3.5 mg/polymyxin B sulfate 10,000 Units/dexamethasone 0.1%/g; susp identical/5 mL **SE:** Local irritation **Notes:** Use under supervision of ophthalmologist

Neomycin-Polymyxin Bladder Irrigant [Neosporin GU Irrigant] [Antibiotic]
Uses: *Continuous irrigant for prophylaxis against bacteriuria & gram(–) bacteremia associated w/ indwelling catheter use* **Action:** Bactericidic; not for Serratia and Streptococci **Dose:** 1 mL irrigant in 1 L of 0.9% NaCl; cont bladder irrigation w/ 1 L of soln/24 h **Caution:** [D] **Contra:** Component allergy **Disp:** Soln neomycin sulfate 40 mg & polymyxin B 200,000 Units/mL; amp 1, 20 mL **SE:** Neomycin-induced ototox or nephrotox (rare) **Notes:** Potential for bacterial or fungal super Infxn; not for irrig

Neomycin, Polymyxin, & Hydrocortisone (Cortisporin Ophthalmic & Otic) [Antibiotic/Anti-inflammatory]
Uses: *Ocular & otic bacterial Infxns* **Action:** Antibiotic & anti-inflammatory **Dose:** *Otic:* 3–4 gtt in the ear(s) tid–qid. *Ophth:* Apply a thin layer to the eye(s) or 1 gt qd–qid **Caution:** [C, ?] **Disp:** Otic susp; ophth soln; ophth oint **SE:** Local irritation

Neomycin, Polymyxin B, & Prednisolone (Poly-Pred Ophthalmic) [Antibiotic/Corticosteroid]
Uses: *Steroid-responsive ocular conditions w/ bacterial Infxn* **Action:** Antibiotic & anti-inflammatory **Dose:** 1–2 gtt in eye(s) q4–6h; apply oint in eye(s) tid–qid **Caution:** [C, ?] **Disp:** Susp neomycin 0.35%/polymyxin B 10,000 Units/mL/prednisolone 0.5%/mL **SE:** Irritation **Notes:** Use under supervision of ophthalmologist

Neomycin Sulfate (Myciguent) [Antibiotic] [OTC]
Uses: *Hepatic coma, bowel prep* **Action:** Aminoglycoside, poorly absorbed PO; ↓ GI bacterial flora **Dose:** *Adults.* 3–12 g/24 h PO in 3–4 ÷ doses. *Peds.* 50–100 mg/kg/24 h PO in 3–4 ÷ doses **Caution:** [C, ?/–] Renal failure, neuromuscular disorders, hearing impair **Contra:** Intestinal obstruction **Disp:** Tabs 500 mg; PO soln 125 mg/5 mL **SE:** Hearing loss w/ long-term use; rash, N/V **Notes:** Do not use parenterally (↑ tox); part of the Condon bowel prep

Nepafenac (Nevanac) [Analgesic, Anti-inflammatory, Antipyretic/NSAID]
Uses: *Inflammation postcataract surgery* **Action:** NSAID **Dose:** *Adults.* 1 gtt in eye(s) TID 1 day before, and 14 days after surgery **Contra:** NSAID or aspirin sensitivity **Caution:** [C,?/–] may ↑ bleeding time, delay healing, cause keratitis **Disp:** Susp 3 mL **SE:** Capsular opacity, visual changes, foreign body sensation, inc. IOP **Interactions:** ↑ effects of oral anticoagulants **NIPE:** Prolonged use ↑ corneal risk; remove contact lenses during use; shake well before use, separate from other drops by > 5 min

Nesiritide (Natrecor) [Vasodilator]
Uses: *Acutely decompensated CHF* **Action:** Human B-type natriuretic peptide **Dose:** 2 mcg/kg IV bolus, then 0.01 mcg/kg/min IV **Caution:** [C, ?/–] When vasodilators are not appropriate **Contra:** SBP <90, cardiogenic shock **Disp:** Vials 1.5 mg **SE:** ↓ BP, HA, GI upset, ar-

rhythmias, ↑ Cr **Notes:** Requires continuous BP monitoring; some studies indicate ↑ in mortality **Interactions:** ↑ Hypotension w/ ACEIs, nitrates **Labs:** ↑ Creatinine

Nevirapine (Viramune) [Antiretroviral/NNRTI] WARNING:
Reports of fatal hepatotox even after short-term use; severe life-threatening skin reactions (Stevens–Johnson, toxic epidermal necrolysis, & allergic Rxns); monitor closely during 1st 8 wk of Rx **Uses:** *HIV Infxn* **Action:** Nonnucleoside RT inhibitor **Dose:** *Adults.* Initial 200 mg/d PO × 14 d, then 200 mg bid. *Peds.* <8 y: 4 mg/kg/d PO × 14 d, then 7 mg/kg bid. >8 y: 4 mg/kg/d × 14 d, then 4 mg/kg bid (w/o regard to food) **Caution:** [C, +/–] OCP **Disp:** Tabs 200 mg; susp 50 mg/5 mL **SE:** Life-threatening rash; HA, fever, D, neutropenia, hepatitis **Notes:** HIV resistance when given as monotherapy; always use in combo w/at least 1 additional antiretroviral agent; give w/out regards to food; not recommended in women if CD4 >250 or men >400 unless benefit >risk of hepatotoxicity **Interactions:** ↑ Effects w/ clarithromycin, erythromycin; ↓ effects w/ rifabutin, rifampin, St. John's wort; ↓ effects OF clarithromycin, indinavir, ketoconazole, methadone, oral contraceptives, protease inhibitors, warfarin **NIPE:** Use barrier contraception

Niacin (Niaspan, Slo-Niacin) [Vitamin/Antilipemic] Uses:
Adjunct in significant hyperlipidemia **Action:** Nicotinic acid, Vit B$_3$; ↓ Lipolysis; ↓ esterification of triglycerides; ↑ lipoprotein lipase **Dose:** 1–6 g + doses PO tid; 9 g/d max (w/ food) **Caution:** [A (C if does >RDA), +] **Contra:** Liver Dz, peptic ulcer, arterial hemorrhage **Disp:** SR caps 125, 250, 300, 400, 500 mg; tabs 25, 50, 100, 250, 500 mg; SR tabs 150, 250, 500, 750 mg; elixir 50 mg/5 mL **SE:** Upper body/facial flushing & warmth; GI upset, flatulence, exacerbate peptic ulcer; HA, paresthesias, liver damage, gout, or altered glucose control in DM. **Notes:** Flushing ↓ by taking aspirin or NSAID 30–60 min prior to dose **Interactions:** ↑ Effects of antihypertensives, anticoagulants; ↓ effects OF hypoglycemics, probenecid, sulfinpyrazone **Labs:** False ↑ urinary catecholamines, false + urine glucose, ↑ LFTs, uric acid **NIPE:** EtOH & hot beverages ↑ flushing

Nicardipine (Cardene) [Antihypertensive, Antianginal/CCB]
Uses: *Chronic stable angina & HTN*; prophylaxis of migraine **Action:** CCB **Dose:** *Adults.* PO: 20–40 mg PO tid. *SR:* 30–60 mg PO bid. *IV:* 5 mg/h IV cont inf; ↑ by 2.5 mg/h q15min to max 15 mg/h. *Peds.* PO: 20–30 mg PO q 8h. *IV:* 0.5–5 mcg/kg/min; ↓ in renal/hepatic impair **Caution:** [C, ?/–] Heart block, CAD **Contra:** Cardiogenic shock **Disp:** Caps 20, 30 mg; SR caps 30, 45, 60 mg; inj 2.5 mg/mL **SE:** Flushing, tachycardia, ↓ BP, edema, HA **Notes:** *PO-to-IV conversion:* 20 mg tid = 0.5 mg/h, 30 mg tid = 1.2 mg/h, 40 mg tid = 2.2 mg/h; take w/ food (not high fat) **Interactions:** ↑ Effects w/ azole antifungals, cimetidine, ranitidine, grapefruit juice; ↑ effects OF cyclosporine, carbamazepine, prazosin, quinidine, tacrolimus; ↑ hypotension w/ antihypertensives, fentanyl, nitrates, quinidine, EtOH; ↑ dysrhythmias w/ digoxin, disopyramide, phenytoin; ↓ effects w/ NSAIDs, rifampin **Labs:** ↑ LFTs **NIPE:** ↑ Risk of photosensitivity—use sunscreen

Nicotine Gum (Nicorette) [Smoking Deterrent] [OTC] Uses: *Aid to smoking cessation for relief of nicotine withdrawal* Action: Systemic delivery of nicotine Dose: Chew 9–12 pieces/d PRN; max 30 pieces/d Caution: [C, ?] Contra: Life-threatening arrhythmias, unstable angina Disp: 2 mg, 4 mg/piece; mint, orange, original flavors SE: Tachycardia, HA, GI upset, hiccups Notes: Must stop smoking & perform behavior modification for max effect Interactions: ↑ Effects w/ cimetidine; ↑ effects OF catecholamines, cortisol; ↑ hemodynamic & A-V blocking effects OF adenosine; ↓ effects w/ coffee, cola NIPE: Chew 30 min for full dose of nicotine; ↓ absorption w/ coffee, soda, juices, wine w/in 15 min

Nicotine Nasal Spray (Nicotrol NS) [Smoking Deterrent] Uses: *Aid to smoking cessation for relief of nicotine withdrawal* Action: Systemic delivery of nicotine Dose: 0.5 mg/actuation; 1–2 sprays/h, 10 sprays/h max Caution: [D, M] Contra: Life-threatening arrhythmias, unstable angina Disp: Nasal inhaler 10 mg/mL SE: Local irritation, tachycardia, HA, taste perversion Notes: Must stop smoking & perform behavior modification for max effect Interactions: ↑ Effects w/ cimetidine, blue cohosh; ↑ effects OF catecholamines, cortisol; ↑ hemodynamic & A-V blocking effects OF adenosine NIPE: ⊘ In pts w/ chronic nasal disorders or severe reactive airway Dz; ↑ incidence of cough

Nicotine Transdermal (Habitrol, Nicoderm CQ [OTC], Nicotrol [OTC]) [Smoking Deterrent] Uses: *Aid to smoking cessation; relief of nicotine withdrawal* Action: Systemic delivery of nicotine Dose: Individualized; 1 patch (14–22 mg/d) & taper over 6 wk Caution: [D, M] Contra: Life-threatening arrhythmias, unstable angina Disp: Habitrol & Nicoderm CQ 7, 14, 21 mg of nicotine/24 h; Nicotrol 5, 10, 15 mg/24 h SE: Insomnia, pruritus, erythema, local site Rxn, tachycardia Notes: Nicotrol worn for 16 h to mimic smoking patterns; others worn for 24 h; must stop smoking & perform behavior modification for max effect Interactions: ↑ Effects w/ cimetidine, blue cohosh; ↑ effects OF catecholamines, cortisol; ↑ hemodynamic & A-V blocking effects OF adenosine; ↑ HTN w/ bupropion NIPE: Change application site daily

Nifedipine (Procardia, Procardia XL, Adalat, Adalat CC) [Antihypertensive, Antianginal/CCB] Uses: *Vasospastic or chronic stable angina & HTN*; tocolytic Action: CCB Dose: *Adults.* SR tabs 30–90 mg/d. *Tocolysis:* 10–20 mg PO q4–6h. *Peds.* 0.6–0.9 mg/kg/24 h ÷ tid–qid Caution: [C, +] Heart block, aortic stenosis Contra: Immediate-release preparation for urgent or emergent HTN; acute MI Disp: Caps 10, 20 mg; SR tabs 30, 60, 90 mg SE: HA common on initial Rx; reflex tachycardia may occur w/ regular release dosage forms; peripheral edema, ↓ BP, flushing, dizziness Notes: Adalat CC & Procardia XL not interchangeable; SL administration not OK Interactions: ↑ Effects w/ antihypertensives, azole antifungals, cimetidine, cisapride, CCBs, diltiazem, famotidine, nitrates, quinidine, ranitidine, EtOH, grapefruit juice; ↑ effects OF digitalis glycosides, phenytoin, vincristine; ↓ effects w/ barbiturates, nafcillin, NSAIDs, phenobarbital, rifampin, St. John's wort, tobacco; ↓ effects OF quinidine

Labs: ↑ LFTs **NIPE:** Take w/o regard to food; ↑ risk of photosensitivity—use sunscreen

Nilutamide (Nilandron) [Antineoplastic/Antiandrogen] WARNING: Interstitial pneumonitis possible; most cases in 1st 3 mo; follow CXR before Rx **Uses:** *Combo w/ surgical castration for metastatic CAP* **Action:** Nonsteroidal antiandrogen **Dose:** 300 mg/d PO in ÷ doses for 30 d, then 150 mg/d **Caution:** [not used in females] **Contra:** Severe hepatic impair or resp insuff **Disp:** Tabs 150 mg **SE:** See warning, Interstitial pneumonitis, hot flashes, loss of libido, impotence, N/V/D, gynecomastia, hepatic dysfunction, interstitial pneumonitis **Notes:** May cause Rxn when taken w/ EtOH **Interactions:** ↑ Effects OF phenytoin, theophylline, warfarin **Labs:** ↑ LFTs (monitor) **NIPE:** Take w/o regard to food; visual adaptation may be delayed

Nimodipine (Nimotop) [CCB] **Uses:** *Prevent vasospasm following subarachnoid hemorrhage* **Action:** CCB **Dose:** 60 mg PO q4h for 21 d; ↓ in hepatic failure **Caution:** [C, ?] **Contra:** Component allergy **Disp:** Caps 30 mg **SE:** ↓ BP, HA, constipation **Notes:** Administered via NG tube if caps cannot be swallowed whole **Interactions:** ↑ Effects w/ antihypertensives, cimetidine, nitrates, omeprazole, protease inhibitors, quinidine, valproic acid, EtOH, grapefruit juice; ↑ effects OF phenytoin **Labs:** ↑ LFTs **NIPE:** ↑ Risk of photosensitivity—use sunscreen

Nisoldipine (Sular) [Antihypertensive/CCB] **Uses:** *HTN* **Action:** CCB **Dose:** 10–60 mg/d PO; do not take w/ grapefruit juice or high-fat meal; ↓ starting doses in elderly or hepatic impair **Caution:** [C, ?] **Disp:** ER tabs 10, 20, 30, 40 mg **SE:** Edema, HA, flushing **Interactions:** ↑ Effects w/ antihypertensives, azole antifungals, cimetidine, famotidine, nitrates, ranitidine, EtOH, high-fat foods; ↑ effects OF tacrolimus; ↓ effects w/ NSAIDs, phenytoin, rifampin **Labs:** ↑ Serum creatine kinase, BUN, creatinine

Nitazoxanide (Alinia) [Antiprotozoal] **Uses:** *Cryptosporidium-* or *Giardia-induced diarrhea in pts 1–11 y* **Action:** Antiprotozoal interferes w/ pyruvate ferredoxin oxidoreductase **Spectrum:** *Cryptosporidium* or *Giardia* **Dose:** *Peds 12–47 mo.* 5 mL (100 mg) PO q 12h × 3 d. *4–11 y:* 10 mL (200 mg) PO q 12h × 3 d; take w/ food **Caution:** [B, ?] **Disp:** 100 mg/5 mL PO susp **SE:** Abdominal pain **Notes:** Susp contains sucrose, interacts w/ highly protein-bound drugs

Nitrofurantoin (Macrodantin, Furadantin, Macrobid) [Urinary Anti-infective] **WARNING:** Pulmonary reactions possible **Uses:** *Prevention & Rx UTI* **Action:** Bacteriostatic; interferes w/ carbohydrate metabolism. **Spectrum:** Susceptible gram(–) & some gram(+) bacteria; *Pseudomonas, Serratia,* & most sp. *Proteus-resistant* **Dose:** *Adults.* Suppression: 50–100 mg/d PO. *Rx:* 50–100 mg PO qid. *Peds.* 4–7 mg/kg/24 h in 4 ÷ doses (w/ food/milk/antacid) **Caution:** [B, +] Avoid if CrCl <50 mL/min, pregnant at term **Contra:** Renal failure, infants < 1 mo **Disp:** Caps/tabs 25, 50, 100 mg; susp 25 mg/5 mL **SE:** GI side effects; dyspnea & a variety of acute/chronic pulmonary reactions, peripheral neuropathy **Notes:** Macrocrystals (Macrodantin) cause < nausea than other forms

Interactions: ↑ Effects w/ anticholinergics, probenecid, sulfinpyrazone; ↓ effects w/ antacids, quinolones **Labs:** False + urine glucose; false ↑ serum bilirubin, creatinine **NIPE:** Take w/ food; may discolor urine

Nitroglycerin (Nitrostat, Nitrolingual, Nitro-Bid Ointment, Nitro-Bid IV, Nitrodisc, Transderm-Nitro, others) [Antianginal, Vasodilator/Nitrate] Uses: *Angina pectoris, acute & prophylactic therapy, CHF, BP control* **Action:** Relaxation of vascular smooth muscle, dilates coronary arteries **Dose:** *Adults.* SL: 1 tab q5min SL PRN for 3 doses. *Translingual:* 1–2 met-doses sprayed onto PO mucosa q3–5min, max 3 doses. *PO:* 2.5–9 mg tid. *IV:* 5–20 mcg/min, titrated to effect. *Topical:* Apply ½ in. of oint to chest wall tid, wipe off at night. *TD:* 0.2–0.4 mg/h/patch qd. *Peds.* 1 mcg/kg/min IV, titrate. **Caution:** [B, ?] Restrictive cardiomyopathy **Contra:** *IV:* Pericardial tamponade, constrictive pericarditis. *PO:* Use w/ sildenafil, tadalafil, vardenafil, head trauma, closed-angle glaucoma **Disp:** SL tabs 0.3, 0.4, 0.6 mg; translingual spray 0.4 mg/dose; SR caps 2.5, 6.5, 9, 13 mg; SR tabs 2.6, 6.5, 9.0 mg; inj 0.5, 5, 10 mg/mL; oint 2%; TD patches 0.1, 0.2, 0.4, 0.6 mg/h; buccal CR 2, 3 mg **SE:** HA, ↓ BP, lightheadedness, GI upset **Notes:** Nitrate tolerance w/ chronic use after 1–2 wk; minimize by providing nitrate-free period qd, using shorter-acting nitrates tid, & removing long-acting patches & oint before sleep to ↓ tolerance **Interactions:** ↑ Hypotensive effects w/ antihypertensives, phenothiazines, sildenafil, EtOH; ↓ effects w/ ergot alkaloids; ↓ effects OF SL tabs & spray w/ antihistamines, phenothiazines, TCAs **Labs:** False ↑ cholesterol, triglycerides **NIPE:** Replace SL tabs q6 mo & keep in original container

Nitroprusside (Nipride, Nitropress) [Antihypertensive/Vasodilator] Uses: *Hypertensive crisis, CHF, controlled ↓ BP periop (↓ bleeding),* aortic dissection, pulmonary edema **Action:** ↓ Systemic vascular resistance **Dose:** *Adults & Peds.* 0.5–10 mcg/kg/min IV inf, titrate; usual dose 3 mcg/kg/min **Caution:** [C, ?] ↓ cerebral perfusion **Contra:** High output failure, compensatory HTN **Disp:** Inj 25 mg/mL **SE:** Excessive hypotensive effects, palpitations, HA **Notes:** Thiocyanate (metabolite w/renal excretion) w/ tox at 5–10 mg/dL, more likely if used for > 2–3 d; w/ aortic dissection use w/ β-blocker **Interactions:** ↑ Effects w/ antihypertensives, anesthetics, guanabenz, guanfacine, sildenafil; ↓ effects w/ estrogens, sympathomimetics **NIPE:** Discard colored soln other than light brown

Nizatidine (Axid, Axic AR [OTC]) [Gastric Antisecretory/H2 Receptor Antagonist] Uses: *Duodenal ulcers, GERD, heartburn* **Action:** H₂-receptor antagonist **Dose:** *Adults.* Active ulcer: 150 mg PO bid or 300 mg PO hs; maint 150 mg PO hs. *GERD:* 300 mg PO bid; maint PO bid. *Heartburn:* 75 mg PO bid. *Peds.* GERD: 10 mg/kg PO bid in ÷ doses, 150 mg bid max ↓ in renal impair **Caution:** [B, +] **Contra:** H₂-receptor antagonist sensitivity **Disp:** Caps 75 [OTC], 150, 300 mg; sol 15 mg/mL **SE:** Dizziness, HA, constipation, D **Interactions:** ↑ Effects OF glipizide, glyburide, nifedipine, nitrendipine, nisoldipine, salicylates, tolbutamide; ↓ effects w/ antacids, tomato/mixed veg juice; ↓ effects OF azole antifungals, delavirdine, didanosine **Labs:** False + urobilinogen **NIPE:** Smoking ↑ gastric acid secretion

Norepinephrine (Levophed) [Vasopressor] Uses: *Acute ↓ BP, cardiac arrest (adjunct)* Action: Peripheral vasoconstrictor acts on arterial/venous beds Dose: *Adults.* 8–12 mcg/min IV, titrate. *Peds.* 0.05 – 0.1 mcg/kg/min IV, titrate Caution: [C, ?] Contra: ↓ BP due to hypovolemia Disp: Inj 1 mg/mL SE: Bradycardia, arrhythmia Notes: Correct volume depletion as much as possible before vasopressors; interaction w/ TCAs leads to severe HTN; infuse into large vein to avoid extravasation; phentolamine 5–10 mg/10 mL NS injected locally for extravasation Interactions: ↑ HTN w/ antihistamines, BBs, ergot alkaloids, guanethidine, MAOIs, methyldopa, oxytocic meds, TCAs; ↑ risk OF arrhythmias w/ cyclopropane, halothane

Norethindrone Acetate/Ethinyl Estradiol (FemHRT) [Progestin & Estrogen] WARNING: Estrogens & progestins should not be used for the prevention of CV Dz; the WHI study reported ↑ risks of MI, breast CA, & DVT in postmenopausal women during 5 y of treatment with estrogens combined with medroxyprogesterone acetate relative to placebo Uses: *Rx of moderate–severe vasomotor Sxs associated w/ menopause; prevent osteoporosis* Action: Hormone replacement Dose: 1 tablet qd Caution: [X, –] Contra: PRG; Hx breast CA; estrogen-dependent tumor; abnormal genital bleeding; Hx DVT, PE, or related disorders; recent (w/in past year) arterial thromboembolic Dz (CVA, MI) Disp: 1 mg norethindrone/5 mcg ethinyl estradiol tablets SE: Thrombosis, dizziness, HA, libido changes Notes: Use in women w/ intact uterus Interactions: ↑ Effects OF caffeine; ↓ effects w/ barbiturates, carbamazepine, fosphenytoin, phenytoin, rifampin Labs: Effects hepatic Fxn tests and endocrine Fxn tests NIPE: ⊘ PRG, cigarette smoking

Norfloxacin (Noroxin, Chibroxin ophthal) [Antibiotic/Fluoroquinolone] Uses: *Complicated & uncomplicated UTI due to gram(–) bacteria, prostatitis, gonorrhea,* & infectious D, conjunctivitis * Action: Quinolone, ↓ DNA gyrase, bactericidal Spectrum: Broad gram (+) and (–) E. faecalis, E. coli, K. pneumoniae, P. mirabilis, P. aeruginosa, S. epidermidis, S. saprophyticus Dose: 400 mg PO bid (↓ in renal impair). Gonorrhea: 800 mg single dose. Prostatitis: 400 mg PO bid; Gastroenteritis, travelers D: 400 mg PO (times) 3–5 d Adults, Peds > 1 y: 1 gt each eye qid for 7 d Caution: [C, –] Tendinitis/tendon rupture, quinolone sensitivity, Contra: Hx of allergy or tendinitis w/ fluoroquinolones Disp: Tabs 400 mg; ophth 3 mg/mL SE: Photosensitivity, HA, GI; ocular burning w/ ophth Notes: Interactions w/ antacids, theophylline, caffeine; good conc in the kidney & urine, poor blood levels; do not use for urosepsis Interactions: ↑ Effects w/ probenecid; ↑ effects OF diazepam, theophylline, caffeine, metoprolol, propranolol, phenytoin, warfarin; ↓ effects w/ antacids, sucralfate, Fe salts, Mg, sucralfate, NaHCO₃, zinc; ↓ effects w/ food; Labs: ↑ LFTs, BUN, SCr NIPE: ⊘ Give to children <18 y; ↑ fluids to 2–3 L/d; may cause photosensitivity—use sunscreen

Norgestrel (Ovrette) [Progestin] Uses: *PO Contraceptive* **Action:** Prevent follicular maturation & ovulation **Dose:** 1 tab/d PO; begin day 1 of menses **Caution:** [X, ?] **Contra:** Thromboembolic disorders, breast CA, PRG, severe hepatic Dz **Disp:** Tabs 0.075 mg **SE:** Edema, breakthrough bleeding, thromboembolism **Notes:** Progestin-only products have ↑ risk of failure in prevention of PRG **Interactions:** ↓ Effects w/ barbiturates, carbamazepine, hydantoins, griseofulvin, penicillins, rifampin, tetracyclines, St. John's wort **NIPE:** Photosensitivity—use sunscreen; D/C drug if suspect PRG—use barrier contraception until confirmed

Nortriptyline (Aventyl, Pamelor) [Antidepressant/TCA] Uses: *Endogenous depression* **Action:** TCA; ↑ synaptic CNS levels of serotonin &/or norepinephrine **Dose:** *Adults.* 25 mg PO tid–qid; >150 mg/d not OK. *Elderly.* 10–25 mg hs. *Peds.* 6–7 y: 10 mg/d. *8–11 y:* 10–20 mg/d. *>11 y:* 25–35 mg/d, ↓ w/ hepatic insuff **Caution:** [D, +/–] NA glaucoma, CV Dz **Contra:** TCA allergy, use w/ MAOI **Disp:** Caps 10, 25, 50, 75 mg; soln 10 mg/5 mL **SE:** Anticholinergic (blurred vision, retention, xerostomia) **Notes:** Max effect seen after 2 wk **Interactions:** ↑ Effects w/ antihistamines, CNS depressants, cimetidine, fluoxetine, oral contraceptives, phenothiazines, quinidine, EtOH; ↑ effects of anticoagulants; ↑ risk of HTN w/ clonidine, levodopa, sympathomimetics; ↓ effects w/ barbiturates, carbamazepine, rifampin **Labs:** ↑ Serum bilirubin, alkaline phosphatase **NIPE:** Concurrent use w/ MAOIs have resulted in HTN, Szs, death; ↑ risk of photosensitivity-use sunscreen

Nystatin (Mycostatin) [Antifungal] Uses: *Mucocutaneous Candida* Infxns (oral, skin, vaginal)* **Action:** Alters membrane permeability. *Spectrum:* Susceptible *Candida* sp **Dose:** *Adults & children.* PO: 400,000–600,000 Units PO "swish & swallow" qid. *Vaginal:* 1 tab vaginally hs × 2 wk. *Topical:* Apply bid–tid to area. *Peds.* Infants: 200,000 Units PO q6h. **Caution:** [B (C PO), +] **Disp:** PO susp 100,000 Units/mL; PO tabs 500,000 Units; troches 200,000 Units; vaginal tabs 100,000 U; topical cream/oint 100,000 Units/g, powder 100,000 units/gram **SE:** GI upset, Stevens–Johnson syndrome **Notes:** Not absorbed PO; not for systemic Infxn **NIPE:** Store susp up to 10 d in refrigerator

Octreotide (Sandostatin, Sandostatin LAR) [Antidiarrheal/ Hormone] Uses: *Suppresses/↓ severe diarrhea associated w/ carcinoid & neuroendocrine GI tumors (eg, VIPoma, ZE syndrome)*; bleeding esophageal varices **Action:** Long-acting peptide; mimics natural hormone somatostatin **Dose:** *Adults.* 100–600 mcg/d SQ/IV in 2–4 ÷ doses; start 50 mcg qd–bid. *Sandostatin LAR (depot):* 10–30 mg IM q4wk *Peds.* 1–10 mcg/kg/24 h SQ in 2–4 ÷ doses. **Caution:** [B, +] Hepatic/renal impair **Disp:** Inj 0.05, 0.1, 0.2, 0.5, 1 mg/mL; 10, 20, 30 mg/5 mL depot **SE:** N/V, abdominal discomfort, flushing, edema, fatigue, cholelithiasis, hyper-/hypoglycemia, hepatitis **Interactions:** ↓ Effects OF cyclosporine **Labs:** Small ↑ LFTs, ↓ serum thyroxine **NIPE:** May alter effects of hypoglycemics

Ofloxacin (Floxin, Ocuflox Ophthalmic) [Antibiotic/Fluoroquinolone] Uses: *Lower resp tract, skin & skin structure, & UTI, prostatitis, uncomplicated gonorrhea, & *Chlamydia* Infxns; topical (bacterial conjunctivitis; otitis externa; if perforated ear drum >12 y)* **Action:** Bactericide; ↓ DNA gyrase. Broad spectrum gram (+) and (–): S. pneumoniae, S. aureus, S. pyogenes, H. influenzae, P. mirabilis, N. gonorrhoeae, C. trachomatis, & E. coli **Dose:** *PO:* **Adults.** 200–400 mg PO bid or IV q12h. *Ophth:* **Adults & Peds >1 y.** 1–2 gtt in eye(s) q2–4h for 2 d, then qid × 5 more d. *Otic:* **Adults & Peds >12 y.** 10 gtt in ear(s) bid for 10 d. **Peds 1–12 y.** 5 gtt in ear(s) bid for 10 d. ↓ in renal impair; (on empty stomach) **Caution:** [C, –] ↓ absorption w/ antacids, sucralfate, Al-, Ca-, Mg-, Fe-, or Zn-containing drugs **Contra:** Quinolone allergy **Disp:** Tabs 200, 300, 400 mg; inj 20, 40 mg/mL; ophth & otic 0.3% **SE:** N/V/D, photosensitivity, insomnia, & HA **Notes:** Use ophth form in ears **Interactions:** ↑ Effects w/ cimetidine, probenecid, St. John's wort; ↑ effects of cyclosporine, procainamide, theophylline, warfarin, caffeine; ↓ effects w/ antacids, antineoplastics, Ca, didanosine, Fe, NaHCO₃, sucralfate, zinc **NIPE:** Take w/o food; use sunscreen; ↑ fluids to 2–3 L/d

Olanzapine (Zyprexa, Zyprexa Zydis) [Antipsychotic/ Thienobenzodiazepine]

WARNING:↑ mortality in elderly w/ dementia-related psychosis **Uses:** *Bipolar mania, schizophrenia, (eit) * psychotic disorders acute agitation in schizophrenia **Action:** Dopamine & serotonin antagonist; p inj 10 mg **Dose:** *Bipolar/Schizophrenia (eit):* 5–10 mg/d, ↑ weekly PRN, 20 mg/d max Agitation: (eit) 10–20mg IMq 2–4h PRN, 40mg day/max **Caution:** [C, –] **Disp:** Tabs 2.5, 5, 7.5, 10, 15, 20 mg; PO disintegrating tabs 5, 10, 15, 20 mg; inj 10 mg **SE:** HA, somnolence, orthostatic ↓ BP, tachycardia, dystonia, xerostomia, constipation **Notes:** Takes weeks to titrate dose; smoking ↓ levels; may be confused w/ Zyrtec **Interactions:** ↑ Effects w/ fluvoxamine, probenecid; ↑ sedation w/ CNS depressants, EtOH; ↑ Szs w/ anticholinergics, CNS depressants; ↑ hypotension w/ antihypertensives, diazepam; ↓ effects w/ activated charcoal, carbamazepine, omeprazole, rifampin, St. John's wort, tobacco; ↓ effects OF dopamine agonists, levodopa **Labs:** ↑ LFTs **NIPE:** ↑ Risk of tardive dyskinesia, photosensitivity—use suncreen, body temp impairment

Olopatadine (Patanol) [Opth Antihistamine]

Uses: *Allergic conjunctivitis* **Action:** H₁-receptor antagonist **Dose:** 1–2 gtt in eye(s) bid q6–8h **Caution:** [C, ?] **Disp:** Soln 0.1% 5 mL **SE:** Local irritation, HA, rhinitis **Notes:** Do not instill w/ contacts in NIPE: ⊘ in children < 3 years; may reinsert contacts 10 min later if eye not red

Olsalazine (Dipentum) [Anti-inflammatory/Aminosalicylic Acid Derivative]

Uses: *Maint remission in ulcerative colitis* **Action:** Topical anti-inflammatory **Dose:** 500 mg PO bid (w/ food) **Caution:** [C, M] Salicylate sensitivity **Disp:** Caps 250 mg **SE:** D, HA, blood dyscrasias, hepatitis **Labs:** ↑ LFTs

Omalizumab (Xolair) [Monoclonal Antibody]

Uses: *Moderate–severe asthma in ≥12 y w/ reactivity to an allergen & when Sxs inadequately controlled w/ inhaled steroids* **Action:** Anti-IgE Ab **Dose:** 150–375 mg SQ q2–4wk (dose/frequency based on serum IgE level & BW—see insert) **Caution:** [B,?/–] **Contra:** Component allergy **Disp:** 75, 150 mg single-use 5-mL vial **SE:** Site Rxn, sinusitis, HA, anaphylaxis reported in 3 pts **Notes:** Continue other asthma medications as indicated **Interactions:** No drug interaction studies done **NIPE:** ⊘ D/C abruptly; not for acute bronchospasm; admin w/in 8 h of reconstitution and store in refrigerator

Omega-3 Fatty Acid [fish oil](Omacor) [Ethyl Ester]   Uses: *Prevent secondary MI, hypertriglyceridemia when diet fails* **Action:** Omega-3-acid ethyl esters, ↓ thrombus, ↓ inflammation, ↓ triglycerides **Dose:** *Post MI:* 1 cap/day; *Hypertriglyceridemia:* 2 caps/d, ↑ to 4/d PRN **Caution:** [?,–] w/ anticoagulant use, w/bleed risk **Contra:** Hypersensitivity to components **Disp:** 1000-mg gelcap **SE:** Dyspepsia, N, GI pain, rash **Interactions:** ↑ effects of anticoagulants **Labs:** Monitor triglycerides, LDL, ALT **NIPE:** Only FDA approved fish oil supplement; not for exogenous hypertriglyceridemia (type 1 hyperchylomicronaemia); many OTC products

Omeprazole (Prilosec, Zegerid) [Proton Pump Inhibitor]   Uses: *Duodenal/gastric ulcers, ZE syndrome, GERD,* H. pylori *Infxns* **Action:** Proton-pump inhibitor **Dose:** 20–40 mg PO qd-bid, Zegerid powder/hac; in small cup w/ 2 Tbsp H2O (not food or other liquids) refill and drink **Caution:** [C, –] **Disp:** DR tabs 20 mg; DR caps 10, 20, 40 mg; Zegerid powder for oral suspension: 20, 40 mg **SE:** HA, D **Notes:** Combo (ie, antibiotic) Rx for H. pylori **Interactions:** ↑ Effects OF carbamazepine, diazepam, digoxin, glipizide, glyburide, nifedipine, nimodipine, nisoldipine, nitrendipine, phenytoin, tolbutamide, warfarin; ↓ effects w/ sucralfate; ↓ effects OF ampicillin, cefpodoxime, cefuroxime, enoxacin, cyanocobalamin, ketoconazole **Labs:** ↑ LFTs **NIPE:** Take w/o food

Ondansetron (Zofran, Zofran ODT) [Antiemetic/5 HT Antagonist]   Uses: *Prevent chemo-associated & postop N/V* **Action:** Serotonin receptor antagonist **Dose:** *Chemo: Adults & Peds.* 0.15 mg/kg/dose IV prior to chemo, then 4 & 8 h after 1st dose or 4–8 mg PO tid; 1st dose 30 min prior to chemo & give on a schedule, not PRN. *Postop. Adults.* 4 mg IV immediately before anesthesia or postop. *Peds.* <40 kg: 0.1 mg/kg. *>40 kg:* 4 mg IV ↓ dose w/ hepatic impair **Caution:** [B, +/–] **Disp:** Tabs 4, 8, 24 mg; soln 4 mg/5 mL; inj 2 mg/mL; 32 mg/50 mL; Zofran ODT tab, 4, 8 mg **SE:** D, HA, constipation, dizziness **Interactions:** ↓ Effects w/ rifampin; **Labs:** ↑ Fibrinogen, AST, ALT, serum bilirubin, ↓ Hmg, serum albumin, transferrin, gamma globulin **NIPE:** Food ↑ absorption

Oprelvekin (Neumega) [Thrombopoetic Growth Factor]   Uses: *Prevent severe thrombocytopenia w/ chemo* **Action:** ↑ Proliferation & maturation of megakaryocytes (interleukin-11) **Dose:** *Adults.* 50 mcg/kg/d SQ for 10–21 d. *Peds.* >12 y: 75–100 mcg/kg/d SQ for 10–21 d. *<12 y:* Use only in clinical trials. **Caution:** [C, ?/–] **Disp:** 5 mg powder for inj **SE:** Tachycardia, palpitations, arrhythmias, edema, HA, dizziness, insomnia, fatigue, fever, nausea, anemia, dyspnea; allergic reactions including anaphylaxis **Interactions:** None noted **Labs:** ↓ Hmg, albumin **NIPE:** Monitor for peripheral edema; use med w/in 3 h of reconstitution

Oral Contraceptives, Biphasic, Monophasic, Triphasic, Progestin Only (Table 7) [Progestin/Hormone] Uses:

Birth control & regulation of anovulatory bleeding **Action:** Birth control: Suppresses LH surge, prevents ovulation; progestins thicken cervical mucus; ↓ fallopian tubule cilia, ↓ endometrial thickness to ↓ chances of fertilization. *Anovulatory bleeding:* Cyclic hormones mimic body's natural cycle & regulate endometrial lining, results in regular bleeding q28d; may also ↓ uterine bleeding & dysmenorrhea **Dose:** 28-d cycle pills take qd; 21-d cycle pills take qd, no pills during last 7 d of cycle (during menses; some available as transdermal patch **Caution:** [X, +] Migraine, HTN, DM, sickle cell Dz, gallbladder Dz **Contra:** Undiagnosed vaginal bleeding, PRG, estrogen-dependent malignancy, hypercoagulation disorders, liver Dz, hemiplegic migraine, smokers >35 y **Disp:** 28-d cycle pills (21 active pills + 7 placebo/Fe supl); 21-d cycle pills (21 active pills) **SE:** Intramenstrual bleeding, oligomenorrhea, amenorrhea, ↑ appetite/weight gain, ↓ libido, fatigue, depression, mood swings, mastalgia, HA, melasma, ↑ vaginal discharge, acne/greasy skin, corneal edema, nausea **Notes:** Taken correctly, 99.9% effective for preventing PRG; no STDs prevention, use additional barrier contraceptive; long term, can ↓ risk of ectopic PRG, benign breast Dz, ovarian & uterine CA. *Rx for menstrual cycle control:* Start w/ monophasic; take for 3 mo before switching to another pill; if bleeding continues, change to pill w/ higher estrogen dose. *Rx for birth control:* Choose pill w/ lowest SE profile for particular pt; SEs numerous, due to Sxs of estrogen excess or progesterone deficiency; each pill's side effect profile is unique (see insert)

Orlistat (Xenical) [GI Lipase Inhibitor] Uses:

Manage obesity w/ BMI ≥ 30 kg/m² or ≥ 27 kg/m² w/ other risk factors; type 2 DM, dyslipidemia **Action:** Reversible inhibitor of gastric & pancreatic lipases. **Dose:** 120 mg PO tid w/ a fat-containing meal **Caution:** [B, ?] May ↓ cyclosporine & ↓ warfarin dose requirements **Contra:** Cholestasis, malabsorption **Disp:** Capsules 120 mg **SE:** Abdominal pain/discomfort, fatty/oily stools, fecal urgency **Notes:** Do not use if meal contains no fat; GI effects ↑ w/ higher-fat meals; supplement w/ fat-soluble vitamins **Interactions:** ↑ Effects OF pravastatin; ↓ effects OF cyclosporine, fat-soluble vitamins **Labs:** Monitor warfarin, ↓ serum glucose, total cholesterol, LDL **NIPE:** ⊘ Administer if meal contains no fat; GI effects ↑ w/ higher-fat meals; supplement w/ fat-soluble vitamins

Orphenadrine (Norflex) [Skeletal Muscle Relaxant] Uses:

Muscle spasms **Action:** Central atropine-like effects cause indirect skeletal muscle relaxation, euphoria, analgesia **Dose:** 100 mg PO bid, 60 mg IM/IV q12h **Caution:** [C, +] **Contra:** Glaucoma, GI obstruction, cardiospasm, MyG **Disp:** Tabs 100 mg; SR tabs 100 mg; inj 30 mg/mL **SE:** Drowsiness, dizziness, blurred vision, flushing, tachycardia, constipation **Interactions:** ↑ CNS depression w/ anxiolytics, butorphanol, hypnotics, MAOIs, nalbuphine, opioids, pentazocine, phenothiazines, tramadol, TCAs, kava kava, valerian, EtOH; ↑ effects w/ anticholinergics **NIPE:** Impaired body temp regulation

Oseltamivir (Tamiflu) [Antiviral/Neuraminidase Inhibitor] **Uses:** *Prevention & Rx influenza A & B* **Action:** ↓ viral neuraminidase **Dose:** *Adults.* 75 mg PO bid for 5 d. *Peds.* PO bid dosing: <14 kg: 30 mg. *16–23 kg:* 45 mg. *24–40 kg:* 60 mg; *>40 kg:* As adults; ↓ in renal impair **Caution:** [C, ?/–] **Contra:** Component allergy **Disp:** Caps 75 mg, powder 12 mg/mL **SE:** N/V, insomnia **Notes:** Initiate w/in 48 h of Sx onset or exposure **Interaction:** ↑ Effects w/ probenecid **NIPE:** Take w/o regard to food

Oxacillin (Bactocill, Prostaphlin) [Antibiotic/Penicillin] **Uses:** *Infxns due to susceptible S. aureus & Streptococcus* **Action:** Bactericidal; ↓ cell wall synthesis. *Spectrum:* Excellent gram(+), poor gram(–) **Dose:** *Adults.* 250–500 mg (1 g severe) IM/IV q4–6h. *Peds.* 150–200 mg/kg/d IV ÷ q4–6h; ↓ in significant renal Dz **Caution:** [B, M] **Contra:** PCN sensitivity **Disp:** Powder for inj 500 mg, 1, 2, 10 g; soln 250 mg/5 mL **SE:** GI upset, interstitial nephritis, blood dyscrasias **Interactions:** ↑ Effects w/ disulfiram, probenecid; ↑ effects OF anticoagulants, MTX; ↓ effects w/ chloramphenicol, tetracyclines, carbonated drinks, fruit juice, food; ↓ effects OF oral contraceptives **Labs:** False + urine and serum protein **NIPE:** Take w/o food

Oxaliplatin (Eloxatin) [Antineoplastic/Alkylating Agent] **WARNING:** Administer w/ supervision of health-care provider experienced in chemo. Appropriate management is possible only w/ adequate diagnostic & Rx facilities. Anaphylactic-like Rxns reported. **Uses:** *Adjuvant Rx stage-III colon CA (primary resected) & metastatic colon CA in combo w/ 5-FU* **Action:** Metabolized to platinum derivatives, crosslinks DNA **Dose:** Per protocol; see insert. *Premedicate:* Antiemetics w/ or w/o dexamethasone **Caution:** [D, –] see Warning **Contra:** Allergy to components or platinum **Disp:** Inj 50, 100 mg **SE:** Anaphylaxis, granulocytopenia, paresthesia, N/V/D, stomatitis, fatigue, neuropathy (common) hepatotox **Notes:** 5-FU & leucovorin are given in combo; epi, corticosteroids, & antihistamines alleviate severe Rxns; **Interactions:** ↑ effects OF nephrotoxic drugs **Labs:** ↑ Bilirubin, creatinine, LFTs; ↓ hmg, K⁺, neutrophils, platelets, WBC **NIPE:** Monitor CBC, platelets, LFTs, BUN & creatinine before each chemotherapy cycle; ↑ acute neurologic symptoms w/ cold exposure/cold liquids

Oxaprozin (Daypro, Daypro ALTA) [Analgesic, Anti-inflammatory, Antipyretic/NSAID] **WARNING:** May ↑ risk of cardiovascular disease & GI bleeding **Uses:** *Arthritis & pain* **Action:** NSAID; ↓ prostaglandins synthesis **Dose:** 600–1200 mg/d (divided dose may help GI tolerance); ↓ in renal/hepatic impair **Caution:** [C (D in 3rd tri or near term), peptic ulcer, bleeding disorders **Contra:** ASA/NSAID sensitivity, peri-operative pain w/CABG Disp: Daypro ALTA tab 600 mg; caplets 600 mg SE: CNS inhibition, sleep disturbance, rash, GI upset, peptic ulcer, edema, renal failure, anaphylactoid reaction with aspirin tried (asthmatic w/rhinitis, nasal polyps and bronchospasm w/NSAID use) Interactions: ↑ Effects OF aminoglycosides, anticoagulants, ASA, diuretics, Li, MTX, ↓ effects OF antihypertensives NIPE: ↑ Risk of photosensitivity—use sunscreen; take w/ food

Oxazepam (Serax) [C-IV] [Anxiolytic/Benzodiazepines]
Uses: *Anxiety, acute EtOH withdrawal,* anxiety w/ depressive Sxs Action: Benzodiazepine Dose: *Adults.* 10–15 mg PO tid–qid; severe anxiety & EtOH withdrawal may require up to 30 mg qid. *Peds.* 1 mg/kg/d in ÷ doses Caution: [D, ?] Disp: Caps 10, 15, 30 mg; tabs 15 mg SE: Sedation, ataxia, dizziness, rash, blood dyscrasias, dependence Notes: Avoid abrupt D/C; metabolite of diazepam (Valium) Interactions: ↑ CNS effects w/ anticonvulsants, antidepressants, antihistamines, barbiturates, MAOIs, opioids, phenothiazines, kava kava, lemon balm, sassafras, valerian, EtOH; ↑ effects w/ cimetidine; ↓ effects w/ oral contraceptives, phenytoin, theophylline, tobacco; ↓ effects OF levodopa Labs: False ↑ serum glucose NIPE: ⊘ D/C abruptly

Oxcarbazepine (Trileptal) [Anticonvulsant/Carbamazepine]
Uses: *Partial Szs,* bipolar disorders Action: Blocks voltage-sensitive Na^+ channels, stabilization of hyperexcited neural membranes Dose: *Adults.* 300 mg PO bid, ↑ weekly to target maint 1200–2400 mg/d. *Peds.* 8–10 mg/kg bid, 500 mg/d max, ↑ weekly to target maint dose; ↓ in renal insuff Caution: [C, –] Cross-sensitivity to carbamazepine; reports of fatal skin and multiorgan hypersensitivity Rxns Contra: Components sensitivity Disp: Tabs 150, 300, 600 mg; susp 300 mg/5 mL SE: ↓ Na^+, HA, dizziness, fatigue, somnolence, GI upset, diplopia, mental concentration difficulties Notes: Do not abruptly D/C, check Na^+ if fatigue reported; advise about symptoms of Steven-Johnson syndrome and topic epidermal necrolysis Interactions: ↑ Effects w/ benzodiazepines, EtOH; ↑ effects OF phenobarbital, phenytoin; ↓ effects w/ barbiturates, carbamazepine, phenobarbital, valproic acid, verapamil; ↓ effects OF CCBs, oral contraceptives Labs: ↓ Thyroid levels, serum Na NIPE: Take w/o regard to food; use barrier contraception

Oxiconazole (Oxistat) [Antifungal] Uses: *Tinea pedis, tinea cruris, & corporis* Action: Antifungal antibiotic. *Spectrum:* Most strains of *Epidermophyton floccosum, Trichophyton mentagrophytes, Trichophyton rubrum, Malassezia furfur* Dose: Apply bid Caution: [B, M] Contra: Component allergy Disp: Cream 1%; lotion SE: Local irritation

Oxybutynin (Ditropan, Ditropan XL) [GU Antispasmodic/ Anticholinergic] Uses: *Symptomatic relief of urgency, nocturia, & incontinence w/ neurogenic or reflex neurogenic bladder* Action: Direct smooth muscle antispasmodic; ↑ bladder capacity Dose: *Adults & Peds > 5 y.* 5 mg PO tid–qid; XL 5 mg PO qd; ↑ to 30 mg/d PO (5 & 10 mg/tab). *Peds 1–5 y.* 0.2 mg/kg/dose bid–qid (syrup 5 mg/5 mL). ↓ in elderly; periodic drug holidays OK Caution:

[B, ? (use w/ caution)] **Contra:** Glaucoma, MyG, GI or GU obstruction, ulcerative colitis, megacolon **Disp:** Tabs 5 mg; XL tabs 5, 10, 15 mg; syrup 5 mg/5 mL **SE:** Anticholinergic (drowsiness, xerostomia, constipation, tachycardia) **Interactions:** ↑ Effects w/ CNS depressants, EtOH; ↑ effects OF atenolol, digoxin, nitrofurantoin; ↑ anticholinergic effects w/ antihistamines, anticholinergics; ↓ effects OF haloperidol, levodopa **NIPE:** ↓ Temp regulation; ↑ photosensitivity—use sunscreen

Oxybutynin Transdermal System (Oxytrol) [GU Antispasmodic/Anticholinergic]
Uses: *Rx OAB* **Action:** Smooth muscle antispasmodic; ↑ bladder capacity **Dose:** One 3.9 mg/d system apply 2×/wk to abdomen, hip, or buttock **Caution:** [B, ?/–] **Contra:** Urinary or gastric retention, uncontrolled NA glaucoma **Disp:** 3.9 mg/d transdermal system **SE:** Anticholinergic effects, itching/redness at application site **Notes:** Avoid reapplication to the same site w/in 7 d **Interactions:** ↑ Effects w/ anticholinergics **NIPE:** Metabolized by the cytochrome P450 CYP3A4 enzyme system

Oxycodone [Dihydrohydroxycodeinone] (OxyContin, OxyIR, Roxicodone) [C-II] [Opioid Analgesic] WARNING:
Swallow whole, do not crush; high abuse potential **Uses:** *Moderate/severe pain, usually in combo w/ nonnarcotic analgesics* **Action:** Narcotic analgesic **Dose:** *Adults.* 5 mg PO q6h PRN. *Peds.* 6–12 y: 1.25 mg PO q6h PRN. *>12 y:* 2.5 mg q6h PRN. ↓ In severe liver Dz **Caution:** [B (D if prolonged use or near term), M] **Contra:** Allergy, resp depression **Disp:** Immediate-release caps (OxyIR) 5 mg; tabs (Percolone) 5 mg; CR (OxyContin) 10, 20, 40, 80 mg; liq 5 mg/5 mL; soln conc 20 mg/mL **SE:** ↓ BP, sedation, dizziness, GI upset, constipation, risk of abuse **Notes:** OxyContin for chronic CA pain; may be sought after as drug of abuse **Interactions:** ↑ CNS & resp. depression w/ amitriptyline, barbiturates, cimetidine, clomipramine, MAOIs, nortriptyline, protease inhibitors, TCAs **Labs:** False ↑ serum amylase, lipase **NIPE:** Take w/ food

Oxycodone & Acetaminophen (Percocet, Tylox) [C-II] [Narcotic Analgesic]
Uses: *Moderate–severe pain* **Action:** Narcotic analgesic **Dose:** *Adults.* 1–2 tabs/caps PO q4–6h PRN (acetaminophen max dose 4 g/d). *Peds.* Oxycodone 0.05–0.15 mg/kg/dose q 4–6h PRN, up to 5 mg/dose **Caution:** [B (D prolonged use or near term), M] **Contra:** Allergy, resp depression **Disp:** Percocet tabs, mg oxycodone/mg APAP: 2.5/325, 5/325, 7.5/325, 10/325, 7.5/500, 10/650; Tylox caps 5 mg oxycodone, 500 mg APAP; soln 5 mg oxycodone & 325 mg APAP/5 mL **SE:** ↓BP, sedation, dizziness, GI upset, constipation **Interactions:** ↑ CNS & resp depression w/ amitriptyline, barbiturates, cimetidine, clomipramine, MAOIs, nortriptyline, protease inhibitors, TCAs **Labs:** False ↑ serum amylase, lipase **NIPE:** Take w/ food

Oxycodone & Aspirin (Percodan, Percodan-Demi) [C-II] [Narcotic Analgesic/Non-Steroidal Analgesic]
Uses: *Moderate–moderately severe pain* **Action:** Narcotic analgesic w/ NSAID **Dose:** *Adults.* 1–2 tabs/caps PO q4–6h PRN. *Peds.* Oxycodone 0.05–0.15 mg/kg/dose q 4–6h

PRN, up to 5 mg/dose; ↓ in severe hepatic failure **Caution:** [B (D prolonged use or near term), M] Peptic ulcer **Contra:** Component allergy **Disp:** Percodan 4.5 mg oxycodone hydrochloride, 0.38 mg oxycodone terephthalate, 325 mg ASA; Percodan-Demi 2.25 mg oxycodone hydrochloride, 0.19 mg oxycodone terephthalate, 325 mg ASA **SE:** Sedation, dizziness, GI upset, constipation **SE:** Sedation, dizziness, GI upset, constipation **Interactions:** ↑ CNS & resp. depression w/ amitriptyline, barbiturates, cimetidine, clomipramine, MAOIs, nortriptyline, protease inhibitors, TCAs; ↑ effects OF anticoagulants **Labs:** False ↑ serum amylase, lipase **NIPE:** Take w/ food

Oxycodone/Ibuprofen (Combunox) [CII] [Narcotic Analgesic/NSAID]

Uses: *Short term (not >7 d) management of acute moderate–severe pain* **Action:** Narcotic w/NSAID **Dose:** Initial **Caution:** [C, –] w/ impaired renal/hepatic Fxn; COPD, CNS depression **Contra:** Paralytic ileus, 3rd tri PRG, allergy to ASA or NSAIDs, where opioids are contraindicated PRG **Disp:** Tabs 5 mg oxycodone /400 mg ibuprofen **SE:** N/V, somnolence, dizziness, sweating, flatulence, ↑ LFTs **Notes:** Monitor renal Fxn; abuse potential w/ oxycodone; **Interactions:** ↑ CNS & resp. depression w/ amitriptyline, barbiturates, cimetidine, clomipramine, MAOIs, nortriptyline, protease inhibitors, TCAs; ↑ effects w/ ASA, corticosteroids, probenecid, EtOH; ↑ effects OF aminoglycosides, anticoagulants, digoxin, hypoglycemics, Li, MTX; ↑ risks of bleeding w/ abciximab, cefotetan, valproic acid, thrombolytic drugs, warfarin, ticlopidine, garlic, ginger, ginkgo biloba; ↓ effects w/ feverfew; ↓ effects OF antihypertensives **Labs:** False ↑ serum amylase, lipase; ↑ BUN, creatinine; ↓ Hmg, Hct, BS, plts **NIPE:** Take w/ food

Oxymorphone (Numorphan) [C-II] [Narcotic Analgesic]

Uses: *Moderate/severe pain, sedative* **Action:** Narcotic analgesic **Dose:** 0.5 mg IM, SQ, IV initial, 1–1.5 mg q4–6h PRN. *PR:* 5 mg q4–6h PRN **Caution:** [B, ?] **Contra:** ↑ ICP, severe resp depression **Disp:** Inj 1, 1.5 mg/mL; supp 5 mg **SE:** ↓ BP, sedation, GI upset, constipation, histamine release **Notes:** Chemically related to hydromorphone **Interactions:** ↑ Effects w/ CNS depressants, cimetidine, neuroleptics, EtOH; ↓ effects w/ phenothiazines **Labs:** False ↑ amylase, lipase

Oxytocin (Pitocin) [Oxytocic/Hormone]

Uses: *Induce labor, control postpartum hemorrhage*; promote milk letdown in lactating women **Action:** Stimulate muscular contractions of the uterus & milk flow during nursing **Dose:** 0.001–0.002 Units/min IV inf; titrate 0.02 Units/min max. *Breast-feeding:* 1 spray in both nostrils 2–3 min before feeding **Caution:** [Uncategorized, no anomalies expected, +/–] **Contra:** Where vaginal delivery not favorable, fetal distress **Disp:** Inj 10 Units/mL; nasal soln 40 Units/mL **SE:** Uterine rupture, fetal death; arrhythmias, anaphylaxis, H_2O intox **Notes:** Monitor vital signs; nasal form for breast-feeding only **Interactions:** ↑ Pressor effects w/ sympathomimetics

Paclitaxel (Taxol, Abraxane) [Antineoplastic]

Uses: *Ovarian & breast CA* CAP **Action:** Mitotic spindle poison promotes microtubule assembly & stabilization against depolymerization **Dose:** Per protocols; use glass or polyolefin containers (eg, nitroglycerin tubing set); PVC sets leach plasticizer; ↓ in hepatic failure; **Caution:** [D, –] **Contra:** Neutropenia <1500 WBC/mm³; solid tumors **Disp:** Inj 6 mg/mL, 5mg/mL albumin bound (Abraxane) **SE:** Myelosuppression, peripheral neuropathy, transient ileus, myalgia, bradycardia, ↓ BP, mucositis, N/V/D, fever, rash, HA, & phlebitis; hematologic tox schedule-dependent; leukopenia dose-limiting by 24-h inf; neurotox limited w/short (1–3 h) inf **Notes:** Hypersensitivity Rxns (dyspnea, hypotension, urticaria, rash) usually w/in 10 min of starting inf; minimize w/ corticosteroid, antihistamine (H₁- and H₂-antagonist) pretreatment. **Interactions:** ↑ Effects w/ BBs, cyclosporine, dexamethasone, diazepam, digoxin, etoposide, ketoconazole, midazolam, quinidine, teniposide, troleandomycin, verapamil, vincristine; ↑ risk OF bleeding w/ anticoagulants, plt inhibitors, thrombolytics; ↑ myelosuppression when cisplatin is admin before paclitaxel; ↓ effects w/ carbamazepine, phenobarbital; ↓ effects of live virus vaccines **Labs:** ↑ ALT, AST, serum bilirubin, alkaline phosphatase **NIPE:** ⊘ PRG, breast-feeding, live virus vaccines; use barrier contraception; maintain hydration

Palivizumab (Synagis) [Antiviral/Monoclonal Antibody]

Uses: *Prevent RSV Infxn* **Action:** MoAb **Dose:** *Peds.* 15 mg/kg IM monthly, typically Nov–Apr **Caution:** [C, ?] Renal/hepatic dysfunction **Contra:** Component allergy **Disp:** Vials 50, 100 mg **SE:** URI, rhinitis, cough, ↑ LFT, local irritation **NIPE:** Use drug w/in 6 h after reconstitution; ⊘ inj in gluteal site; for prophylaxis

Palifermin (Kepivance)

Uses: Oral mucositis w/ BMT * **Action:** Synthetic keratinocyte GF **Dose:** *Phase 1:* 60 mcg/kg IV qd ×3, 3rd dose 24–48 h before chemo *Phase 2:* 60 mcg/kg IV qd ×3, immediately after stem cell infusion **Caution:** [C, ?/–] **Contra:** None **Disp:** Inj 6.25 mg **SE:** Unusual mouth sensations, tongue thickening, rash, **Notes:** *E coli*-derived; separate phases by 4 d; safety unknown w/ nonhematologic malignancies **LABS:** ↑ Amylase, lipase **NIPE:** Evaluate for rash & taste alterations

Palonosetron (Aloxi) [Antiemetic/5 HT3 Antagonist]

WARNING: May ↑ QT$_{C INTERVAL}$ **Uses:** *Prevention acute & delayed N/V w/ emetogenic chemo* **Action:** 5HT3-receptor antagonist **Dose:** 0.25 mg IV 30 min prior to chemo; do not repeat w/in 7 d **Caution:** [B, ?] **Contra:** Component allergy **Disp:** 0.25 mg/5mL vial **SE:** HA, constipation, dizziness, abdominal pain, anxiety **Interactions:** Potential for drug interactions low

Pamidronate (Aredia) [Antihypercalcemic/Bisphosphonate]

Uses: *↑ Ca²⁺ of malignancy, Paget's Dz, palliate symptomatic bone metastases* **Action:** ↓ Nl & abnormal bone resorption **Dose:** ↑ Ca²⁺: 60 mg IV over 4 h or 90 mg IV over 24 h. *Paget's Dz:* 30 mg/d IV slow inf for 3 d **Caution:** [C, ?/–] Avoid invasive dental procedures in pt **Contra:** PRG **Disp:** Powder for inj 30, 60, 90 mg **SE:** Fever, inj site Rxn, uveitis, fluid overload, HTN, abdominal pain, N/V, constipation, UTI, bone pain,↓ K⁺, ↓Ca²⁺,↓Mg²⁺, hypophosphatemia; jaw osteonecrosis, dental exam pre-therapy **Interactions:** ↓ Serum Ca levels w/ foscarnet; ↓ effects w/ Ca, vitamin D **NIPE:** ⊘ Ingest food w/ Ca or vitamins w/ minerals before or 2–3 h after admin of drug

Pancrelipase (Pancrease, Cotazym, Creon, Ultrase) [Pancreatic Enzyme] **Uses:** *Exocrine pancreatic secretion deficiency (eg, CF, chronic pancreatitis, pancreatic insuff), steatorrhea of malabsorption* **Action:** Pancreatic enzyme supl **Dose:** 1–3 caps (tabs) w/ meals & snacks; ↑ to 8 caps (tabs); do not crush or chew EC products; dose-dependent on digestive requirements of pt; avoid antacids **Caution:** [C, ?/–] **Contra:** Pork product allergy **Disp:** Caps, tabs **SE:** N/V, abdominal cramps **Notes:** Individualize therapy **Interactions:** ↓ Effects w/ antacids w/ Ca or Mg; ↓ effects OF Fe **Labs:** ↑ Serum and urine uric acid **NIPE:** Take w/ food; stress adherence to diet (usually low-fat, high-protein, high-calorie)

Pancuronium (Pavulon) [Skeletal Muscle Relaxant/Nondepolarizing Neuromuscular Blocking Agent] **Uses:** *Paralysis w/ mechanical ventilation* **Action:** Nondepolarizing neuromuscular blocker **Dose:** **Adults.** 2–4 mg IV q2–4h PRN. **Peds.** 0.02–0.1 mg/kg/dose q2–4h PRN; ↓ in renal/hepatic impair; intubate pt & keep on controlled ventilation; use adequate sedation or analgesia **Caution:** [C, ?/–] **Contra:** Component or bromide sensitivity **Disp:** Inj 1, 2 mg/mL **SE:** Tachycardia, HTN, pruritus, other histamine reactions **Interactions:** ↑ Effects w/ aminoglycosides, bacitracin, clindamycin, enflurane, K-depleting diuretics, isoflurane, lidocaine, Li, metocurine, quinine, sodium colistimethate, succinylcholine, tetracycline, trimethaphan, tubocurarine, verapamil; ↓ effects w/ carbamazepine, phenytoin, theophylline

Pantoprazole (Protonix) [Gastric Acid Suppressant/Proton Pump Inhibitor] **Uses:** *GERD, erosive gastritis,* ZE syndrome, PUD **Action:** Proton-pump inhibitor **Dose:** 40 mg/d PO; do not crush/chew tabs; 40 mg IV/d (not >3 mg/min, use Protonix filter) **Caution:** [B, ?/–] **Disp:** Tabs, delayed release 20, 40 mg; powder for inj 40 mg; **SE:** Chest pain, anxiety, GI upset, ↑ LFTs **Interactions:** ↑ effects OF warfarin; ↑ effects OF photosensitivity w/ St. John's wort; ↓ effects OF ketoconazole; **Labs:** ↑ serum glucose, lipids, LFTs; monitor PT, INR **NIPE:** ⊘ sun exposure—use sunscreen; take w/o regard to food; antacids will not effect drug absorption

Paregoric [Camphorated Tincture of Opium] [C-III] [Narcotic Antidiarrheal] **Uses:** *Diarrhea,* pain, & neonatal opiate withdrawal syndrome **Action:** Narcotic **Dose:** **Adults.** 5–10 mL PO qd–qid PRN. **Peds.** 0.25–0.5 mL/kg qd–qid. *Neonatal withdrawal:* 3–6 gtt PO q3–6 h PRN to relieve Sxs for 3–5 d, then taper over 2–4 wk **Caution:** [B (D w/ prolonged use/high dose near term, +] **Contra:** Tincture in children; convulsive disorder **Disp:** Liq 2 mg morphine = 20 mg/opium/5 mL **SE:** ↓ BP, sedation, constipation **Notes:** Contains anhydrous morphine from opium; short-term use only **Interactions:** ↑ Effects OF ampicillin esters, azole antifungals, Fe salts **Labs:** ↑ LFTs, SCr **NIPE:** Take w/o regard to food

Paroxetine (Paxil, Paxil CR) [Antidepressant/SSRI] **WARNING:** Closely monitor for worsening depression or emergence of suicidality, particularly in ped pts **Uses:** *Depression, OCD, panic disorder, social anxiety disorder,* PMDD **Action:** SSRI **Dose:** 10–60 mg PO single daily dose in AM; CR 25 mg/d PO; ↑ 12.5 mg/wk (max range 26–62.5 mg/d) **Caution:** [B, ?/] **Contra:** MAOI **Disp:** Tabs 10, 20, 30, 40 mg; susp 10 mg/5 mL; CR 12.5, 25, 37.5 mg **SE:** Sexual dysfunction, HA, somnolence, dizziness, GI upset, D, xerostomia, tachycardia **Interactions:** ↑ Effects w/ cimetidine; ↑ effects OF BBs, dexfenfluramine, dextromethorphan, fenfluramine, haloperidol, MAOIs, theophylline, thioridazine, TCAs, warfarin, St. John's wort, EtOH; ↓ effects w/ cyproheptadine, phenobarbital, phenytoin; ↓ effects OF digoxin, phenytoin **Labs:** ↑ LFTs **NIPE:** Take w/o regard to food, may take up to 4 wk for full effect

Pegfilgrastim (Neulasta) [Colony Stimulating Factor] **Uses:** *↓ Frequency of Infxn in pts w/ nonmyeloid malignancies receiving myelosuppressive anti-CA drugs that cause febrile neutropenia* **Action:** Granulocyte and macrophage stimulating factor **Dose:** *Adults.* 6 mg SQ × 1/chemo cycle. *Peds.* 100 mcg/kg SQ × 1/chemo cycle **Caution:** [C, M] in sickle cell **Contra:** Allergy *E. coli* derived proteinsor to filgrastim **Disp:** *Syringes:* 6 mg/0.6 mL **SE:** Splenic rupture, HA, fever, weakness, fatigue, dizziness, insomnia, edema, N/V/D, stomatitis, anorexia, constipation, taste perversion, dyspepsia, abdominal pain, granulocytopenia, neutropenic fever, arthralgia, myalgia, bone pain, ARDS, alopecia, aggravation of sickle cell Dz **Notes:** Never give between 14 d before & 24 h after dose of cytotoxic chemo **Interactions:** ↑ Effects w/ Li **Labs:** ↑ LFTs, uric acid, alkaline phosphatase, LDH **NIPE:** ⊘ Exposure to infection

Peg Interferon Alfa-2a (Pegasys) [Antiviral/Immunomodulator] **Uses:** *Chronic hepatitis C w/ compensated liver Dz* **Action:** Biologic response modifier **Dose:** 180 mcg (1 mL) SQ qwk × 48 wk; ↓ in renal impair **Caution:** [C, /?–] **Contra:** Autoimmune hepatitis, decompensated liver Dz **Disp:** 180 mcg/mL inj **SE:** Depression, insomnia, suicidal behavior, GI upset, neutropenia & thrombocytopenia, alopecia, pruritus **Notes:** May aggravate neuropsychiatric, autoimmune, ischemic, & infectious disorders; Copegus is ribavirin product **NIPE:** ⊘ Exposure to infection, use barrier contraception

Peg Interferon Alfa-2b (PEG-Intron) [Antiviral/Immunomodulator] **WARNING:** Can cause or aggravate fatal or life-threatening neuropsychiatric, autoimmune, ischemic, and infectious disorders. Monitor patients closely **Uses:** *Rx hepatitis C* **Action:** Immune modulation **Dose:** 1 mcg/kg/wk SQ; 1.5 mcg/kg/wk combined w/ribavirin **Caution:** [C, ?/–] w/psychiatric Hx **Contra:** Autoimmune hepatitis, decompensated liver Dz, hemoglobinopathy **Disp:** Vials 50, 80, 120, 150 mcg/0.5 mL; Redipen 50, 80, 120, 150 mcg/5 mL; reconstitute w/0.7 mL provided sterile water diluent **SE:** Depression, insomnia, suicidal behavior, GI upset, neutropenia, thrombocytopenia, alopecia, pruritus **Notes:** Give hs or w/APAP to ↓ flu-like Sxs **Interactions:** ↑ Myelosuppression w/ antineoplastics; ↑ effects OF doxorubicin, theophylline; ↑ neurotoxicity w/ vinblastine **Labs:** ↑ ALT, ↓ neutrophils, plts; monitor CBC/platelets **NIPE:** Maintain hydration; use barrier contraception

Pemetrexed (Alimta) [Antineoplastic] Uses: *W/ cisplatin in nonresectable mesothelioma* NSCLC **Action:** Antifolate antineoplastic **Dose:** 500 mg/m² IV over 10 min every 3 wk; hold if CrCl <45 mL/min; give w/ vitamin B₁₂ (1000 mcg IM every 9 wk) & folic acid (350–1000 mcg PO qd); start 1 wk before; dexamethasone 4 mg PO bid × 3 start 1 d before each Rx **Caution:** [D, –] Renal/hepatic/BM impair **Contra:** Component sensitivity **Disp:** 500-mg vial **SE:** Neutropenia, thrombocytopenia, N/V/D, anorexia, stomatitis, renal failure, neuropathy, fever, fatigue, mood changes, dyspnea, anaphylactic reactions **Interactions:** ↑ effects w/ NSAIDs, probenecid due to decreased pemetrexed clearance **Labs:** ↑ Creatinine, LFTs; ↓ hmg, hct; monitor CBC/ platelets **NIPE:** ⊘ pregnancy & lactation; ⊘ use NSAIDs 5 days before, during, or 5 days after treatment

Pemirolast (Alamast) [Mast Cell Stabilizer] Uses: *Allergic conjunctivitis* **Action:** Mast cell stabilizer **Dose:** 1–2 gtt in each eye qid **Caution:** [C, ?/–] **Disp:** 0.1% (1 mg/mL) in 10-mL bottles **SE:** HA, rhinitis, cold/flu symptoms, local irritation **NIPE:** Wait 10 min before inserting contacts

Penbutolol (Levatol) [Antihypertensive/BB] Uses: *HTN* **Action:** β-adrenergic receptor blocker, β₁, β₂ **Dose:** 20–40 mg/d; ↓ in hepatic insuff **Caution:** [C (1st tri); D if 2nd/3rd tri), M] **Contra:** Asthma, cardiogenic shock, cardiac failure, heart block, bradycardia **Disp:** Tabs 20 mg **SE:** Flushing, ↓ BP, fatigue, hyperglycemia, GI upset, sexual dysfunction, bronchospasm **Interactions:** ↑ Effects w/ CCBs, fluoroquinolones; ↑ bradycardia w/ adenosine, amiodarone, digitalis, dipyridamole, epinephrine, neuroleptics, phenylephrine, physostigmine, tacrine; ↑ effects OF lidocaine, verapamil; ↓ effects w/ antacids, NSAIDs; ↓ effects OF insulin, hypoglycemics, theophylline **Labs:** ↑ Serum glucose, BUN, K⁺, lipoprotein, triglycerides, uric acid **NIPE:** ↑ Cold sensitivity

Penciclovir (Denavir) [Antiviral] Uses: *Herpes simplex (herpes labialis/cold sores)* **Action:** Competitive inhibitor of DNA polymerase **Dose:** Apply at 1st sign of lesions, then q2h for 4 d **Caution:** [B, ?/–] **Contra:** Allergy **Disp:** Cream 1% [OTC] **SE:** Erythema, HA **NIPE:** ⊘ Recommended in lactation or in children; ⊘ apply to mucous membranes or near eyes

Penicillin G, Aqueous (Potassium or Sodium) (Pfizerpen, Pentids) [Antibiotic/Penicillin] Uses: *Bacteremia, endocarditis, pericarditis, resp tract Infxns, meningitis, neurosyphilis, skin/skin structure Infxns* **Action:** Bactericide; ↓ cell wall synthesis. *Spectrum:* Most gram(+) (not staphylococci, streptococci, *N. meningitidis*, syphilis, clostridia, & anaerobes (not *Bacteroides*) **Dose:** *Adults.* 400,000–800,000 Units PO qid; IV doses vary depending on indications; range 0.6–24 MU/d in ÷ doses q4h. *Peds.* Newborns <1 wk: 25,000–50,000 Units/kg/dose IV q12h. *Infants 1 wk–<1 mo:* 25,000–50,000 Units/kg/dose IV q8h. *Children:* 100,000–300,000 Units/kg/24h IV ÷ q4h; ↓ in renal impair **Caution:** [B, M] **Contra:** Allergy **Disp:** Tabs 200,000, 250,000, 400,000, 800,000 Units; susp 200,000, 400,000 Units/5 mL; powder for inj **SE:** Allergic Rxns; interstitial nephritis, D, Szs **Notes:** Contains 1.7 mEq of K⁺/MU **Interactions:** ↑ Effects w/ probenecid; ↑ effects of MTX; ↑ risk OF bleeding w/ anticoagulants; ↓ effects w/ chloramphenicol, macrolides, tetracyclines; ↓ effects OF oral contraceptives **Labs:** ↑ LFTs, ↓ serum albumin, folate **NIPE:** Monitor for superinfection; use barrier contraception

Penicillin G Benzathine (Bicillin) [Antibiotic/Penicillin]
Uses: *Single-dose regimen for streptococcal pharyngitis, rheumatic fever, glomerulonephritis prophylaxis, & syphilis* **Action:** Bactericide; ↓ cell wall synthesis. *Spectrum:* See Penicillin G **Dose:** *Adults.* 1.2–2.4 million units deep IM inj q2–4wk. *Peds.* 50,000 Units/kg/dose, 2.4 million units/dose max; deep IM inj q2–4 wk **Caution:** [B, M] **Contra:** Allergy **Disp:** Inj 300,000, 600,000 Units/mL; Bicillin L-A benzathine salt only; Bicillin C-R combo of benzathine & procaine (300,000 Units procaine w/ 300,000 Units benzathine) or 900,000 Units benzathine w/ 300,000 Units procaine/2 mL) **SE:** Inj site pain, acute interstitial nephritis, anaphylaxis **Notes:** Sustained action, detectable levels up to 4 wk; drug of choice for noncongenital syphilis **Interactions:** See Penicillin G

Penicillin G Procaine (Wycillin, others) [Antibiotic/Penicillin]
Uses: *Infxns of respir tract, skin/soft tissue, scarlet fever, syphilis* **Action:** Bactericidal; ↓ cell wall synthesis. *Spectrum:* PCN G-sensitive organisms that respond to low, persistent serum levels **Dose:** *Adults.* 0.6–4.8 MU/d in ÷ doses q12–24h; give probenecid at least 30 min prior to PCN to prolong action. *Peds.* 25,000–50,000 Units/kg/d IM ÷ qd–bid **Caution:** [B, M] **Contra:** Allergy **Disp:** Inj 300,000, 500,000, 600,000 Units/mL **SE:** Pain at inj site, interstitial nephritis, anaphylaxis **Interactions:** See Penicillin G, Aqueous **NIPE:** Long-acting parenteral PCN; levels up to 15 h

Penicillin V (Pen-Vee K, Veetids, others) [Antibiotic/Penicillin]
Uses: *Susceptible streptococci Infxns, otitis media, URIs, skin/soft tissue Infxns (PCN-sensitive staph)* **Action:** Bactericidal; ↓ cell wall synthesis. *Spectrum:* Most gram(+), including strep **Dose:** *Adults.* 250–500 mg PO q6h, q8h, q12h. *Peds.* 25–50 mg/kg/25h PO in 4 doses; ↓ in renal Dz; on empty stomach **Caution:** [B, M] **Contra:** Allergy **Disp:** Tabs 125, 250, 500 mg; susp 125, 250 mg/5 mL **SE:** GI upset, interstitial nephritis, anaphylaxis, convulsions **Interactions:** See Penicillin G, Aqueous **NIPE:** Well-tolerated PO PCN; 250 mg = 400,000 units of PCN G

Pentamidine (Pentam 300, NebuPent) [Antiprotozoal]
Uses: *Rx & prevention of PCP* **Action:** ↓ DNA, RNA, phospholipid, & protein synthesis **Dose:** *Rx: Adults & Peds.* 4 mg/kg/24 h IV qd for 14–21 d. *Prevention:* *Adults & Peds >5 y.* 300 mg once q4wk, give via Respigard II neb; ↓ w/IV in renal impair **Caution:** [C, ?] **Contra:** Component allergy **Disp:** Inj 300 mg/vial; aerosol 300 mg **SE:** Associated w/ pancreatic cell necrosis w/ hyperglycemia; pan-

reatitis, CP, fatigue, dizziness, rash, GI upset, renal impair, blood dyscrasias leukopenia & thrombocytopenia) **Notes:** Follow CBC, glucose, pancreatic Fxn monthly for the 1st 3 mo; monitor for ↓ BP following IV administration **Interactions:** ↑ Nephrotoxic effects w/ aminoglycosides, amphotericin B, capreomycin, idofovir, cisplatin, cyclosporine, colistin, ganciclovir, methoxyflurane, polymyxin B, vancomycin; ↑ bone marrow suppression w/ antineoplastics, radiation therapy **Labs:** ↑ LFTs, serum K+ **NIPE:** Reconstitute w/ sterile H_2O only, inhalation may ause metallic taste; ↑ fluids to 2–3 L/d

Pentazocine (Talwin, Talwin Compound, Talwin NX) [C-IV] Narcotic Analgesic] Uses: *Moderate–severe pain* **Action:** Partial narotic agonist–antagonist **Dose:** *Adults.* 30 mg IM or IV; 50–100 mg PO q3–4h PRN. *Peds.* 5–8 y: 15 mg IM q4h PRN. *8–14 y:* 30 mg IM q4h PRN; ↓ in renal/heatic impair **Caution:** [C (1st tri, D w/ prolonged use/high dose near term), +/–] **Contra:** Allergy **Disp:** Talwin Compound tab 12.5 mg + 325 mg ASA; Talwin NX 0 mg + 0.5 mg naloxone; inj 30 mg/mL **SE:** Considerable dysphoria; drowsiness, GI upset, xerostomia, Szs **Notes:** 30–60 mg IM = 10 mg of morphine IM **Interactions:** ↑ CNS depression w/ antihistamines, barbiturates, hypnotics, phenothiazines, EtOH; ↑ effects w/ cimetidine; ↑ effects OF digitoxin, phenytoin, rifampin; ↓ effects of opioids **Labs:** ↑ Serum amylase, lipase **NIPE:** May cause withdrawal in ts using opioids; Talwin NX has naloxone to curb abuse by nonoral route

Pentobarbital (Nembutal, others) [C-II] [Anticonvulsant, Sedative/Hypnotic/Barbiturate] Uses: *Insomnia, convulsions,* induced coma following severe head injury **Action:** Barbiturate **Dose:** *Adults. Sedative:* 20–40 mg PO or PR q6–12h. *Hypnotic:* 100–200 mg PO or PR hs PRN. *Induced coma:* Load 5–10 mg/kg IV, then maint 1–3 mg/kg/h IV inf (keep serum evel 20–50 mg/mL). *Peds.* Hypnotic: 2–6 mg/kg/dose PO hs PRN. *Induced coma:* As adult **Caution:** [D, +/–] Severe hepatic impair **Contra:** Allergy **Disp:** Caps 50, 00 mg; elixir 18.2 mg/5 mL (= 20 mg pentobarbital); supp 30, 60, 120, 200 mg; nj 50 mg/mL **SE:** Resp depression, ↓ BP w/ aggressive IV use for cerebral edema; bradycardia, ↓ BP, sedation, lethargy, hangover, rash, Stevens–Johnson yndrome, blood dyscrasias, resp depression **Interactions:** ↑ Effects w/ chloramphenicol, MAOIs, narcotic analgesics, kava kava, valerian, EtOH; ↓ effects OF Bs, CCBs, corticosteroids, cyclosporine, digitoxin, disopyramide, doxycycline, estrogen, griseofulvin, neuroleptics, oral anticoagulants, oral contraceptives, propafenone, quinidine, tacrolimus, theophylline, TCAs **Labs:** ↑ Ammonia; ↓ bilirubin **NIPE:** Tolerance to sedative–hypnotic effect w/in 1–2 wk

Pentosan Polysulfate Sodium (Elmiron) [Urinary Analgesic] Uses: * Relief of pain/discomfort associated w/ interstitial cystitis* **Action:** Bladder wall buffer **Dose:** 100 mg PO tid on empty stomach w/ H_2O 1 h ac or 2 h pc **Caution:** [B, ?/–] **Contra:** Allergy **Disp:** Caps 100 mg **SE:** Alopecia, N/D, HA, hrombocytopenia **Notes:** Reassess after 3 mo **Interactions:** Risk OF ↑ anticoagulation w/ anticoagulants, ASA, thrombolytics; **Labs:** ↑ LFTs

Pentoxifylline (Trental) [Hemorheologic/Xanthine Derivative] Uses: *Symptomatic management of peripheral vascular Dz* Action: ↓ Blood cell viscosity by restoring erythrocyte flexibility Dose: *Adults.* 400 mg PO tid pc; Rx for at least 8 wk for full effect; ↓ to bid w/ GI/CNS SEs Caution: [C, +/–] Contra: Cerebral/retinal hemorrhage Disp: Tabs CR 400 mg; Tabs ER 400 mg SE: Dizziness, HA, GI upset Interactions: ↑ Effects w/ cimetidine, fluoroquinolones, H₂ antagonists, warfarin; ↑ effects OF antihypertensives, theophylline Labs: ↓ Serum Ca²⁺, Mg²⁺ NIPE: Take w/ food

Pergolide (Permax) [Antiparkinson Agent/Dopaminergic Agonist] Uses: *Parkinson Dz* Action: Centrally active dopamine receptor agonist Dose: Initial, 0.05 mg PO tid, titrated q2–3d to effect; maint 2–3 mg/d in ÷ doses Caution: [B, ?/–] Contra: Ergot sensitivity Disp: Tabs 0.05, 0.25, 1.0 mg SE: Dizziness, somnolence, confusion, nausea, constipation, dyskinesia, rhinitis, MI Notes: May cause ↓ BP during initiation of therapy Interactions: ↑ Risk OF dyskinesia w/ levodopa; ↑ hypotension w/ antihypertensives; ↓ effects w/ antipsychotics, butyrophenones, haloperidol, metoclopramide, phenothiazines, thioxanthenes Labs: ↓ Prolactin NIPE: Take w/ food

Perindopril Erbumine (Aceon) [Antihypertensive/ACEI] Uses: *HTN,* CHF, DN, post-MI Action: ACE inhibitor Dose: 4–8 mg/d; avoid w/ food; ↓ in elderly/renal impair Caution: [C (1st tri, D 2nd & 3rd tri), ?/–] ACE inhibitor-induced angioedema Contra: Bilateral renal artery stenosis, primary hyperaldosteronism Disp: Tabs 2, 4, 8 mg SE: HA, ↓ BP, dizziness, GI upset, cough Notes: OK w/ diuretics Interactions: ↑ Effects w/ antihypertensives, diuretics; ↑ effects OF cyclosporine, insulin, Li, sulfonylureas, tacrolimus; ↓ effects w/ NSAIDs Labs: ↑ Serum K⁺, LFTs, uric acid, cholesterol, creatinine NIPE: ↓ Effects if taken w/ food; risk of persistent cough

Permethrin (Nix, Elimite) [Scabicides/Pediculicides] [OTC] Uses: *Eradication of lice/scabies* Action: Pediculicide Dose: *Adults & Peds.* Saturate hair & scalp; allow 10 min before rinsing Caution: [B, ?/–] Contra: Allergy Disp: Topical lotion 1%; cream 5% SE: Local irritation Notes: Disinfect clothing, bedding, combs & brushes Notes: Disinfect clothing, bedding, combs/brushes NIPE: Drug remains on hair up to 2 wk, reapply in 1 wk if live lice

Perphenazine (Trilafon) [Antipsychotic, Antiemetic/ Phenothiazine] Uses: *Psychotic disorders, severe nausea,* intractable hiccups* Action: Phenothiazine; blocks brain dopaminergic receptors Dose: *Antipsychotic.* 4–16 mg PO tid; max 64 mg/d. *Hiccups:* 5 mg IM q6h PRN or 1 mg IV at intervals not <1–2 mg/min, 5 mg max. *Peds.* 1–6 y: 4–6 mg/d PO in ÷ doses. *6–12 y:* 6 mg PO in ÷ doses. >*12 y:* 4–16 mg PO bid–qid; ↓ in hepatic insuff Caution: [C, ?/–] NA glaucoma, severe hyper-/↓ BP Contra: Phenothiazine sensitivity, BM depression, severe liver or cardiac Dz Disp: Tabs 2, 4, 8, 16 mg; PO conc 16 mg/5 mL; inj 5 mg/mL SE: ↓ BP, tachycardia, bradycardia, EPS, drowsiness, Szs, photosensitivity, skin discoloration, blood dyscrasias, constipation Interactions: ↑ Effects w/ antidepressants; ↑ effects OF anticholinergics, antidepressants, propranolol, phenytoin; ↑ CNS effects w/ CNS depressants, EtOH; ↓ effects w/ antacids, Li, phenobarbital, caffeine, tobacco; ↓ effects OF levodopa, Li **Labs:** ↑ Serum cholesterol, glucose; ↓ uric acid, false + urine PRG test **NIPE:** Take oral dose w/ food; risk of photosensitivity—use sunscreen

Phenazopyridine (Pyridium, others) [Urinary Analgesic]

Uses: *Lower urinary tract irritation* **Action:** Local anesthetic on urinary tract mucosa **Dose:** *Adults.* 100–200 mg PO tid. *Peds 6–12 y.* 12 mg/kg/24 h PO in 3 ÷ doses; ↓ in renal insuff **Caution:** [B, ?] Hepatic Dz **Contra:** Renal failure **Disp:** Tabs 95, 97.2, 100, 200 mg; **SE:** GI disturbances; HA, dizziness, acute renal failure, methemoglobinemia **Labs:** Interferes w/ urinary tests for glucose, ketones, bilirubin, protein, steroids **NIPE:** Urine may turn red-orange in color and can stain clothing; take pc

Phenelzine (Nardil) [Antidepressant/MAOI]

WARNING: Antidepressants increase the risk of suicidal thinking and behavior in children and adolescents w/ major depressive disorder and other psychiatric disorders **Uses:** *Depression* **Action:** MAOI **Dose:** 15 mg PO tid. *Elderly:* 15–60 mg/d ÷ doses **Caution:** [C, −] Interacts w/ SSRI, ergots, triptans **Contra:** CHF, Hx liver Dz **Disp:** Tabs 15 mg **SE:** Postural ↓ BP; edema, dizziness, sedation, rash, sexual dysfunction, xerostomia, constipation, urinary retention **Interactions:** ↑ HTN Rxn w/ amphetamines, fluoxetine, levodopa, metaraminol, phenylephrine, phenylpropanolamine, pseudoephedrine, reserpine, sertraline, tyramine, EtOH, foods w/ tyramine, caffeine, tryptophan; ↑ effects OF barbiturates, narcotics, sedatives, sumatriptan, TCAs, ephedra, ginseng **Labs:** ↓ Glucose, false + ↑ in bilirubin & uric acid **NIPE:** May take 2–4 wk for effect; avoid tyramine-containing foods (eg, cheeses)

Phenobarbital [C-IV] [Anticonvulsant, Sedative/Hypnotic/Barbiturate]

Uses: *Sz disorders,* insomnia, anxiety **Action:** Barbiturate **Dose:** *Adults.* Sedative–hypnotic: 30–120 mg/d PO or IM PRN. *Anticonvulsant:* Load 10–12 mg/kg in 3 ÷ doses, then 1–3 mg/kg/24 h PO, IM, or IV. *Peds.* Sedative–hypnotic: 2–3 mg/kg/24 h PO or IM hs PRN. *Anticonvulsant:* Load 15–20 mg/kg ÷ in 2 equal doses 4 h apart, then 3–5 mg/kg/24h PO ÷ in 2–3 doses. **Caution:** [D, M] **Contra:** Porphyria, liver dysfunction **Disp:** Tabs 8, 15, 16, 30, 32, 60, 65, 100 mg; elixir 15, 20 mg/5 mL; inj 30, 60, 65, 130 mg/mL **SE:** Bradycardia, ↓ BP, hangover, Stevens–Johnson syndrome, blood dyscrasias, resp depression **Notes:** Tolerance develops to sedation; paradoxic hyperactivity seen in ped pts; long half-life allows single daily dosing (Table 2) **Interactions:** ↑ CNS depression w/ CNS depressants, anesthetics, antianxiety meds, antihistamines, narcotic analgesics, EtOH, Indian snakeroot, kava kava; ↑ effects w/ chloramphenicol, MAOIs, procarbazine, valproic acid; ↓ effects w/ rifampin; ↓ effects OF anticoagulants, BBs, carbamazepine, clozapine, corticosteroids, doxorubicin, doxycycline, estrogens, felodipine, griseofulvin, haloperidol, methadone, metronidazole, oral contraceptives, phenothiazines, quinidine, TCAs, theophylline, verapamil **Labs:** ↑ LFTs, creatinine, ↑ or ↓ bilirubin **NIPE:** May take 2–3 wk for full effects, ⊘ D/C abruptly

Phenylephrine, nasal (Neo-Synephrine Nasal) (OTC) [Vasopressor/Decongestant]

Uses: *Nasal congestion* **Action:** α-adrenergic agonist **Dose:** *Adults.* 2–3 drops or 1–2 sprays/nostril q4h (usual 0.25%) PRN. *Peds. 6 mo–2 yr:* 0.125% 1–2 drops/nostril q3–4h, *2–6 yr:* 0.125% 2–3 drops/nostril q3–4h *6–12 yr:* 1–2 sprays/nostril q4h or 0.125% 2–3 drops/nostril q4h or 0.25% 2–3 drops **Caution:** [C, +/–] HTN, acute pancreatitis, hepatitis, coronary Dz, NA glaucoma, hyperthyroidism **Contra:** Bradycardia, arrhythmias **Disp:** Nasal soln 0.125, 0.25, 0.5, 1%; liquid 7.5 mg/5 mL; drops 2.5 mg/mL; tabs 10 mg; chew tabs 10 mg; tabs OD 10 mg; strips 10 mg **SE:** Arrhythmias, HTN, nasal irritation, dryness, sneezing, rebound congestion w/ prolonged use, HA **NIPE:** Do not use > 3 days

Phenylephrine, ophthalmic (Neo-Synephrine Ophthalmic, AK-Dilate, Zincfrin [OTC]) [Vasopressor/Decongestant]

Uses: *Mydriasis, ocular redness [OTC], periop mydriasis, posterior synechiae, uveitis w/posterior Synechiae* **Action:** α-Adrenergic agonist **Dose:** *Adults. Redness:* 1 gtt 0.12% Q 3–4h PRN; *Exam mydriasis:* 1 gtt 2.5% (15 min–1 h for effect); Preop 1 gtt 2.5–10% 30–60 min preop; *Ocular disorders:* 1 gtt 2.5–10% QD–TID *Peds.* As adult, only use 2.5% for exam, preop, and ocular conditions **Caution:** [C] may cause late-term fetal anoxia/bradycardia, +/–] HTN, w/ elderly w/ CAD, **Contra:** Narrow-angle glaucoma **Disp:** Ophth soln 0.12% (Zincfrin OTC), 2.5, 10%; **SE:** Tearing, HA, irritation, eye pain, photophobia, arrhythmia, tremor

Phenylephrine, oral (Sudafed PE, SudoGest PE, Nasop, Lusonal, AH-chew D, Sudafed PE quick dissolve) (OTC) [Vasopressor/Decongestant]

Uses: *Nasal congestion* **Action:** α-Adrenergic agonist **Dose:** *Adults.* 10 mg PO Q4H PRN, Max 60 mg/d *Peds.* 10 mg PO q4h prn, max 60 mg/day **Caution:** [C, +/–] HTN, acute pancreatitis, hepatitis, coronary Dz, NA glaucoma, hyperthyroidism **Contra:** MAOI w/in 14 d, narrow-angle glaucoma, severe ↑ (BP or CAD, urinary retention **Disp:** Liquid 7.5 mg/5 mL; drops 2.5 mg/mL; tabs 10 mg; chew tabs 10 mg; tabs OD 10 mg; strips 10 mg **SE:** Arrhythmias, HTN, HA, agitation, anxiety, tremor, palpitations **Interactions:** ↑ risk of HTN crisis w/ MAOIs; ↑ risk of pressor effects w/ BB; ↑ risk of arrhythmias w/epinephrine, isoproterenol; ↓ effects OF guanethidine, methyldopa, reserpine

Phenylephrine, systemic (Neo-Synephrine) [Vasopressor]

Uses: *Vascular failure in shock, allergy, or drug-induced ↓ BP;* **Action:** Stimulates α-Adrenergic agonist **Dose:** *Adults.* Mild–moderate ↓ BP: 2–5 mg IM or SQ ↑ BP for 2 h; 0.1–0.5 mg IV elevates BP for 15 min. *Severe ↓ BP/shock:* Cont inf at 100–180 mg/min; after BP stabilized, maint 40–60 mg/min *Peds.* ↓ BP: 5–20 mcg/kg/dose IV q10–15 min or 0.1–0.5 mg/kg/min IV inf, titrate to effect. **Caution:** [C, +/–] HTN, acute pancreatitis, hepatitis, coronary Dz, NA glaucoma, hyperthyroidism **Contra:** Bradycardia, arrhythmias **Disp:** Inj 10 mg/mL **SE:** Arrhythmias, HTN, peripheral vasoconstriction activity potentiated by oxytocin, MAOIs, & TCAs; HA, weakness, necrosis, ↓ renal perfusion **Notes:** Promptly restore blood volume if loss has occurred; use large veins to avoid extravasation; phentolamine 10 mg in 10–15 mL of NS for local inj as antidote for extravasation **Interactions:** ↑ HTN w/ BBs, MAOIs; ↑ pressor response w/ guanethidine, methyldopa, reserpine, TCAs

Phenytoin (Dilantin) [Anticonvulsant/Hydantoin] Uses: *Sz disorders* **Action:** ↓ Sz spread in the motor cortex **Dose:** *Load: Adults & Peds.* 15–20 mg/kg IV, 25 mg/min max or PO in 400-mg doses at 4-h intervals. *Maint: Adults.* Initial, 200 mg PO or IV bid or 300 mg hs; then follow levels. *Peds.* 4–7 mg/kg/24h PO or IV ÷ qd–bid; avoid PO susp (erratic absorption) **Caution:** [D, +] **Contra:** Heart block, sinus bradycardia **Disp:** Dilantin Infatab chew 50 mg; Dilantin/Phenytek capsules 100 mg; capsules, ER 30, 100, 200, 300 mg; suspension 125 mg/5 mL; inj 50 mg/mL **SE:** Nystagmus/ataxia early signs of tox; gum hyperplasia w/ long-term use. *IV:* ↓ BP, bradycardia, arrhythmias, phlebitis; peripheral neuropathy, rash, blood dyscrasias, Stevens–Johnson syndrome **Notes:** Follow levels (Table 2); phenytoin albumin bound & levels reflect bound & free phenytoin; w/ ↓ albumin & azotemia, low levels may be therapeutic (nl free levels); do not change dosage (↑ or ↓ at intervals <7–10 d) **Interactions:** ↑ Effects w/ amiodarone, allopurinol, chloramphenicol, disulfiram, INH, omeprazole, sulfonamides, quinolones, trimethoprim; ↑ effects OF Li; ↓ effects w/ cimetidine, cisplatin, diazoxide, folate, pyridoxine, rifampin; ↓ effects OF azole antifungals, benzodiazepines, carbamazepine, corticosteroids, cyclosporine, digitalis glycosides, doxycycline, furosemide, levodopa, oral contraceptives, quinidine, tacrolimus, theophylline, thyroid meds, valproic acid **Labs:** ↑ Serum cholesterol, glucose, alkaline phosphatase **NIPE:** Take w/ food; may alter urine color; use barrier contraception; ⊘ D/C abruptly

Physostigmine (Antilirium) [Antimuscarinic Antidote/Reversible Cholinesterase Inhibitor] Uses: *Antidote for TCA, atropine, & scopolamine OD; glaucoma* **Action:** Reversible cholinesterase inhibitor **Dose:** *Adults.* 2 mg IV or IM q 20 min. *Peds.* 0.01–0.03 mg/kg/dose IV q15–30 min up to 2 mg total if needed **Caution:** [C, ?] **Contra:** GI/GU obstruction, CV Dz **Disp:** Inj 1 mg/mL; ophth oint 0.25% **SE:** Rapid IV admin associated w/SZs; cholinergic side effects; sweating, salivation, lacrimation, GI upset, asystole, changes in heart rate **Notes:** Excessive readministration can result in cholinergic crisis; crisis reversed w/ atropine **Interactions:** ↑ Resp depression w/ succinylcholine, ↑ effects w/ cholinergics, jaborandi tree, pill-bearing spurge **Labs:** ↑ ALT, AST, serum amylase

Phytonadione [Vitamin K] (AquaMEPHYTON, others) [Blood Modifier/Vitamin K] Uses: *Coagulation disorders due to faulty formation of factors II, VII, IX, X*; hyperalimentation **Action:** Cofactor for production of factors II, VII, IX, & X **Dose:** *Adults & Children.* Anticoagulant-induced prothrombin deficiency: 1–10 mg PO or IV slowly. *Hyperalimentation:* 10 mg IM or IV qwk. *Infants.* 0.5–1 mg/dose IM, SQ, or PO **Caution:** [C, +] **Contra:** Allergy **Disp:** Tabs 5 mg; inj 2, 10 mg/mL **SE:** Anaphylaxis from IV dosage give IV slowly; GI upset (PO), inj site Rxns **Notes:** W/ parenteral Rx, 1st change in PT usually seen in 12–24 h; use makes re-coumadinization more difficult **Interactions:** ↓ Effects w/ antibiotics, cholestyramine, colestipol, salicylates, sucralfate; ↓ effects OF oral anticoagulants **Labs:** Falsely ↑ urine steroids

Pimecrolimus (Elidel) [Topical Immunomodulator] Uses:
Atopic dermatitis refractory, severe perianal itching **Action:** Inhibits T-lymphocytes **Dose:** Apply bid; use at least 1 wk following resolution **Caution:** [C, ?/–] w/ local Infxn, lymphadenopathy; immunocompromise; avoid < 2 yrs of age **Contra:** Allergy **Disp:** Cream 1%; 30-g, 60-g, 100-g tubes **SE:** Phototox, local irritation/burning, flu-like Sxs, may ↑ malignancy **NIPE:** Apply to dry skin only; wash hands after use; theoretical cancer risk; second-line/short-term use only

Pindolol (Visken) [Antihypertensive/BB] Uses:
HTN **Action:** β-Adrenergic receptor blocker, β₁, β₂, ISA **Dose:** 5–10 mg bid, 60 mg/d max; ↓ in hepatic/renal failure **Caution:** [B (1st tri; D if 2nd or 3rd tri), +/–] **Contra:** Uncompensated CHF, cardiogenic shock, bradycardia, heart block, asthma, COPD **Disp:** Tabs 5, 10 mg **SE:** Insomnia, dizziness, fatigue, edema, GI upset, dyspnea; fluid retention may exacerbate CHF **Interactions:** ↑ Effects w/ amiodarone, antihypertensives, diuretics; ↓ effects w/ NSAIDs; ↓ effect OF hypoglycemics **Labs:** ↑ LFTs, uric acid **NIPE:** ⊘ D/C abruptly; ↑ cold sensitivity

Pioglitazone HCL/Glimepiride (Duetact) [Hypoglycemic/ Thiazolidinedione & Sulfonylurea] Uses:
Type 2 DM as adjunct to diet and exercise **Action:** Combined ↑ insulin resistance, ↑ pancreatic insulin secretion, ↓ hepatic glucose output and production; **Dose:** Initially one tab PO OD with the first main meal **Caution:** [C, –] **Contra:** Hepatic impair, DKA; **Disp:** Tabs pioglitazone HCL/glimepiride: 30 mg/2 mg, 30 mg/4 mg **SE:** ↑ Risk of CV mortality, hypoglycemia, weight gain, HA, edema, N, URI **Interactions:** ↑ effects w/ ASA, BB, chloramphenicol, ketoconazole, MAOIs, NSAIDs, probenecid, salicylates, sulfonamides, ↓ effects w/ corticosteroids, diuretics, estrogens, isoniazid, phenothiazines, phenytoin, sympathomimetics, thyroid drugs ↓ effects OF oral contraceptives **Labs:** ↑ LFTs, ↓ Hmg, Hct **NIPE:** Take w/first main meal of the day; use barrier contraception; ⊘ use in type 1 DM

Pioglitazone/Metformin (ActoPlus Met) [Hypoglycemic/ Thiazolidinedione & Biguanide] WARNING:
Can cause lactic acidosis which is fatal in 50% of cases. **Uses:** *Type 2 DM as adjunct to diet and exercise* **Action:** Combined ↑ insulin sensitivity w/ ↓ hepatic glucose release **Dose:** Initial 1 tab PO qd or bid, titrate; max daily pioglitazone 45 mg & metformin 2550 mg **Caution:** [C, –] stop w/ radiologic contrast agents **Contra:** Renal impair, aci-

dosis **Disp:** Tabs pioglitazone mg/metformin mg: 15/500, 15/850 **SE:** Lactic acidosis, hypoglycemia, edema, weight gain, URI, HA, GI upset, liver damage **Interactions:** ↑ Effects w/ amiloride, cimetidine, digoxin, furosemide, ketoconazole, MAOIs, morphine, procainamide, quinidine, quinine, ranitidine, triamterene, trimethoprim, vancomycin; ↓ effects OF oral contraceptives; ↓ effects w/ corticosteroids, CCBs, diuretics, estrogens, INH, oral contraceptives, phenothiazines, phenytoin, sympathomimetics, thyroid drugs, tobacco **Labs:** ↑ LFTs, ↓ Hmg, Hct; monitor serum glucose **NIPE:** Take w/o regard to food; use barrier contraception; ⊘ dehydration, EtOH; follow LFTs, BS, Hmg, Hct

Pioglitazone (Actos) [Hypoglycemic/Thiazolidinedione]
Uses: *Type 2 DM* **Action:** ↑ Insulin sensitivity **Dose:** 15–45 mg/d PO **Caution:** [C, –] **Contra:** Hepatic impair **Disp:** Tabs 15, 30, 45 mg **SE:** Weight gain, URI, HA, hypoglycemia, edema **Interactions:** ↑ Effects w/ ketoconazole; ↓ effects OF oral contraceptives **Labs:** ↑ LFTs, ↓ Hmg, Hct **NIPE:** Take w/o regard to food; use barrier contraception

Piperacillin (Pipracil) [Antibiotic/Penicillin-4th gen]
Uses: *Infxns of skin, bone, resp &, urinary tract, abdomen, sepsis* **Action:** 4th-gen PCN; bactericidal; ↓ cell wall synthesis. *Spectrum:* Primarily gram(+), better Enterococcus, H. influenza, not staph; gram(–) E. coli, Proteus, Shigella, Pseudomonas, not β-lactamase-producing **Dose:** *Adults.* 3 g IV q4–6h. *Peds.* 200–300 mg/kg/d IV ÷ q4–6h; ↓ in renal failure **Caution:** [B, M] PCN sensitivity **Disp:** Powder for inj: 2, 3, 4, 40 g **SE:** ↑ Plt aggregation, interstitial nephritis, renal failure, anaphylaxis, hemolytic anemia **Notes:** Often used w/ aminoglycoside **Interactions:** ↑ Effects w/ probenecid; ↑ effects OF anticoagulants, MTX; ↓ effects w/ macrolides, tetracyclines; ↓ effects OF oral contraceptives **Labs:** ↑ LFTs, BUN, creatinine, ↑ direct Coombs' test, ↓ K⁺ **NIPE:** Inactivation of aminoglycosides if drugs given together—admin at least 1 h apart

Piperacillin–Tazobactam (Zosyn) [Antibiotic/Extended Spectrum Penicillin, beta-lactamase inhibitor]
Uses: *Infxns of skin, bone, resp & urinary tract, abdomen, sepsis* **Action:** PCN plus β-lactamase inhibitor; bactericidal; ↓ cell wall synthesis. *Spectrum:* Good gram(+), excellent gram(–); covers anaerobes & β-lactamase producers **Dose:** *Adults.* 3.375–4.5 g IV q6h; ↓ in renal insuff **Caution:** [B, M] PCN or β-lactam sensitivity **Disp.:** Powder for inj: 2.25, 3.373, 4.5 g; inj 2.35, 3.375, 4.5 g **SE:** D, HA, insomnia, GI upset, serum sickness-like reaction, pseudomembranous colitis **Notes:** Often used in combo w/ aminoglycoside See Piperacillin Interactions **Additional Labs:** ↓ Hmg, Hct, protein, albumin

Pirbuterol (Maxair) [Bronchodilator/Sympathomimetic]
Uses: *Prevention & Rx reversible bronchospasm* **Action:** β₂-Adrenergic agonist **Dose:** 2 inhal q4–6h; max 12 inhal/d **Caution:** [C, ?/–] **Disp:** Aerosol 0.2 mg/actuation; **SE:** Nervousness, restlessness, trembling, HA, taste changes, tachycardia **Interactions:** ↑ Effects w/ epinephrine, sympathomimetics; ↑ vascular effects w/ MAOIs, TCAs; ↓ effects w/ BBs **NIPE:** Rinse mouth after use; shake well before use

Piroxicam (Feldene) [Bronchodilator/Beta Adrenergic Agonist]   WARNING: May ↑ risk of cardiovascular events & GI bleeding Uses: *Arthritis & pain* Action: NSAID; ↓ prostaglandins Dose: 10–20 mg/d Caution: [B (1st tri; D if 3rd tri or near term), +] GI bleeding Contra: ASA or NSAID sensitivity Disp: Caps 10, 20 mg SE: Dizziness, rash, GI upset, edema, acute renal failure, peptic ulcer Interactions: ↑ Effects w/ probenecid; ↑ effects OF aminoglycosides, anticoagulants, hypoglycemics, Li, MTX; ↑ risk OF bleeding w/ ASA, corticosteroids, NSAIDs, feverfew, garlic, ginger, ginkgo biloba, EtOH; ↓ effect w/ ASA, antacids, cholestyramine; ↓ effect OF BBs, diuretics Labs: ↑ BUN, LFTs, serum Cl, serum Na, PT NIPE: Take w/ food, full effect after 2 wk admin, ↑ risk of photosensitivity—use sunscreen

Plasma Protein Fraction (Plasmanate, others) [Plasma Volume Expander]   Uses: *Shock & ↓ BP* Action: Plasma volume expander Dose: Initial, 250–500 mL IV (not >10 mL/min); subsequent inf based on response. Peds. 10–15 mL/kg/dose IV; subsequent inf based on response Caution: [C, +] Contra: Renal insuff, CHF Disp: Inj 5% SE: ↓ BP associated w/ rapid inf; hypocoagulability, metabolic acidosis, PE NIPE: 130–160 mEq Na/L; not substitute for RBC

Pneumococcal 7-Valent Conjugate Vaccine (Prevnar) [Vaccine]   Uses: *Immunization against pneumococcal Infxns in infants & children* Action: Active immunization Dose: 0.5 mL IM/dose; series of 3 doses; 1st dose 2 mo of age w/ subsequent doses q2mo Caution: [C, +] Thrombocytopenia Contra: Diphtheria toxoid sensitivity, febrile illness Disp: Inj SE: Local reactions, arthralgia, fever, myalgia

Pneumococcal Vaccine, Polyvalent (Pneumovax-23) [Vaccine/Inactive Bacteria]   Uses: *Immunization against pneumococcal Infxns in pts at high risk (eg, all ≥65 y of age)* Action: Active immunization Dose: 0.5 mL IM. Caution: [C, ?] Contra: Do not vaccinate during immunosuppressive therapy Disp: Inj 0.5 mL SE: Fever, inj site Rxn, hemolytic anemia, thrombocytopenia, anaphylaxis Interactions: ↓ Effects w/ corticosteroids, immunosuppressants

Podophyllin (Podocon-25, Condylox Gel 0.5%, Condylox) [Antimitotic Effect]   Uses: *Topical therapy of benign growths (genital & perianal warts [condylomata acuminata],* papillomas, fibromas) Action: Direct antimitotic effect; exact mechanism unknown Dose: Condylox gel & Condylox: Apply 3 consecutive d/wk for 4 wk. Podocon-25: Use sparingly on the lesion, leave on for 1–4 h, then thoroughly wash off Caution: [C, ?] Immunosuppression Contra: DM, bleeding lesions Disp: Podocon-25 (w/ benzoin) 15-mL bottles; Condylox gel 0.5% 35 g clear gel; Condylox soln 0.5% 35 g clear SE: Local reactions, significant absorption; anemias, tachycardia, paresthesias, GI upset, renal/hepatic damage NIPE: Podocon-25 applied only by the clinician; do not dispense directly to patient NIPE: ⊘ use on warts on mucous membranes; ⊘ use near eyes

Polyethylene Glycol [PEG]–Electrolyte Solution (GoLYTELY, CoLyte) [Laxative] Uses: *Bowel prep prior to examination or surgery* **Action:** Osmotic cathartic **Dose:** *Adults.* Following 3–4-h fast, drink 240 mL of soln q10min until 4 L consumed. *Peds.* 25–40 mL/kg/h for 4–10 h **Caution:** [C, ?] **Contra:** GI obstruction, bowel perforation, megacolon, ulcerative colitis **Disp:** Powder for reconstitution to 4 L **SE:** Cramping or nausea, bloating **Notes:** 1st BM should occur in approximately 1 h **Interactions:** Drugs taken within 1 hr of polyethylene glycol administration may not be absorbed **NIPE:** Instruct pt to drink solution rapidly q10 min until finished

Polyethylene Glycol [PEG] 3350 (MiraLax) [Laxative] Uses: *Occasional constipation* **Action:** Osmotic laxative **Dose:** 17 g powder (1 heaping Tbsp) in 8 oz (1 cup) of H_2O & drink; max 14 d **Contra:** GI obstruction, allergy to PEG **Disp:** Powder for reconstitution; bottle cap holds 17 g **SE:** Upset stomach, bloating, cramping, gas, severe D, hives **Notes:** Can add to H_2O, juice, soda, coffee, or tea **NIPE:** may take 2–4 days for BM

Polymyxin B & Hydrocortisone (Otobiotic Otic) [Antibiotic/Anti-inflammatory] Uses: *Superficial bacterial Infxns of external ear canal* **Action:** Antibiotic/anti-inflammatory combo **Dose:** 4 gtt in ear(s) tid–qid **Caution:** [B, ?] **Disp:** Soln polymyxin B 10,000 Units/hydrocortisone 5 mg/mL **SE:** Local irritation **Notes:** Useful in neomycin allergy **NIPE:** Clean ear before instillation of gtts; ⊘ use w/perforated eardrum

Posaconazole (Noxafil) [Antifungal] Uses: Prophylaxis against invasive aspergillus & candida infections in severely immunocompromised pts **Action:** Antifungal, which inhibits a component of the fungal cell membrane **Dose:** > 13 y take w/food or liquid supl, for invasive fungal prophylaxis: 200 mg PO OD; for oropharyngeal candidiasis: 100 mg PO BID for day 1 then 100 mg PO OD for 13 days **Caution:** [C,–] with pts who cannot eat a full meal/supl, severe renal impair, D, V; **Contra:** Concomitant ergots, drugs that cause QU prolongation, drugs metabolized by CYP3A4 such as astemizole, cisapride, halofantrine, pimozide, quinidine, terfenadine **Disp:** oral suspension 40 mg/mL; **SE:** Fever, HA, GI distress, anorexia, fatigue, abdominal pain, rash, somnolence **Interactions:** ↑ Effects of CCB, cyclosporine, midazolam, sirolimus, statins, tacrolimus, vinca alkaloids; ↓ effects w/ cimetidine, phenytoin, rifabutin **Labs:** Monitor LFTs, electrolytes, bilirubin **NIPE:** Monitor for breakthrough fungal infections; ⊘ for children < 13 y

Potassium Citrate (Urocit-K) [Urinary Alkalinizer] Uses: *Alkalinize urine, prevention of urinary stones (uric acid, calcium stones if hypocitraturic)* **Action:** Urinary alkalinizer **Dose:** 10–20 mEq PO tid w/ meals, max 100 mEq/d **Caution:** [A, +] **Contra:** Severe renal impair, dehydration, ↑ K^+, peptic ulcer; use of K^+-sparing diuretics or salt substitutes **Disp:** 540-, 1080-mg tabs **SE:** GI upset, ↓ Ca^{2+}, ↑ K^+, metabolic alkalosis **Notes:** Tabs 540 mg = 5 mEq, 1080 mg = 10 mEq **Interactions:** ↑ Risk of hyperkalemia w/ ACEIs, K-sparing diuretics **NIPE:** Take within 30 min of meals or hs snack

Potassium Citrate & Citric Acid (Polycitra-K) [Urinary Alkalinizer] Uses: *Alkalinize urine, prevent urinary stones (uric acid, Ca stones if hypocitraturic)* Action: Urinary alkalinizer Dose: 10–20 mEq PO tid w/ meals, max 100 mEq/d Caution: [A, +] Contra: Severe renal impair, dehydration, ↑ K⁺, peptic ulcer; use of K⁺-sparing diuretics or salt substitutes Disp: Soln 10 mEq/5 mL; powder 30 mEq/packet SE: GI upset, ↓ Ca²⁺, ↑ K⁺, metabolic alkalosis Interactions: ↑ Risk OF hyperkalemia w/ ACEIs, K-sparing diuretics

Potassium Iodide [Lugol Solution] (SSKI, Thyro-Block) [Iodine Supl] Uses: *Thyroid storm,* ↓ vascularity before thyroid surgery, block thyroid uptake of radioactive iodine, thin bronchial secretions Action: Iodine supl Dose: *Adults & Peds >2 y.* Preop thyroidectomy: 50–250 mg PO tid (2–6 gtt strong iodine soln); give 10 d preop. *Peds 1 y.* Thyroid crisis: 300 mg (6 gtt SSKI q8h). *Peds <1 y:* ½ adult dose Caution: [D, +] ↑ K⁺, TB, PE, bronchitis, renal impair Contra: Iodine sensitivity Disp: Tabs 130 mg; soln (SSKI) 1 g/mL; Lugol soln, strong iodine 100 mg/mL; syrup 325 mg/5 mL SE: Fever, HA, urticaria, angioedema, goiter, GI upset, eosinophilia Interactions: ↑ Risk OF hypothyroidism w/ antithyroid drugs and Li; ↑ risk OF hyperkalemia w/ ACEIs, K-sparing diuretics, K supls Labs: May alter TFTs NIPE: Take pc w/ food or milk

Potassium Supplements (Kaon, Kaochlor, K-Lor, Slow-K, Micro-K, Klorvess, others) [K⁺ Supl/Electrolyte] Uses: *Prevention or Rx of ↓ K⁺* (eg, diuretic use) Action: K⁺ supl Dose: *Adults.* 20–100 mEq/d PO ÷ qd–bid; IV 10–20 mEq/h, max 40 mEq/h & 150 mEq/d (monitor K⁺ levels frequently w/ high-dose IV). *Peds.* Calculate K⁺ deficit; 1–3 mEq/kg/d PO ÷ qd–qid; IV max dose 0.5–1 mEq/kg/h Caution: [A, +] Renal insuff, use w/ NSAIDs & ACE inhibitors Contra: ↑ K⁺ Disp: PO forms (Table 8); injectable forms SE: Can cause GI irritation; bradycardia, ↑ K⁺, heart block Notes: Mix powder & liq w/ beverage (unsalted tomato juice, etc); follow K⁺; Cl⁻ salt OK w/ alkalosis; w/ acidosis use acetate, bicarbonate, citrate, or gluconate salt Interactions: ↑ Effects w/ ACEI, K-sparing diuretics, salt substitutes NIPE: Take w/ food

Pramipexole (Mirapex) [Antiparkinson Agent/Dopamine Agonist] Uses: *Parkinson Dz* Action: Dopamine agonist Dose: 1.5–4.5 mg/d PO, initial 0.375 mg/d in 3 ÷ doses; titrate slowly Caution: [C, ?/–] Contra: Component allergy Disp: Tabs 0.125, 0.25, 0.5, 1, 1.5 mg SE: Postural ↓ BP, asthenia, somnolence, abnormal dreams, GI upset, EPS Interactions: ↑ Effects w/ cimetidine, diltiazem, quinidine, quinine, ranitidine, triamterene, verapamil; ↑ effects OF levodopa; ↑ CNS depression w/ CNS depressants, EtOH; ↓ effects w/ antipsychotics, butyrophenones, metoclopramide, phenothiazines, thioxanthenes NIPE: May take w/ food; ⊘ D/C abruptly

Pramoxine (Anusol Ointment, Proctofoam-NS, others) [Topical Anesthetic] Uses: *Relief of pain & itching from hemorrhoids, anorectal surgery*; topical for burns & dermatosis Action: Topical anesthetic Dose: Apply freely to anal area q3h Caution: [C, ?] Disp: [OTC] All 1%; foam (Proctofoam-NS), cream, oint, lotion, gel, pads, spray **SE:** Contact dermatitis, mucosal thinning w/ chronic use **NIPE:** ⊘ Use on large areas

Pramoxine + Hydrocortisone (Enzone, Proctofoam-HC) [Topical Anesthetic/Anti-inflammatory] **Uses:** *Relief of pain & itching from hemorrhoids* **Action:** Topical anesthetic, anti-inflammatory **Dose:** Apply freely to anal area tid–qid **Caution:** [C, ?/–] **Disp:** Cream pramoxine 1% acetate 0.5/1%; foam pramoxine 1% hydrocortisone 1%; lotion pramoxine 1% hydrocortisone 0.25/1/2.5%, pramoxine 2.5% & hydrocortisone 1% **SE:** Contact dermatitis, mucosal thinning with chronic use **NIPE:** ⊘ Use on large areas

Pravastatin (Pravachol) [Antilipemic/HMG-CoA Reductase Inhibitor] **Uses:** ↓ Cholesterol **Action:** HMG-CoA reductase inhibitor **Dose:** 10–80 mg PO hs; ↓ in significant renal/hepatic insuff **Caution:** [X, –] w/gemfibrozil **Contra:** Liver Dz or persistent LFT ↑ **Disp:** Tabs 10, 20, 40, 80 mg **SE:** Use caution w/ concurrent gemfibrozil; HA, GI upset, hepatitis, myopathy, renal failure **Interactions:** ↑ Risk OF myopathy & rhabdomyolysis w/ clarithromycin, clofibrate, cyclosporine, danazol, erythromycin, fluoxetine, gemfibrozil, niacin, nefazodone, troleandomycin; ↑ effects w/ azole antifungals, cimetidine, grapefruit juice; ↓ effects w/ cholestyramine, isradipine **Labs:** ↑ LFTs **NIPE:** ⊘ PRG, breast-feeding; take w/o regard to food; full effect may take up to 4 wks; ↑ risk of photosensitivity—use sunscreen

Prazosin (Minipress) [Antihypertensive/Alpha Blocker] **Uses:** * HTN* **Action:** Peripherally acting α-adrenergic blocker **Dose:** *Adults.* 1 mg PO tid; can ↑ to 20 mg/d max. *Peds.* 5–25 mcg/kg/dose q6h, to 25 mcg/kg/dose max **Caution:** [C, ?] **Contra:** Component allergy **Disp:** Caps 1, 2, 5 mg; tabs ER 2.5, 5 mg extended release **SE:** Dizziness, edema, palpitations, fatigue, GI upset **Notes:** Can cause orthostatic ↓ BP, take the 1st dose hs; tolerance develops to this effect; tachyphylaxis may result **Interactions:** ↑ Hypotension w/ antihypertensives, diuretics, nitrates, EtOH; ↓ effects w/ NSAIDs, butcher's broom **Labs:** ↑ Serum Na levels, vanillylmandelic acid level; alters test for pheochromocytoma **NIPE:** ⊘ D/C abruptly

Prednisolone [Corticosteroid] [See Steroids page 249 and Table 4, page 308], **Interactions:** ↑ Effects w/ clarithromycin, erythromycin, estrogen, ketoconazole, oral contraceptives, troleandomycin; ↓ effects w/ antacids, aminoglutethimide, barbiturates, cholestyramine, colestipol, phenytoin, rifampin; ↓ effects OF anticoagulants, hypoglycemics, INH, salicylates, vaccine toxoids **Labs:** False – skin allergy tests; false ↑ cortisol, digoxin, theophylline **NIPE:** ⊘ Use live virus vaccines, ⊘ D/C abruptly; take w/ food

Prednisone [Corticosteroid] [See Steroids page 249 and Table 4, page 308] **Interactions:** ↑ Effects w/ clarithromycin, cyclosporine, erythromycin, estrogen, ketoconazole, oral contraceptives, troleandomycin; ↓ effects w/ antacids, aminoglutethimide, barbiturates, carbamazepine, cholestyramine, colestipol, phenytoin, rifampin; ↓ effects OF anticoagulants, hypoglycemics, INH, salicylates,

vaccine toxoids **Labs:** False – skin allergy tests, false ↑ cortisol, digoxin, theophylline **NIPE:** Take w/ food; ⊘ use live virus vaccine, ⊘ D/C abruptly, infection may be masked

Pregabalin (Lyrica) [Antinociceptive/Antiseizure]   Uses: *DM peripheral neuropathy pain; postherpetic neuralgia; adjunct Rx adult partial onset seizures* **Action:** Nerve transmission modulator, antinociceptive and antiseizure effect; mechanism ? **Dose:** *Neuropathic pain:* 50 mg tid PO, ↑ to 300 mg/d w/in 1 wk based on response (300 mg/d max) *Postherpetic neuralgia:* 75–150 mg bid, or 50–100 mg tid; start 75 mg bid or 50 mg tid; ↑to 300 mg/d w/in 1 wk based on response; if pt still has pain after 2–4 wk, ↑ to 600 mg/d; *Epilepsy:* Start 150 mg/d (75 mg bid or 50 mg tid) may ↑ to max 600 mg/d; ↓ w/ renal insuffic; w/ or w/o food **Caution:** [X, –] with significant renal impair, see insert for dosing; w/ elderly, severe CHF **Contra:** PRG **Disp:** Caps 25, 50, 75, 100, 150, 200, 225, 300 mg **SE:** Dizziness, drowsiness, xerostomia, peripheral edema, blurred vision, weight gain, difficulty concentrating **Notes:** Related to gabapentin **NIPE:** Avoid abrupt D/C; w/ D/C, taper over at least 1 wk

Probenecid (Benemid, others) [Urocosuric/Analgesic]   Uses: *Prevent gout & hyperuricemia; prolongs levels of PCNs & cephalosporins* **Action:** Urocosuric, renal tubular blocking for organic anions **Dose:** *Adults.* Gout: 250 mg bid × 1 wk, then 0.5 g PO bid; can ↑ by 500 mg/mo up to 2–3 g/d. *Antibiotic effect:* 1–2 g PO 30 min before dose. *Peds >2 y.* 25 mg/kg, then 40 mg/kg/d PO ÷ qid **Caution:** [B, ?] **Contra:** High-dose ASA, moderate–severe renal impair, age <2 y **Disp:** Tabs 500 mg **SE:** HA, GI upset, rash, pruritus, dizziness, blood dyscrasias **Notes:** Do not use during acute gout attack **Interactions:** ↑ Effects OF acyclovir, allopurinol; ↑ effects of benzodiazepines, cephalosporins, ciprofloxacin, clofibrate, dapsone, dyphylline, MTX, NSAIDs, olanzapine, rifampin, sulfonamides, sulfonylureas zidovudine; ↓ effects w/ niacin, EtOH; ↓ effects OF penicillamine **Labs:** False + urine glucose; false ↑ level of theophylline **NIPE:** Take w/ food, ↑ fluids to 2–3 L/d; ⊘ ASA, NSAIDs, salicylates

Procainamide (Pronestyl, Procan) [Antiarrhythmic]   Uses: *Supraventricular/ventricular arrhythmias* **Action:** Class 1A antiarrhythmic **Dose:** *Adults.* Recurrent VF/VT: 20 mg/min IV (max total 17 mg/kg). *Maint:* 1–4 mg/min. *Stable wide-complex tachycardia of unknown origin, AF w/ rapid rate in WPW:* 20 mg/min IV until arrhythmia suppression, ↓ BP, QRS widens >50%, then 1–4 mg/min. *Chronic dosing:* 50 mg/kg/d PO in ÷ doses q4–6h. *Peds.* Chronic maint: 15–50 mg/kg/24 h PO ÷ q3–6h; ↓ in renal/hepatic impair **Caution:** [C, +] **Contra:** Complete heart block, 2nd- or 3rd-degree heart block w/o pacemaker, torsades de pointes, SLE **Disp:** Tabs & caps 250, 375, 500 mg; SR tabs 250, 500, 750, 1000 mg; inj 100, 500 mg/mL **SE:** ↓ BP & a lupus-like syndrome; GI upset, taste perversion, arrhythmias, tachycardia, heart block, angioneurotic edema **Notes:** Follow levels (Table 2) **Interactions:** ↑ Effects w/ acetazolamide, amiodarone, cimetidine, ranitidine, trimethoprim; ↑ effects OF anticholinergics, antihypertensives;

↓ effects w/ procaine, EtOH **Labs:** ↑ LFTs, + Coombs' test **NIPE:** Take w/ food if GI upset, ⊘ crush SR tab

Procarbazine (Matulane) [Antineoplastic/Alkylating Agent]

WARNING: Highly toxic; handle w/ care **Uses:** *Hodgkin Dz,* NHL, brain & lung tumors **Action:** Alkylating agent; ↓ DNA & RNA synthesis **Dose:** Per protocol **Caution:** [D, ?] W/ EtOH ingestion **Contra:** Inadequate BM reserve **Disp:** Caps 50 mg **SE:** Myelosuppression, hemolytic reactions (w/ G6PD deficiency) N/V/D; disulfiram-like Rxn; cutaneous & constitutional Sxs, myalgia, arthralgia, CNS effects, azoospermia, cessation of menses **Interactions:** ↑ CNS depression w/ antihistamines, antihypertensives, barbiturates, CNS depressants, narcotics, phenothiazines; ↑ effects OF hypoglycemics; ↑ risk of HTN w/ guanethidine, levodopa, MAOIs, methyldopa, sympathomimetics, TCAs, tyramine-containing foods; ↓ effects OF digoxin **NIPE:** Disulfiram-like Rxn w/ EtOH; ↑ fluids to 2–3 L/d; ↑ risk of photosensitivity—use sunscreen; ⊘ exposure to infection

Prochlorperazine (Compazine) [Antiemetic, Antipsychotic/Phenothiazine]

Uses: *N/V, agitation, & psychotic disorders* **Action:** Phenothiazine; blocks postsynaptic dopaminergic CNS receptors **Dose:** *Adults.* Antiemetic: 5–10 mg PO tid–qid or 25 mg PR bid or 5–10 mg deep IM q4–6h. *Antipsychotic:* 10–20 mg IM acutely or 5–10 mg PO tid–qid for maint; ↑ doses may be required for antipsychotic effect. *Peds.* 0.1–0.15 mg/kg/dose IM q4–6h or 0.4 mg/kg/24 h PO ÷ tid–qid **Caution:** [C, +/–] NA glaucoma, severe liver/cardiac Dz **Contra:** Phenothiazine sensitivity, BM suppression **Disp:** Tabs 5, 10, 25 mg; SR caps 10, 15 mg; syrup 5 mg/5 mL; supp 2.5, 5, 25 mg; inj 5 mg/mL **SE:** EPS common; Rx w/ diphenhydramine **Interactions:** ↑ Effects w/ chloroquine, indomethacin, narcotics, procarbazine, SSRIs, pyrimethamine; ↑ effects OF antidepressants, BBs, EtOH; ↓ effects w/ antacids, anticholinergics, barbiturates, tobacco; ↓ effects OF guanethidine, levodopa, Li **Labs:** False + urine bilirubin, amylase, phenylketonuria, ↑ serum prolactin **NIPE:** ⊘ D/C abruptly; ↑ risk of photosensitivity—use sunscreen; urine may turn pink/red

Promethazine (Phenergan) [Antihistamine, Antiemetic, Sedative/Phenothiazine]

Uses: *N/V, motion sickness* **Action:** Phenothiazine; blocks CNS postsynaptic mesolimbic dopaminergic receptors **Dose:** *Adults.* 12.5–50 mg PO, PR, or IM bid–qid PRN. *Peds.* 0.1–0.5 mg/dose PO or IM q2–6h PRN **Caution:** [C, +/–] use w/ agents w/ respiratory depressant effects **Contra:** Component allergy, NA glaucoma, age < 2 yrs **Disp:** Tabs 12.5, 25, 50 mg; syrup 6.25 mg/5 mL, 25 mg/5 mL; supp 12.5, 25, 50 mg; inj 25, 50 mg/mL **SE:** Drowsiness, tardive dyskinesia, EPS, lowered Sz threshold, ↓ BP, GI upset, blood dyscrasias, photosensitivity; respiratory depression in children **Interactions:** ↑ Effects w/ CNS depressants, MAOIs, EtOH; ↑ effects OF antihypertensives; ↓ effects w/ anticholinergics, barbiturates, tobacco; ↓ effect OF levodopa **NIPE:** Effects skin allergy tests; use sunscreen for photosensitivity

Propafenone (Rythmol) [Antiarrhythmic]

Uses: *Life-threatening ventricular arrhythmias, AF* **Action:** Class IC antiarrhythmic (Table 12) **Dose:**

Adults. 150–300 mg PO q8h. **Peds.** 8–10 mg/kg/d ÷ in 3–4 doses; may ↑ 2 mg/kg/d, to max of 20 mg/kg/d **Caution:** [C, ?] w/ amprenavir, ritonavir **Contra:** Uncontrolled CHF, bronchospasm, cardiogenic shock, conduction disorders **Disp:** Tabs 150, 225, 300 mg, extended release caps 225, 325, 425 mg **SE:** Dizziness, unusual taste, 1st-degree heart block, arrhythmias, prolongs QRS & QT intervals; fatigue, GI upset, blood dyscrasias **Interactions:** ↑ Effects w/ cimetidine, quinidine; ↑ effects OF anticoagulants, BBs, digitalis glycosides, theophylline; ↓ effects w/ rifampin, phenobarbital, rifabutin **Labs:** ↑ ANA titers **NIPE:** Take w/o regard to food

Propantheline (Pro-Banthine) [Antimuscarinic] Uses: *PUD,* symptomatic Rx of small intestine hypermotility, spastic colon, ureteral spasm, bladder spasm, pylorospasm **Action:** Antimuscarinic **Dose:** ***Adults.*** 15 mg PO ac & 30 mg PO hs; ↓ in elderly. **Peds.** 2–3 mg/kg/24h PO ÷ tid–qid **Caution:** [C, ?] **Contra:** NA glaucoma, ulcerative colitis, toxic megacolon, GI/GU obstruction **Disp:** Tabs 7.5, 15 mg **SE:** Anticholinergic (eg, xerostomia, blurred vision) **Interactions:** ↑ Anticholinergic effects w/ antihistamines, antidepressants, atropine, haloperidol, phenothiazines, quinidine, TCAs; ↑ effects OF atenolol, digoxin; ↓ effects w/ antacids **NIPE:** May cause heat intolerance, ↑ risk of photosensitivity—use sunscreen

Propofol (Diprivan) [Anesthetic] Uses: *Induction & maint of anesthesia; sedation in intubated pts* **Action:** Sedative–hypnotic; mechanism unknown **Dose:** ***Adults.*** Anesthesia: 2–2.5 mg/kg induction, then 0.1–0.2 mg/kg/min inf. *ICU sedation:* 5 mcg/kg/min IV (times) 5 min, ↑ PRN 5–10 mcg/kg/min q5–10 min, 5–50 mcg/kg/min cont inf; ↓ in elderly, debilitated, ASA II/IV pts **Peds.** Anesthesia: 2.5–3.5 mg/kg induction; then 125–300 mcg/kg/min **Caution:** [B, +] **Contra:** If general anesthesia contraindicated **Disp:** Inj 10 mg/mL **SE:** May ↑ triglycerides w/ extended dosing; ↓ BP, pain at site, apnea, anaphylaxis **Notes:** 1 mL of propofol has 0.1 g fat **Interactions:** ↑ Effects w/ antihistamines, opioids, hypnotics, EtOH **Labs:** ↓ Serum cortisol levels

Propoxyphene (Darvon); Propoxyphene & Acetaminophen (Darvocet); & Propoxyphene & Aspirin (Darvon Compound-65, Darvon-N + Aspirin) [C-IV] [Narcotic Analgesic] Uses: *Mild–moderate pain* **Action:** Narcotic analgesic **Dose:** 1–2 PO q4h PRN; ↓ in hepatic impair, elderly **Caution:** [C (D if prolonged use), M] Hepatic impair (APAP), peptic ulcer (ASA); severe renal impair **Contra:** Allergy **Disp:** *Darvon:* Propoxyphene HCl caps 65 mg. *Darvon-N:* Propoxyphene napsylate 100 mg tabs. *Darvocet-N:* Propoxyphene napsylate 50 mg/APAP 325 mg. *Darvocet-N 100:* Propoxyphene napsylate 100 mg/APAP 650 mg. *Darvon Compound-65:* Propoxyphene HCl caps 65-mg/ASA 389 mg/caffeine 32 mg. *Darvon-N w/ ASA:* Propoxyphene napsylate 100 mg/ASA 325 mg **SE:** OD can be lethal; ↓ BP, dizziness, sedation, GI upset, ↑ levels on LFTs **Interactions:** ↑ CNS depression w/ antidepressants, antihistamines, barbiturates, glutethimide, methocarbamol, protease inhibitors, EtOH, St. John's wort; ↑ effects OF BBs, carbamazepine, MAOIs, phenobarbital, TCAs, warfarin; ↓ effects w/ tobacco **Labs:** ↑ LFTs, serum amylase, lipase **NIPE:** Take w/ food if GI upset

Propranolol (Inderal) [Antihypertensive, Antianginal, Antiarrhythmic/BB]
Uses:*HTN, angina, MI, hyperthyroidism, essential tremor, hypertropic subaortic stenosis, pheochromocytoma; prevents migraines & atrial arrhythmias* **Action:** β-Adrenergic receptor blocker, β₁, β₂; only β-blocker to block conversion of T_4 to T_3 **Dose:** *Adults.* Angina: 80–320 mg/d PO ÷ bid–qid or 80–160 mg/d SR. *Arrhythmia:* 10–80 mg PO tid–qid or 1 mg IV slowly, repeat q 5 min, 5 mg max. *HTN:* 40 mg PO bid or 60–80 mg/d SR, ↑ weekly to max 640 mg/d. *Hypertrophic subaortic stenosis:* 20–40 mg PO tid–qid. *MI:* 180–240 mg PO ÷ tid–qid. *Migraine prophylaxis:* 80 mg/d ÷ tid–tid, ↑ weekly 160–240 mg/d ÷ tid–qid max; wean if no response in 6 wk. *Pheochromocytoma:* 30–60 mg/d ÷ tid–qid. *Thyrotoxicosis:* 1–3 mg IV × 1; 10–40 mg PO q6h. *Tremor:* 40 mg PO bid, ↑ PRN 320 mg/d max. *Peds.* Arrhythmia: 0.5–1.0 mg/kg/d ÷ tid–qid, ↑ PRN q3–7d to 60 mg/d max; 0.01–0.1 mg/kg IV over 10 min, 1 mg max. *HTN:* 0.5–1.0 mg/kg ÷ bid–qid, ↑ PRN q3–7d to 2 mg/kg/d max; ↓ in renal impair **Caution:** [C (1st tri), D if 2nd or 3rd tri), +] **Contra:** Uncompensated CHF, cardiogenic shock, bradycardia, heart block, PE, severe resp Dz **Disp:** Tabs 10, 20, 40, 60, 80 mg; SR caps 60, 80, 120, 160 mg; oral soln 4, 8, 80 mg/mL; inj 1 mg/mL **SE:** Bradycardia, ↓ BP, fatigue, GI upset, ED **Interactions:** ↑ Effects w/ antihypertensives, cimetidine, fluvoxamine, flecainide, hydralazine, methimazole, neuroleptics, nitrates, propylthiouracil, quinidine, quinolones, theophylline, EtOH; ↑ effects OF digitalis, glycosides, hypoglycemics, hydralazine, lidocaine, neuroleptics, rizatriptan; ↓ effects w/ NSAIDs, phenobarbital, phenytoin, rifampin, tobacco **Labs:** ↑ LFTs, BUN, K⁺, serum lipoprotein, triglycerides, uric acid; ↑ or ↓ serum glucose **NIPE:** ⊘ D/C abruptly; ↑ cold sensitivity

Propylthiouracil [PTU] [Antithyroid Agent/Thyroid Hormone Antagonist]
Uses: *Hyperthyroidism* **Action:** ↓ Production of T_3 & T_4 & conversion of T_4 to T_3 **Dose:** *Adults.* Initial: 100 mg PO q8h (may need up to 1200 mg/d); after pt euthyroid (6–8 wk), taper dose by ½ q4–6wk to maint, 50–150 mg/24 h; can usually D/C in 2–3 y; in elderly *Peds.* Initial: 5–7 mg/kg/24 h PO ÷ q8h. *Maint:* ⅓ - {2/3} of initial dose **Caution:** [D, –] **Contra:** Allergy **Disp:** Tabs 50 mg **SE:** Fever, rash, leukopenia, dizziness, GI upset, taste perversion, SLE-like syndrome **Notes:** Monitor pt clinically, check TFT **Interactions:** ↑ Effects w/ iodinated glycerol, Li, KI, NaI **Labs:** ↑ LFTs, PT; ↑ effects of anticoagulants **NIPE:** Take w/ food for GI upset; omit dietary sources of I; full effects take 6–12 wk

Protamine (generic) [Heparin Antagonist]
Uses: *Reverse heparin effect* **Action:** Neutralize heparin by forming a stable complex **Dose:** Based on degree of heparin reversal; give IV slowly; 1 mg reverses approx. 100 Units of heparin given in the preceding 3–4 h, 50 mg max **Caution:** [C, ?] **Contra:** Allergy

Disp: Inj 10 mg/mL **SE:** Follow coags; anticoag effect if given w/o heparin; ↓ BP, bradycardia, dyspnea, hemorrhage **Interactions:** Incompatible w/ many penicillins & cephalosporins—⊘ mix

Pseudoephedrine (Sudafed, Novafed, Afrinol, others) [Decongestant/Sympathomimetic] [OTC]

Uses: *Decongestant* **Action:** Stimulates α-adrenergic receptors w/ vasoconstriction **Dose:** *Adults.* 30–60 mg PO q6–8h; *Peds.* 4 mg/kg/24 h PO ÷ qid; ↓ in renal insuff **Caution:** [C, +] **Contra:** Poorly controlled HTN or CAD, w/ MAOIs **Disp:** Tabs 30, 60 mg; caps 60 mg; SR tabs 120, 240 mg; liq 7.5 mg/0.8 mL, 15, 30 mg/5 mL **SE:** HTN, insomnia, tachycardia, arrhythmias, nervousness, tremor **Notes:** Found in many OTC cough/cold preparations; OTC restricted distribution **Interactions:** ↑ Risk of HTN crisis w/ MAOIs; ↑ effects w/ BBs, sympathomimetics; ↓ effects w/ TCAs; ↓ effect OF methyldopa, reserpine

Psyllium (Metamucil, Serutan, Effer-Syllium) [OTC] [Laxative]

Uses: *Constipation & colonic diverticular Dz* **Action:** Bulk laxative **Dose:** 1 tsp (7 g) in glass of H_2O PO qd–tid **Caution:** [B, ?] Effer-Syllium (effervescent Psyllium) usually contains K^+; caution w/ renal failure; phenylketonuria (in products w/ aspartame) **Disp:** Suspected bowel obstruction **Disp:** Granules 4, 25 g/tsp; powder 3.5 g/packet; caps 0.52 g (3 g/6 caps); wafers 3.4 g/dose **SE:** D, abdominal cramps, bowel obstruction, constipation, bronchospasm **Interactions:** ↓ Effects OF digitalis glycosides, K-sparing diuretics, nitrofurantoin, salicylates, tetracyclines, warfarin **NIPE:** Psyllium dust inhalation may cause wheezing, runny nose, watery eyes

Pyrazinamide (generic) [Antitubercular]

Uses: *Active TB in combo w/ other agents* **Action:** unknown mechanism **Dose:** *Adults.* 15–30 mg/kg/24 h PO ÷ tid–qid; max 2 g/d. *Peds.* 15–30 mg/kg/d PO ÷ qd–bid; ↓ w/ renal/hepatic impair **Caution:** [C, +/–] **Contra:** Severe hepatic damage, acute gout **Disp:** Tabs 500 mg **SE:** Hepatotox, malaise, GI upset, arthralgia, myalgia, gout, photosensitivity **Notes:** Use in combo w/ other anti-TB drugs; consult *MMWR* for the latest TB recommendations; dosage regimen differs for "directly observed" therapy **Interactions:** ↓ Effects OF cyclosporine, tacrolimus **Labs:** False + urine ketones **NIPE:** ↑ Risk of photosensitivity—use sunscreen; ↑ fluids to 2 L/d

Pyridoxine [Vitamin B₆] [Vitamin B Supl]

Uses: *Rx & prevention of vitamin B_6 deficiency* **Action:** Vitamin B_6 supl **Dose:** *Adults.* Deficiency: 10–20 mg/d PO. *Drug-induced neuritis:* 100–200 mg/d; 25–100 mg/d prophylaxis. *Peds.* 5–25 mg/d × 3 wk **Caution:** [A (C if doses exceed RDA), +] **Contra:** Component allergy **Disp:** Tabs 25, 50, 100 mg; inj 100 mg/mL **SE:** Allergic Rxns, HA, N **Interactions:** ↑ Pyridoxine needs w/ chloramphenicol, cycloserine, hydralazine, immunosuppressant drugs, INH, oral contraceptives, penicillamine, high-protein diet; ↓ effects OF levodopa, phenobarbital, phenytoin **Labs:** False ↑ urobilinogen **NIPE:** Lactation suppressed w/ pyridoxine

Quadrivalent Human Papillomavirus (HPV types 6, 11, 16, 18) Recombinant Vaccine (Gardasil) [Vaccine] Uses: prevent cervical CA, genital warts, cervical adenocarcinoma in situ, cervical intraepithelial neoplasia grades 2 & 3, vulvar intraepithelial neoplasia grades 2 & 3, vaginal intraepithelial neoplasia grades 2 & 3, cervical intraepithelial neoplasia grade 1 caused by HPV types 6, 11, 16, 18 Dose: 0.5 mL IM inj in deltoid or upper thigh; Peds. < 9 y not recommended; Females 9–26 yrs. give 1st dose, 2nd dose 2 mon > 1st dose, 3rd dose 6 mon > 1st dose Caution: [B, –] Disp: 0.5 mL IM inj; SE: Inj site reaction, fever Interactions: ↓ Response w/ immunosuppressants NIPE: May not protect all recipients; not a substitute for routine cervical screening

Quazepam (Doral) [C-IV] [Sedative/Hypnotic/Benzodiazepine] Uses: *Insomnia* Action: Benzodiazepine Dose: 7.5–15 mg PO hs PRN; ↓ in elderly & hepatic failure Caution: [X, ?/–] NA glaucoma Contra: PRG, sleep apnea Disp: Tabs 7.5, 15 mg SE: Sedation, hangover, somnolence, resp depression[sic] Interactions: ↑ Effects w/ azole antifungals, cimetidine, digoxin, disulfiram, INH, levodopa, macrolides, neuroleptics, phenytoin, quinolones, SSRIs, verapamil, grapefruit juice, EtOH; ↓ effects w/ carbamazepine, rifampin, rifabutin, tobacco NIPE: ⊘ Breast-feed, PRG; ⊘ D/C abruptly; use barrier contraception

Quetiapine (Seroquel) [Antipsychotic] WARNING: mortality in elderly with dementia-related psychosis Uses: *Acute exacerbations of schizophrenia* Action: Serotonin & dopamine antagonism Dose: 150–750 mg/d; initiate at 25–100 mg bid–tid; slowly ↑ dose; ↓ dose for hepatic & geriatric pts Caution: [C, –] Contra: Component allergy Disp: Tabs 25, 50, 100, 200, 300, 400 mg SE: Reports of confusion w/ nefazodone; HA, somnolence, weight gain, orthostatic ↓ BP, dizziness, cataracts, neuroleptic malignant syndrome, tardive dyskinesia, QT prolongation Interactions: ↑ Effects w/ azole antifungals, cimetidine, macrolides, EtOH; ↑ effects OF antihypertensives, lorazepam; ↓ effects w/ barbiturates, carbamazepine, glucocorticoids, phenytoin, ↑ rifampin, thioridazine; ↓ effects OF dopamine antagonists, levodopa Labs: ↑ LFTs, cholesterol, triglycerides NIPE: ↑ risk of cataract formation, tardive dyskinesia; take w/o regard to food; ↓ body temp regulation

Quinapril (Accupril) [Antihypertensive/ACEI] WARNING: ACE inhibitors used during the 2nd & 3rd tri of PRG can cause fetal injury & death Uses: *HTN, CHF, DN, post-MI* Action: ACE inhibitor Dose: 10–80 mg PO qd; ↓ in renal impair Caution: [D, +] Contra: ACE inhibitor sensitivity or angioedema Disp: Tabs 5, 10, 20, 40 mg SE: Dizziness, HA, ↓ BP, impaired renal Fxn, angioedema, taste perversion, cough Interactions: ↑ Effects w/ diuretics, antihypertensives; ↑ effects OF insulin, Li; ↓ effects w/ ASA, NSAIDs; ↓ effects OF quinolones, tetracyclines Labs: ↑ BUN, SCr NIPE: ↓ Absorption w/ high-fat foods; ↑ risk of cough

Quinidine (Quinidex, Quinaglute) [Antiarrhythmic/antimalarial] Uses: *Prevention of tachydysrhythmias, malaria* Action: Class 1A antiarrhythmic **Dose:** *Adults.* AF/flutter conversion: After digitalization, 200 mg q2–3h × 8 doses;↑ qd to 3–4 g max or nl rhythm. *Peds.* 15–60 mg/kg/24 h PO in 4–5 ÷ doses; ↓ in renal impair **Caution:** [C, +] w/ ritonavir **Contra:** Digitalis tox & AV block; conduction disorders **Disp:** *Sulfate:* Tabs 200, 300 mg; SR tabs 300 mg. *Gluconate:* SR tabs 324 mg; inj 80 mg/mL **SE:** Extreme ↓ BP may be seen w/ IV administration; syncope, QT prolongation, GI upset, arrhythmias, fatigue, cinchonism (tinnitus, hearing loss, delirium, visual changes), fever, hemolytic anemia, thrombocytopenia, rash **Notes:** Check levels (Table 2); sulfate salt 83% quinidine; gluconate salt 62% quinidine; use in combo w/ drug that slows AV conduction (eg, digoxin, diltiazem, β-blocker) **Interactions:** ↑ Effects w/ acetazolamide, antacids, amiodarone, azole antifungals, cimetidine, K, macrolides, NaHCO₃, thiazide diuretics, lily-of-the-valley, pheasant's eye herb, scopolia root, squill; ↑ effects OF anticoagulants, dextromethorphan, digitalis glycosides, disopyramide, haloperidol, metoprolol, nifedipine, procainamide, propafenone, propranolol, TCAs, verapamil; ↓ effects w/ barbiturates, disopyramide, nifedipine, phenobarbital, phenytoin, rifampin, sucralfate **NIPE:** Take w/ food, ↑ risk of photosensitivity—use sunscreen

Quinupristin–Dalfopristin (Synercid) [Antibiotic/Streptogramin]
Uses: *Vancomycin-resistant Infxns due to *E. faecium* & other gram(+)'s* **Action:** ↓ Ribosomal protein synthesis. *Spectrum:* Vancomycin-resistant *Enterococcus faecium*, methicillin-susceptible *Staphylococcus aureus*, *Streptococcus pyogenes;* not active against *Enterococcus faecalis* **Dose:** *Adults & Peds.* 7.5 mg/kg IV q8–12h (use central line if possible); incompatible w/ NS or heparin; flush IV w/ dextrose; ↓ in hepatic failure **Caution:** [B, M] Multiple drug interactions (eg, cyclosporine) **Contra:** Component Allergy **Disp:** Inj 500 mg (150 mg quinupristin/350 mg dalfopristin) **SE:** Hyperbilirubinemia, inf site Rxns & pain, arthralgia, myalgia **Interactions:** ↑ Effects OF CCBs, carbamazepine, cyclosporine, diazepam, disopyramide, docetaxel, lovastatin, methylprednisolone, midazolam, paclitaxel, protease inhibitors, quinidine, tacrolimus, vinblastine **Labs:** ↑ LFTs, BUN, creatinine, Hct; ↑ or ↓ serum glucose, K

Rabeprazole (Aciphex) [Antiulcer Agent/Proton Pump Inhibitor]
Uses: *PUD, GERD, ZE* *H. pylori* **Action:** Proton-pump inhibitor **Dose:** 20 mg/d; may ↑ to 60 mg/d; *H. pylori* 20 mg PO bid (times) 7 days (w/ amoxicillin and clarithromycin); do not crush tabs **Caution:** [B, ?/–] **Disp:** Tabs 20 mg delayed release **SE:** HA, fatigue, GI upset **Interactions:** ↑ Effects OF cyclosporine, digoxin; ↓ effects OF ketoconazole **Labs:** ↑ LFTs, TSH **NIPE:** Take w/o regard to food; ↑ risk of photosensitivity—use sunscreen

Raloxifene (Evista) [Selective Estrogen Receptor Modulator]
Uses: *Prevent osteoporosis* **Action:** Partial antagonist of estrogen, behaves like estrogen **Dose:** 60 mg/d **Caution:** [X, –] **Contra:** Thromboembolism, PRG **Disp:** Tabs 60 mg **SE:** Chest pain, insomnia, rash, hot flashes, GI upset, muscle dysfunction **Interactions:** ↓ Effects w/ ampicillin, cholestyramine **NIPE:** ⊘ PRG, breastfeeding; take w/o regard to food; ↑ risk of venous thromboembolic effects

Ramelteon (Rozerem) [Hypnotic] Uses:
Short-term RX of insomnia esp w/difficulty of sleep onset **Action:** Hypnotic agent **Dose:** 8 mg tab PO within 30 min of bedtime **Caution:** [C, –] **Contra:** Severe hepatic impair; concurrent use of fluvoxamine **Disp:** 8 mg tabs **SE:** HA, N, somnolence, fatigue, dizziness, URI, depression, D, myalgia, arthralgia **Interactions:** ↑ effects w/ CYP1A2 inhibitors (fluvoxamine), CYP3A4 inhibitors (ketoconazole), and CYP2C9 inhibitors (fluconazole); ↓ effects w/ CYP450 inducers (rifampin) **Labs:** ↓ testosterone levels & ↑ prolactin levels noted; **NIPE:** high-fat foods delay effect; ⊘ use in pts w/ severe sleep apnea & severe COPD

Ramipril (Altace) [Antihypertensive/ACEI] WARNING:
ACE inhibitors used during the 2nd & 3rd tri of PRG can cause fetal injury & death **Uses:** *HTN, CHF, DN, post-MI* **Action:** ACE inhibitor **Dose:** 2.5–20 mg/d PO ÷ qd-bid; ↓ in renal failure **Caution:** [D, +] **Contra:** ACE-inhibitor–induced angioedema **Disp:** Caps 1.25, 2.5, 5, 10 mg **SE:** Cough, HA, dizziness, ↓ BP, renal impair, angioedema **Notes:** OK in combo w/ diuretics **Interactions:** ↑ effects w/ α-adrenergic blockers, loop diuretics; ↑ effects of insulin, Li; ↑ risk OF hyperkalemia w/ K⁺, K-sparing diuretics, K salt substitutes, trimethoprim, ↓ effects w/ ASA, NSAIDs, food **Labs:** ↑ BUN, creatinine, K⁺, ↓ Hmg, Hct, cholesterol **NIPE:** ↑ Risk of photosensitivity—use sunscreen; ↑ risk of cough esp w/ capsaicin; take w/o food

Ranitidine Hydrochloride (Zantac) [Antiulcer Agent/H2 Receptor Antagonist] Uses:
Duodenal ulcer, active benign ulcers, hypersecretory conditions, & GERD **Action:** H₂-receptor antagonist **Dose:** *Adults.* Ulcer: 150 mg PO bid, 300 mg PO hs, or 50 mg IV q6–8h; or 400 mg IV/d cont inf, then maint of 150 mg PO hs. *Hypersecretion:* 150 mg PO bid, up to 600 mg/d. *GERD:* 300 mg PO bid; maint 300 mg PO hs. Dyspepsia: 75 mg PO qd-bid **Peds.** 0.75–1.5 mg/kg/dose IV q6–8h or 1.25–2.5 mg/kg/dose PO q12h; ↓ in renal insuff/failure **Caution:** [B, +] **Contra:** Component allergy **Disp:** Tabs 75 [OTC], 150, 300 mg; caps 150, 300 mg; effervescent tabs 150 mg; syrup 15 mg/mL; inj 25 mg/mL **SE:** Dizziness, sedation, rash, GI upset **Notes:** PO & parenteral doses differ **Interactions:** ↑ Effects OF glipizide, glyburide, lidocaine, nifedipine, nitrendipine, nisoldipine, procainamide, TCAs, theophylline, tolbutamide, warfarin; ↓ effects w/ antacids, tobacco; ↓ effects OF cefuroxime, cefpodoxime, diazepam, enoxacin, ketoconazole, itraconazole, oxaprozin **Labs:** ↑ SCr, LFTs, false + urine protein **NIPE:** ASA, NSAIDs, EtOH, caffeine ↑ stomach acid production

Ranolazine (Ranexa) [Antianginal] Uses:
Chronic angina **Action:** ↓ Ischemia-related Na⁺ entry into myocardium **Dose:** *Adults.* 500 mg PO bid, to 1000 mg PO bid **Contra:** CYP3A inhibitors (Table 13); w/ agents that ↑ QT interval **Caution:** [C, ?/–] QT interval prolongation; hepatic impairment; HTN may develop w/renal impairment **Disp:** SR tabs 500 mg **SE:** Dizziness, HA, constipation, arrhythmias **NIPE:** Must use w/ amlodipine, nitrates, beta blockers

Rasagiline Mesylate (Azilect) [Antiparkinson Agent/MAO B Inhibitor] Uses: *Early Parkinson disease as monotherapy; levodopa adjunct in advanced dz* **Action:** MAO B inhibitor **Dose:** *Adults.* Early dz: 1 PO daily, start 0.5 mg PO daily w/ levodopa, ↓ CYP1A2 inhibitors or hepatic impair **Contra:** MAOIs, sympathomimetic amines, meperidine, methadone, tramadol, propoxyphene, dextromethorphan, mirtazapine, cyclobenzaprine, St. John's wort, sympathomimetic vasoconstrictors, general anesthetics, SSRIs **Caution:** [C, ?] Avoid tyramine-containing foods; moderate/severe hepatic impairment **Disp:** Tabs 0.5, 1 mg **SE:** Arthralgia, indigestion, dyskinesia, hallucinations, ↓ weight, postural ↓ BP, N, V, constipation, xerostomia, rash, sedation, CV conduction disturbances; **Notes:** Initial ↓ levodopa dose recommended **Interactions:** ↑ Risk of HTN crisis W/ tyramine containing foods; ↑ effects W/ ciprofloxacin; ↑ CNS toxicity/death w/ TCA, SSRIs, MAOIs; **Labs:** monitor LFTs **NIPE:** Rare melanoma reported; do periodic dermatologic exams; D/C 14 days prior to elective surgery; D/C fluoxetine 5 weeks before starting rasagiline

Rasburicase (Elitek) [Antigout Agent/Antimetabolite] Uses: *Reduce ↑ uric acid due to tumor lysis (peds)* **Action:** Catalyzes uric acid **Dose:** *Peds.* 0.15 or 0.20 mg/kg IV over 30 min, qd × 5 **Caution:** [C, ?/–] Falsely ↓ uric acid values **Contra:** Anaphylaxis, screen for G6PD deficiency to avoid hemolysis, methemoglobinemia **Disp:** 1.5 mg inj **SE:** Fever, neutropenia, GI upset, HA, rash

Repaglinide (Prandin) [Hypoglycemic/Meglitinide] Uses: *Type 2 DM* **Action:** ↑ pancreatic insulin release **Dose:** 0.5–4 mg ac, PO start 1–2 mg, ↑ to 16 mg/d max; take pc **Caution:** [C, ?/–] **Contra:** DKA, type 1 DM **Disp:** Tabs 0.5, 1, 2 mg **SE:** HA, hyper-/hypoglycemia, GI upset **Interactions:** ↑ Effects w/ ASA, BBs, chloramphenicol, erythromycin, ketoconazole, miconazole, MAOIs, NSAIDs, probenecid, sulfa drugs, warfarin, celery, coriander, dandelion root, fenugreek, garlic, ginseng, juniper berries; ↓ effects w/ barbiturates, carbamazepine, CCBs, corticosteroids, diuretics, estrogens, INH, oral contraceptives, phenytoin, phenothiazines, rifampin, sympathomimetics, thiazide diuretics, thyroid drugs **NIPE:** Take 15 min before meal; skip drug if meal skipped

Reteplase (Retavase) [Tissue Plasminogen Activator] Uses: *Post-AMI* **Action:** Thrombolytic agent **Dose:** 10 Units IV over 2 min, 2nd dose in 30 min, 10 Units IV over 2 min **Caution:** [C, ?/–] **Contra:** Internal bleeding, spinal surgery/trauma, Hx CNS vascular malformations, uncontrolled ↓ BP, sensitivity to thrombolytics **Disp:** Inj 10.8 Units/2 mL **SE:** Bleeding, allergic reactions **Interactions:** ↑ Risk of bleeding w/ ASA, abciximab, dipyridamole, heparin, NSAIDs, oral anticoagulants, vitamin K antagonists **Labs:** ↓ Fibrinogen, plasminogen **NIPE:** Monitor ECG during Rx for ↑ risk of reperfusion arrhythmias

Ribavirin (Virazole, Copegus) [Antiviral/Nucleoside Analogue] Uses: *RSV Infxn in infants; hepatitis C (in combo w/ interferon alfa-2b Copegus)* **Action:** Unknown **Dose:** *RSV:* 6 g in 300 mL sterile H_2O, inhale over 12–18 h. *Hep C:* 600 mg PO bid in combo w/ interferon alfa-2b (see Rebetron, page 157) **Caution:** [X, ?] May accumulate on soft contact lenses **Contra:** PRG, autoimmune hepatitis, CrCl <50 mL/min **Disp:** Powder for aerosol 6 g; Tabs 200, 400, 600 mg, caps 200 mg, solution 40 mg/mL; **SE:** fatigue, HA, GI upset, anemia, myalgia, alopecia, bronchospasm **Notes:** Aerosolized by a SPAG; **Interactions:** ↓ Effects w/ Al, Mg, simethicone; ↓ effect OF zidovudine **Labs:** ↑ Bilirubin, uric acid, ↓ Hmg; monitor labs **NIPE:** ⊘ PRG, breast-feeding; PRG test monthly; ↑ risk of photosensitivity—use sunscreen; take w/o regard to food

Rifabutin (Mycobutin) [Antibiotic/Antitubercular]

Uses: *Prevent *M. avium* complex Infxn in AIDS pts w/ CD4 count <100* **Action:** ↓ DNA-dependent RNA polymerase activity **Dose:** *Adults.* 150–300 mg/d PO. *Peds.* 1 y: 15–25 mg/kg/d PO; *y:* 4.4–18.8 mg/kg/d PO. *14–16 y:* 2.8–5.4 mg/kg/d PO **Caution:** [B; ?/–] WBC <1000/mm³ or platelets <50,000/mm³; ritonavir **Contra:** Allergy **Disp:** Caps 150 mg **SE:** Discolored urine, rash, neutropenia, leukopenia, myalgia, ↑ LFTs **Notes:** SEs/interactions similar to rifampin **Interactions:** ↑ Effects w/ ritonavir; ↓ effects OF anticoagulants, anticonvulsants, barbiturates, benzodiazepines, BBs, clofibrate, corticosteroids, cyclosporine, dapsone, delavirdine, digoxin, eprosartan, fluconazole, hypoglycemics, ketoconazole, nifedipine, oral contraceptives, propafenone, protease inhibitors, quinidine, tacrolimus, theophylline **Labs:** ↑ ALT, AST, alkaline phosphatase **NIPE:** Urine and body fluids may turn reddish brown in color, discoloration of soft contact lenses, use barrier contraception, take w/o food

Rifampin (Rifadin) [Antibiotic/Antitubercular]

Uses: *TB & Rx & prophylaxis of *N. meningitidis, H. influenzae,* or *S. aureus* carriers* adjunct for severe *S. aureus* **Action:** ↓ DNA-dependent RNA polymerase **Dose:** *Adults.* *N. meningitidis* & *H. influenzae* carrier: 600 mg/d PO for 4 d. *TB:* 600 mg PO or IV qd or 2 ×/wk w/ combo regimen. *Peds.* 10–20 mg/kg/dose PO or IV qd–bid; ↓ in hepatic failure **Caution:** [C, +] Amprenavir, multiple drug interactions **Contra:** Allergy, presence of active *N. meningitidis* Infxn, concomitant use of saquinavir/ritonavir **Disp:** Caps 150, 300 mg; inj 600 mg **SE:** Orange-red discoloration of bodily fluids, ↑ LFTs, flushing, HA **Notes:** Never use as single agent w/ active TB **Interactions:** ↓ Effects w/ aminosalicylic acid; ↓ effects OF acetaminophen, aminophylline, amiodarone, anticoagulants, barbiturates, BBs, CCBs, chloramphenicol, clofibrate, delavirdine, digoxin, disopyramide, doxycycline, enalapril, estrogens, haloperidol, hypoglycemics, hydantoins, methadone, morphine, nifedipine, ondansetron, oral contraceptives, phenytoin, protease inhibitors, quinidine, repaglinide, sertraline, sulfapyridine, sulfones, tacrolimus, theophylline, thyroid drugs, tocainide, TCAs, theophylline, verapamil, zidovudine, zolpidem **Labs:** ↑ LFTs, uric acid; affects serum folate and vit B_{12} levels **NIPE:** Use barrier contraception, take w/o food, reddish brown color in urine and body fluids, stains soft contact lenses

Rifapentine (Priftin) [Antibiotic/Antitubercular]

Uses: *Pulmonary TB* **Action:** ↓ DNA-dependent RNA polymerase. *Spectrum: M. tuberculosis*

Dose: *Intensive phase:* 600 mg PO 2×/wk for 2 mo; separate doses by 3 or more days. *Continuation phase:* 600 mg/wk for 4 mo; part of 3–4 drug regimen **Caution:** [C, red-orange breast milk] ↓ protease inhibitor efficacy, antiepileptics, β-blockers, CCBs **Contra:** Allergy to rifamycins **Disp:** 150-mg tabs **SE:** Neutropenia, hyperuricemia, HTN, HA, dizziness, rash, GI upset, blood dyscrasias, ↑ LFTs, hematuria, discolored secretions **Interactions:** ↓ Effects OF anticoagulants, BBs, CCBs, corticosteroids, cyclosporine, digoxin, fluoroquinolones, methadone, metoprolol, oral contraceptives, phenytoin, propranolol, protease inhibitors, rifampin, sulfonylureas, TCAs, theophylline, verapamil, warfarin **Labs:** ↑ LFTs, platelets, uric acid; ↓ hmg, neutrophil, WBCs; inhibits folate & B_{12} levels **NIPE:** May take with food; body fluids, teeth, tongue, feces may become orange-red; may permanently discolor soft contact lenses; use barrier contraception; monitor LFTs.

Rifaximin (Xifaxan) [Antibiotic/Rifamycin Antibacterial]
Uses: *Travelers' diarrhea (noninvasive strains of *E coli*) in patients > 12 y* **Action:** Not absorbed, derivative of rifamycin. **Spectrum:** *E coli* **Dose:** 1 tab PO qd × 3 d **Caution:** [C, ?/–] Allergy (rash, angioedema, urticaria); pseudomembranous colitis **Contra:** Allergy to rifamycins **Disp:** Tabs 200 mg **SE:** Flatulence, HA, abdominal pain, GI distress, fever **Notes:** D/C if Sx worsen or persist > 24–48 h, or w/ fever or blood in stool; **Interactions:** None significant **Labs:** None noted **NIPE:** May be taken w/o regard to food; ⊘ crush/chew tabs—swallow whole

Rimantadine (Flumadine) [Antiviral]
Uses: *Prophylaxis & Rx of influenza A viral Infxns* **Action:** Antiviral **Dose:** *Adults & Peds >9 y.* 100 mg PO bid. *Peds 1–9 y.* 5 mg/kg/d PO, 150 mg/d max; qd w/ severe renal/hepatic impair & elderly; initiate w/in 48 h of Sx onset **Caution:** [C, –] w/ cimetidine; avoid in PRG or breast-feeding **Contra:** Component & amantadine allergy **Disp:** Tabs 100 mg; syrup 50 mg/5 mL **SE:** Orthostatic ↓ BP, edema, dizziness, GI upset, ↓ Sz threshold **Interactions:** ↑ Effects w/ cimetidine; ↓ effects w/ acetaminophen, ASA

Rimexolone (Vexol Ophthalmic) [Steroid]
Uses: *Postop inflammation & uveitis* **Action:** Steroid **Dose:** *Adults & Peds >2 y.* Uveitis: 1–2 gtt/h daytime & q2h at night, taper to 1 gtt q4h. *Postop:* 1–2 gtt qid ≤ 2 wk **Caution:** [C, ?/–] Ocular Infxns **Disp:** Susp 1%; **SE:** Blurred vision, local irritation **Notes:** Taper dose **NIPE:** Shake well, ⊘ touch eye w/ dropper

Risedronate (Actonel) [Bisphosphonate/Hormone]
Uses: *Paget's Dz; treat/prevent glucocorticoid-induced/postmenopausal osteoporosis* **Action:** Bisphosphonate; ↓ osteoclast-mediated bone resorption **Dose:** *Paget Dz:* 30 mg/d PO for 2 mo. *Osteoporosis Rx/prevention:* 5 mg qd or 35 mg qwk; 30 min before 1st food/drink of the day; stay upright for at least 30 min after **Caution:** [C, ?/–] Ca supls & antacids ↓ absorption **Contra:** Allergy, ↓ Ca^{2+}, esophageal abnormalities, unable to stand/sit for 30 min, CrCl < 30 mL/min **Disp:** Tabs 5, 30, 35 mg **SE:** HA, D, abdominal pain, arthralgia; flu-like Sxs, rash, esophagitis, bone pain **Interactions:** ↓ Effects w/ antacids, Ca^{2+}, food **Labs:** Interference w/ bone-imaging agents; **Labs:** Monitor LFT, Ca^{2+}, PO^{3+}, K^+ **NIPE:** EtOH intake and cigarette smoking promote osteoporosis

Risperidone (Risperdal) [Antipsychotic] WARNING: ↑ mortality in elderly with dementia-related psychosis **Uses:** *Psychotic disorders (schizophrenia),* dementia of the elderly, bipolar disorder, mania, Tourette disorder, autism **Action:** Benzisoxazole antipsychotic **Dose:** *Adults.* 0.5–6 mg PO bid. *Peds/Adolescents.* 0.25 mg PO bid, ↑ q5–7d; ↓ start dose w/ elderly, renal/hepatic impair **Caution:** [C, –], ↑ ↓ BP w/ antihypertensives, clozapine **Contra:** Component allergy **Disp:** Tabs 0.25, 0.5, 1, 2, 3, 4, 5 mg; soln 1 mg/mL; orally disintegrating tabs 0.5, 1, 2, 3, 4 mg **SE:** Orthostatic ↓ BP, EPS w/ high dose, tachycardia, arrhythmias, sedation, dystonias, neuroleptic malignant syndrome, sexual dysfunction, constipation, xerostomia, blood dyscrasias, cholestatic jaundice, weight gain **Interactions:** ↑ Effects w/ clozapine, CNS depressants, EtOH; ↑ effects OF antihypertensives; ↓ effects w/ carbamazepine; ↓ effects OF levodopa **Labs:** ↑ LFTs, serum prolactin **NIPE:** ↑ Risk photosensitivity—use sunscreen, extrapyramidal effects; may alter body temp regulation; several weeks to see effect

Ritonavir (Norvir) [Antiretroviral/Protease Inhibitor] Uses: *HIV* **Actions:** Protease inhibitor; ↓ maturation of immature noninfectious virions to mature infectious virus **Dose:** *Adults.* Initial 300 mg PO bid, titrate over 1 wk to 600 mg PO bid (titration will ↓ GI SE). *Peds* ≥2 y. 250 mg/m² titrate to 400 mg bid (dose adjust w/ amprenavir, indinavir, nelfinavir, & saquinavir); (w/ food) **Caution:** [B, +] w/ ergotamine, amiodarone, bepridil, flecainide, propafenone, quinidine, pimozide, midazolam, triazolam **Contra:** W/ ergotamine, amiodarone, bepridil, flecainide, propafenone, quinidine, pimozide, midazolam, triazolam **Disp:** Caps 100 mg; soln 80 mg/mL **SE:** N/V/D/C, abdominal pain, taste perversion, anemia, weakness, HA, fever, malaise, rash, paresthesias **Notes:** Refrigerate **Interactions:** ↑ Effects w/ erythromycin, interleukins, grapefruit juice, food; ↑ effects OF amiodarone, astemizole, atorvastatin, barbiturates, bepridil, bupropion, cerivastatin, cisapride, clorazepate, clozapine, clarithromycin, desipramine, diazepam, encainide, ergot alkaloids, estazolam, flecainide, flurazepam, indinavir, ketoconazole, lovastatin, meperidine, midazolam, nelfinavir, phenytoin, pimozide, piroxicam, propafenone, propoxyphene, quinidine, rifabutin, saquinavir, sildenafil, simvastatin, SSRIs, TCAs, terfenadine, triazolam, troleandomycin, zolpidem; ↓ effects w/ barbiturates, carbamazepine, phenytoin, rifabutin, rifampin, St. John's wort, tobacco; ↓ effects OF didanosine, hypnotics, methadone, oral contraceptives, sedatives, theophylline, warfarin **Labs:** ↑ Serum glucose, LFTs, triglycerides, uric acid **NIPE:** Food ↑ absorption; use barrier contraception; disulfiram-like Rxn w/ disulfiram, metronidazole

Rivastigmine (Exelon) [Cholinesterase Inhibitor/Anti-Alzheimer's Agent] Uses: *Mild–moderate dementia in Alzheimer Dz* **Action:** Enhances cholinergic activity **Dose:** 1.5 mg bid; ↑ to 6 mg bid, w/ ↑ at 2-wk intervals (w/ food) **Caution:** [B, ?] β-Blockers, CCBs, smoking, neuromuscular blockade, digoxin **Contra:** Allergy to rivastigmine or carbamates **Disp:** Caps 1.5, 3, 4.5, 6 mg; soln 2 mg/mL **SE:** Dose-related GI effects, N/V/D; dizziness, insomnia, fatigue, tremor, diaphoresis, HA **Interactions:** ↑ Risk OF GI bleed w/ NSAIDs; ↓ effects w/ nicotine; ↓ effects of anticholinergics **NIPE:** Take w/ food; swallow capsules whole, do not break, chew, or crush; avoid EtOH

Rizatriptan (Maxalt, Maxalt MLT) [Antimigraine Agent/5 HT1 Agonist] (See Table 11)

Rocuronium (Zemuron) [Skeletal Muscle Relaxant] Uses: *Skeletal muscle relaxation during rapid-sequence intubation, surgery, or mechanical ventilation* **Action:** Nondepolarizing neuromuscular blocker **Dose:** *Rapid sequence intubation:* 0.6–1.2 mg/kg IV. *Continuous inf:* 4–16 mcg/kg/min IV; ↓ in hepatic impair **Caution:** [C, ?] Aminoglycosides, vancomycin, tetracycline, polymyxins enhance blockade **Contra:** Component or pancuronium allergy **Disp:** Inj preservative free 10 mg/mL 5,10 mL vials **SE:** BP changes, tachycardia **Interactions:** ↑ Effects w/ MAOIs, propranolol; ↑ vasospastic Rxn w/ ergot-containing drugs; ↑ risk OF hyperreflexia, incoordination, weakness w/ SSRIs **NIPE:** Food delays drug action; ⊘ take > 30 mg/24 h

Ropinirole (Requip) [Dopamine Agonist/Antiparkinson Agent] Uses: *Rx of Parkinson Dz* **Action:** Dopamine agonist **Dose:** Initial 0.25 mg PO tid, weekly ↑ 0.25 mg/dose, to 3 mg max **Caution:** [C, ?/–] Severe CV, renal, or hepatic impair **Contra:** Component allergy **Disp:** Tabs 0.25, 0.5, 1, 2, 3, 4, 5 mg **SE:** Syncope, postural ↓ BP, N/V, HA, somnolence, hallucinations, dyskinesias **Interactions:** ↑ Risk OF bleeding w/ ASA, NSAIDs, feverfew, garlic, ginger, horse chestnut, red clover, EtOH, tobacco; ↑ effects OF amitriptyline, Li, MTX, theophylline, warfarin; ↑ risk OF photosensitivity w/ dong quai—use sunscreen, St. John's wort; ↓ effects w/ antacids, rifampin; ↓ effects OF ACEIs, diuretics **Labs:** ↑ ALT, AST **NIPE:** Take w/ food; D/C w/ 7-d taper

Rosiglitazone (Avandia) [Hypoglycemic/Thiazolidinedione] Uses: *Type 2 DM * **Action:** ↑ insulin sensitivity **Dose:** 4–8 mg/d PO or in 2 ÷ doses (w/o regard to meals) **Caution:** [C, –] Not for DKA; w/ ESRD (renal elimination) **Contra:** Active liver Dz **Disp:** Tabs 2, 4, 8 mg **SE:** Weight gain, hyperlipidemia, HA, edema, fluid retention, exacerbated CHF, hyper-/hypoglycemia, hepatic damage **Interactions:** ↑ Risk of hypoglycemia w/ insulin, ketoconazole, oral hypoglycemics, fenugreek, garlic, ginseng, glucomannan; ↓ effects OF oral contraceptives **Labs:** ↑ ALT, total cholesterol, LDL, HDL, ↓ Hmg, Hct **NIPE:** Use barrier contraception

Rosiglitazone/Metformin (Avandamet) [Hypoglycemic/thiazolidinedione & Biguanide] **WARNING:** Associated w/ lactic acidosis Uses: Type 2 DM **Action:** ↓ Hepatic glucose production & intestinal absorption of glucose; ↑ insulin sensitivity **Dose:** *Adults.* Initial: 2 mg/500 mg PO OD or BID with AM and PM meal; increase by 2 mg/500 mg per day after 4 wks; max 8 mg/2000 mg per day. *Peds.* Not recommended **Caution:** [C, –] hold dose before & 48 h after ionic contrast; not for DKA; w/ ESRD (renal elimination) **Contra:** SCr > 1.4 in females or > 1.5 in males; hypoxemic conditions (eg, acute

CHF/sepsis); active liver dis; metabolic acidosis **Disp:** Tabs rosiglitazone/ metformin: 2 mg/500 mg, 4 mg/500 mg, 2 mg/1000 mg, 4 mg/1000 mg **SE:** Weight gain, hyperlipidemia, HA, edema, fluid retention, exacerbated CHF, hyper-/hypoglycemia, hepatic damage, anorexia, N/V, rash, lactic acidosis (rare, but serious) **Interactions:** ↑ Risk of hypoglycemia w/ insulin, ketoconazole, fenugreek, garlic, ginseng, glucomannan; ↑ effects w/ amiloride, cimetidine, digoxin, furosemide, MAOIs, morphine, procainamide, quinidine, quinine, ranitidine, triamterene, trimethoprim, vancomycin; ↓ effects w/ corticosteroids, CCBs, diuretics, estrogens, INH, oral contraceptives, phenothiazines, phenytoin, sympathomimetics, thyroid drugs, tobacco; ↓ effects OF oral contraceptives **Labs:** ↑ LFTs, lipids, SCr ↓ Hmg, Hct; monitor LFTs, SCr baseline & periodically **NIPE:** Use barrier contraception; take w/ food; ⊘ dehydration, EtOH, before surgery

Rosuvastatin (Crestor) [Antilipemic/HMG-CoA Reductase Inhibitor]
Uses: *Rx primary hypercholesterolemia & mixed dyslipidemia* **Action:** HMG-CoA reductase inhibitor **Dose:** 5–40 mg PO qd; max 5 mg/d w/ cyclosporine, 10 mg/d w/ gemfibrozil or CrCl < 30 mL/min (avoid Al-/Mg-based antacids for 2 h after) **Caution:** [X, ?/–] **Contra:** Active liver Dz or unexplained ↑ LFT Disp: Tabs 5, 10, 20, 40 mg **SE:** Myalgia, constipation, asthenia, abdominal pain, nausea, myopathy, rarely rhabdomyolysis **Interactions:** ↑ Effects OF warfarin; ↑ risk of myopathy w/ cyclosporine, fibrates, niacin, statins **Labs:** ↑ warfarin; ↑ LFTs; monitor LFTs at baseline, 12 wk, then q6mo; ↑ urine protein, Hmg **NIPE:** ⊘ PRG or breast-feeding; ↓ dose in Asian patients

Rotavirus vaccine, live, oral, pentavalent (RotaTeq) [Vaccine]
Uses: *Prevent rotavirus gastroenteritis* **Action:** Active immunization **Dose:** *Peds.* Single dose PO at 2, 4, and 6 mo **Caution:** [?, ?] **Disp:** Oral susp 2-mL single-use tubes **SE:** D, V, otitis **Interactions:** ↓ Effects w/ immunosuppressants such as irradiation, chemotherapy, or high-dose steroids **NIPE:** Begin series by 12 wks and conclude by 32 wks of age; ⊘ take with oral polio vaccine

Salmeterol (Serevent) [Bronchodilator/Sympathomimetic]
Uses: *Asthma, exercise-induced asthma, COPD* **Action:** Sympathomimetic bronchodilator, β$_2$-agonist **Dose:** *Adults & Peds ≥12 y.* 1 diskus-dose inhaled bid **Caution:** [C, ?/–] **Contra:** Acute asthma; w/in 14 d of MAOI **Disp:** Dry powder discus; metered dose inhaler **SE:** HA, pharyngitis, tachycardia, arrhythmias, nervousness, GI upset, tremors **Notes:** Not for acute attacks; also prescribe short-acting β-agonist **Interactions:** ↑ Effects w/ MAOIs, TCAs; ↓ effects w/ BBs **Labs:** ↓ serum K$^+$ **NIPE:** Shake canister before use, inhale q12h, not for acute exacerbations

Saquinavir (Fortovase, Invirase) [Antiretroviral/Protease Inhibitor]
Uses: *HIV Infxn* **Action:** HIV protease inhibitor **Dose:** 1200 mg PO tid w/in 2 h pc (dose adjust w/ ritonavir, delavirdine, lopinavir, & nelfinavir) **Caution:** [B, +] w/ rifampin, ketoconazole, statins, sildenafil **Contra:** Allergy, sun exposure w/o sunscreen/clothing, triazolam, midazolam, ergots; rifampin **Disp:**

Caps 200 mg, tabs 500 mg **SE:** Dyslipidemia, lipodystrophy, rash, hyperglycemia, GI upset, weakness, hepatic dysfunction **Notes:** Take 2h after meal, avoid direct sunlight **Interactions:** ↑ Effects w/ clarithromycin, delavirdine, erythromycin, indinavir, ketoconazole, nelfinavir, ritonavir, grapefruit juice, food; ↑ effects OF astemizole, cisapride, clarithromycin, ergot alkaloids, erythromycin, lovastatin, midazolam, phenytoin, sildenafil, simvastatin, terfenadine, triazolam; ↓ effects w/ barbiturates, carbamazepine, dexamethasone, efavirenz, phenytoin, rifabutin, rifampin, St. John's wort; ↓ effects OF oral contraceptives **Labs:** ↑ LFTs, ↓ neutrophils **NIPE:** Use barrier contraception; ↑ risk of photosensitivity—use sunscreen

Sargramostim [GM-CSF] (Leukine) [Colony Stimulating Factor]
Uses: *Myeloid recovery following BMT or chemo* **Action:** Recombinant GF, Activates mature granulocytes & macrophages **Dose:** *Adults & Peds.* 250 mcg/m^2/d IV for 21 d (BMT) **Caution:** [C, ?/–] Lithium, corticosteroids **Contra:** >10% blasts, allergy to yeast, concurrent chemo/RT **Disp:** Inj 250, 500 mcg **SE:** Bone pain, fever, ↓ BP, tachycardia, flushing, GI upset, myalgia **Notes:** use APAP PRN for pain **Interactions:** ↑ Effects w/ corticosteroids, Li **Labs:** ↑ Serum glucose, BUN, creatinine, LFTs; ↓ albumin, Ca^{2+} **NIPE:** ⊘ Exposure to infection; rotate inj sites

Scopolamine, Scopolamine Transdermal and Ophthalmic (Scopace, Transderm-Scop) [Antiemetic/Antivertigo/Anticholinergic]
Uses: *Prevent N/V associated w/ motion sickness, anesthesia, opiates; mydriatic,* cycloplegic, Rx uveitis, iridocyclitis **Action:** Anticholinergic, inhibits iris and ciliary bodies, antiemetic **Dose:** 1 mg/72 hr, 1 patch behind ear q3d; apply > 4 h before exposure; 0.4–0.8 PO, repeat PRN q4–6h; cycloplegic 1–2 gtt 1 h pre, uveitis 1–2 gtt up to QID max; ↓ in elderly **Caution:** [C, +] APAP, levodopa, ketoconazole, digitalis, KCl **Contra:** NA glaucoma, GI or GU obstruction, thyrotoxicosis, paralytic ileus **Disp:** Patch 1.5 mg, tabs 0.4 mg, ophth 0.25% **SE:** Xerostomia, drowsiness, blurred vision, tachycardia, constipation **Interactions:** ↑ Effects w/ antihistamines, amantadine, antidepressants, disopyramide, opioids, procainamide, quinidine, TCAs, EtOH; ↓ effects OF acetaminophen, digoxin, ketoconazole, levodopa, K$^+$, phenothiazines, riboflavin **NIPE:** Do not blink excessively after eye gtt, wait 5 min before dosing other eye; activity w/ patch requires several hours; ⊘ D/C abruptly; wash hands after applying patch; may cause heat intolerance

Secobarbital (Seconal) [C-II] [Anticonvulsant, Sedative/Hypnotic/Barbiturate]
Uses: *Insomnia, short-term use,* preanesthetic agent **Action:** Rapid-acting barbiturate **Dose:** *Adults.* Caps 50, 100 mg, 100–200 mg HS, 100–300 mg preop. *Peds.* 2–6 mg/kg/dose, 100 mg/max, ↓ in elderly **Caution:** [D, +] CYP2C9, 3A3/4, 3A5/7 inducer (Table 13); ↑ tox w/ other CNS depressants **Contra:** Porphyria, PRG **Disp.:** Caps 50, 100 mg **SE:** Resp depression, CNS depression, porphyria **Interactions:** ↑ Effects w/ MAOIs, valproic acid, EtOH, kava kava, valerian; ↑ effects OF meperidine; ↓ effects OF anticoagulants,

BBs, CCBs, CNS depressants, chloramphenicol, corticosteroids, cyclosporine, digitoxin, disopyramide, doxycycline, estrogen, griseofulvin, methadone, neuroleptics, oral contraceptives, propafenone, quinidine, tacrolimus, theophylline **NIPE:** Tolerance in 1–2 wk; photosensitivity; ⊘ PRG, breast-feeding; use barrier contraception

Selegiline (Eldepryl) [Antiparkinson Agent/MAO B Inhibitor] **Uses:** Parkinson Dz **Action:** MAOI **Dose:** 5 mg PO bid; ↓ in elderly **Caution:** [C, ?] Meperidine, SSRI, TCAs **Contra:** w/ concurrent meperidine **Disp:** Tabs/caps 5 mg **SE:** Nausea, dizziness, orthostatic ↓ BP, arrhythmias, tachycardia, edema, confusion, xerostomia **Notes:** ↓ carbidopa/levodopa if used in combo; see transdermal form; **Interactions:** ↑ Risk of serotonin syndrome w/ dextroamphetamine, dextromethorphan, fenfluramine, meperidine, methylphenidate, sibutramine, venlafaxine; ↑ risk OF hypertension w/ dextroamphetamine, levodopa, methylphenidate, SSRIs, tyramine containing foods, EtOH, ephedra, ginseng, ma-huang, St. John's wort **Labs:** False ↑ uric acid, urine protein; false + urine ketones, urine glucose

Selegiline HCL (Zelapar, orally disintegrating tabs) [Antiparkinson Agent/MAO B Inhibitor] **Use:** Parkinson's disease, adjunct to levodopa/carbidopa **Action:** MAOI **Dose:** 1.25 mg PO OD for at least 6 weeks before increasing dose **Caution:** [C, –] renal impair, hepatic impair **Contra:** Within 2 wks of meperidine, SSRIs, TCA, Phenobarbital, phenytoin, carbamazepine, nafcillin, rifampin or concomitant tramadol, methadone, propoxyphene, dextromethorphan **Disp:** Orally disintegrating tablets dissolve on tongue 1.25, 2.5 mg **SE:** Postural hypotension, dizziness, GI distress, HA, insomnia, HTN, rhinitis, ECG abnormality, hallucinations **Interactions:** ↑ Risk of serotonin syndrome w/ dextroamphetamine, dextromethorphan, fenfluramine, meperidine, methylphenidate, sibutramine, venlafaxine; ↑ risk OF hypertension w/ dextroamphetamine, levodopa, methylphenidate, SSRIs, EtOH, ephedra, ginseng, ma-huang, St. John's wort; wait 5 wks after D/C fluoxetine **NIPE:** When taken in recommended doses no need to restrict tyramine-containing foods; ⊘ swallow product ↑ risk of HTN crisis; ⊘ use in children < 16 y

Selegiline, Transdermal (Emsam) [Antiparkinson Agent/ MAO B Inhibitor] **Uses:** *Depression* **Action:** MAOI **Dose:** *Adults.* Apply patch daily to upper torso, upper thigh, or outer upper arm **Contra:** Tyramine-containing foods w/ 9- or 12-mg doses; serotonin-sparing agents **Caution:** [C, –] ↑ carbamazepine and oxcarbazepine levels **Disp:** ER patches 6, 9, 12 mg **SE:** Local reactions requiring topical steroids; HA, insomnia, orthostatic hypotension, serotonin syndrome, suicide risk **Interactions:** ↑ Risk of serotonin syndrome w/ dextroamphetamine, dextromethorphan, fenfluramine, meperidine, methylphenidate, sibutramine, venlafaxine; ↑ risk OF hypertension w/ dextroamphetamine, levodopa, methylphenidate, SSRIs, tyramine containing foods, EtOH, ephedra, ginseng, ma-huang, St. John's wort **NIPE:** ⊘ ETOH & tyramine-containing foods; rotate site; see oral form

Selenium Sulfide (Exsel Shampoo, Selsun Blue Shampoo, Selsun Shampoo) [Antiseborrheic]   Uses: *Scalp seborrheic dermatitis,* scalp itching & flaking due to *dandruff;* tinea versicolor **Action:** Antiseborrheic **Dose:** *Dandruff, seborrhea:* Massage 5–10 mL into wet scalp, leave on 2–3 min, rinse, repeat; use 2×/wk, then once q1–4wk PRN. *Tinea versicolor:* Apply 2.5% qd for 7 d on area & lather w/ small amounts of water; leave on skin 10 min, then rinse **Caution:** [C, ?] **Contra:** Open wounds **Disp:** Shampoo [OTC] 1, 2.5% **SE:** Dry or oily scalp, lethargy, hair discoloration, local irritation **NIPE:** ⊘ Use on excoriated skin; may cause reversible hair loss; rinse thoroughly after use; DO NOT use more than 2 (times)/wk

Sertaconazole (Ertaczo) [Antifungal]   Uses: *Topical Rx interdigital tinea pedis* **Action:** Imidazole antifungal. *Spectrum: Trichophyton rubrum, T. mentagrophytes, Epidermophyton floccosum* **Dose:** *Adults & Peds > 12.* Apply between toes & immediate surrounding healthy skin bid × 4 wk **Caution:** [C, ?] **Contra:** Component allergy **Disp:** 2% cream **SE:** Contact dermatitis, dry/burning skin, tenderness **Notes:** Use in immunocompetent pts **NIPE:** Avoid occlusive dressings; avoid contact with mucous membranes

Sertraline (Zoloft) [Antidepressant/SSRI]   WARNING: Closely monitor pts for worsening depression or emergence of suicidality, particularly in ped pts **Uses:** *Depression, panic disorders, obsessive–compulsive disorder (OCD), posttraumatic stress disorders (PTSD),* social anxiety disorder, eating disorders, premenstrual disorders **Action:** ↓ neuronal uptake of serotonin **Dose:** *Adults.* Depression: 50–200 mg/d PO. *PTSD:* 25 mg PO qd ×1 wk, then 50 mg PO qd, 200 mg/d max. *Peds.* 6–12 y: 25 mg PO qd. *13–17 y:* 50 mg PO qd **Caution:** [C, ?/–] w/ haloperidol (serotonin syndrome), sumatriptan, linezolid, hepatic impair **Contra:** MAOI use w/in 14 d; concomitant pimozide **Disp:** Tabs 25, 50, 100 mg; 20 mg/mL oral **SE:** Can activate manic/hypomanic state; weight loss; insomnia, somnolence, fatigue, tremor, xerostomia, N/D, dyspepsia, ejaculatory dysfunction, ↓ libido, hepatotox **Interactions:** ↑ Effects w/ cimetidine, MAOIs, tryptophan, St. John's wort; ↑ effects OF clozapine, diazepam, hydantoins, sumatriptan, tolbutamide, TCAs, warfarin, EtOH; ↓ effects w/ carbamazepine, rifampin **Labs:** ↑ LFTs, triglycerides, ↓ uric acid

Sevelamer (Renagel) [Phosphate Binder]   Uses: ↓ serum phosphorus in ESRD **Action:** Binds intestinal PO_4^{3+} **Dose:** 2–4 capsules PO tid w/ meals; adjust based on PO_4^{3+} max 4 g/dose **Caution:** [C, ?] **Contra:** Hypophosphatemia; bowel obstruction **Disp:** Capsules 403 mg, tabs 400, 800 mg **SE:** BP changes, N/V/D, dyspepsia, thrombosis **Notes:** 800 mg sevelamer = 667 mg Ca acetate **Interactions:** ↓ Effects Of antiarrhythmics, anticonvulsants when given w/ sevelamer **Labs:** Monitor serum bicarbonate, Ca, Cl, P **NIPE:** Must be admin with meals; take daily multivitamin, may ↓ fat-soluble vitamin absorption; take 1 h before or 3 h after other meds; do not open or chew capsules

Sibutramine (Meridia) [C-IV] [Anorexic/CNS Stimulant]   Uses: *Obesity* **Action:** Blocks uptake of norepinephrine, serotonin, dopamine

Dose: 10 mg/d PO, may ↓ to 5 mg after 4 wk **Caution:** [C, –] SSRIs, lithium, dextromethorphan, opioids **Contra:** MAOI w/in 14 d, uncontrolled HTN, arrhythmias **Disp:** Caps 5, 10, 15 mg **SE:** HA, insomnia, xerostomia, constipation, rhinitis, tachycardia, HTN **Notes:** Use w/ low-calorie diet, monitor BP & HR **Interactions:** ↑ Risk OF serotonin syndrome w/ dextromethorphan, ergots, fentanyl, Li, meperidine, MAOIs, naratriptan, pentazocine, rizatriptan, sumatriptan, SSRIs, tromethorphan, tryptophan, zolmitriptan, St. John's wort; ↑ effects w/ cimetidine, erythromycin, ketoconazole; ↑ CNS depression w/ EtOH **NIPE:** ⊘ EtOH; take early in the day to avoid insomnia

Sildenafil (Viagra, Revatio) [Anti-impotence Agent/PDE 5]

Uses: *Viagra:* *Erectile dysfunction,* *Revatio:* *Pulmonary artery HTN* **Action:** ↓ Phosphodiesterase type 5 (responsible for cGMP breakdown); ↑ cGMP activity, causing smooth muscle relaxation & ↑ flow to the corpus cavernosum and pulmonary vasculature; possible antiproliferative effect on pulmonary artery smooth muscle; **Dose:** 25–100 mg PO 1 h before sexual activity, max 1/day; ↓ if >65 y; avoid fatty foods w/ dose; Revatio 20 mg PO tid **Caution:** [B, ?] CYP3A4 inhibitors (Table 13) **Contra:** W/ nitrates; retinitis pigmentosa; hepatic/severe renal impair **Disp:** Tabs 25, 50, 100 mg, tabs (Revatio) 20 mg **SE:** HA; flushing; dizziness; blue haze visual disturbance (usually reversible) **Notes:** Cardiac events in absence of nitrates debatable **Interactions:** ↑ Effects w/ amlodipine, cimetidine, erythromycin, indinavir, itraconazole, ketoconazole, nelfinavir, protease inhibitors, ritonavir, saquinavir, grapefruit juice; ↑ risk OF hypotension w/ antihypertensives, nitrates; ↓ effects w/ rifampin **NIPE:** High-fat food delays absorption; ↑ risk of cardiac arrest if used w/ nitrates

Silver Nitrate (Dey-Drop, others) [Antiseptic/Astringent]

Uses: *Removal of granulation tissue & warts; prophylaxis in burns* **Action:** Caustic antiseptic & astringent **Dose:** *Adults & Peds.* Apply to moist surface 2–3×/wk for several wks or until effect **Caution:** [C, ?] **Contra:** Do not use on broken skin **Disp:** Topical impregnated applicator sticks, soln 10, 25, 50%; ophth 1% amp **SE:** May stain tissue black, usually resolves; local irritation, methemoglobinemia **NIPE:** D/C if redness or irritation develop; no longer used in US for newborn prevention of GC conjunctivitis

Silver Sulfadiazine (Silvadene, others) [Antibiotic]

Uses: *Prevention & Rx of Infxn in 2nd- & 3rd-degree burns* **Action:** Bactericidal **Dose:** *Adults & Peds.* Aseptically cover the area w/ {1/16}-in. coating bid **Caution:** [B unless near term, ?/–] **Contra:** Infants < 2 mo, PRG near term **Disp:** Cream 1% **SE:** Itching, rash, skin discoloration, blood dyscrasias, hepatitis, allergy **Notes:** Systemic absorption w/ extensive application **Interactions:** May inactivate topical proteolytic enzymes **Labs:** ↓ WBCs; monitor LFTs, BUN, Creatinine **NIPE:** photosensitivity—use sunscreen

Simethicone (Mylicon, others) [OTC] [Antiflatulent]

Uses: Flatulence **Action:** Defoaming, alters gas bubble surface tension action **Dose:** *Adults*

& *Peds.* 40–125 mg PO pc & hs PRN; 500 mg/D max; *Peds.* < 2 yr: 20 mg PO QID PRN; 2–12 yr: 40 mg PO QID PRN ; > 12 yr–adult **Caution:** [C, ?] **Contra:** GI Intestinal perforation or obstruction **Disp:** [OTC] Tabs 80, 125 mg; caps 125 mg; softgels 125, 166, 180 mg; suspension 40 mg/0.6 mL; chew tabs 80, 125 mg **SE:** N/D **Notes:** Available in combo products OTC **Interactions:** ↓ Effects OF topical proteolytic enzymes

Simvastatin (Zocor) [Antilipemic/HMG-CoA Reductase Inhibitor]
Uses: ↓ Cholesterol **Action:** HMG-CoA reductase inhibitor **Dose:** 5–80 mg PO; w/ meals; ↓ in renal insuff **Caution:** [X, –] Avoid concurrent use of gemfibrozil **Contra:** PRG, liver Dz **Disp:** Tabs 5, 10, 20, 40, 80 mg **SE:** HA, GI upset, myalgia, myopathy (muscle pain, tenderness or weakness with creatine kinase 10× ULN), hepatitis **Interactions:** ↑ Effects w/ amprenavir, azole antifungals, cyclosporine, danazol, diltiazem, gemfibrozil, indinavir, macrolides, nefazodone, nelfinavir, ritonavir, saquinavir, verapamil, grapefruit juice; ↑ effects OF digoxin, warfarin; ↓ effects w/ cholestyramine, colestipol, fluvastatin, isradipine **Labs:** ↑ LFTs, monitor **NIPE:** Take w/ food and in the evening; ⊘ PRG, breast-feeding

Sirolimus [Rapamycin] (Rapamune) [Immunosuppressant]
WARNING: Can cause immunosuppression & Infxns **Uses:** Prophylaxis of organ rejection **Action:** ↓ T-lymphocyte activation **Dose:** *Adults >40 kg.* 6 mg PO on day 1, then 2 mg/d PO. *Adults <40 kg & Peds ≥13 y.* 3 mg/m² load, then 1 mg/m²/d in H₂O/orange juice; no grapefruit juice while on sirolimus); take 4 h after cyclosporine; ↓ in hepatic impair **Caution:** [C, ?/–] Grapefruit juice, ketoconazole **Contra:** Component allergy **Disp:** Soln 1 mg/mL, tab 1, 2 mg **SE:** HTN, edema, CP, fever, HA, insomnia, acne, rash, ↑ cholesterol, GI upset, ↑ or ↓ K⁺, Infxns, blood dyscrasias, arthralgia, tachycardia, renal impair, hepatic artery thrombosis, graft loss & death in de novo liver transplant **Notes:** Levels not needed except in liver failure (trough 9–17 ng/mL) **Interactions:** ↑ Effects w/ azole antifungals, cimetidine, cyclosporine, diltiazem, macrolides, nicardipine, protease inhibitors, verapamil, grapefruit juice; ↓ effects w/ carbamazepine, phenobarbital, phenytoin, rifabutin, rifapentine, rifampin; ↓ effects OF live virus vaccines **Labs:** ↑ LFTs, BUN, creatinine, cholesterol, triglycerides **NIPE:** Take w/o regard to food; ⊘ PRG while taking drug and for 12 wk after drug D/C

Sitagliptin Phosphate (Januvia) [Hypoglycemic/DPP-4 Inhibitor]
Uses: Type 2 DM combined w/ diet & exercise; monotherapy or combined w/ metformin or a thiazolidinedione **Action:** Dipeptidyl peptidase-4 (DPP-4) inhibitor; drug responds to elevated glucose levels by promoting release of insulin & ↓ of glucagon **Dose:** 100 mg PO OD; if CrCl > 30–50 mL/min use 50 mg PO OD; if CrCl < 30 mL/min or on dialysis use 25 mg PO OD **Caution:** [B, –]; **Contra:** ⊘ type 1 DM, DKA **Disp:** tabs 25, 50, 100 mg; **SE:** HA, URI, nasal congestion, pharyngitis **Interactions:** Monitor digoxin levels **Labs:** monitor LFTs, BUN/Crea **NIPE:** ⊘ children < 18 yr; monitor renal function < start drug & periodically.

Smallpox Vaccine (Dryvax) [Vaccine] Uses: Immunization against smallpox (variola virus) Action: Active immunization (live attenuated vaccinia virus) Dose: *Adults (routine nonemergency)* or all ages (emergency): 2–3 punctures w/ bifurcated needle dipped in vaccine into deltoid, posterior triceps muscle; check site for Rxn in 6–8; if major Rxn, site scabs, & heals, leaving scar; if mild/equivocal Rxn, repeat w/ 15 punctures Caution: [X, N/A] Contra: *Nonemergency use:* Febrile illness, immunosuppression, Hx eczema & their household contacts; *Emergency:* No absolute contraindications Disp: Vial for reconstitution: 100 million pock-forming Units/mL SE: Malaise, fever, regional lymphadenopathy, encephalopathy, rashes, spread of inoculation to other sites administered; Stevens–Johnson syndrome, eczema vaccinatum w/ severe disability NIPE: Virus transmission possible until scab separates from skin (14–21 days); avoid infant contact for 14 d

Sodium Bicarbonate [NaHCO$_3$] [Alkalinizing Agent] Uses: *Alkalinization of urine,* RTA, *metabolic acidosis, ↑ K⁺, TCA OD* Action: Alkalinizing agent Dose: *Adults.* Cardiac arrest: Initiate ventilation, 1 mEq/kg/dose IV; repeat 0.5 mEq/kg in 10 min once or based on acid–base status. *Metabolic acidosis:* 2–5 mEq/kg IV over 8 h & PRN based on acid–base status. *Alkalinize urine:* 4 g (48 mEq) PO, then 1–2 g q4h; adjust based on urine pH; 2 amp/1 L D$_5$W at 100–250 mL/h IV, monitor urine pH & serum bicarbonate. *Chronic renal failure:* 1–3 mEq/kg/d. *Distal RTA:* 1 mEq/kg/d PO. *Peds >1 y:* Cardiac arrest: See Adult dosage. *Peds <1 y:* ECC: Initiate ventilation, 1:1 dilution 1 mEq/mL dosed 1 mEq/kg IV; can repeat w/ 0.5 mEq/kg in 10 min ×1 or based on acid–base status. *Chronic renal failure:* See Adult dosage. *Distal RTA:* 2–3 mEq/kg/d PO. *Proximal RTA:* 5–10 mEq/kg/d; titrate based on serum bicarbonate. *Urine alkalinization:* 84–840 mg/kg/d (1–10 mEq/kg/d) in ÷ doses; adjust based on urine pH Caution: [C, ?] Contra: Alkalosis, ↑ Na⁺, severe pulmonary edema, ↓ Ca²⁺ Disp: Powder, tabs; 300 mg = 3.6 mEq; 325 mg = 3.8 mEq; 520 mg = 6.3 mEq; 600 mg = 7.3 mEq; 650 mg = 7.6 mEq; inj 1 mEq/1 mL, 4.2% (5 mEq/10 mL), 7.5% 8.92 mEq/mL, 8.4% (10 mEq/10 mL) vial or amp SE: Belching, edema, flatulence, ↑ Na⁺, metabolic alkalosis Notes: 1 g neutralizes 12 mEq of acid; 50 mEq bicarb = 50 mEq Na; can make 3 amps in 1 L D$_5$W = D$_5$NS w/ 150 mEq bicarb Interactions: ↑ Effects OF anorexiants, amphetamines, ephedrine, flecainide, mecamylamine, pseudoephedrine, quinidine, sympathomimetics; ↓ effects OF BBs, cefpodoxime, cefuroxime, ketoconazole, Li, MTX, quinolones, salicylates, sulfonylureas, tetracyclines Labs: False + urinary protein NIPE: ⊘ Take w/in 2 h of other drugs; ↑ risk of milk-alkali syndrome w/ long-term use or when taken w/ milk

Sodium Citrate/Citric Acid (Bicitra) [Alkalinizing Agent] Uses: Chronic metabolic acidosis; alkalinize urine; dissolve uric acid & cysteine stones Action: Urinary alkalinizer Dose: *Adults.* 2–6 tsp (10–30 mL) diluted in 1–3 oz H$_2$O pc & hs. *Peds.* 1–3 tsp (5–15 mL) diluted in 1–3 oz H$_2$O pc & hs; best after meals **Caution:** [C, +] **Contra:** Aluminum-based antacids; severe renal impair or Na-restricted diets **Disp:** 15- or 30-mL unit dose: 16 (473 mL) or 4 (118 mL) fl oz **SE:** Cramp, metabolic alkalosis, ↑ K+, GI upset; avoid use of multiple 50-mL amps; can cause ↓ Na+/hyperosmolar **Notes:** 1 mL = 1 mEq Na & 1 mEq bicarb **Interactions:** ↑ Effects OF amphetamines; ephedrine, flecainide, pseudoephedrine, quinidine; ↓ effects OF barbiturates, chlorpropamide, Li, salicylates **NIPE:** Dilute w/ water; take pc to ⊘ laxative effect

Sodium Oxybate (Xyrem) [C-III] [Inhibitory Neurotransmitter]
Uses: *Narcolepsy-associated cataplexy* **Action:** Inhibitory neurotransmitter **Dose:** *Adults & Peds ≥ 16 y:* 2.25 g PO qhs, second dose 2.5–4 h later; may ↑ 9 g/d max **Caution:** [B, ?/−] **Contra:** Succinic semialdehyde dehydrogenase deficiency; potentiates EtOH **Disp:** 500 mg/mL 180-mL PO soln **SE:** Confusion, depression, diminished level of consciousness, incontinence, significant vomiting, resp depression, psychiatric Sxs **Notes:** May lead to dependence; synonym for {g}-hydroxybutyrate (GHB), abused as a "date rape drug"; controlled distribution (prescriber & pt registration); must be administered when pt in bed **Interactions:** ↑ Risk OF CNS depression w/ sedatives, hypnotics, EtOH **NIPE:** Dilute w/ 2 oz water, ⊘ eat w/in 2 h of taking this drug

Sodium Phosphate (Visicol) [Laxative]
Uses: Bowel prep prior to colonoscopy **Action:** Hyperosmotic laxative **Dose:** 3 tabs PO w/ at least 8 oz clear liq every 15 min (20 tabs total night before procedure); 3–5 h before colonoscopy, repeat) **Caution:** [C, ?] Renal impair, electrolyte disturbances **Contra:** Megacolon, bowel obstruction, CHF, ascites, unstable angina, gastric retention, bowel perforation, colitis, hypomotility **Disp:** Tablets 0.398, 1.102, 2 g **SE:** QT prolongation, D, ↑ Na+, flatulence, cramps **Interactions:** May bind with Al- & Mg-containing antacids and sucralfate; ↑ risk OF hypoglycemia w/ bisphosphonates; ↓ absorption OF other meds **Labs:** Monitor electrolytes; **NIPE:** Drink clear liq 12 h before start of this med; ⊘ take w/ drugs that prolong QT interval, ⊘ take other laxatives

Sodium Polystyrene Sulfonate (Kayexalate) [Potassium removing resin]
Uses: *↑ K+* **Action:** Na+/K+ ion-exchange resin **Dose:** *Adults.* 15–60 g PO or 30–60 g PR q6h based on serum K+. *Peds.* 1 g/kg/dose PO or PR q6h based on serum K+ (given w/ agent, eg, sorbitol, to promote movement through the bowel) **Caution:** [C, M] **Contra:** ↑ Na+ **Disp:** Powder; susp 15 g/60 mL sorbitol **SE:** Can cause ↑ Na+, ↓ K+, Na retention, GI upset, fecal impaction **Notes:** Enema acts more quickly than PO; PO most effective **Interactions:** ↑ Risk OF systemic alkalosis w/ Ca- or Mg-containing antacids **NIPE:** Mix w/ chilled fluid other than orange juice

Solifenacin (VESIcare) [Antispasmodic/Muscarinic Receptor Antagonist]
Uses: OAB **Action:** Antimuscarinic; ↓ detrusor contractions **Dose:** 5 mg PO qd, 10 mg/d max; ↓ w/ renal/hepatic impair **Caution:** [C, ?/−] Bladder outflow or GI obstruction, ulcerative colitis, MyG, renal/hepatic impair, QT prolongation risk **Contra:** NA glaucoma, urinary/gastric retention **Disp:** Tabs

, 10 mg **SE:** Constipation, xerostomia **Notes:** Do not ↑ dose w/ severe renal/moderate hepatic impair **Interactions:** ↑ Effects OF azole antifungals & other CYP3A4 inhibitors; ↑ risk OF prolonged QT interval w/ amiodarone, amitriptyline, bepridil, disopyramide, erythromycin, gatifloxacin, haloperidol, imipramine, moxifloxacin, quinidine, pimozide, procainamide, sparfloxacin, thioridazine; other drugs that prolong QT **Labs:** monitor BUN, Creatinine, LFTs **NIPE:** take w/ or w/o food, swallow whole w/ H₂0

orafenib (Nexavar) [Kinase Inhibitor] **Uses:** *Advanced RCC* metastatic liver cancer **Action:** Kinase inhibitor **Dose:** *Adults.* 400 mg PO bid on empty stomach **Caution:** [D,–] w/ irinotecan or doxorubicin **Disp:** Tabs 200 mg **SE:** Hand-foot syndrome; treatment-emergent hypertension; bleeding, ↑ INR, cardiac infarction/ischemia; ↑ pancreatic enzymes, hypophosphatemia, lymphopenia, anemia, fatigue, alopecia, pruritus, D, GI upset, HA, neuropathy **NIPE:** Monitor BP during first 6 wks; may require ↓ dose (QD or every other day); impaired metabolism w/Asian descent; unknown effect on wound healing, D/C for major surgery

orbitol (generic) [Laxative] **Uses:** *Constipation* **Action:** Laxative **Dose:** 30–60 mL PO of a 20–70% soln PRN **Caution:** [B, +] **Contra:** Anuria **Disp:** Liq 70% **SE:** Edema, electrolyte losses, lactic acidosis, GI upset, xerostomia **Notes:** May be vehicle for many liq formulations (eg, zinc, Kayexalate) **NIPE:** ⊘ Use unless soln clear

otalol (Betapace) [Antiarrhythmic, Antihypertensive/BB] **WARNING:** Monitor pts for 1st 3 d of Rx to ↓ risks of arrhythmia **Uses:** *Ventricular arrhythmias, AF* **Action:** β-Adrenergic-blocking agent **Dose:** *Adults.* 80 mg PO bid; may be ↑ to 240–320 mg/d. *Peds.* Neonates: 9 mg/m² tid. *1–19 mo:* 20 mg/m² tid. *20–23 mo:* 29.1 mg/m² tid. *≥ 2 y:* 30 mg/m² tid; ↓ in renal failure **Caution:** [B (1st tri) (D if 2nd or 3rd tri), +] **Contra:** Asthma, bradycardia, prolonged QT interval, 2nd- or 3rd-degree heart block w/o pacemaker, cardiogenic shock, uncontrolled CHF, CrCl <40 mL/min **Disp:** Tabs 80, 120, 160, 240 mg **SE:** Bradycardia, CP, palpitations, fatigue, dizziness, weakness, dyspnea **Notes:** Betapace should not be substituted for Betapace AF because of significant differences in labeling **Interactions:** ↑ Effects w/ ASA, antihypertensives, nitrates, oral contraceptives, fluoxetine, prazosin, sulfinpyrazone, verapamil, EtOH; ↑ risk OF prolonged QT interval w/ amiodarone, amitriptyline, bepridil, disopyramide, erythromycin, gatifloxacin, haloperidol, imipramine, moxifloxacin, quinidine, pimozide, thioridazine; ↑ effects OF lidocaine; ↓ effects w/ antacids, clonidine, NSAIDs, thyroid drugs; ↓ effects OF hypoglycemics, terbutaline, theophylline **Labs:** ↑ BUN, serum glucose, lipoprotein, triglycerides, K⁺, uric acid **NIPE:** May ↑ sensitivity to cold; D/C MAOIs 14 d before drug; take w/o food

otalol (Betapace AF) [Antiarrhythmic, Antihypertensive/BB] **WARNING:** To minimize risk of induced arrhythmia, pts initiated/

reinitiated on Betapace AF should be placed for a minimum of 3 d (on their mair dose) in a facility that can provide cardiac resuscitation, continuous ECG monitor ing, & calculations of CrCl; Betapace should not be substituted for Betapace AF be cause of labeling differences **Uses:** *Maintain sinus rhythm for symptomatic A fib/flutter* **Action:** β-Adrenergic-blocking agent **Dose:** *Adults.* Initial CrCl >6(mL/min: 80 mg PO q12h. *CrCl 40–60 mL/min:* 80 mg PO q2h; ↑ to 120 mg during hospitalization; monitor QT interval 2–4 h after each dose, w/ dose reduction or D/C if QT interval >500 ms. *Peds.* Neonates: 9 mg/m² tid. *1–19 mo:* 20 mg/m² tid. *20–23 mo:* 29.1 mg/m² tid. ≥ 2 y: 30 mg/m² tid; can double all dosages as max daily dose; allow ≥ 36 h between dosage titrations **Caution:** [B (1st tri; D if 2nd or 3r tri), +] if converting from previous antiarrhythmic therapy **Contra:** Asthma, brady cardia, prolonged QT interval, 2nd- or 3rd-degree heart block w/o pacemaker, car diogenic shock, uncontrolled CHF, CrCl <40 mL/min **Disp:** Tabs 80, 120, 160 mg **SE:** Bradycardia, CP, palpitations, fatigue, dizziness, weakness, dyspnea **Notes** Follow renal Fxn & QT interval **Interactions:** ↑ risk of prolonged QT interval w amiodarone, amitriptyline, bepridil, disopyramide, erythromycin, gatifloxacin haloperidol, imipramine, moxifloxacin, quinidine, pimozide, procainamide sparfloxacin, TCAs, thioridazine; ↑ effects w/ general anesthesia, phenytoin admin istered IV, verapamil; ↓ effects of insulin, oral hypoglycemics; ↑ risk of hypoten sion w/ antihypertensives, ASA, bismuth sub-salicylate, magnesium salicylate sulfinpyrazone, nitrates, oral contraceptives, ETOH; ↑ CV reactions w/ CCB digoxin; ↑ risk OF severe HTN if used within 14 days of MAOIs; ↓ effects w antacids; ↓ effects OF beta-adrenergic bronchodilators, dopamine, dobutamine theophylline **Labs:** ↑ ANA titers, BUN, K⁺,serum glucose, serum lipoprotein triglycerides, uric acid; may effect GTT **NIPE:** ⊘ D/C abruptly after long-term use; take w/o food; administer antacids 2 hr < or > sotalol

Sparfloxacin (Zagam) [Antibiotic/Fluoroquinolone] Uses

Community-acquired pneumonia, acute exacerbations of chronic bronchitis **Ac tion:** Quinolone; ↓ DNA gyrase **Dose:** 400 mg PO day 1, then 200 mg q24h × 10 d; ↓ in renal impair **Caution:** [C, ?/–] W/ theophylline, caffeine, sucralfate warfarin, & antacids **Contra:** w/QT prolongation & drugs that prolong QT inter val **Disp:** Tabs 200 mg **SE:** restlessness, N/V/D, rash, sleep disorders, confusion convulsions **Interactions:** ↑ Effects w/ cimetidine, probenecid; ↑ effects OF cy closporine, diazepam, metoprolol, theophylline, warfarin, caffeine; ↑ risk OF pro longed QT interval w/ amiodarone, bepridil, disopyramide, erythromycin pentamidine, phenothiazines, procainamide, propranolol, quinidine, sotalol, TCAs ↓ effects w/ antacids, antineoplastics, didanosine, sucralfate **Labs:** ↑ LFTs **NIPE:** ↑ Risk of tendon rupture; photosensitivity—use sunscreen, Protect from sunlight up to 5 d after last dose; take w/o food; ↑ fluids to 2–3 L/d

Spironolactone (Aldactone) [Potassium Sparing Diuretic

Uses: *Hyperaldosteronism, ascites from CHF or cirrhosis* **Action:** Aldosterone antagonist; K⁺-sparing diuretic **Dose:** *Adults.* 25–100 mg PO qid; CHF (NYHA class III–IV) 25–50 mg/d. *Peds.* 1–3.3 mg/kg/24 h PO ÷ bid–qid. *Neonates:* 0.5–1 mg/kg/dose q8h; w/ food **Caution:** [D, +] **Contra:** ↑ K+, renal failure, anuria **Disp:** Tabs 25, 50, 100 mg **SE:** arrhythmia, sexual dysfunction, confusion, dizziness **Interactions:** ↑ Risk OF hyperkalemia w/ACEIs, K supls, K-sparing diuretics, ↑ K diet; ↑ effects OF Li; ↓ effects w/ salicylates; ↓ effects OF anticoagulants **Labs:** ↑ K+, false ↑ of corticosteroids, digoxin **NIPE:** Take w/ food; ↑ risk of gynecomastia; maximum effects of drug may take 2–3 wk

Stavudine (Zerit) [Antiretroviral/Reverse Transcriptase Inhibitor] **WARNING:** Lactic acidosis & severe hepatomegaly w/ steatosis & pancreatitis reported **Uses:** *Advanced HIV* **Action:** Reverse transcriptase inhibitor **Dose:** *Adults.* >60 kg: 40 mg bid. *<60 kg:* 30 mg bid. *Peds.* Birth–13 d: 0.5 mg/kg q12h. *>14 d & <30 kg:* 1 mg/kg q12h. *≥30 kg:* Adult dose; ↓ in renal insuff/failure **Caution:** [C, +] **Contra:** Allergy **Disp:** Caps 15, 20, 30, 40 mg; soln 1 mg/mL **SE:** Peripheral neuropathy, HA, chills, fever, malaise, rash, GI upset, anemias, lactic acidosis, pancreatitis **Interactions:** ↑ Risk of pancreatitis w/ didanosine; ↑ effects w/ probenecid; ↓ effects w/ zidovudine **Labs:** ↑ LFTs **NIPE:** Take w/o regard to food; Take w/ plenty of H_2O

Steroids, Systemic [Glucocorticoid] (See also Table 4) The following relates only to the commonly used systemic glucocorticoids **Uses:** *Endocrine disorders* (adrenal insuff), *rheumatoid disorders, collagen–vascular Dzs, dermatologic Dzs, allergic states, cerebral edema,* nephritis, nephrotic syndrome, immunosuppression for transplantation, ↑ Ca^{2+}, malignancies (breast, lymphomas), preop (in any pt who has been on steroids in the previous year, known hypoadrenalism, preop for adrenalectomy); inj into joints/tissue **Action:** Glucocorticoid **Dose:** Varies w/ use & institutional protocols. *Adrenal insuff, acute:* **Adults.** Hydrocortisone: 100 mg IV; then 300 mg/d ÷ q6h; convert to 50 mg PO q8h ×6 doses, taper to 30–50 mg/d ÷ bid. **Peds.** Hydrocortisone: 1–2 mg/kg IV, then 150–250 mg/d ÷ tid. *Adrenal insuff, chronic (physiologic replacement):* May need mineralocorticoid supl such as Florinef. **Adults.** Hydrocortisone 20 mg PO qAM, 10 mg PO qPM; cortisone 0.5–0.75 mg/kg/d ÷ bid; cortisone 0.25–0.35 mg/kg/d IM; dexamethasone 0.03–0.15 mg/kg/d or 0.6–0.75 mg/m²/d ÷ q6–12h PO, IM, IV. **Peds.** Hydrocortisone: 0.5–0.75 mg/kg/d PO tid; hydrocortisone succinate 0.25–0.35 mg/kg/d IM. *Asthma, acute:* **Adults.** Methylprednisolone 60 mg PO/IV q6h or dexamethasone 12 mg IV q6h. **Peds.** Prednisolone 1–2 mg/kg/d or prednisone 1–2 mg/kg/d ÷ qd–bid for up to 5 d; methylprednisolone 1 mg/kg IV q6h ÷ tid; dexamethasone 0.1–0.3 mg/kg/d divided q6h. *Congenital adrenal hyperplasia:* **Peds.** Initial hydrocortisone 30–36 mg/m²/d PO ÷ ⅓ dose qAM, {2/3} dose qPM; maint 20–25 mg/m²/d ÷ bid. *Extubation/airway edema:* **Adults.** Dexamethasone 0.5–1 mg/kg/d IM/IV ÷ q6h (start 24 h prior to extubation; continue × 4 more doses). **Peds.** Dexamethasone 0.1–0.3 mg/kg/d ÷ q6h × 3–5 d (start 48–72h before extubation) *Immunosuppressive/antiinflammatory:* **Adults & Older Peds.** Hydrocortisone: 15–240 mg PO, IM, IV q12h; *methylprednisolone:* 4–48 mg/d PO, taper to lowest effective dose;

methylprednisolone Na succinate: 10–80 mg/d IM. *Adults.* Prednisone or pred-nisolone: 5–60 mg/d PO ÷ qd–qid. *Infants & Younger Children.* Hydrocortisone 2.5–10 mg/kg/d PO ÷ q6–8h; 1–5 mg/kg/d IM/IV ÷ bid. *Nephrotic syndrome Peds.* Prednisolone or prednisone 2 mg/kg/d PO tid–qid until urine is protein-free for 5 d, use up to 28 d; for persistent proteinuria, 4 mg/kg/dose PO qod max 120 mg/d for an additional 28 d; maint 2 mg/kg/dose qod for 28 d; taper over 4–6 wk (max 80 mg/d). *Septic shock* (controversial): *Adults.* Hydrocortisone 500 mg–1 g IM/IV q2–6h. *Peds.* Hydrocortisone 50 mg/kg IM/IV, repeat q4–24 h PRN. *Status asthmaticus: Adults & Peds.* Hydrocortisone 1–2 mg/kg/dose IV q6h; then ↓ by 0.5–1 mg/kg q6h. *Rheumatic Dz: Adults.* Intraarticular: Hydrocortisone acetate 25–37.5 mg large joint, 10–25 mg small joint; methylprednisolone acetate 20–80 mg large joint, 4–10 mg small joint. *Intrabursal:* Hydrocortisone acetate 25–37.5 mg. *Intraganglial:* Hydrocortisone acetate 25–37.5 mg. *Tendon sheath:* Hydrocortisone acetate 5–12.5 mg. *Periop steroid coverage:* Hydrocortisone 100 mg IV night before surgery, 1 h preop, intraop, & 4, 8, & 12 h postop; postop d #1 100 mg IV q6h; postop d #2 100 mg IV q8h; postop d #3 100 mg IV q12h; postop d #4 50 mg IV q12h; postop d #5 25 mg IV q12h; resume prior PO dosing if chronic use or D/C if only periop coverage required. *Cerebral edema:* Dexamethasone 10 mg IV then 4 mg IV q4–6h **Caution:** [C, ?/–] **Contra:** Active varicella Infxn, serious Infxn except TB, fungal Infxns **Disp:** See Table 4, **SE:** All can cause ↑ appetite, hyperglycemia, ↓ K⁺, osteoporosis, nervousness, insomnia, "steroid psychosis," adrenal suppression **Notes:** Hydrocortisone succinate for systemic, acetate for in-traarticular **NIPE:** Never abruptly D/C steroids, especially in chronic Rx; taper dose

Streptokinase (Streptase, Kabikinase) [Thrombolytic En-zyme]

Uses: *Coronary artery thrombosis, acute massive PE, DVT, & some occluded vascular grafts* **Action:** Activates plasminogen to plasmin that degrades fibrin **Dose:** *Adults.* PE: Load 250,000 Units peripheral IV over 30 min, then 100,000 Units/h IV for 24–72 h. *Coronary artery thrombosis:* 1.5 million Units IV over 60 min. *DVT or arterial embolism:* Load as w/ PE, then 100,000 Units/h for 72 h. *Peds.* 3500–4000 Units/kg over 30 min, followed by 1000–1500 Units/kg/h. *Occluded catheter* (controversial): 10,000–25,000 Units IN NS to final volume of catheter (leave in place for 1h, aspirate & flush catheter w/ NS) **Caution:** [C, +] **Contra:** Streptococcal Infxn or streptokinase in last 6 mo, active bleeding, CVA, TIA, spinal surgery, or trauma in last month, vascular anomalies, severe hepatic or renal Dz, endocarditis, pericarditis, severe uncontrolled HTN **Disp:** Powder for inj 250,000, 750,000, 1,500,000 units **SE:** Bleeding, ↓ BP, fever, bruising, rash, GI upset, hemorrhage, anaphylaxis **Notes:** If maint inf inadequate to maintain throm-bin clotting time 2–5× control, see package insert for adjustments; antibodies re-main 3–6 mo following dose **Interactions:** ↑ Risk OF bleeding w/ anticoagulants, ASA, heparin, indomethacin, NSAIDs, dong quai, feverfew, garlic, ginger, horse chestnut, red clover; ↓ effects w/ aminocaproic acid **Labs:** ↑ PT, PTT

Streptomycin [Antibiotic/Aminoglycoside] Uses: *TB,* streptococcal or enterococcal endocarditis **Action:** Aminoglycoside; interferes w/ protein synthesis **Dose:** *Adults.* Endocarditis: 1 g q12h 1–2 wk, then 500 mg q12h 1–4 wk; *TB:* 15 mg/kg/d (up to 1 g), directly observed therapy (DOT) 2×wk 20–30 mg/kg/dose (max 1.5gm), DOT 3×wk 25–30 mg/kg/dose (max 1g). *Peds.* 15 mg/kg/d; DOT 2×wk 20–40 mg/kg/dose (max 1 g); DOT 3×wk 25–30 mg/kg/dose (max 1 g); ↓ in renal failure insuff, either IM or IV over 30–60 min **Caution:** [D, +] **Contra:** PRG **Disp:** Inj 400 mg/mL (1-g vial) **SE:** ↑ incidence of vestibular & auditory tox, neurotox, nephrotox **Notes:** Monitor levels: peak 20–30 mcg/mL, trough < 5 mcg/mL; toxic peak > 50, trough > 10; IV over 30–60 min **Interactions:** ↑ Risk OF nephrotoxicity w/ amphotericin B, cephalosporins, cisplatin, methoxyflurane, polymyxin B, vancomycin; ↑ risk OF ototoxicity w/ carboplatin, furosemide, mannitol, urea; ↑ effects OF anticoagulants **Labs:** False + urine glucose, false ↑ urine protein **NIPE:** ↑ Fluid intake

Streptozocin (Zanosar) [Alkylating Agent/Nitrosourea] Uses: *Pancreatic islet cell tumors* & carcinoid tumors **Action:** DNA–DNA (interstrand) cross-linking; DNA, RNA, & protein synthesis inhibitor **Dose:** Per protocol; ↓ in renal failure **Caution:** w/renal failure [D, ?/–] **Contra:** Caution in PRG **Disp:** Inj 1 g **SE:** N/V, duodenal ulcers; myelosuppression rare (20%) & mild; nephrotox (proteinuria & azotemia often heralded by hypophosphatemia) dose-limiting; hypo-/hyperglycemia; inj site Rxns **Interactions:** ↑ Risk OF nephrotoxicity w/ aminoglycosides, amphotericin B, cisplatin, vancomycin; ↑ effects OF doxorubicin; ↓ effects w/ phenytoin **Labs:** Monitor Cr. **NIPE:** ⊘ PRG, breast-feeding; ↑ fluid intake to 2–3 L/d

Succimer (Chemet) [Chelating Agent] Uses: *Lead poisoning (levels >45 mcg/mL)* **Action:** Heavy-metal chelating agent **Dose:** *Adults & Peds.* 10 mg/kg/dose q8h × 5 d, then 10 mg/kg/dose q12h for 14 d; ↓ in renal impair **Caution:** [C, ?] **Contra:** Allergy **Disp:** Caps 100 mg **SE:** Rash, fever, GI upset, hemorrhoids, metallic taste, drowsiness, **Notes:** Monitor lead levels, maintain hydration, may open capsules **Labs:** ↑ LFTs; false + urinary ketones, false ↑ serum CPK, false ↓ uric acid **NIPE:** ⊘ Take w/ other chelating agents; ↑ fluid intake to 2–3 L/d

Succinylcholine (Anectine, Quelicin, Sucostrin, others) [Skeletal Muscle Relaxant] WARNING: Risk of cardiac arrest from hyperkalemic rhabdomyolysis Uses: *Adjunct to general anesthesia to facilitate ET intubation & to induce skeletal muscle relaxation during surgery or mechanical ventilation* **Action:** Depolarizing neuromuscular blocking agent **Dose:** *Adults.* 1–1.5 mg/kg IV over 10–30 s, then followed by 0.04–0.07 mg/kg or 10-100 mcg/kg/min inf. *Peds.* 1–2 mg/kg/dose IV, then followed by 0.3–0.6 mg/kg/dose q5min use of CI not OK; ↓ w/ severe liver/hepatic impair **Caution:** See warning [C, M] **Contra:** If risk for malignant hyperthermia; myopathy; skeletal myopathy in children; recent major burn, multiple trauma, extensive skeletal muscle denervation; pseudocholinesterase deficiency **Disp:** Inj 20, 50, 100 mg/mL; **SE:** May precipitate malignant hyperthermia, resp depression, or prolonged apnea; multiple drugs potentiate; observe for CV effects (arrhythmias, ↓ BP, brady/tachycardia), ↑ intraocular pressure, postop stiffness, salivation, myoglobinuria **Notes:** May be given IVP or inf or IM in the deltoid; hyperkalemic rhabdomyolysis in children with undiagnosed myopathy such as Duchenne muscular dystrophy **Interactions:** ↑ Effects w/ amphotericin B, aprotinin, BBs, clindamycin, lidocaine, Li, metoclopramide, oral contraceptives, oxytocin, phenothiazines, procainamide, procaine, quinidine, quinine, trimethaphan; ↓ effect w/ diazepam **Labs:** ↑ Serum K+

Sucralfate (Carafate) [Antiulcer Agent/pepsin inhibitor]
Uses: *Duodenal ulcers,* gastric ulcers, stomatitis, GERD, preventing stress ulcers, esophagitis **Action:** Forms ulcer-adherent complex that protects against acid, pepsin, & bile acid **Dose:** *Adults.* 1 g PO qid, 1 h prior to meals & hs. *Peds.* 40–80 mg/kg/d ÷ q6h; continue 4–8 wk unless healing demonstrated by x-ray or endoscopy; separate from other drugs by 2 h; on empty stomach ac **Caution:** [B, +] **Contra:** Component allergy **Disp:** Tabs 1 g; susp 1 g/10 mL **SE:** Constipation frequent; D, dizziness, xerostomia **Notes:** Aluminum may accumulate in renal failure **Interactions:** ↓ Effects OF cimetidine, digoxin, levothyroxine, phenytoin, quinolones, quinidine, ranitidine, tetracyclines, theophylline, warfarin **NIPE:** Take w/o food

Sulfacetamide (Bleph-10, Cetamide, Sodium Sulamyd) [Antibiotic] **Uses:** *Conjunctival Infxns* **Action:** Sulfonamide antibiotic **Dose:** 10% oint apply qid & hs; soln for keratitis apply q2–3h based on severity **Caution:** [C, M] **Contra:** Sulfonamide sensitivity; age <2 mo **Disp:** Oint 10%; soln 10, 15, 30% **SE:** Irritation, burning; blurred vision, brow ache, Stevens–Johnson syndrome, photosensitivity **Interactions:** ↓ Effects w/ tetracyclines **NIPE:** Not compatible w/ Ag-containing preps; purulent exudate inactivates drug; ↑ risk OF photosensitivity—use sunscreen

Sulfacetamide & Prednisolone (Blephamide, others) [Antibiotic, Anti-inflammatory] **Uses:** *Steroid-responsive inflammatory ocular conditions w/ Infxn or a risk of Infxn* **Action:** Antibiotic & antiinflammatory **Dose:** *Adults & Peds >2 y.* Apply oint to lower conjunctival sac qd–qid; soln 1–3 gtt 2–3 h while awake **Caution:** [C, ?/–] Sulfonamide sensitivity; age <2 mo **Disp:** Oint sulfacetamide 10%/prednisolone 0.5%, sulfacetamide 10%/prednisolone 0.2%, sulfacetamide 10%/prednisolone 0.25%; susp sulfacetamide 10%/prednisolone 0.25%, sulfacetamide 10%/prednisolone 0.5%, sulfacetamide 10%/prednisolone 0.2% **SE:** Irritation, burning, blurred vision, brow ache, Stevens–Johnson syndrome, photosensitivity **Notes:** Ophth susp can be used as an otic agent **Interactions:** ↓ Effects w/ tetracyclines **NIPE:** Not compatible w/ Ag-containing preps; purulent exudate inactivates drug; ↑ risk of sensitivity to light; ① D/C abruptly

Sulfasalazine (Azulfidine, Azulfidine EN) [Anti-inflammatory, Antirheumatic (DMARD)/Sulfonamide] **Uses:** *Ulcerative colitis, RA, juvenile RA,* active Crohn Dz, ankylosing spondylitis, psoriasis **Action:** Sulfonamide; actions unclear **Dose:** *Adults.* Initial, 1 g PO tid–qid; ↑ to a max of 8 g/d in 3–4 ÷ doses; maint 500 mg PO qid. *Peds.* Initial, 40–60 mg/kg/24 h PO ÷ q4–6h; maint, 20–30 mg/kg/24 h PO ÷ q6h. *RA >6 y:* 30–50 mg/kg/d in 2 doses, start w/ ¼-⅓ maint dose, ↑ weekly until dose reached at 1 mo, 2 g/d max; ↓ in renal failure **Caution:** [B (D if near term), M] **Contra:** Sulfonamide or salicylate sensitivity, porphyria, GI or GU obstruction; avoid in hepatic impair **Disp:** Tabs 500 mg; EC tabs 500 mg; EC delayed release tabs 500 mg; PO susp 250 mg/5 mL **SE:** Can cause severe GI upset; discolors urine; dizziness, HA, photosensitivity, oligospermia, anemias, Stevens–Johnson syndrome **Interactions:** ↑ Effects OF anticoagulants, hypoglycemics, MTX, phenytoin, zidovudine; ↓ effects w/ antibiotics; ↓ effects OF digoxin, folic acid, Fe, procaine, proparacaine, sulfonylureas, tetracaine **Labs:** False + urinary glucose; false ↑ serum conjugated bilirubin, creatinine; false ↓ serum unconjugated bilirubin, K⁺ **NIPE:** Take pc; ↑ fluids to 2–3 L/d; ↑ risk of photosensitivity—use sunscreen; skin & urine may become yellow-orange; may stain contact lenses

Sulfinpyrazone (Anturane) [Uricosuric/Antigout Agent]
Uses: *Acute & chronic gout* **Action:** ↓ renal tubular absorption of uric acid **Dose:** 100–200 mg PO bid for 1 wk, ↑ PRN to maint of 200–400 mg bid; max 800 mg/d; take w/ food or antacids, & plenty of fluids; avoid salicylates **Caution:** [C (D if near term), ?/–] **Contra:** Renal impair, avoid salicylates; peptic ulcer; blood dyscrasias, near term PRG, allergy **Disp:** Tabs 100 mg; caps 200 mg **SE:** N/V, stomach pain, urolithiasis, leukopenia **Interactions:** ↑ Effects OF anticoagulants, hypoglycemics, MTX; ↓ effects w/ ASA, cholestyramine, niacin, salicylates, EtOH; ↓ effects OF acetaminophen, BBs, nitrofurantoin, theophylline, verapamil **Labs:** ↓ Serum uric acid **NIPE:** Take w/ food, ↑ fluids to 2–3 L/d

Sulindac (Clinoril) [Analgesic, Anti-inflammatory, Antipyretic/NSAID]
WARNING: May ↑ risk of cardiovascular events & GI bleeding **Uses:** *Arthritis & pain* **Action:** NSAID; ↓ prostaglandins **Dose:** 150–200 mg bid w/ food **Caution:** [B (D if 3rd tri or near term), ?] **Contra:** NSAID or ASA sensitivity, ulcer, GI bleeding **Disp:** Tabs 150, 200 mg **SE:** Dizziness, rash, GI upset, pruritus, edema, ↓ renal blood flow, renal failure (May have fewer renal effects than other NSAIDs), peptic ulcer, GI bleeding **Interactions:** ↑ Effects w/ NSAIDs, probenecid; ↑ effects OF aminoglycosides, anticoagulants, cyclosporine, digoxin, Li, MTX, K-sparing diuretics; ↑ risk of bleeding w/ ASA, NSAIDs, EtOH, dong quai, feverfew, garlic, ginger, horse chestnut, red clover; ↓ effects w/ antacids, ASA; ↓ effects OF BBs, captopril, diuretics, hydralazine **Labs:** ↑ Serum Cl, Na, glucose, LFTs, PT **NIPE:** Take w/ food; ↑ risk of photosensitivity—use sunscreen; may take several weeks for full drug effect

Sumatriptan (Imitrex) [Antimigraine Agent/Selective 5 HT1 Receptor Agonist]
Uses: Rx acute migraine attacks **Action:** Vascular serotonin receptor agonist **Dose:** *Adults.* SQ: 6 mg SQ as a single dose PRN; repeat

PRN in 1 h to a max of 12 mg/24 h. *PO:* 25 mg, repeat in 2 h, PRN, 100 mg/d max PO dose; max 300 mg/d. *Nasal spray:* 1 spray into 1 nostril, repeat in 2 h to 40 mg/24 h max. **Peds.** Nasal spray: 6–9 y: 5–20 mg/d. *12–17 y:* 5–20 mg, up to 40 mg/d **Caution:** [C, M] **Contra:** Angina, ischemic heart Dz, uncontrolled HTN, ergot use, MAOI use w/in 14 d **Disp:** Inj 6, 8, 12 mg/mL; orally disintegrating tabs 25, 50, 100 mg; nasal spray 5, 10, 20 mg/spray **SE:** Pain & bruising at site; dizziness, hot flashes, paresthesias, CP, weakness, numbness, coronary vasospasm, HTN **Interactions:** ↑ Effects OF weakness, incoordination and hyperreflexia w/ ergots, MAOIs, and SSRIs, horehound, St. John's wort **NIPE:** Admin drug as soon as possible after onset of migraine

Sunitinib (Sutent) [Kinase Inhibitor]
Uses: *Advanced GI stromal tumor refractory/intolerant of imatinib; advanced RCC* **Action:** Kinase inhibitor **Dose:** *Adults.* 50 mg PO daily (times) 4 wks, followed by 2 wk holiday = 1 cycle; ↓ to 37.5 mg w/CYP3A4 inhibitors (Table 13), to ↑ 87.5 mg w/CYP3A4 inducers (PRN) **Caution:** [D,–] Multiple interactions require dose modification (eg, St. John's wort) **Disp:** Caps 12.5, 25, 50 mg **SE:** ↑ WBC & plt, bleeding, ↑ BP, ↓ ejection fraction, ↑ QT interval, pancreatitis, DVT, seizures, adrenal insufficiency, N, V, D, skin discoloration, oral ulcers, taste perversion, hypothyroidism **LABS:** Monitor CBC, platelets, chemistries at cycle onset; baseline cardiac fxn recommended **NIPE:** ↓ dose in 12.5-mg increments if not tolerated

Tacrine (Cognex) [Anti-Alzheimer Agent/Centrally Acting Reversible Cholinesterase Inhibitor]
Uses: *Mild–moderate Alzheimer dementia* **Action:** Cholinesterase inhibitor **Dose:** 10–40 mg PO qid to 160 mg/d; separate doses from food **Caution:** [C, ?] **Contra:** Previous tacrine-induced jaundice **Disp:** Caps 10, 20, 30, 40 mg **SE:** LFT, HA, dizziness, GI upset, flushing, confusion, ataxia, myalgia, bradycardia **Interactions:** ↑ Effects w/ cimetidine, quinolones, SSRIs, ↑ effects OF BBs, cholinergics, cholinesterase inhibitors, succinylcholine, theophylline; ↓ effects w/ tobacco, food; ↓ effects OF anticholinergics, levodopa **Labs:** ↑ LFTs **NIPE:** If taken w/ food ↓ drug plasma levels by 30%; may take up to 6 wk for ALT elevations–monitor LFTs; serum conc > 20 mg/mL have more SE

Tacrolimus [FK 506] (Prograf, Protopic) [Immunosuppressant]
Uses: *Prevent organ rejection, eczema* **Action:** Macrolide immunosuppressant **Dose:** *Adults.* IV: 0.05–0.1 mg/kg/d cont inf. *PO:* 0.15–0.3 mg/kg/d ÷ 2 doses. **Peds.** IV: 0.03–0.05 mg/kg/d as cont inf. *PO:* 0.15–0.2 mg/kg/d PO ÷ q 12 h. **Adults & Peds.** Eczema: Apply bid, continue 1 wk after clearing; ↓ in hepatic/renal impair **Caution:** [C, –] Do not use w/ cyclosporine; avoid topical if < 2 yrs of age **Contra:** Component allergy **Disp:** Caps 1, 5 mg; inj 5 mg/mL; oint 0.03, 0.1% **SE:** Neurotox & nephrotox, HTN, edema, HA, insomnia, fever, pruritus, ↓ K+/↑ K+, hyperglycemia, GI upset, anemia, leukocytosis, tremors, paresthesias, pleural effusion, Szs, lymphoma **Lab:** Monitor levels **NIPE:** reports of ↑ cancer risk; topical use for short term & second line

Tadalafil (Cialis) [Anti-impotence Agent/PDE 5] Uses: *Erectile dysfunction **Action:** Phosphodiesterase 5 inhibitor; increases cGMP and NO levels; relaxes smooth muscles, dilates cavernosal arteries **Dose:** *Adults.* 10 mg PO before sexual activity w/o regard to meals (range 5–20 mg max); ↓ 5 mg (10 mg max) w/ renal/& hepatic insuff **Caution:** [B, –] 1 dose/72h w/CYP3A4 inhibitor (Table 13) **Contra:** Nitrates, α-blockers (except tamsulosin), severe hepatic insuff **Disp:** 5-, 10-, 20-mg tabs **SE:** HA, flushing, dyspepsia, rhinitis, back pain, myalgia **Notes:** Longest acting of class (36 h) **Interactions:** ↑ Effects w/ ketoconazole, ritonavir, and other cytochrome P450 CYP3A4 inhibitors; ↑ hypotension w/ antihypertensives, EtOH; ↓ effects w/ P450 CYP3A4 inducers such as rifampin, antacids **NIPE:** ↑ Risk of priapism; use barrier contraception to prevent STDs

Talc (Sterile Talc Powder) [Sclerosing Agent] Uses: *↓ recurrence of malignant pleural effusions (pleurodesis) **Action:** Sclerosing agent **Dose:** Mix slurry: 50 mL NS w/ 5-g vial, mix, distribute 25 mL into two 60-mL syringes, volume to 50 mL/syringe w/ NS. Infuse each into chest tube, flush w/ 25 mL NS. Keep tube clamped; have pt change positions q15min for 2 h, unclamp tube **Caution:** [X, –] **Contra:** Planned further surgery on site **Disp:** 5 g powder **SE:** Pain, Infxn **Notes:** May add 10–20 mL 1% lidocaine/syringe; must have chest tube placed, monitor closely while tube clamped (tension pneumothorax), not antineoplastic **NIPE:** Monitor for MI, PE, respiratory distress

Tamoxifen (Nolvadex) [Antineoplastic/Antiestrogen] WARNING: Cancer of the uterus, stroke, and blood clots can occur Uses: *Breast CA [postmenopausal, estrogen receptor(+)], reduction of breast CA in high-risk women, metastatic male breast CA,* Ductal carcinoma in situ, mastalgia, pancreatic CA, gynecomastia, ovulation induction **Action:** Nonsteroidal antiestrogen; mixed agonist–antagonist effect **Dose:** 20–40 mg/d (typically 10 mg bid or 20 mg/d); prevention: 10 mg PO bid (times) 5 y **Caution:** [D, –] leukopenia, thrombocytopenia, hyperlipidemia **Contra:** PRG, undiagnosed vag bleeding, h/o thromboembolism **Disp:** Tabs 10, 20 mg **SE:** Uterine malignancy & thrombotic events noted in breast CA prevention trials; menopausal Sxs (hot flashes, N/V) in premenopausal pts; vaginal bleeding & menstrual irregularities; skin rash, pruritus vulvae, dizziness, HA, peripheral edema; acute flare of bone metastasis pain & ↑ Ca^{2+}; retinopathy reported (high dose) **Notes:** ↑ risk of PRG in premenopausal women by inducing ovulation; brand Nolvadex suspended in US **Interactions:** ↑ Effects w/ bromocriptine, grapefruit juice; ↑ effects OF warfarin, cyclosporine, warfarin; ↓ effects w/ antacids, aminoglutethimide, letrozole, medroxyprogesterone, rifamycins **Labs:** ↑ Ca^{2+}, T_4, BUN, creatinine, LFTs **NIPE:** ⊘ PRG or breast-feeding; use barrier contraception; ↑ risk of photosensitivity—use sunscreen

Tamsulosin (Flomax) [Smooth Muscle Relaxant/Antiadrenergic] Uses: *BPH* **Action:** Antagonist of prostatic α-receptors **Dose:** 0.4 mg/d PO; do not crush, chew, or open caps **Caution:** [B, ?] **Contra:** Female gender **Disp:** Caps 0.4 mg **SE:** HA, dizziness, syncope, somnolence, ↓ libido, GI upset, retrograde ejaculation, rhinitis, rash, angioedema, IFIS **Notes:** Not for use as antihypertensive **Interactions:** ↑ Effects w/ cimetidine; ↑ hypotension w/ doxazosin, prazosin, terazosin **NIPE:** Ensure – test results for prostate CA before drug admin

Tazarotene (Tazorac) [Keratolytic/Retinoid] **Uses:** *Facial acne vulgaris; stable plaque psoriasis up to 20% body surface area* **Action:** Keratolytic **Dose:** *Adults & Peds >12 y.* Acne: Cleanse face, dry, & apply thin film qd hs on acne lesions. *Psoriasis:* Apply hs **Caution:** [X, ?/–] **Contra:** Retinoid sensitivity **Disp:** Gel 0.05, 0.1%; cream 0.05%, 0.1% **SE:** Burning, erythema, irritation, rash, photosensitivity, desquamation, bleeding, skin discoloration **Notes:** D/C w/ excessive pruritus, burning, skin redness or peeling occur until Sxs resolve **Interactions:** ↑ Risk OF photosensitivity w/ quinolones, phenothiazines, sulfonamides, tetracyclines, thiazide diuretics **NIPE:** ⊘ PRG or breast-feeding; use contraception; use sunscreen for ↑ photosensitivity risk

Tegaserod (Zelnorm) [Anti-irritable Bowel Agent/5-HT4 Receptor Agonist] **WARNING:** Drug sales have been suspended since 3/31/07 due to CV risks. Rare reports of ischemic colitis **Uses:** *Short-term Rx of constipation-predominant IBS in women; chronic idiopathic constipation in pts < 65 y* **Action:** 5HT4 serotonin agonist **Dose:** 6 mg PO bid pc for 4–6 wk; may continue for 2nd course **Caution:** Do not administer if D present, as GI motility ↑; [B, ?/–] **Contra:** Severe renal, moderate–severe hepatic impair, Hx of bowel obstruction, gallbladder Dz, sphincter of Oddi dysfunction, abdominal adhesions **Disp:** Tabs 2, 6 mg **SE:** Do not administer if D present, as GI motility ↑; D/C if abdominal pain worsens; **Labs:** Monitor bun, creatinine, LFTs; **NIPE:** Take ac; maintain hydration

Telbivudine (Tyzeka) [Antiretroviral, NRTI] **WARNING:** Lactic acidosis, severe hepatomegaly w/ steatosis, and myopathy reported; risk of hepatitis B reactivation **Uses:** Chronic hepatitis B **Action:** Nucleoside analogue reverse transcriptase inhibitor, resulting in viral DNA chain termination **Dose:** > 16 yr (CrCl > 50 mL/min) 600 mg PO OD; in renal impairment (CrCl 30–49 mL/min) 600 mg PO q 48 hrs; not on dialysis (CrCl < 30 mL/min) 600 mg PO q 72 hrs; ESRD 600 mg PO q 96 hrs given after dialysis; **Caution:** [B, –]; **Contra:** ⊘ in children < 16 yrs; **Disp:** Tabs 600 mg; **SE:** Fatigue, malaise, fever, joint pain, URI, HA, myalgia, myopathy **Interactions:** ↑ Risk of myopathy w/ azole antifungals, chloroquine, corticosteroids, cyclosporine, erythromycin, fibrates, hydroxychloroquine, niacin, penicillamine, statins, zidovudine; ↑ risk of renal impair w/ cyclosporine, tacrolimus; **Labs:** ↑ CPK; **NIPE:** Not a cure for hepatitis B, does not reduce transmission of hepatitis B by sexual contact or blood contamination

Telithromycin (Ketek) [Antibiotic/Macrolide Derivative] **WARNING:** May be associated with pseudomembranous colitis and hepatic failure **Uses:** *Acute bacterial exacerbations of chronic bronchitis, acute bacterial sinusitis; mild–moderate community-acquired pneumonia* **Action:** Unique macrolide, blocks protein synthesis; bacteriocidal. *Spectrum:* Staphylococcus aureus, Streptococcus pneumoniae, H. influenzae, M. catarrhalis, Chlamydophila pneumoniae, M. pneumoniae **Dose:** *Chronic bronchitis/sinusitis:* 800 mg (2 tabs) PO qd ×5; *Pneumonia:* 800 mg (2 tabs) PO qd × 7–10 d **Caution:** [C, M] pseudomembranous colitis, QTc interval prolongation, MyG exacerbations, visual disturbances, hepatic dysfunction; dosing in renal impair unknown **Contra:** Macrolide allergy, use w/ cisapride or pimozide **Disp:** Tabs 300, 400 mg **SE:** N/V/D, dizziness **Notes:** CYP450 inhibitor; multiple drug interactions **Interactions:** ↑ QT interval & arrhythmias w/ antiarrhythmics, mesoridazine, quinolone antibiotics, thioridazine; ↑ effects OF alprazolam, atorvastatin, benzodiazepines, CCBs, carbamazepine, cisapride, colchicine, cyclosporine, digoxin, ergot alkaloids, felodipine, lovastatin, mirtazapine, midazolam, nateglinide, nefazodone, pimozide, sildenafil, simvastatin, sirolimus, tacrolimus, tadalafil, triazolam, vardenafil, venlafaxine, verapamil; ↑ effects w/ azole antifungals, ciprofloxin, clarithromycin, diclofenac, doxycycline, erythromycin, imatinib, INH, nefazodone, nicardipine, propofol, protease inhibitors, quinidine, verapamil; ↓ effect w/ aminoglutethimide, carbamazepine, nafcillin, nevirapine, phenobarbital, phenytoin, rifampin, rifamycins **NIPE:** Take w/o regard to food; ⊘ chew or crush tablets

Telmisartan (Micardis) [Antihypertensive/ARB] Uses: *HTN, CHF,* DN **Action:** Angiotensin II receptor antagonist **Dose:** 40–80 mg/d **Caution:** [C (1st tri; D 2nd & 3rd tri). ?/–) **Contra:** Angiotensin II receptor antagonist sensitivity **Disp:** Tabs 20, 40, 80 mg **SE:** Edema, GI upset, HA, angioedema, renal impair, orthostatic ↓ BP **Interactions:** ↑ Effects w/ EtOH; ↑ effects OF digoxin; ↓ effects OF warfarin **Labs:** ↑ Creatinine, ↓ Hmg **NIPE:** Take w/o regard to food; ⊘ PRG; use barrier contraception

Temazepam (Restoril) [Sedative/Hypnotic/Benzodiazepine] [C-IV] Uses: *Insomnia,* anxiety, depression, panic attacks **Action:** Benzodiazepine **Dose:** 15–30 mg PO hs PRN; ↓ in elderly **Caution:** [X, ?/–] Potentiates CNS depressive effects of opioids, barbs, EtOH, antihistamines, MAOIs, TCAs **Contra:** NA glaucoma **Disp:** Caps 7.5, 15, 30 mg **SE:** Confusion, dizziness, drowsiness, hangover **Notes:** Abrupt D/C after >10 d use may cause withdrawal **Interactions:** ↑ Effects w/ cimetidine, disulfiram, kava kava, valerian; ↑ CNS depression w/ anticonvulsants, CNS depressants, EtOH; ↑ effects OF haloperidol, phenytoin; ↓ effects w/ aminophylline, dyphylline, oral contraceptives, oxtriphylline, rifampin, theophylline, tobacco; ↓ effects OF levodopa **NIPE:** ⊘ D/C abruptly after prolonged use, use in PRG or breast-feeding

Tenecteplase (TNKase) [Thrombolytic/Recombinant Tissue Plasminogen Activator] Uses: *Restore perfusion & ↓ mortality w/ AMI* **Action:** Thrombolytic; TPA **Dose:** 30–50 mg; see following table:

Tenecteplase Dosing

Weight (kg)	TNKase (mg)	TNKase[a] Volume (mL)
<60	30	6
≥60–70	35	7
≥70–80	40	8
≥80–90	45	9
≥90	50	10

[a]From one vial of reconstituted TNKase.

Caution: [C, ?], ↑ bleeding w/ NSAIDs, ticlopidine, clopidogrel, GPIIb/IIIa antagonists **Contra:** Bleeding, CVA, major surgery (intracranial, intraspinal) or trauma w/in 2 mo **Disp:** Inj 50 mg, reconstitute w/ 10 mL sterile H_2O **SE:** Bleeding, allergy **Notes:** Do not shake when reconstituting; do *not* use D_5W either in the IV line or to reconstitute **Interactions:** ↑ Risk OF bleeding w/ anticoagulants, ASA, clopidogrel, dipyridamole, ticlopidine, vitamin K antagonists; ↓ effects w/ aminocaproic acid **NIPE:** Eval for S/Sxs bleeding

Tenofovir (Viread) [Antiretroviral/NRTI] Uses: *HIV Infxn* **Action:** Nucleotide RT inhibitor **Dose**: 300 mg PO qd w/ a meal **Caution:** [B, ?/–] Didanosine (separate admin times), lopinavir, ritonavir w/ known risk factors for liver Dz **Contra:** CrCl <60 mL/min; **Disp:** Tabs 300 mg **SE:** GI upset, metabolic syndrome, hepatotox; separate didanosine doses by 2 h **Notes:** Take w/ fatty meal; combination product w/ emtricitabine known as Truvada **Interactions:** ↑ Effects w/ acyclovir, cidofovir, ganciclovir, indinavir, lopinavir, ritonavir, valacyclovir, food; ↓ effects OF didanosine, lamivudine, ritonavir **Labs:** ↑ LFTs, triglycerides, serum and urine glucose **NIPE:** Take w/ food, take 2 h before or 1 h after didanosine, lopinavir/ritonavir

Tenofovir/Emtricitabine (Truvada) [Antiretroviral, Dual NRTI] **WARNING:** Lactic acidosis & severe hepatomegaly with steatosis, including fatal cases, have been reported with the use of nucleoside analogs alone or in combo w/ other antiretrovirals. Not OK w/ chronic hepatitis; effects in patients co-infected with hepatitis B & HIV unknown **Uses:** *HIV Infxn* **Action:** Dual nucleotide RT inhibitor **Dose:** 300 mg PO qd w/ or w/o a meal **Caution:** W/ known risk factors for liver Dz [B, ?/–] **Contra:** CrCl <30 mL/min; **Disp:** Tabs 200 mg emtricitabine/300 mg tenofovir **SE:** GI upset, metabolic syndrome, hepatotox; **NIPE:** Take w/ fatty meal **Interactions:** ↑ Effects w/ acyclovir, cidofovir, ganciclovir, indinavir, lopinavir, ritonavir, valacyclovir, food; ↓ effects OF didanosine, lamivudine, ritonavir **Labs:** ↑ LFTs, triglycerides, serum and urine glucose **NIPE:** Take w/ food, take 2 h before or 1 h after didanosine, lopinavir/ritonavir; causes redistribution and accumulation of body fat; take w/ other antiretrovirals; not a cure for HIV or prevention of opportunistic infections

Terazosin (Hytrin) [Antihypertensive/Peripherally Acting Antiadrenergic] Uses: *BPH & HTN* Action: α₁-Blocker (blood vessel & bladder neck/prostate) **Dose:** Initial, 1 mg PO hs; ↑ 20 mg/d max **Caution:** [C, ?] ↑ ↓ BP w/ BB, CCB, ACEI **Contra:** α-Antagonist sensitivity **Disp:** Tabs 1, 2, 5, 10 mg; caps 1, 2, 5, 10 mg **SE:** ↓ BP & syncope following 1st dose; dizziness, weakness, nasal congestion, peripheral edema common; palpitations, GI upset **Notes:** Caution w/ 1st dose syncope; if for HTN, combine w/ thiazide diuretic **Interactions:** ↑ Effects w/ antihypertensives, diuretics; ↑ effects OF finasteride; ↓ effects w/ NSAIDs, α-blockers, ephedra, garlic, ginseng, saw palmetto, yohimbe; ↓ effects OF clonidine **Labs:** ↓ Albumin, Hmg, Hct, WBCs **NIPE:** Take w/o regard to food, ⊘ D/C abruptly

Terbinafine (Lamisil) [Antifungal] Uses: *Onychomycosis, athlete's foot, jock itch, ringworm,* cutaneous candidiasis, pityriasis versicolor Action: ↓ squalene epoxidase resulting in fungal death **Dose:** *PO:* 250 mg/d PO for 6–12 wk. *Topical:* Apply to area; ↓ in renal/hepatic impair **Caution:** [B, –] May ↑ effects of drug metab by CYP2D6 **Contra:** Liver Dz or kidney failure **Disp:** Tabs 250 mg; cream, gel, soln 1% **SE:** HA, dizziness, rash, pruritus, alopecia, GI upset, taste perversion, neutropenia, retinal damage, Stevens–Johnson syndrome **Notes:** Effect may take months due to need for new nail growth; do not use occlusive dressings **Interactions:** ↑ Effects w/ cimetidine; ↑ effects OF dextromethorphan, theophylline, caffeine; ↓ effects w/ rifampin; ↓ effects OF cyclosporine **Labs:** LFT abnormalities

Terbutaline (Brethine) [Bronchodilator/Sympathomimetic] Uses: *Reversible bronchospasm (asthma, COPD); inhibits labor* Action: Sympathomimetic; tocolytic **Dose:** *Adults.* Bronchodilator: 2.5–5 mg PO qid or 0.25 mg SQ; may repeat in 15 min (max 0.5 mg in 4 h). *Met-dose inhaler:* 2 inhal q4–6h. *Premature labor:* Acutely 2.5–10 mg/min/IV, gradually ↑ as tolerated q10–20min; maint 2.5–5 mg PO q4–6h until term *Peds.* PO: 0.05–0.15 mg/kg/dose PO tid; max 5 mg/24h; ↓ in renal failure **Caution:** [B, +] ↑ tox w/ MAOIs, TCAs; diabetes, HTN, hyperthyroidism **Contra:** Tachycardia, component allergy **Disp:** Tabs 2.5, 5 mg; inj 1 mg/mL; met-dose inhaler **SE:** HTN, hyperthyroidism; β₁-adrenergic effects w/ high dose; nervousness, trembling, tachycardia, HTN, dizziness **Interactions:** ↑ Effects w/ MAOIs, TCAs; ↓ effects w/ BBs **Labs:** ↑ LFTs, serum glucose **NIPE:** Take oral soln w/ food

Terconazole (Terazol 7) [Antifungal] Uses: *Vaginal fungal Infxns* **Action:** Topical antifungal **Dose:** 1 applicatorful or 1 supp intravag hs for 3–7 d **Caution:** [C, ?] **Contra:** Component allergy **Disp:** Vaginal cream 0.4%, 0.8%, vaginal supp 80 mg **SE:** Vulvar/vaginal burning **NIPE:** Insert cream or supp high into vagina, complete full course of Rx, ⊘ intercourse during drug Rx, ↑ risk of breakdown of latex condoms & diaphragms w/ drug

Teriparatide (Forteo) [Antiosteoporotic/Parathyroid Hormone] Uses: *Severe/refractory osteoporosis* **Action:** PTH (recombinant) **Dose:** 20 mcg SQ qd in thigh or abdomen **Caution:** [C, ?/–] **Contra:** w/ Paget's Dz, prior radiation, bone metastases, ↑ Ca²⁺; caution in urolithiasis **Disp:** 3-mL prefilled device (discard after 28 d) **SE:** Symptomatic orthostatic ↓ BP on administration, N/D, ↑ Ca, leg cramps **Notes:** OK for use > 2 y; osteosarcoma in animals **Labs:** ↑ Serum Ca²⁺, uric acid, urine Ca²⁺ **NIPE:** ⊘ Take if Hx Paget's Dz, bone mets or malignancy, or Hx radiation therapy; take w/o regard to food; not used to prevent osteoporosis

Testosterone (AndroGel, Androderm, Striant, Testim, Testoderm) [CIII] [Androgen Replacement] Uses: *Male hypogonadism* **Action:** Testosterone replacement; ↑ lean body mass, libido **Dose:** All daily AndroGel: 5 g gel. Androderm: two 2.5-mg or one 5-mg patch qd. Striant: 30-mg buccal tabs bid. Testim: one 5-g gel tube. Testoderm: one 4- or 6-mg scrotal patch **Caution:** [N/A, N/A] **Disp:** AndroGel, Testim: 5-gm gel (50-mg test). Androderm: 2.5-, 5-mg patches; Striant: 30-mg buccal tabs; Testoderm: 4- or 6-mg scrotal patch **SE:** Site Rxns, acne, edema, weight gain, gynecomastia, HTN, ↑ sleep apnea, prostate enlargement **Notes:** Injectable testosterone enanthate (Delatestryl; Testro-L.A.) & cypionate (Depo-Testosterone) require inj every 14–28 d with highly variable serum levels; PO agents (methyltestosterone & oxandrolone) associated w/ hepatitis/hepatic tumors; transdermal/mucosal forms preferred **Interactions:** OF Effects of anticoagulants, cyclosporine, insulin, hypoglycemics, oxyphenbutazone; ↑ effects w/ grapefruit juice; ↓ effects w/ St. John's wort **Labs:** ↑ AST, creatinine, Hgb, Hct, LDL, serum alkaline phosphatase, bilirubin, Ca, K & Na; ↓ HDL, thyroid hormones **NIPE:** Wear gloves if handling transdermal patches; topical drug may cause virilization in female partners. Apply Testoderm to dry shaved scrotal skin (⊘ use chemical depilatories), Androderm to nonscrotal skin, AndroGel to shoulder and upper arms, buccal system, on gum above incisors

Tetanus Immune Globulin [Tetanus Prophylaxis/Immune Serum] Uses: *Passive tetanus immunization* (suspected contaminated wound w/ unknown immunization status, see also Table 9) **Action:** Passive immunization **Dose:** *Adults & Peds.* 250–500 Units IM (higher dose w/ delayed Rx) **Caution:** [C, ?] **Contra:** Thimerosal sensitivity **Disp:** Inj 250-unit vial or syringe **SE:** Pain, tenderness, erythema at inj site; fever, angioedema, muscle stiffness, anaphylaxis **Notes:** May begin active immunization series at different inj site if required **Interactions:** ↓ Immune response when admin w/ Td **NIPE:** Drug does not cause AIDs or hepatitis

Tetanus Toxoid [Tetanus Prophylaxis/Vaccine] Uses: *Tetanus prophylaxis* (See also Table 9) **Action:** Active immunization **Dose:** Based on previous immunization (Table 9) **Caution:** [C, ?] **Contra:** Chloramphenicol use, neurologic Sxs w/ previous use, active Infxn (for routine primary immunization) **Disp:** Inj tetanus toxoid, fluid, 4–5 Lf Units/0.5 mL; tetanus toxoid, adsorbed, 5, 10 Lf Units/0.5 mL **SE:** Local erythema, induration, sterile abscess; chills, fever, neurologic disturbances **Interactions:** Delay of active immunity if given w/ tetanus immune globulin; ↓ immune response if given to pts taking corticosteroids or immunosuppressive drugs **NIPE:** Stress the need of timely completion of immunization series

Tetracycline (Achromycin V, Sumycin) [Antibiotic/Tetracycline] Uses: *Broad-spectrum antibiotic* **Action:** Bacteriostatic; ↓ protein synthesis. *Spectrum:* Gram(+): *Staphylococcus, Streptococcus.* Gram(–): *H. pylori.* Atypicals: *Chlamydia, Rickettsia, & Mycoplasma* **Dose:** *Adults.* 250–500 mg PO bid-qid. *Peds >8 y.* 25–50 mg/kg/24 h PO q6–12h; ↓ in renal/hepatic impair **Caution:** [D, +] **Contra:** PRG, antacids, dairy products; children ≤ 8 y **Disp:** Caps 100, 250, 500 mg; tabs 250, 500 mg; PO susp 250 mg/5 mL **SE:** Photosensitivity, GI upset, renal failure, pseudotumor cerebri, hepatic impair **Notes:** Can stain tooth enamel & depress bone formation in children **Interactions:** ↑ Effects OF anticoagulants, digoxin; ↓ effects w/ antacids, cimetidine, laxatives, penicillin, Fe supl, dairy products; ↓ effects OF oral contraceptives **Labs:** False – of urinary glucose, serum folate; false ↑ serum glucose **NIPE:** ⊘ Take w/ dairy products, take w/o food; use barrier contraception

Thalidomide (Thalomid) [Immunomodulatory Agent] Uses: *Erythema nodosum leprosum (ENL),* graft-versus-host Dz, aphthous ulceration in HIV(+) pts **Action:** ↓ Neutrophil chemotaxis, ↓ monocyte phagocytosis **Dose:** *GVHD:* 100–1600 mg PO qd. *Stomatitis:* 200 mg bid for 5 d, then 200 mg qd up to 8 wk. *ENL:* 100–300 mg PO qhs **Cautions:** [X, –] May ↑ HIV viral load; Hx Szs **Contra:** PRG; sexually active males not using latex condoms, or females not using 2 forms of contraception **Disp:** 50, 100, 200 mg cap; **SE:** Dizziness, drowsiness, rash, fever, orthostasis, Stevens–Johnson syndrome, peripheral neuropathy, Szs **Notes:** Health-care provider must register w/ STEPS risk management program; informed consent necessary; immediately D/C if rash develops **Interactions:** ↑ Effects OF barbiturates, CNS depressants, chlorpromazine, reserpine, ETOH; ↑ peripheral neuropathy w/ INH, Li, metronidazole, phenytoin **Labs:** Monitor LFTs, WBC, differential, PRG test before start of therapy & monthly during therapy **NIPE:** If also taking drugs that ↓ hormonal contraceptives (carbamazepine, griseofulvin, phenytoin, rifabutin, rifampin) use two other contraceptive methods; take 1 h pc—food will affect absorption; photosensitivity—use sunscreen; ⊘ PRG & breast-feeding

Theophylline (Theo24, TheoChron) [Bronchodilator/Xanthine Derivative] Uses: *Asthma, bronchospasm* **Action:** Relaxes smooth muscle of the bronchi & pulmonary blood vessels **Dose:** *Adults.* 900 mg PO ÷ q6h; SR products may be ÷ q8–12h (maint). *Peds.* 16–22 mg/kg/24 h PO ÷ q6h; SR products may be ÷

q8–12h (maint); ↓ in hepatic failure **Caution:** [C, +] Multiple interactions (eg, caffeine, smoking, carbamazepine, barbiturates, β-blockers, ciprofloxacin, E-mycin, INH, loop diuretics) **Contra:** Arrhythmia, hyperthyroidism, uncontrolled Szs **Disp:** Elixir 80 mg/15 mL; syrup 80, 150 mg/15 mL; caps 100, 200, 250 mg; tabs 100, 125, 200, 225, 250, 300 mg; SR caps 50, 75, 100, 125, 200, 250, 260, 300 mg; SR tabs 100, 125, 200, 250, 260, 300, SR tabs 100, 200, 300, 400, 450, 600 mg **SE:** N/V, tachycardia, & Szs; nervousness, arrhythmias **Notes:** See levels, Table 2 **Interactions:** ↑ effects w/ allopurinol, BBs, CCBs, cimetidine, corticosteroids, macrolide antibiotics, oral contraceptives, quinolones, rifampin, tacrine, tetracyclines, verapamil, zileuton; ↑ effects OF digitalis; ↓ effects w/ barbiturates, loop diuretics, thyroid hormones, tobacco, St. John's wort; ↓ effects OF benzodiazepines, Li, phenytoin **Labs:** False + ↑ uric acid, ↑ bilirubin, ESR **NIPE:** Use barrier contraception; take w/ food if GI upset; caffeine foods ↑ drug effects; smoking ↓ drug effects

Thiamine [Vitamin B₁] [Vitamin] Uses: *Thiamine deficiency (beriberi), alcoholic neuritis, Wernicke encephalopathy* **Action:** Dietary supl **Dose:** *Adults.* Deficiency: 100 mg/d IM for 2 wk, then 5–10 mg/d PO for 1 mo. *Wernicke encephalopathy:* 100 mg IV single dose, then 100 mg/d IM for 2 wk. *Peds.* 10–25 mg/d IM for 2 wk, then 5–10 mg/24 h PO for 1 mo **Caution:** [A (C if doses exceed RDA), +] **Contra:** Component allergy **Disp:** Tabs 5, 10, 25, 50, 100, 250, 500 mg; inj 100, 200 mg/mL **SE:** Angioedema, paresthesias, rash, anaphylaxis w/ rapid IV **Notes:** IV use associated w/ anaphylactic Rxn; **Interactions:** ↑ Effects OF neuromuscular blocking drugs **Labs:** False + uric acid; interference w/ theophylline levels **NIPE:** Give IV slowly

Thiethylperazine (Torecan) [Antiemetic] Uses: *N/V* **Action:** Antidopaminergic antiemetic **Dose:** 10 mg PO, PR, or IM qd–tid; ↓ in hepatic failure **Caution:** [X, ?] **Contra:** Phenothiazine & sulfite sensitivity, PRG **Disp:** Tabs 10 mg; supp 10 mg; inj 5 mg/mL **SE:** EPS, xerostomia, drowsiness, orthostatic ↓ BP, tachycardia, confusion **Interactions:** ↑ Effects w/ atropine, CNS depressants, epinephrine, Li, MAOIs, TCAs, EtOH; ↑ effects OF antihypertensives, phenytoin; ↓ effects OF bromocriptine, cabergoline, levodopa **Labs:** ↑ Serum prolactin level, interferes w/ PRG test **NIPE:** May cause tardive dyskinesia; ↑ risk of photosensitivity—use sunscreen

6-Thioguanine [6-TG] (Tabloid) [Purine Antimetabolite] Uses: *AML, ALL, CML* **Action:** Purine-based antimetabolite (substitutes for natural purines interfering w/ nucleotide synthesis) **Dose:** 2–3 mg/kg/d; ↓ in severe renal/hepatic impair **Caution:** [D, –] **Contra:** Resistance to mercaptopurine **Disp:** Tabs 40 mg **SE:** Myelosuppression (leucopenia/thrombocytopenia), N/V/D, anorexia, stomatitis, rash, hyperuricemia, rare hepatotox **Interactions:** ↑ Bleeding w/ anticoagulants, NSAIDs, salicylates, thrombolytics **Labs:** ↑ Serum and urine uric acid **NIPE:** Take w/o food; ↑ fluids to 2–3 L/d; ⊘ exposure to infection

Thioridazine (Mellaril) [Antipsychotic/Phenothiazine] WARN-ING: Dose-related QT prolongation Uses: *Schizophrenia,* psychosis **Action:**

Phenothiazine antipsychotic **Dose:** *Adults.* Initial, 50–100 mg PO tid; maint 200–800 mg/24 h PO in 2–4 ÷ doses. *Peds >2 y.* 0.5–3 mg/kg/24 h PO in 2–3 ÷ doses **Caution:** [C, ?] Phenothiazines, QT$_c$-prolonging agents, aluminum **Contra:** Phenothiazine sensitivity **Disp:** Tabs 10, 15, 25, 50, 100, 150, 200 mg; PO conc 30, 100 mg/mL **SE:** Low incidence of EPS; ventricular arrhythmias; ↓ BP, dizziness, drowsiness, neuroleptic malignant syndrome, Szs, skin discoloration, photosensitivity, constipation, sexual dysfunction, blood dyscrasias, pigmentary retinopathy, hepatic impair **Interactions:** ↑ Effects w/ BBs; ↑ effects OF anticholinergics, antihypertensives, antihistamines, CNS depressants, nitrates, EtOH; ↓ effects w/ barbiturates, Li, tobacco; ↓ effects OF levodopa **Labs:** False + and − urinary PRG test; false + urine bilirubin and amylase; ↑ serum LFTs **NIPE:** ↑ Risk of photosensitivity—use sunscreen, take w/ food; ⊘ D/C abruptly; ↓ temp regulation; urine color change to reddish brown; avoid EtOH, dilute PO conc in 2–4 oz liq

Thiothixene (Navane) [Antipsychotic/Thioxanthene]

Uses: *Psychotic disorders* **Action:** Antipsychotic **Dose:** *Adults & Peds >12 y.* Mild–moderate psychosis: 2 mg PO tid, up to 20–30 mg/d. *Severe psychosis:* 5 mg PO bid; ↑ to a max of 60 mg/24 h PRN. *IM use:* 16–20 mg/24 h ÷ bid–qid; max 30 mg/d. *Peds <12 y.* 0.25 mg/kg/24 h PO ÷ q6–12h **Caution:** [C, ?] **Contra:** Phenothiazine sensitivity **Disp:** Caps 1, 2, 5, 10, 20 mg; PO conc 5 mg/mL; inj 10 mg/mL **SE:** Drowsiness, EPS most common; ↓ BP, dizziness, drowsiness, neuroleptic malignant syndrome, Szs, skin discoloration, photosensitivity, constipation, sexual dysfunction, blood dyscrasias, pigmentary retinopathy, hepatic impair **Notes:** Dilute PO conc immediately before administration **Interactions:** ↑ Effects w/ BBs; ↑ effects OF anticholinergics, antihistamines, BBs, CNS depressants, nitrates, EtOH; ↓ effects w/ barbiturates, Li, tobacco, caffeine; ↓ effects OF levodopa **Labs:** ↑ Serum glucose, cholesterol; ↓ serum uric acid; false + urinary PRG test **NIPE:** ↑ risk of photosensitivity—use sunscreen; take w/ food; ⊘ D/C abruptly; ↓ temp regulation; darkens urine color

Tiagabine (Gabitril) [Anticonvulsant]

Uses: *Adjunct in Rx of partial Szs,* bipolar disorder **Action:** Inhibition of GABA **Dose:** *Adults & Peds ≥12 y.* Initial 4 mg/d PO, ↑ by 4 mg during 2nd wk; ↑ PRN by 4–8 mg/d based on response, 56 mg/d max **Caution:** [C, M] **Contra:** Component allergy **Disp:** Tabs 2, 4, 6, 8, 10, 12, 16, 20 mg **SE:** Dizziness, HA, somnolence, memory impair, tremors **Notes:** Use gradual withdrawal; used in combo w/ other anticonvulsants **Interactions:** ↑ Effects w/ valproate; ↑ effects OF CNS depressants, EtOH; ↓ effects w/ barbiturates, carbamazepine, phenobarbital, phenytoin, primidone, rifampin, ginkgo biloba **NIPE:** Take w/ food; ⊘ D/C abruptly

Ticarcillin (Ticar) [Antibiotic/Penicillin]

Uses: Infxns due to gram(−) bacteria (*Klebsiella, Proteus, E. coli, Enterobacter, P. aeruginosa, & Serratia*) involving the skin, bone, resp & urinary tract, abdomen, sepsis **Action:** 4th-gen PCN, bactericidal; ↓ cell wall synthesis. *Spectrum:* Some gram(+) (strep, fair enterococcus, not MRSA), gram(−); enhanced w/aminoglycoside use, good anaerobes

(*Bactericides*) **Dose:** *Adults.* 3 g IV q4–6h. *Peds.* 200–300 mg/kg/d IV ÷ q4–6h; ↓ in renal insuff/failure **Caution:** [B, +] PCN sensitivity, renal impair, Sz hx, Na restriction **Contra:** Allergy to class; **Disp:** Inj 1, 3, 6, 20, 30 g **SE:** Interstitial nephritis, anaphylaxis, bleeding, rash, hemolytic anemia **Notes:** Used in combo w/ aminoglycosides **Interactions:** ↑ Effects w/ probenecid; ↑ effects OF anticoagulants, MTX; ↓ effects w/ tetracyclines, ↓ effects of aminoglycosides **Labs:** False ↑ urine glucose, ↑ serum AST, ALT, alkaline phosphatase **NIPE:** Monitor for S/Sxs superinfection; frequent loose stools may be due to pseudomembranous colitis

Ticarcillin/Potassium Clavulanate (Timentin) [Antibiotic/Penicillin, Beta-lactamase Inhibitor]
Uses: *Infxns of the skin, bone, resp & urinary tract, abdomen, sepsis* **Action:** 4th-gen PCN; bactericidal; ↓ cell wall synthesis; clavulanic acid blocks β-lactamase. *Spectrum:* Good gram(+), not MRSA; good gram(−) & anaerobes **Dose:** *Adults.* 3.1 g IV q4–6h. *Peds.* 200–300 mg/kg/d IV ÷ q4–6h; ↓ in renal failure **Caution:** [B, +/−] PCN sensitivity **Disp:** Inj 3 g/1 g vial; **SE:** Hemolytic anemia, false + proteinuria **Notes:** Often used in combo w/ aminoglycosides; penetrates CNS with meningeal irritation; also see ticarcillin **Interactions:** ↑ Effects w/ probenecid; ↑ effects OF anticoagulants, MRX; ↓ effects w/ tetracyclines, ↓ effects OF aminoglycosides, oral contraceptives **Labs:** False ↑ urine glucose, false + urine proteins **NIPE:** Monitor for S/Sxs superinfection; frequent loose stools may be due to pseudomembranous colitis; use barrier contraception

Ticlopidine (Ticlid) [Antiplatelet]
WARNING: Neutropenia/agranulocytosis, TTP, aplastic anemia reported **Uses:** *↓ risk of thrombotic stroke,* protect grafts status post CABG, diabetic microangiopathy, ischemic heart Dz, DVT prophylaxis, graft prophylaxis after renal transplant **Action:** Plt aggregation inhibitor **Dose:** 250 mg PO bid w/ food **Caution:** [B, ?/−], ↑ tox of ASA, anticoagulation, NSAIDs, theophylline **Contra:** Bleeding, hepatic impair, neutropenia, thrombocytopenia **Disp:** Tabs 250 mg **SE:** Bleeding, GI upset, rash, ↑ on LFTs **Interactions:** ↑ Effects w/ anticoagulants, cimetidine, dong quai, evening primrose oil, feverfew, garlic, ginkgo biloba, ginseng, grapeseed extract, red clover; ↑ effects OF ASA, carbamazepine, phenytoin, theophylline; ↓ effects w/ antacids; ↓ effects OF cyclosporine, digoxin **Labs:** ↑ LFTs, cholesterol, triglycerides; monitor CBC for 1st 3 mo **NIPE:** Take w/ food

Tigecycline (Tygacil) [Antibiotic/related to Tetracycline]
Uses: *Rx complicated skin & soft tissue Infxns, & complicated intraabdominal Infxns* **Action:** New class: related to tetracycline; *Spectrum:* Broad gram(+), gram(−), anaerobic, some mycobacterial; *E. coli, Enterococcus faecalis* (vanco-susceptible isolates), *Staphylococcus aureus* (meth-susceptible/resistant), *Streptococcus* (*agalactiae, anginosus* grp, *pyogenes*), *Citrobacter freundii, Enterobacter cloacae, B. fragilis* group, *C. perfringens, Peptostreptococcus* **Dose:** *Adults.* 100 mg, then 50 mg q12h IV over 30–60 min every 12 h **Caution:** [D, ?] hepatic impair, monotherapy w/ intestinal perf, not OK in peds **Contra:** Component sensitivity **Disp:** Inj 50-mg vial; **SE:** N/V, inj site Rxn **NIPE:** ⊘ with children

Timolol (Blocadren) [Antihypertensive/BB] **WARNING:** Exacerbation of ischemic heart Dz w/ abrupt D/C **Uses:** *HTN & MI* **Action:** β-Adrenergic receptor blocker, $β_1$, $β_2$ **Dose:** *HTN:* 10–20 mg bid, up to 60 mg/d. *MI:* 10 mg bid **Caution:** [C (1st tri; D if 2nd or 3rd tri), +] **Contra:** CHF, cardiogenic shock, bradycardia, heart block, COPD, asthma **Disp:** Tabs 5, 10, 20 mg **SE:** Sexual dysfunction, arrhythmia, dizziness, fatigue, CHF **Interactions:** ↑ Effects w/ antihypertensives, ciprofloxacin, fentanyl, quinidine, ↑ bradycardia and myocardial depression w/ cardiac glycosides, diltiazem, tacrine, verapamil; ↑ effects OF epinephrine, ergots, flecainide, lidocaine, nifedipine, phenothiazines, prazosin, verapamil; ↓ effects w/ barbiturates, cholestyramine, colestipol, NSAIDs, penicillin, rifampin, salicylates, sulfinpyrazone; ↓ effect OF hypoglycemics, sulfonylureas, theophylline **Labs:** ↑ Serum glucose, BUN, K^+, lipoprotein, triglycerides, uric acid **NIPE:** ⊘ D/C abruptly; ↑ cold sensitivity

Timolol, Ophthalmic (Timoptic) [Anti-glaucoma Agent/BB] **Uses:** *Glaucoma* **Action:** β-Blocker **Dose:** 0.25% 1 gt bid; ↓ to qd when controlled; use 0.5% if needed; 1 gt/d gel **Caution:** [C (1st tri; D 2nd or 3rd), ?/+] **Disp:** Soln 0.25/0.5%; Timoptic XE (0.25, 0.5%) gel-forming soln **SE:** Local irritation See Timolol, above **Additional NIPE:** Depress lacrimal sac 1 min after admin to lessen systemic absorption, admin other drops 10 min before gel

Tinidazole (Tindamax) [Antiprotozoal] **WARNING:** Off-label use discouraged (animal carcinogenicity w/ other drugs in class) **Uses:** *Adults/children >3 y.* *Trichomoniasis & giardiasis; intestinal amebiasis or amebic liver abscess* **Action:** Antiprotozoal nitroimidazole *Spectrum:* Trichomonas vaginalis, Giardia duodenalis, Entamoeba histolytica **Dose:** *Adults.* Trichomoniasis: 2 g PO; treat partner; *Giardiasis:* 2 g PO; *Amebiasis:* 2 g PO qd ×3; *Amebic liver abscess:* 2 g PO qd ×3–5; *Peds.* Trichomoniasis: 50 mg/kg PO, 2 g/day max; *Giardiasis:* 50 mg/kg PO, 2 g max; *Amebiasis:* 50 mg/kg PO qd ×3, 2 g/day max; *Amebic liver abscess:* 50 mg/kg PO qd ×3–5, 2 g/day max (w/food) **Caution:** [C, D in 1st trimester; –] May be cross-resistant with metronidazole; Sz/peripheral neuropathy may require D/C; w/CNS/hepatic impair **Contra:** Metronidazole allergy, 1st trimester PRG, w/ EtOH use **Disp:** Tabs 250, 500 **SE:** CNS disturbances; blood dyscrasias, taste disturbances, N/V, darkens urine **Interactions:** ↑ Effects OF anticoagulants, cyclosporine, fluorouracil, lithium, phenytoin IV, tacrolimus; ↑ effects w/ cimetidine, ketoconazole; ↑ effects OF abdominal cramping, N/V, HA w/ disulfiram, EtOH; ↓ effects w/ cholestyramine, oxytetracycline, phenobarbital, rifampin, phenytoin; ↓ effects OF fluorouracil **NIPE:** crush & disperse in cherry syrup for peds; removed by HD

Tinzaparin (Innohep) [Anticoagulant/LMW Heparin] **Uses:** *Rx of DVT w/ or w/o PE* **Action:** LMW heparin **Dose:** 175 Units/kg SQ qd at least 6 d until warfarin dose stabilized **Caution:** [B, ?] Pork allergy, active bleeding, mild–moderate renal dysfunction **Contra:** Allergy to sulfites, heparin, benzyl alcohol, HIT **Disp:** Inj. 20,000 Units/mL **SE:** Bleeding, bruising, thrombocytopenia,

Notes: Monitor via Anti-Xa levels; no effect on: bleeding time, plt Fxn, PT, aPTT **Interactions:** ↑ Bleeding w/ anticoagulants, cephalosporins, dextran, NSAIDs, penicillins, salicylates, thrombolytics **Labs:** ↑ LFTs **NIPE:** ⊘ Rub inj site, admin deep SQ inj, rotate abdominal inj sites; causes inj site pain

Tioconazole (Vagistat) [Antifungal] Uses: *Vaginal fungal Infxns* **Action:** Topical antifungal **Dose:** 1 applicatorful intravag hs (single dose) **Caution:** [C, ?] **Contra:** Component allergy **Disp:** Vaginal oint 6.5% **SE:** Local burning, itching, soreness, polyuria **Interactions:** Risk OF inactivation of nonoxynol-9 spermicidal **NIPE:** Insert high into vaginal canal; may cause staining of clothing; refrain from intercourse during drug therapy; risk of latex breakdown of condoms and diaphragm

Tiotropium (Spiriva) [Bronchodilator/Anticholinergic] Uses: Bronchospasm w/ COPD, bronchitis, emphysema **Action:** Synthetic anticholinergic like atropine **Dose:** 1 cap/d inhaled using HandiHaler, *do not* use w/ spacer **Caution:** [C, ?/–] BPH, NA glaucoma, MyG, renal impair **Contra:** Acute bronchospasm **Disp:** Inhalation Caps 18 mcg **SE:** URI, xerostomia **Notes:** Monitor FEV$_1$ or peak flow **Interactions:** ↑ Effects w/ other anticholinergic drugs **Labs:** Monitor peak flow & PFT **NIPE:** ⊘ For acute resp episode; take daily at same time each day

Tipranavir (Aptivus) [Antiretroviral/Protease Inhibitor] **WARNING:** Co-administration w/ ritonavir assoc w/ hepatitis & hepatic decomp w/ fatalities. D/C w/ s/s of hepatitis **Uses:** HIV 1 infection w/ highly treatment-experienced pts or HIV 1 strains resistant to multiple protease inhibitors. Must be used w/ ritonavir 200 mg. **Action:** Antiretroviral HIV-1 protease inhibitor **Dose:** 500 mg PO BID w/food, administer w/ ritonavir 200 mg PO BID **Caution:** [C, –] sulfa allergy, liver dis **Contra:** Moderate to severe hep insuf; concomitant use w/ amiodarone, astemizole, bepridil, cisapride, ergots, flecainide, lovastatin, midazolam, pimozide, propafenone, quinidine, rifampin, simvastatin, terfenadine, triazolam, St. John's wort **Disp:** Soft gel cap 250 mg **SE:** HA, GI distress, rash, fatigue, fat redistribution, hyperglycemia, hepatitis, liver dis, lipid elevations **Interactions:** ↑ Effects OF anticoagulants, antiplatelets, azole antifungals, CCB, clarithromycin, NNRTIs, rifabutin, sildenafil, statins, tadalafil, vardenafil; ↓ effects w/ antacids, didanosine; ↓ effects OF estrogens, methadone **Labs:** ↑ BS, LFTs, lipids, monitor baseline and periodically **NIPE:** ↑ Bioavailability w/ high fat meals; monitor for bleeding in pts w/hemophilia

Tirofiban (Aggrastat) [Antiplatelet Agent] Uses: *Acute coronary syndrome* **Action:** Glycoprotein IIB/IIIa inhibitor **Dose:** Initial 0.4 mcg/kg/min for 30 min, followed by 0.1 mcg/kg/min; use in combo w/ heparin; ↓ in renal insuff **Caution:** [B, ?/–] **Contra:** Bleeding, intracranial neoplasm, vascular malformation, stroke/surgery/trauma w/in last 30 d, severe HTN **Disp:** Inj 50, 250 mcg/mL **SE:** Bleeding, bradycardia, coronary dissection, pelvic pain, rash **Interactions:** ↑ Bleeding risks w/ anticoagulants, antiplatelets, NSAIDs, salicylates, dong quai, feverfew, garlic, ginger, ginkgo, horse chestnut; ↓ effects w/ levothyroxine, omeprazole **Labs:** ↓ Hmg, Hct, plts **NIPE:** ⊘ Breast-feeding

Tobramycin (Nebcin) [Antibiotic/Aminoglycoside]
Uses: *Serious gram(–) Infxns* **Action:** Aminoglycoside; ↓ protein synthesis. **Spectrum:** Gram(–) bacteria (including *Pseudomonas*) **Dose:** *Adults.* 1–2.5 mg/kg/dose IV q8–24h. *Peds.* 2.5 mg/kg/dose IV q8h; ↓ w/ renal insuff **Caution:** [C, M] **Contra:** Aminoglycoside sensitivity **Disp:** Inj 10, 40 mg/mL **SE:** Nephrotox & ototox **Notes:** Follow CrCl & levels for dosage adjustments (Table 2) **Interactions:** ↑ Effects w/ carbenicillin, NSAIDs, ticarcillin; ↑ nephrotoxic, neurotoxic, and/or ototoxic effects w/ aminoglycosides, amphotericin B, cephalosporins, cisplatin, furosemide, mannitol, methoxyflurane, polymyxin B, urea, vancomycin **Labs:** ↑ LFTs, BUN, creatinine, serum protein; ↓ serum K⁺, Na⁺, Ca²⁺, Mg²⁺ **NIPE:** ↑ Fluids to 2–3 L/d; monitor for superinfection

Tobramycin Ophthalmic [Antibiotic/Aminoglycoside] (AKTob, Tobrex)
Uses: *Ocular bacterial Infxns* **Action:** Aminoglycoside **Dose:** 1–2 gtt q4h; oint bid–tid; if severe, use oint q3–4h, or 2 gtt q30–60min, then less frequently **Caution:** [C, M] **Contra:** Aminoglycoside sensitivity **Disp:** Oint & soln tobramycin 0.3% **SE:** Ocular irritation **Additional NIPE:** Depress lacrimal sac for 1 min to prevent systemic absorption; ↑ risk of blurred vision & burning

Tobramycin & Dexamethasone Ophthalmic (TobraDex) [Antibiotic/Anti-inflammatory]
Uses: *Ocular bacterial Infxns associated w/ significant inflammation* **Action:** Antibiotic w/ antiinflammatory **Dose:** 0.3% oint apply q3–8h or soln 0.3% apply 1–2 gtt q1–4h **Caution:** [C, M] **Contra:** Aminoglycoside sensitivity **Disp:** Oint & suspension 2.5, 5, & 10 mL, tobramycin 0.3% & dexamethasone 0.1% **SE:** Local irritation/edema **Notes:** Use under ophthalmologist's direction **Additional NIPE:** Eval intraocular pressure and lens if prolonged use

Tolazamide (Tolinase) [Hypoglycemic/Sulfonylurea]
Uses: *Type 2 DM* **Action:** Sulfonylurea; ↑ pancreatic insulin release; ↑ peripheral insulin sensitivity; ↓ hepatic glucose output **Dose:** 100–500 mg/d (no benefit >1 g/d) **Caution:** [C, +/–] Elderly, hepatic or renal impair **Disp:** Tabs 100, 250, 500 mg; **SE:** HA, dizziness, GI upset, rash, hyperglycemia, photosensitivity, blood dyscrasias **Interactions:** ↑ Effects w/ chloramphenicol, cimetidine, clofibrate, insulin, MAOIs, phenylbutazone, probenecid, salicylates, sulfonamides, garlic, ginseng; ↓ effects w/ diuretics **NIPE:** Risk of disulfiram-type Rxn w/ EtOH; take w/ food; use sunscreen

Tolazoline (Priscoline) [Alpha Adrenergic Antagonist]
Uses: *Peripheral vasospastic disorders* **Action:** Competitively blocks α-adrenergic receptors **Dose:** *Adults.* 10–50 mg IM/IV/SQ qid. *Neonates.* 1–2 mg/kg IV over 10–15 min, then 1–2 mg/kg/h (adjust w/ ↓ renal Fxn) **Caution:** [C, ?] **Contra:** CAD **Disp:** Inj 25 mg/mL **SE:** ↓ BP, peripheral vasodilation, tachycardia, arrhythmias, GI

upset & bleeding, blood dyscrasias, renal failure **Interactions:** ↓ BP w/ epinephrine, norepinephrine, phenylephrine **NIPE:** Risk of disulfiram-type Rxn w/ EtOH

Tolbutamide (Orinase) [Hypoglycemic/Sulfonylurea]

Uses: *Type 2 DM* **Action:** Sulfonylurea; ↑ pancreatic insulin release; ↑ peripheral insulin sensitivity; ↓ hepatic glucose output **Dose:** 500–1000 mg bid; ↓ in hepatic failure **Caution:** [C, +] **Contra:** Sulfonylurea sensitivity **Disp:** Tabs 250, 500 mg **SE:** HA, dizziness, GI upset, rash, photosensitivity, blood dyscrasias, hypoglycemia **Interactions:** ↑ Effects w/ anticoagulants, antidepressants, chloramphenicol, insulin, H_2 antagonists, MAOIs, metformin, NSAIDs, phenylbutazone, probenecid, salicylates; ↓ effects w/ BBs, CCBs, cholestyramine, corticosteroids, hydantoins, INH, oral contraceptives, phenothiazines, phenytoin, rifampin, sympathomimetics, thiazides, thyroid drugs **NIPE:** Risk of disulfiram-type Rxn w/ EtOH; take w/ food; use barrier contraception; ↑ risk of photosensitivity—use sunscreen

Tolcapone (Tasmar) [Antiparkinson Agent/COMT Inhibitor]

Uses: *Adjunct to carbidopa/levodopa in Parkinson Dz* **Action:** Catechol-*O*-methyltransferase inhibitor slows metabolism of levodopa **Dose:** 100 mg PO w/ first daily levodopa/carbidopa dose, then dose 6 & 12 h later; ↓ in renal impair **Caution:** [C, ?] **Contra:** Hepatic impair; nonselective MAOI **Disp:** Tablets 100 mg, 200 mg **SE:** Constipation, xerostomia, vivid dreams, anorexia, N/D, orthostasis, liver failure **Interactions:** ↑ Effects OF apomorphine, dobutamine, CNS depressants, desipramine, isoproterenol, levodopa, methyldopa, SSRIs, TCAs, warfarin, EtOH, gout kola, kava kava, St. John's wort, valerian; ↑ risk OF hypertensive crisis with nonselective MAO inhibitors (phenelzine, tranylcypromine) **Labs:** Monitor LFTs **NIPE:** May give w/o regard to food but food ↑ bioavailability of drug, may experience hallucinations; do not abruptly D/C or ↓ dose

Tolmetin (Tolectin) [Analgesic, Anti-inflammatory, Antipyretic/NSAID]

WARNING: May ↑ risk of cardiovascular events & GI bleeding **Uses:** *Arthritis & pain* **Action:** NSAID; ↓ prostaglandins **Dose:** 200–600 mg PO tid; 2000 mg/d max **Caution:** [C (D in 3rd tri or near term), +] **Contra:** NSAID or ASA sensitivity **Disp:** Tabs 200, 600 mg; caps 400 mg **SE:** Dizziness, rash, GI upset, edema, GI bleeding, renal failure **Interactions:** ↑ Effect OF aminoglycosides, anticoagulants, cyclosporine, digoxin, insulin, Li, MRX, K-sparing diuretics, sulfonylureas; ↓ effect w/ ASA, food; ↓ effect OF furosemide, thiazides **Labs:** ↑ ALT, AST, serum K⁺, BUN, ↓ Hmg, Hct **NIPE:** Take w/ food if GI upset; ↑ risk of photosensitivity—use sunscreen

Tolnaftate (Tinactin) [Antifungal] [OTC]

Uses: *Tinea pedis, t. cruris, t. corporis, t. manus, t. versicolor* **Action:** Topical antifungal **Dose:** Apply to area bid for 2–4 wk **Caution:** [C, ?] **Contra:** Nail & scalp Infxns **Disp:** OTC 1% liq; gel; powder; topical cream; ointment, spray soln **SE:** Local irritation **NIPE:** Avoid ocular contact, Infxn should improve in 7–10 d; ⊘ with children < 2 years

Tolterodine (Detrol, Detrol LA) [Anticholinergic/Muscarinic Antagonist]

Uses: *OAB (frequency, urgency, incontinence)* Action: Anticholinergic Dose: Detrol 1–2 mg PO bid; Detrol LA 2–4 mg/d Caution: [C, ?/–] w/ CYP2D6 & 3A3/4 inhibitor (Table 13) Contra: Urinary retention, gastric retention, or uncontrolled NA glaucoma Disp: Tabs 1, 2 mg; Detrol LA tabs 2, 4 mg SE: Xerostomia, blurred vision Interactions: ↑ Effects w/ azole antifungals, macrolides, grapefruit juice, food; ↑ anticholinergic effects w/ amantadine, amoxapine, bupropion, clozapine, cyclobenzaprine, disopyramide, olanzapine, phenothiazines, TCAs NIPE: May cause blurred vision

Topiramate (Topamax) [Anticonvulsant]

Uses: *Adjunctive Rx for complex partial Szs & tonic–clonic Szs,* bipolar disorder, neuropathic pain; migraine prophylxis Action: Anticonvulsant Dose: *Adults.* Seizures: Total dose 400 mg/d; see insert for 8-wk titration schedule. Migraine prophylaxis: titrate 100 m/d total *Peds 2–16 y:* Initial, 1–3 mg/kg/d PO qhs; titrate per insert to 5–9 mg/kg/d; ↓ in renal impair Caution: [C, ?/–] Contra: Component allergy Disp: Tabs 25, 50, 100, 200 mg; caps sprinkles 15, 25, 50 mg SE: Metabolic acidosis, kidney stones; fatigue, dizziness, psychomotor slowing, memory impair, GI upset, tremor, nystagmus; weight loss, acute secondary glaucoma requiring drug D/C Interactions: ↑ CNS effects w/ CNS depressants, EtOH; ↑ effects OF phenytoin; ↓ effects w/ carbamazepine, phenytoin, valproate, ginkgo biloba; ↓ effects OF digoxin, oral contraceptives Labs: ↑ LFTs NIPE: Take w/o regard to food; ⊘ D/C abruptly; use barrier contraception; ↑ fluids to 2–3 L/d; metabolic acidosis responsive to dose ↓ or D/C; D/C requires taper

Topotecan (Hycamtin) [Antineoplastic]

WARNING: Chemo precautions, BM suppression possible Uses: *Ovarian CA (cisplatin-refractory), small-cell lung CA,* sarcoma, ped non-small-cell lung CA Action: Topoisomerase I inhibitor; ↓ DNA synthesis Dose: 1.5 mg/m²/d as a 1-h IV inf ×5 days, repeat q3wk; ↓ in renal failure Caution: [D, –] Contra: PRG, breast-feeding Disp: Inj 4-mg vials SE: Myelosuppression, N/V/D, drug fever, skin rash Interactions: ↑ Myelosuppression w/ cisplatin, other neoplastic drugs, radiation therapy; ↑ in duration OF neutropenia w/ filgrastim Labs: ↑ AST, ALT, bilirubin NIPE: Monitor CBC; ⊘ PRG, breast-feeding, immunizations; ⊘ exposure to infection; use barrier contraception

Torsemide (Demadex) [Antihypertensive/Loop Diuretic]

Uses: *Edema, HTN, CHF, & hepatic cirrhosis* Action: Loop diuretic; ↓ reabsorption of Na⁺ & Cl⁻ in ascending loop of Henle & distal tubule Dose: 5–20 mg/d PO or IV Caution: [B, ?] Contra: Sulfonylurea sensitivity Disp: Tabs 5, 10, 20, 100 mg; inj 10 mg/mL SE: Orthostatic ↓ BP, HA, dizziness, photosensitivity, electrolyte imbalance, blurred vision, renal impair Notes: 20 mg torsemide = 40 mg furosemide Interactions: ↑ Risk of ototoxicity w/ aminoglycosides, cisplatin; ↑ effects w/ thiazides; ↑ effects OF anticoagulants, antihypertensives, Li, salicylates; ↓ effects w/ barbiturates, carbamazepine, cholestyramine, NSAIDs, phenytoin, phenobarbital, probenecid, dandelion **NIPE:** Monitor electrolytes, BUN, creatinine, glucose, uric acid; take w/o regard to food; monitor for S/Sxs tinnitus

Tramadol (Ultram) [Centrally Acting Analgesic/Non-narcotic]
Uses: *Moderate–severe pain* **Action:** Centrally acting analgesic **Dose:** *Adults.* 50–100 mg PO q4–6h PRN, 400 mg/d max. *Peds.* 0.5–1 mg/kg PO q 4–6h PRN **Caution:** [C, ?/–] **Contra:** Opioid dependency; w/MAOIs; sensitivity to codeine **Disp:** Tabs 50 mg **SE:** Dizziness, HA, somnolence, GI upset, resp depression, anaphylaxis **Interactions:** ↑ Effects w/ cimetidine, CNS depressants, MAOIs, phenothiazines, quinidine, TCAs, EtOH, St. John's wort; ↑ effects OF digoxin, warfarin; ↓ effects w/ carbamazepine **Labs:** ↑ Creatinine, LFTs, ↓ Hmg **NIPE:** Take w/o regard to food; ↓ Szz threshold; tolerance or dependence may develop

Tramadol/Acetaminophen (Ultracet) [Centrally Acting Analgesic/Non-narcotic]
Uses: *Short-term Rx acute pain (<5 d)* **Action:** Centrally acting analgesic; nonnarcotic analgesic **Dose:** 2 tabs PO q4–6h PRN; 8 tabs/d max. *Elderly/renal impair:* Lowest possible dose; 2 tabs q12h max if CrCl <30 **Caution:** [C, –] Szs, hepatic/renal impair, or Hx addictive tendencies **Contra:** Acute intox **Disp:** Tab 37.5 mg tramadol/325 mg APAP **SE:** SSRIs, TCAs, opioids, MAOIs ↑ risk of Szs; dizziness, somnolence, tremor, HA, N/V/D, constipation, xerostomia, liver tox, rash, pruritus, ↑ sweating, physical dependence **Interactions:** ↑ Effects w/ cimetidine, CNS depressants, MAOIs, phenothiazines, quinidine, TCAs, EtOH, St. John's wort; ↑ effects OF digoxin, warfarin; ↓ effects w/ carbamazepine **Labs:** ↑ Creatinine, LFTs, ↓ Hmg **NIPE:** Take w/o regard to food; ⊘ take other acetaminophen-containing drugs; avoid EtOH

Trandolapril (Mavik) [Antihypertensive/ACEI]
WARNING: Use in PRG in 2nd/3rd tri can result in fetal death **Uses:** *HTN,* CHF, LVD, post-AMI **Action:** ACE inhibitor **Dose:** *HTN:* 2–4 mg/d. *CHF/LVD:* 4 mg/d; ↓ in severe renal/hepatic impair **Caution:** [D, +] ACE inhibitor sensitivity, angioedema w/ ACE inhibitors **Disp:** Tabs 1, 2, 4 mg **SE:** ↓ BP, bradycardia, dizziness, ↑ K⁺, GI upset, renal impair, cough, angioedema **Notes:** Afro-Americans, min. dose is 2 mg vs 1 mg in Caucasians **Interactions:** ↑ Effects w/ diuretics; ↑ effects OF insulin, Li; ↓ effects w/ ASA, NSAIDs **NIPE:** ⊘ Take if PRG or breast-feeding; ⊘ K-containing salt substitutes

Trastuzumab (Herceptin) [Antineoplastic/Monoclonal Antibody]
Uses: *Metastatic breast CAs that overexpress the HER2/neu overexpression protein* breast cancer, adjuvant, w/ doxorubicin, cyclophosphamide, and paclitaxel if pt HER2/neu(+) **Action:** MoAb; binds human epidermal GF receptor 2 protein (HER2); mediates cellular cytotox **Dose:** Per protocol **Caution:** [B, ?] CV dysfunction, allergy/inf Rxns **Contra:** None known **Disp:** Inj form 21 mg/mL **SE:** Anemia, cardiomyopathy, nephrotic syndrome, pneumonitis **Notes:** Inf related Rxns minimized w/ acetaminophen, diphenhydramine, & meperidine **Interactions:** ↑ Risk OF cardiac dysfunction w/ anthracyclines, cyclophosphamide, dox-

orubicin, epirubicin **Labs:** Monitor cardiac function **NIPE:** ⊘ Use dextrose inf soln; ⊘ breast-feed for 6 mo following drug therapy

Trazodone (Desyrel) [Antidepressant]

Uses: *Depression,* hypnotic, augment other antidepressants **Action:** Antidepressant; ↓ reuptake of serotonin & norepinephrine **Dose:** *Adults & Adolescents.* 50–150 mg PO qd–qid; max 600 mg/d. *Sleep:* 50 mg PO, qhs, PRN **Caution:** [C, ?/–] **Contra:** Component allergy **Disp:** Tabs 50, 100, 150, 300 mg **SE:** Dizziness, HA, sedation, nausea, xerostomia, syncope, confusion, tremor, hepatitis, EPS **Notes:** Takes 1–2 wk for symptom improvement; may interact with CYP3A4 inhibitors to ↑ trazodone concentrations, carbamazepine to ↓ trazodone concentrations **Interactions:** ↑ Effects w/ fluoxetine, phenothiazines; ↑ risk of serotonin syndrome w/ MAOIs, SSRIs, venlafaxine, St. John's wort; ↑ CNS depression w/ barbiturates, CNS depressants, opioids, sedatives, EtOH; ↑ hypotension w/ antihypertensive, neuroleptics; nitrates, EtOH; ↑ effects OF clonidine, digoxin, phenytoin; ↓ effects w/ carbamazepine **NIPE:** Take w/ food; ↑ fluids to 2–3 L/d; ⊘ D/C abruptly; ↑ risk of priapism

Treprostinil Sodium (Remodulin) [Antihypertensive/Vasodilator]

Uses: *NYHA class II–IV pulmonary arterial HTN* **Action:** Vasodilation, inhibits plt aggregation **Dose:** 0.625–1.25 ng/kg/min cont inf **Caution:** [B, ?/–] **Contra:** Component allergy **Disp:** 1, 2.5, 5, 10 mg/mL inj **SE:** Additive effects w/ anticoagulants, antihypertensives; inf site Rxns **Notes:** Initiate in monitored setting; do not D/C or ↓ dose abruptly **Interactions:** ↑ Effects w/ antihypertensives; ↑ effects OF anticoagulants **NIPE:** Teach care of inf site and pump; use barrier contraception; once med vial used discard after 14 d

Tretinoin, Topical [Retinoic Acid] (Retin-A, Avita, Renova) [Retinoid]

Uses: *Acne vulgaris, sun-damaged skin, wrinkles* (photo aging), some skin CAs **Action:** Exfoliant retinoic acid derivative **Dose:** *Adults & Peds >12 y.* Apply qd hs (w/ irritation, ↓ frequency). *Photoaging:* Start w/ 0.025%, ↑ to 0.1% over several months (apply only q3d if on neck area; dark skin may require bid application) **Caution:** [C, ?] **Contra:** Retinoid sensitivity **Disp:** Cream 0.02, 0.025, 0.05, 0.1%; gel 0.01, 0.025%; microformulation gel 0.1, 0.04%; liq 0.05% **SE:** Avoid sunlight; edema; skin dryness, erythema, scaling, changes in pigmentation, stinging, photosensitivity **Interactions:** ↑ photosensitivity w/ quinolones, phenothiazines, sulfonamides, tetracyclines, thiazides, dong quai, St. John's wort; ↑ skin irritation w/ topical sulfur, resorcinol, benzoyl peroxide, salicylic acid; ↑ effects w/ vitamin A supl and foods w/ excess vitamin A such as fish oils **NIPE:** ⊘ Apply to mucous membranes, wash skin and apply med after 30 min, wash hands after application; ⊘ breast-feeding, PRG use contraception; use sunscreen

Triamcinolone (Azmacort) [Anti-inflammatory/Corticosteroid]

Uses: *Chronic asthma* **Actions:** Topical steroid **Dose:** Two inhalations tid–qid or 4 inhal bid **Caution:** [C, ?] **Contra:** Component allergy **Disp:** Aerosol, metered inhaler 100 mcg spray; **SE:** Cough, oral candidiasis **Interactions:** ↑ Effects w/ salmeterol, troleandomycin; ↓ effects w/ barbiturates, hydantoins, phenytoin, rifampin; ↓ effects OF diuretics, insulin, oral hypoglycemics, K supl, salicylates, somatrem, live virus vaccines **Labs:** ↑ Serum glucose, lipids, amylase, sodium; ↓ skin test reaction, serum Ca, K⁺, thyroxine **NIPE:** Use bronchodilator several minutes before triamcinolone; allow 1 min between repeated inhalations; instruct pts to rinse mouth after use; not for acute asthma

Triamcinolone & Nystatin (Mycolog-II) [Anti-inflammatory, Antifungal/Corticosteroid]

Uses: *Cutaneous candidiasis* **Action:** Antifungal & antiinflammatory **Dose:** Apply lightly to area bid; max 25 mg/d **Caution:** [C, ?] **Contra:** Varicella; systemic fungal Infxns **Disp:** Cream & oint 15, 30, 60, 120 mg **SE:** Local irritation, hypertrichosis, changes in pigmentation **Notes:** For short-term use (<7 d) **Interactions:** ↓ Effects w/ barbiturates, phenytoin, rifampin; ↓ effects OF salicylates, vaccines **NIPE:** ⊘ Eyes; ⊘ apply to open skin/wounds, eyes, mucous membranes

Triamterene (Dyrenium) [Diuretic/Potassium-sparing Agent]

Uses: *Edema associated w/ CHF, cirrhosis* **Action:** K⁺-sparing diuretic **Dose:** *Adults.* 100–300 mg/24 h PO ÷ qd-bid. *Peds.* 2–4 mg/kg/d in 1–2 ÷ doses; ↓ in renal/hepatic impair **Caution:** [B (manufacturer; D expert opinion), ?/–] **Contra:** ↑ K⁺, renal impair, DM; caution w/ other K⁺-sparing diuretics **Disp:** Caps 50, 100 mg **SE:** ↓ K⁺, blood dyscrasias, liver damage, other Rxns **Interactions:** ↑ Risk of hyperkalemia w/ ACEIs, K supls, K-sparing drugs, K-containing drugs, K salt substitutes; ↑ effects w/ cimetidine, indomethacin; ↑ effects OF amantadine, antihypertensives, Li; ↓ effects OF digitalis **Labs:** False ↑ serum digoxin **NIPE:** Take w/ food, blue discoloration of urine, ↑ risk of photosensitivity—use sunscreen

Triazolam (Halcion) [C-IV] [Sedative/Hypnotic/Benzodiazepine]

Uses: *Short-term management of insomnia* **Action:** Benzodiazepine **Dose:** 0.125–0.25 mg/d PO hs PRN; ↓ in elderly **Caution:** [X, ?/–] **Contra:** NA glaucoma; cirrhosis; concurrent amprenavir, ritonavir, or nelfinavir **Disp:** Tabs 0.125, 0.25 mg **SE:** Tachycardia, CP, drowsiness, fatigue, memory impair, GI upset **Interactions:** Additive CNS depression w/ EtOH & other CNS depressants **Interactions:** ↑ Effects w/ azole antifungals, cimetidine, clarithromycin, ciprofloxin, CNS depressants, disulfiram, digoxin, erythromycin, fluvoxamine, INH, protease inhibitors, troleandomycin, verapamil, EtOH, grapefruit juice, kava kava, valerian; ↓ effects OF levodopa; ↓ effects w/ carbamazepine, phenytoin, rifampin, theophylline **NIPE:** ⊘ PRG or breast-feeding; ⊘ D/C abruptly after long-term use

Triethanolamine (Cerumenex) [Ceruminolytic Agent] [OTC]

Uses: *Cerumen (ear wax) removal* **Action:** Ceruminolytic agent **Dose:** Fill ear canal & insert cotton plug; irrigate w/ H₂O after 15 min; repeat PRN **Caution:** [C, ?] **Contra:** Perforated tympanic membrane, otitis media **Disp:** Soln 6, 12 mL **SE:** Local dermatitis, pain, erythema, pruritus **NIPE:** Warm soln to body temp before use for better effect

Triethylenetriphosphamide (Thio-Tepa, Tespa, TSPA) [Alkylating Agent] Uses: *Hodgkin Dz & NHLs; leukemia; breast, ovarian CAs, preparative regimens for allogeneic & ABMT w/ high doses, intravesical for bladder CA* Action: Polyfunctional alkylating agent Dose: 0.5 mg/kg q1–4wk, 6 mg/m² IM or IV ×4 d q2–4wk, 15–35 mg/m² by cont IV inf over 48 h; 60 mg into the bladder & retained 2 h q1–4wk; 900–125 mg/m² in ABMT regimens (highest dose w/o ABMT is 180 mg/m²); 1–10 mg/m² (typically 15 mg) IT 1 or 2 ×/wk; 0.8 mg/kg in 1–2 L of soln may be instilled intraperitoneally; ↓ in renal failure Caution: [D, −] Contra: Component allergy Disp: Inj 15, 30 mg SE: Myelosuppression, N/V, dizziness, HA, allergy, paresthesias, alopecia Notes: Intravesical use in bladder Ca infrequent today Interactions: ↑ Risk OF bleeding w/ anticoagulants, ASA, NSAIDs; ↑ effects OF myelosuppressives; ↑ risk OF muscular paralysis w/ neuromuscular blockers; ↑ risk OF apnea w/ pancuronium Labs: ↑ Uric acid; ↓ hmg, lymphocytes, neutrophils, platelets, RBCs, WBCs NIPE: ⊘ in pregnancy, lactation, bone marrow suppression, hepatic dysfunction, renal dysfunction; ⊘ ASA or NSAIDs; report S/Sys of infection.

Trifluoperazine (Stelazine) [Antipsychotic/Phenothiazine] Uses: *Psychotic disorders* Action: Phenothiazine; blocks postsynaptic CNS dopaminergic receptors Dose: *Adults.* 2–10 mg PO bid. *Peds 6–12 y.* 1 mg PO qd–bid initial, gradually ↑ to 15 mg/d; ↓ in elderly/debilitated pts Caution: [C, ?/−] Contra: Hx blood dyscrasias; phenothiazine sensitivity Disp: Tabs 1, 2, 5, 10 mg; PO conc 10 mg/mL; inj 2 mg/mL SE: Orthostatic ↓ BP, EPS, dizziness, neuroleptic malignant syndrome, skin discoloration, lowered Sz threshold, photosensitivity, blood dyscrasias Notes: PO conc must be diluted to 60 mL or more prior to administration; requires several weeks for onset of effects Interactions: ↑ CNS depression w/ barbiturates, benzodiazepines, TCAs, ETOH; ↑ effects OF antihypertensives, propranolol, ↓ effects OF anticoagulants ↓ effects w/ antacids Labs: ↑ LFTs; ↓ WBCs NIPE: ↑ Risk of photosensitivity—use sunscreen; urine color may change to pink to reddish-brown

Trifluridine (Viroptic) [Antiviral] Uses: *Herpes simplex keratitis & conjunctivitis* Action: Antiviral Dose: 1 gt q2h (max 9 gtt/d); ↓ to 1 gt q4h after healing begins; Rx up to 14 d Caution: [C, M] Contra: Component allergy Disp: Soln 1% SE: Local burning, stinging Interactions: ↑ Hypotensive effects w/ antihypertensives, nitrates, sulfadoxine-pyrimethamine, EtOH; ↑ effects OF anticholinergics; ↑ CNS depression w/ antihistamines, CNS depressants, narcotics, EtOH; ↓ effects w/ barbiturates, Li, caffeine, tobacco); ↓ effects OF guanadrel, guanethidine, levodopa Labs: ↑ LFTs, serum prolactin levels, ↓ Hmg, Hct, plts, false PRG test results + or − NIPE: Use sunscreen due to photosensitivity; affects body temperature regulation; reddish brown urine color change; ⊘ D/C abruptly after long-term use

Trihexyphenidyl (Artane) [Antiparkinson Agent/Anticholinergic] Uses: *Parkinson Dz* Action: Blocks excess acetylcholine at cerebral synapses **Dose:** 2–5 mg PO qd–qid **Caution:** [C, +] **Contra:** NA glaucoma, GI obstruction, MyG, bladder obstructions **Disp:** Tabs 2, 5 mg; SR caps 5 mg; elixir 2 mg/5 mL **SE:** Dry skin, constipation, xerostomia, photosensitivity, tachycardia, arrhythmias **Interactions:** ↑ Effects w/ MAOIs, phenothiazines, quinidine, TCAs; ↑ effects OF amantadine, anticholinergics, digoxin; ↓ effects w/ antacids, tacrine; ↓ effects OF chlorpromazine, haloperidol, tacrine **Labs:** False ↑ T3, T4 **NIPE:** Take w/ food; monitor for urinary hesitancy or retention; ⊘ D/C abruptly; ↑ risk of heat stroke

Trimethobenzamide (Tigan) [Antiemetic/Anticholinergic] Uses: *N/V* **Action:** ↓ medullary chemoreceptor trigger zone **Dose:** *Adults.* 250 mg PO or 200 mg PR or IM tid–qid PRN. *Peds.* 20 mg/kg/24 h PO or 15 mg/kg/24 h PR or IM in 3–4 ÷ doses **Caution:** [C, ?] **Contra:** Benzocaine sensitivity **Disp:** Caps 100, 250 mg; supp 100, 200 mg; inj 100 mg/mL **SE:** Drowsiness, ↓ BP, dizziness; hepatic impair, blood dyscrasias, Szs, parkinsonian-like syndrome **Interactions:** ↑ CNS depression w/ antidepressants, antihistamines, opioids, sedatives, EtOH; ↑ risk OF extrapyramidal effects **NIPE:** In the presence of viral Infxns, may mask emesis or mimic CNS effects of Reye's syndrome

Trimethoprim (Trimpex, Proloprim) [Antibiotic/Folate Antagonist] Uses: *UTI* due to susceptible gram(+) & gram(−) organisms;* suppression of UTI **Action:** ↓ dihydrofolate reductase. *Spectrum:* Many gram(+) & (−) except *Bacteroides, Branhamella, Brucella, Chlamydia, Clostridium, Mycobacterium, Mycoplasma, Nocardia, Neisseria, Pseudomonas,* & *Treponema* **Dose:** *Adults.* 100 mg/d PO bid or 200 mg/d PO. *Peds.* 4 mg/kg/d in 2 ÷ doses; ↓ in renal failure **Caution:** [C, +] **Contra:** Megaloblastic anemia due to folate deficiency **Disp:** Tabs 100, 200 mg; PO soln 50 mg/5 mL **SE:** Rash, pruritus, megaloblastic anemia, hepatic impair, blood dyscrasias **Notes:** Take w/ plenty of H₂O bd] **Interactions:** ↑ Effects w/ dapsone; ↑ effects OF dapsone, phenytoin, procainamide; ↓ efficacy w/ rifampin **Labs:** ↑ LFTs, BUN, creatinine **NIPE:** ↑ Fluids to 2–3 L/d; ↑ risk of folic acid deficiency

Trimethoprim (TMP)–Sulfamethoxazole (SMX) [Co-Trimoxazole] (Bactrim, Septra) [Antibiotic/Folate Antagonist] Uses: *UTI Rx & prophylaxis, otitis media, sinusitis, bronchitis* **Action:** SMX-inhibiting synthesis of dihydrofolic acid; TMP-inhibiting dihydrofolate reductase to impair protein synthesis. *Spectrum:* Includes *Shigella, P. jiroveci* (formerly *carinii*), & *Nocardia* Infxns, *Mycoplasma, Enterobacter* sp, *Staphylococcus, Streptococcus,* & more **Dose:** *Adults.* 1 DS tab PO bid or 5–20 mg/kg/24 h (based on TMP) IV in 3–4 ÷ doses. *P. jiroveci:* 15–20 mg/kg/d IV or PO (TMP) in 4 ÷ doses. *Nocardia:* 10–15 mg/kg/d IV or PO (TMP) in 4 ÷ doses. *UTI prophylaxis:* 1 PO qd. *Peds.* 8–10 mg/kg/24 h (TMP) PO ÷ into 2 doses or 3–4 doses IV; do not use in newborns; ↓ in renal failure; maintain hydration **Caution:** [B (D if near term), +] **Contra:** Sulfonamide sensitivity, porphyria, megaloblastic anemia w/ folate deficiency, significant hepatic impair **Disp:** Regular tabs 80 mg TMP/400 mg SMX; DS tabs

160 mg TMP/800 mg SMX; PO susp 40 mg TMP/200 mg SMX/5 mL; inj 80 mg TMP/ 400 mg SMX/5 mL **SE:** Allergic skin Rxns, photosensitivity, GI upset, Stevens–Johnson syndrome, blood dyscrasias, hepatitis **Notes:** Synergistic combo, interacts w/ warfarin **Interactions:** ↑ Effect OF dapsone, MTX, phenytoin, sulfonylureas, warfarin, zidovudine; ↓ effects w/ rifampin; ↓ effect OF cyclosporine **Labs:** ↑ Serum bilirubin, alkaline phosphatase, creatinine **NIPE:** ↑ Risk of photosensitivity—use sunscreen; ↑ fluids to 2–3 L/d

Trimetrexate (Neutrexin) [Antiinfective, Antiprotozoal/Folic Acid Antimetabolite] **WARNING:** Must be used w/ leucovorin to avoid tox **Uses:** *Moderate–severe PCP* **Action:** ↓ dihydrofolate reductase **Dose:** 45 mg/m² IV q24h for 21 d; administer w/ leucovorin 20 mg/m² IV q6h for 24 d; ↓ in hepatic impair **Caution:** [D, ?/–] **Contra:** MTX sensitivity **Disp:** Inj 25, 200 mg/25 mg/vial **SE:** Sz, fever, rash, GI upset, anemias, ↑ LFTs, peripheral neuropathy, renal impair **Notes:** Use cytotoxic cautions; inf over 60 min **Interactions:** ↑ Effects w/ azole antifungals, cimetidine, erythromycin; ↓ effects w/ rifabutin, rifampin; ↓ effects OF pneumococcal immunization **Labs:** ↑ LFTs, SCr **NIPE:** ⊘ PRG, breast-feeding use contraception; ⊘ exposure to infection

Triptorelin (Trelstar Depot, Trelstar LA) [Antineoplastic/Gonadotropin-releasing Hormone] **Uses:** *Palliation of advanced CAP* **Action:** LHRH analog; ↓ GNRH w/ continuous dosing; transient ↑ in LH, FSH, testosterone, & estradiol 7–10 d after first dose; w/ chronic/continuous use (usually 2–4 wk); sustained ↓ LH & FSH w/ ↓ testicular & ovarian steroidogenesis similar to surgical castration **Dose:** 3.75 mg IM monthly or 11.25 mg IM q3mo **Caution:** [X, N/A] **Contra:** Not indicated in females **Disp:** Inj depot 3.75 mg; LA 11.25 mg **SE:** Dizziness, emotional lability, fatigue, HA, insomnia, HTN, D, vomiting, ED, retention, UTI, pruritus, anemia, inj site pain, musculoskeletal pain, osteoporosis, allergic Rxns **Interactions:** ↑ Risk OF severe hyperprolactinemia w/ antipsychotics, metoclopramide **Labs:** Suppression of pituitary-gonadal Fxn **NIPE:** ⊘ PRG or breast-feeding; may cause hot flashes; initial ↑ bone pain

Trospium Chloride (Sanctura) [Antispasmodic/Anticholinergic] **Uses:** * OAB * **Action:** Antimuscarinic, antispasmodic **Dose:** 20 mg PO bid, ↓ w/renal impair or >75 y (on empty stomach or 1 h ac) **Caution:** [C, ?/–] BOO, GI obstruction, ulcerative colitis, MyG, renal/hepatic impair **Contra:** NA glaucoma, urinary/gastric retention **Disp:** Tabs 20 mg **SE:** Constipation, xerostomia **Interactions:** ↑ Effects may be seen when used w/ amiloride, digoxin, morphine, metformin, procainamide, quinidine, quinine, ranitidine, tenofovir, triamterene, trimethoprim, vancomycin; ↑ effects OF these drugs may be seen amiloride, digoxin, morphine, metformin, procainamide, quinidine, quinine, ranitidine, tenofovir, triamterene, trimethoprim, vancomycin **NIPE:** Take w/o food 1 h ac

Trovafloxacin (Trovan) [Antibiotic/Fluoroquinolonee] **WARNING:** Trovan has been associated w/ serious liver injury leading to need for liver transplantation &/or death. **Uses:** *Life-threatening Infxns* including pneumonia, complicated intraabdominal, gynecologic/pelvic, or skin Infxns **Action:** Fluoro-quinolone antibiotic; ↓ DNA gyrase. *Spectrum:* Broad-spectrum gram(+) & gram(−), including anaerobes; TB typically resistant **Dose:** 200 mg/d; ↓ w/hepatic impair **Caution:** [C, −] in children **Contra:** Hepatic impair **Disp:** Inj 5 mg/mL in 40 & 60 mL; tabs 100, 200 mg **SE:** Liver failure, dizziness, HA, nausea, rash **Notes:** Use restricted to hospitals; hepatotox led to restricted availability **Interactions:** ↑ Risk OF photosensitivity w/ dong quai, St. John's wort; ↑ risk of tendon rupture if used w/ corticosteroids ↓ effects w/ antacids containing Al or Mg, Fe salts, Mg, sucralfate, vitamins/minerals containing Fe, zinc; IV morphine; dairy products **Labs:** Monitor LFTs **NIPE:** Admin antacids or IV morphine 2 h after trovafloxacin on empty stomach, take w/o regard to food and w/ 8 oz water, risk of photosensitivity—use sunscreen

Urokinase (Abbokinase) [Thrombolytic Enzyme]

Uses: *PE, DVT, restore patency to IV catheters* **Action:** Converts plasminogen to plasmin; causes clot lysis **Dose:** *Adults & Peds.* Systemic effect: 4400 Units/kg IV over 10 min, then by 4400–6000 Units/kg/h for 12 h. *Restore catheter patency:* Inject 5000 Units into catheter & aspirate **Caution:** [B, +] **Contra:** Do not use w/in 10 d of surgery, delivery, or organ biopsy; bleeding, CVA, vascular malformation **Disp:** Powder for inj, 250,000-unit vial **SE:** Bleeding, ↓ BP, dyspnea, bronchospasm, anaphylaxis, cholesterol embolism **Interactions:** ↑ Risk OF bleeding w/ anticoagulants, ASA, heparin, indomethacin, NSAIDs, phenylbutazone, feverfew, garlic, ginger, ginkgo biloba; ↓ effects w/ aminocaproic acid **Labs:** ↑ PT, PTT; ↓ fibrinogen, plasminogen

Valacyclovir (Valtrex) [Antiviral/Synthetic Purine Nucleoside]

Uses: *Herpes zoster; genital herpes* **Action:** Prodrug of acyclovir; ↓ viral DNA replication. *Spectrum:* Herpes simplex I & II **Dose:** 1 g PO tid. *Genital herpes:* 500 mg bid × 7 d. *Herpes prophylaxis:* 500–1000 mg/d; ↓ w/renal failure **Caution:** [B, +] **Disp:** Caplets 500, 1000 mg **SE:** HA, GI upset, dizziness, pruritus, photophobia **Interactions:** ↑ Effects w/ cimetidine, probenecid **Labs:** ↑ LFTs, creatinine **NIPE:** Take w/o regard to food; ↑ fluids to 2–3 L/d; begin drug at first sign of S/Sxs

Valganciclovir (Valcyte) [Antiviral/Synthetic Nucleoside]

Uses: *CMV* **Action:** Ganciclovir prodrug; ↓ viral DNA synthesis **Dose:** Induction, 900 mg PO bid w/ food × 21 d, then 900 mg PO qd; ↓ in renal dysfunction **Caution:** [C, ?/−] Use w/ imipenem/cilastatin, nephrotoxic drugs **Contra:** Allergy to acyclovir, ganciclovir, valganciclovir; ANC < 500/mm²; plt < 25 K; Hgb < 8 g/dL **Disp:** Tabs 450 mg **SE:** BM suppression **Interactions:** ↑ Effects w/ cytotoxic drugs, immunosuppressive drugs, probenecid; ↑ risks of nephrotoxicity w/ amphotericin B, cyclosporine; ↑ effects w/ didanosine **Labs:** ↑ Cr; monitor CBC & Cr **NIPE:** Take w/ food; ⊘ PRG, breast-feeding, EtOH, NSAIDs; use contraception for at least 3 mo after drug Rx

Valproic Acid (Depakene, Depakote) [Anticonvulsant]

Uses: *Rx epilepsy, mania; prophylaxis of migraines,* Alzheimer behavior disorder **Ac-**

tion: Anticonvulsant; ↑ availability of GABA *Dose: Adults & Peds.* Szs: 30–60 mg/kg/24 h PO ÷ tid (after initiation of 10–15 mg/kg/24 h). *Mania:* 750 mg in 3 ÷ doses, ↑ 60 mg/kg/d max. *Migraines:* 250 mg bid, ↑ 1000 mg/d max; ↓ in hepatic impair **Caution:** [D, +] **Contra:** Severe hepatic impair **Disp:** Caps 250 mg; syrup 250 mg/5 mL **SE:** Somnolence, dizziness, GI upset, diplopia, ataxia, rash, thrombocytopenia, hepatitis, pancreatitis, prolonged bleeding times, alopecia, weight gain, hyperammonemic encephalopathy reported in pts w/ urea cycle disorders **Interactions:** ↑ Effects w/ clarithromycin, erythromycin, felbamate, INH, phenytoin, salicylates, troleandomycin; ↑ effects OF anticoagulants, lamotrigine, nimodipine, phenobarbital, phenytoin, primidone, zidovudine; ↑ CNS depression w/ CNS depressants, haloperidol, loxapine, maprotiline, MAOIs, phenothiazines, thioxanthenes, TCAs, EtOH; ↓ effects w/ cholestyramine, colestipol; ↓ effects OF clozapine, rifampin **Labs:** ↑ LFTs; altered TFTs, false + urinary ketones; monitor LFTs and serum levels (Table 2) **NIPE:** Take w/ food for GI upset; ⊘ PRG, breast-feeding; D/C abruptly

Valsartan (Diovan) [Antihypertensive/ARB] WARNING: Use during 2nd/3rd tri of PRG can cause fetal harm

Uses: HTN, CHF, DN **Action:** Angiotensin II receptor antagonist **Dose:** 80–160 mg/d given **Caution:** [C (1st tri; D 2nd & 3rd tri), ?/–] W/ K⁺-sparing diuretics or K⁺ supls **Contra:** Severe hepatic impair, biliary cirrhosis/obstruction, primary hyperaldosteronism, bilateral renal artery stenosis **Disp:** Caps 40, 80, 160, 320 mg **SE:** ↓ BP, dizziness **Interactions:** ↑ Effects w/ diuretics, Li; ↑ risk OF hyperkalemia w/ K-sparing diuretics, K supls, trimethoprim **Labs:** ↑ LFTs, K⁺, ↓ Hmg, Hct **NIPE:** Take w/o regard to food; ⊘ PRG, breast-feeding; use contraception

Vancomycin (Vancocin, Vancoled) [Antibiotic]

Uses: *Serious MRSA Infxns; enterococcal Infxns; PO Rx of C. difficile pseudomembranous colitis* **Action:** ↓ Cell wall synthesis. *Spectrum:* Gram(+) bacteria & some anaerobes (includes MRSA, *Staphylococcus* sp, *Enterococcus* sp, *Streptococcus* sp, *C. difficile*) **Dose:** *Adults.* 1 g IV q12h; for colitis 125–500 mg PO q6h. *Peds.* 40–60 mg/kg/24 h IV in ÷ doses q6–12 h. *Neonates.* 10–15 mg/kg/dose q12h; (↓ in renal insuff) **Caution:** [C, M] **Contra:** Component allergy; avoid in Hx hearing loss **Disp:** Caps 125, 250 mg; powder 250 mg/5 mL, 500 mg/6 mL for PO soln; powder for inj 500 mg, 1000 mg, 10 g/vial **SE:** Ototoxic & nephrotoxic; GI upset (PO), neutropenia **Notes:** See drug levels (Table 2); not absorbed PO, local effect in gut only; give IV dose slowly (over 1–3 h) to prevent "red-man syndrome" (red flushing of head, neck, upper torso); IV product may be given PO for colitis **Interactions:** ↑ Ototoxicity and nephrotoxicity w/ ASA, aminoglycosides, cyclosporine, cisplatin, loop diuretics; ↓ effects OF MRX **Labs:** ↑ BUN; **NIPE:** Take w/ food, ↑ fluid to 2–3 L/d

Vardenafil (Levitra) [Anti-impotence Agent/PDE 5] WARNING: May prolong QT_c interval

Uses: *ED* **Action:** Phosphodiesterase 5 inhibitor; increases cGMP and NO levels; relaxes smooth muscles, dilates cavernosal arteries **Dose:** 10 mg PO 60 min before sexual activity; 2.5 mg if administered w/ CYP3A4 inhibitors (Table 13); max ×1 ≤20 mg **Caution:** [B, –] W/ CV, hepatic, or renal Dz **Contra:** Nitrates; ↑ Qtc interval **Disp:** 2.5-mg, 5-mg, 10-mg, 20-mg tabs **SE:** ↓ BP, HA, dyspepsia, priapism **Notes:** Concomitant α-blockers may cause ↓ BP **Interactions:** ↑ Effects w/ erythromycin, ketoconazole, indinavir, ritonavir; ↑ effects Of α-blockers, nitrates; ↓ effects Of indinavir, ritonavir **NIPE:** Take w/o regard to food; ↑ risk of priapism

Varenicline (Chantix) [Nicotinic Acetylcholine Receptor Partial Agonist] Uses: *Smoking cessation* Action: Nicotine receptor partial

agonist **Dose:** *Adults.* 0.5 mg PO daily × 3 d, 0.5 mg bid × 4 d, then 1 mg PO BID for 12 wks total; after meal w/ glass of water **Caution:** [C, ?/—] ↓ dose w/renal impair **Disp:** Tabs 0.5, 1 mg **SE:** N, V, insomnia, flatulence, unusual dreams **Interactions:** May affect metabolism of warfarin, theophylline, insulin; ↑ effects with nicotine replacement drugs **NIPE:** Slowly ↑ dose to ↓ N; initiate 1 wk before desired smoking cessation date

Varicella Virus Vaccine (Varivax) [Vaccine] Uses: *Prevent vari-

cella (chickenpox)* **Action:** Active immunization; live attenuated virus **Dose:** *Adults & Peds.* 0.5 mL SQ, repeat 4–8 wk **Caution:** [C, M] **Contra:** Immunocompromise; neomycin-anaphylactoid Rxn, blood dyscrasias; immunosuppressive drugs; avoid PRG for 3 mo after **Disp:** Powder for inj **SE:** Mild varicella Infxn; fever, local Rxns, irritability, GI upset **Notes:** OK for all children & adults who have not had chickenpox **Interactions:** ↓ Effects w/ acyclovir, immunosuppressant drugs **NIPE:** ⊘ Salicylates for 6 wk after immunization; ⊘ PRG for 3 mo after immunization

Vasopressin [Antidiuretic Hormone, ADH) (Pitressin) [Antidiuretic Hormone/Posterior Pituitary Hormone] Uses: *DI; Rx

postop abdominal distension*; adjunct Rx of GI bleeding & esophageal varices; asystole and PEA pulseless VT & VF, adjunct systemic vasopressor (IV drip) **Action:** Posterior pituitary hormone, potent GI peripheral vasoconstrictor, potent peripheral vasoconstrictor **Dose:** *Adults & Peds.* DI: 2.5–10 Units SQ or IM tid–qid *GI hemorrhage:* 0.2–0.4 Units/min; ↓ in cirrhosis; caution in vascular Dz. *VT/VF:* 40 Units IVP × 1. *Vasopressor:* 0.01–0.1 Units/kg/min **Caution:** [B, +] **Contra:** Allergy **Disp:** Inj 20 Units/mL **SE:** HTN, arrhythmias, fever, vertigo, GI upset, tremor **Notes:** Addition of vasopressor to concurrent norepinephrine or epi infs **Interactions:** ↑ Vasopressor effects w/ guanethidine, neostigmine; ↑ antidiuretic effects w/ carbamazepine, chlorpropamide, clofibrate, phenformin urea, TCAs; ↓ antidiuretic effects w/ demeclocycline, epinephrine, heparin, Li, phenytoin, EtOH **Labs:** ↑ cortisol level **NIPE:** Take 1–2 glasses H₂O w/ drug

Vecuronium (Norcuron) [Skeletal Muscle Relaxant/Nondepolarizing Neuromuscular Blocker] Uses: *Skeletal muscle relax-

ation during surgery or mechanical ventilation* **Action:** Nondepolarizing neuromuscular blocker **Dose:** *Adults & Peds.* 0.08–0.1 mg/kg IV bolus; maint

.010–0.015 mg/kg after 25–40 min; additional doses q12–15min PRN; ↓ in severe renal/hepatic impair **Caution:** [C, ?] Drug interactions cause ↑ effect (eg, aminoglycosides, tetracycline, succinylcholine) **Disp:** Powder for inj 10, 20 mg **SE:** Bradycardia, ↓ BP, itching, rash, tachycardia, CV collapse **Notes:** Fewer cardiac effects than pancuronium **Interactions:** ↑ Neuromuscular blockade w/ aminoglycosides, BBs, CCBs, clindamycin, furosemide, lincomycin, quinidine, tetracylines, thiazide diuretics, verapamil; ↑ resp depression w/ opioids; ↓ effects w/ phenytoin **NIPE:** Will not provide pain relief or sedation

Venlafaxine (Effexor, Effexor XR) [Antidepressant/Serotonin, Norepinephrine, & Dopamine Reuptake Inhibitor] WARN-ING: Closely monitor for worsening depression or emergence of suicidality, particularly in ped pts **Uses:** *Depression, generalized anxiety, panic disorder* anxiety disorder; obsessive–compulsive disorder, chronic fatigue syndrome, ADHD, autism **Action:** Potentiation of CNS neurotransmitter activity **Dose:** 75–375 mg/d ÷ into 2–3 equal doses; ↓ in renal/hepatic impair; extended release caps—one cap PO, **OD Caution:** [C, ?/–] **Contra:** MAOIs **Disp:** Tabs 25, 37.5, 50, 75, 100 mg; XR caps 37.5, 75, 150 mg **SE:** HTN, arthralgia↑ HR, HA, somnolence, GI upset, sexual dysfunction, confusion; actuates mania or Szs **Interactions:** ↑ Effects w/ cimetidine, desipramine, haloperidol, MAOIs; ↑ risk of serotonin syndrome w/ buspirone, Li, meperidine, sibutramine, sumatriptan, SSRIs, TCAs, trazodone, St. John's wort **Labs:** ↑ LFTs, creatinine **NIPE:** XR caps swallow whole—⊘ chew; take w/ food; ⊘ use ETOH; ⊘ D/C abruptly; D/C MAOI 14 days before start of this drug; ↑ fluids to ~3 L/d; may take 2–3 wk for full effects; frequent edema & wt. gain

Verapamil (Calan, Isoptin) [Antihypertensive, Antianginal, Antiarrhythmic/CCB] **Uses:** *Angina, HTN, PSVT, AF, atrial flutter,* migraine prophylaxis, hypertrophic cardiomyopathy, bipolar Dz **Action:** CCB **Dose:** **Adults.** Arrhythmias: 2nd line for PSVT w/ narrow QRS complex & adequate BP .5–5 mg IV over 1–2 min; repeat 5–10 mg in 15–30 min PRN (30 mg max). *Angina:* 80–120 mg PO tid, ↑ 480 mg/24 h max. *HTN:* 80–180 mg PO tid or SR tabs 120–240 mg PO qd to 240 mg bid. **Peds.** <1 y: 0.1–0.2 mg/kg IV over 2 min may repeat in 30 min). *1–16y:* 0.1–0.3 mg/kg IV over 2 min (may repeat in 30 min); 5 mg max. *PO: 1–5 y:* 4–8 mg/kg/d in 3 ÷ doses. *>5 y:* 80 mg q6–8h; ↓ in renal/hepatic impair **Caution:** [C, +] Amiodarone/β-blockers/flecainide can cause bradycardia; statins, midazolam, tacrolimus, theophylline levels may be ↑ **Contra:** Conduction disorders, cardiogenic shock; caution w/ elderly pts **Disp:** Tabs 40, 80, 120 mg; SR tabs 120, 180, 240 mg; SR caps 120, 180, 240, 360 mg; inj 5 mg/2 mL **SE:** Gingival hyperplasia, constipation, ↓ BP, bronchospasm, heart rate or conduction disturbances **Interactions:** ↑ Effects w/ antihypertensives, nitrates, quinidine, EtOH, grapefruit juice; ↑ effects OF buspirone, carbamazepine, cyclosporine, digoxin, prazosin, quinidine, theophylline, warfarin; ↑ effects w/ antineoplastics, barbiturates, NSAIDs, ↓ effects OF Li, rifampin **Labs:** ↑ ALT, AST, alkaline phosphatase **NIPE:** Take w/ food; ↑ fluids and bulk foods to prevent constipation

Vinblastine (Velban, Velbe) [Antineoplastic/Vinca Alkaloid]
WARNING: Chemotherapeutic agent; **Uses:** *Hodgkin Dz &
NHLs, mycosis fungoides, CAs (testis, renal cell, breast, non-small-cell lung
AIDS-related Kaposi sarcoma,* choriocarcinoma), histiocytosis **Action:** ↓ micro
tubule assembly **Dose:** 0.1–0.5 mg/kg/wk (4–20 mg/m²); ↓ in hepatic failure **Cau**
tion: [D, ?] **Contra:** Intrathecal use **Disp:** Inj 1 mg/mL in 10-mg vial **SE**
Myelosuppression (especially leukopenia), N/V, constipation, neurotox, alopecia
rash; myalgia, tumor pain **Interactions:** ↑ Effects w/ erythromycin, itraconazole
↓ effects w/ glutamic acid, tryptophan; ↓ effects OF phenytoin **Labs:** ↑ Uric acid
NIPE: ↑ Fluids to 2–3 L/d; ⊘ PRG or breast-feeding; use contraception for at leas
2 mo after drug; photosensitivity—use sunscreen; ⊘ admin immunizations

Vincristine (Oncovin, Vincasar PFS) [Antineoplastic/Vince
Alkaloid] **WARNING:** Chemotherapeutic agent; handle w/ caution***Fata**
if administered intrathecally* **Uses:** *ALL, breast & small-cell lung CA
sarcoma (eg, Ewing tumor, rhabdomyosarcoma), Wilms tumor, Hodgkin Dz &
NHLs, neuroblastoma, multiple myeloma* **Action:** Promotes disassembly of mi
totic spindle, causing metaphase arrest **Dose:** 0.4–1.4 mg/m² (single dose
2 mg/max); ↓ in hepatic failure **SE:** Neurotox commonly dose limiting, jaw pain (trigemina
neuralgia), fever, fatigue, anorexia, constipation & paralytic ileus, bladder atony
no significant myelosuppression w/ standard doses; tissue necrosis w/ extravasa
tion **Interactions:** ↑ Effects w/ CCBs; ↑ effects OF MTX; ↑ risk OF bron
chospasm w/ mitomycin; ↓ effects OF digoxin, phenytoin **NIPE:** ↑ Fluids to 2–
L/d; reversible hair loss; ⊘ exposure to infection; ⊘ admin immunizations

Vinorelbine (Navelbine) [Antineoplastic/Vinca Alkaloid
WARNING: Chemotherapeutic agent; handle w/ caution **Uses:** *Breast & non
small-cell lung CA* (alone or w/ cisplatin) **Action:** ↓ polymerization of micro
tubules, impairing mitotic spindle formation; semisynthetic vinca alkaloid **Dose**
30 mg/m²/wk; ↓ in hepatic failure **Caution:** [D, ?] **Contra:** Intrathecal use **Disp**
Inj 10 mg **SE:** Myelosuppression (leukopenia), mild GI effects, infrequent neuro
tox (6–29%); constipation & paresthesias (rare); tissue damage from extravasation
Interactions: ↑ Risk OF granulocytopenia w/ cisplatin, ↑ pulmonary effects w
mitomycin, paclitaxel **Labs:** ↑ LFTs **Disp:** ⊘ PRG or breast-feeding; use contra
ception; ⊘ infectious environment; ↑ fluids to 2–3 L/d

Vitamin B₁ See Thiamine (page 262)
Vitamin B₆ See Pyridoxine (page 230)
Vitamin B₁₂ See Cyanocobalamin (page 86)
Vitamin K See Phytonadione (page 219)
Vitamin, multi See Multivitamins (Table 15)
Voriconazole (VFEND) [Antifungal] **Uses:** *Invasive aspergillosis
serious fungal Infxns* **Action:** ↓ ergosterol synthesis. *Spectrum:* Several types o
fungus: *Aspergillus, Scedosporium* sp, *Fusarium* sp **Dose:** *Adults & Peds ≥ 12 y*

V: 6 mg/kg q12h × 2, then 4 mg/kg bid; may ↓ to 3 mg/kg/dose. *PO:* <40 kg: 100 ng q12h, up to 150 mg; >40 kg: 200 mg q 12 h, up to 300 mg; ↓ in mild–moderate hepatic impair; IV only one dose w/ renal impair (PO empty stomach) **Caution:** D, ?/–] **Contra:** Severe hepatic impair **Disp:** Tabs 50, 200 mg; susp 200 mg/5 mL; 200-mg inj **SE:** Visual changes, fever, rash, GI upset, ↑ LFTs **Notes:** Screen for multiple drug interactions (eg, ↑ dose w/ phenytoin) **Interactions:** ↑ Effects w/ delavirdine, efavirenz; ↑ effects OF benzodiazepines, buspirone, CCBs, cisapride, cyclosporine, ergots, pimozide, quinidine, sirolimus, sulfonylureas, tacrolimus; ↓ effects w/ carbamazepine, mephobarbital, phenobarbital, rifampin, rifabutin **NIPE:** Take w/o food; ↑ risk of photosensitivity—use sunscreen; ⊘ PRG or breast-feeding

Warfarin (Coumadin) [Anticoagulant] Uses: *Prophylaxis & Rx of PE & DVT, AF w/ embolization,* other postop indications **Action:** ↓ Vitamin K-dependent production of clotting factors in this order: VII-IX-X-II **Dose:** *Adults.* Titrate to keep INR 2.0–3.0 for most; mechanical valves INR is 2.5–3.5. ACCP guidelines: 5 mg initial (unless rapid therapeutic INR needed), may use 7.5–10 mg; ↓ if pt elderly or has other bleeding risk factors; *Alternative:* 10–15 mg PO, IM, or IV qd for 1–3 d; maint 2–10 mg/d PO, IV, or IM; follow daily INR initial to adjust dosage (see Table 10). *Peds.* 0.05–0.34 mg/kg/24 h PO, IM, or IV; follow PT/INR to adjust dosage; monitor vitamin K intake; ↓ in hepatic impair/elderly **Caution:** [X, +] **Contra:** Severe hepatic/renal Dz, bleeding, peptic ulcer, PRG **Disp:** Tabs 1, 2, 2.5, 3, 4, 5, 6, 7.5, 10 mg; inj **SE:** Bleeding due to overanticoagulation (PT >3× control or INR >5.0–6.0) or injury & INR w/in therapeutic range; bleeding, alopecia, skin necrosis, purple toe syndrome Interactions: *Common warfarin interactions:* ↑ Action with APAP, EtOH (w/ liver Dz), amiodarone, cimetidine, ciprofloxacin, cotrimoxazole, erythromycin, fluconazole, flu vaccine, isoniazid, itraconazole, metronidazole, omeprazole, phenytoin, propranolol, quinidine, tetracycline. ↓ Action with barbiturates, carbamazepine, chlordiazepoxide, cholestyramine, dicloxacillin, nafcillin, rifampin, sucralfate, high-vitamin K foods Labs: ↑ PTT; false ↑ serum theophylline levels NIPE: INR preferred test; to rapidly correct overanticoagulation, use vitamin K, FFP, or both; Reddish discoloration of urine; ⊘ PRG or breast-feeding; use barrier contraception; highly teratogenic; caution pt on taking w/ other meds, especially ASA; monitor for bleeding

Zafirlukast (Accolate) [Bronchodilator/Leukotriene Receptor Antagonist] Uses: *Adjunctive Rx of asthma* **Action:** Selective & competitive inhibitor of leukotrienes **Dose:** *Adults & Peds ≥ 12 y.* 20 mg bid. *Peds 5–11 y.* 10 mg PO bid (empty stomach) **Caution:** [B, –] Interacts w/ warfarin, ↑ INR **Contra:** Component allergy **Disp:** Tabs 10, 20 mg **SE:** Hepatic dysfunction, usually reversible on D/C; HA, dizziness, GI upset; Churg–Strauss syndrome **Interactions:** ↑ Effects w/ ASA; ↑ effects of CCBs, cyclosporine; ↑ risk of bleeding w/ warfarin; ↓ effects w/ erythromycin, theophylline, food **Labs:** ↑ ALT **NIPE:** Take w/o food; ⊘ use for acute asthma attack

Zalcitabine (Hivid) [Antiretroviral/NRTI] **WARNING:** Use w caution in pts w/ neuropathy, pancreatitis, lactic acidosis, hepatitis **Uses:** *HIV* **Action:** Antiretroviral agent **Dose:** *Adults.* 0.75 mg PO tid. *Peds.* 0.015–0.04 mg/kg PO q 6h; ↓ in renal failure **Caution:** [C, +] **Contra:** Component allergy **Disp:** Tabs 0.375, 0.75 mg **SE:** Peripheral neuropathy, pancreatitis, fever, malaise anemia, hypo/hyperglycemia, hepatic impair **Notes:** May be used in combo w/ zi dovudine **Interactions:** ↑ Risk OF peripheral neuropathy w/ amphotericin B aminoglycosides, cisplatin, didanosine, disulfiram, foscarnet, INH, phenytoin, ribavirin, vincristine; ↑ effects w/ cimetidine, metoclopramide; probenecid; ↓ effects w/ antacids **Labs:** ↑ LFTs, lipase, triglycerides **NIPE:** Use barrier contraception take w/o regard to food

Zaleplon (Sonata) [Sedative/Hypnotic] [C-IV] **Uses:** *Insomnia* **Action:** A nonbenzodiazepine sedative/hypnotic, a pyrazolopyrimidine **Dose:** 5–2 mg hs PRN; ↓ in renal/hepatic insuff, elderly **Caution:** [C, ?/–] w/ mental/psycho logical conditions **Contra:** Component allergy **Disp:** Caps 5, 10 mg **SE:** HA edema, amnesia, somnolence, photosensitivity **Notes:** Take immediately before de sired onset **Interactions:** ↑ CNS depression w/ cimetidine, CNS depressants imipramine, thioridazine, EtOH; ↓ effects w/ carbamazepine, phenobarbital phenytoin, rifampin **NIPE:** Rapid effects of drug; take w/o food ⊘ D/C abruptly

Zanamivir (Relenza) [Antiviral/Neuramidase Inhibitor] **Uses:** *Influenza A & B* **Action:** ↓ viral neuraminidase **Dose:** *Adults & Peds >7 y* 2 inhal (10 mg) bid for 5 d; initiate w/in 48 h of Sxs **Caution:** [C, M] **Contra:** Pul monary Dz **Disp:** Powder for inhal 5 mg **SE:** Bronchospasm, HA, GI upset **Notes** Uses a Diskhaler for administration **Labs:** ↑LFTs, CPK **NIPE:** Does not reduce risk of transmitting virus

Ziconotide (Prialt) [Pain Control Agent/Nonnarcotic] **WARNING:** Psychiatric, cognitive, neurologic impair may develop over severa weeks; monitor frequently; may necessitate D/C **Uses:** * IT Rx of severe, refrac tory, chronic pain* **Action:** N-type CCB in spinal cord **Dose:** 2.6 mcg/d IT at 0. mcg/h; may ↑ 0.8 mcg/d to total 19.2 mcg/d by day 21 **Caution:** [C, ?/–] Re versible psychiatric/neurologic impair **Contra:** Psychosis **Disp:** Inj 25, 10 mg/mL **SE:** Dizziness, N/V, confusion, abnormal vision; may require dosage ad justment **NIPE:** May D/C abruptly; uses specific pumps; do not ↑ more frequently than 2–3 ×/wk; monitor for S/Sys psychotic behavior & meningitis

Zidovudine (Retrovir) [Antiretroviral/NRTI] **WARNING:** Neu tropenia, anemia, lactic acidosis, & hepatomegaly w/ steatosis **Uses:** *HIV Infxn prevention of maternal transmission of HIV* **Action:** ↓ RT **Dose:** *Adults.* 200 m PO tid or 300 mg PO bid or 1–2 mg/kg/dose IV q4h. *PRG:* 100 mg PO 5×/d unti labor starts; during labor 2 mg/kg over 1 h followed by 1 mg/kg/h until clamping o the cord. *Peds.* 160 mg/m²/dose q8h; ↓ in renal failure **Caution:** [C, ?/–] **Contra** Allergy **Disp:** Caps 100 mg; tabs 300 mg; syrup 50 mg/5 mL; inj 10 mg/mL **SE:** Hematologic tox, HA, fever, rash, GI upset, malaise **Interactions:** ↑ Effects w/ flu conazole, phenytoin, probenecid, trimethoprim, valproic acid, vinblastine, vincristine; ↑ hematologic toxicity w/ adriamycin, dapsone, ganciclovir, interferon-α; ↓ effects w/ rifampin, ribavirin, stavudine **NIPE:** Take w/o food monitor for S/Sxs opportunistic infection; monitor for anemia

Zidovudine & Lamivudine (Combivir) [Antiretroviral/NRTI]
WARNING: Neutropenia, anemia, lactic acidosis, & hepatomegaly w/ steatosis **Uses:** *HIV Infxn* **Action:** Combo of RT inhibitors **Dose:** *Adults & Peds >12 y.* 1 tab PO bid; ↓ in renal failure **Caution:** [C, ?/–] **Contra:** Component allergy **Disp:** Caps zidovudine 300 mg/lamivudine 150 mg **SE:** Hematologic tox, HA, fever, rash, GI upset, malaise, pancreatitis **Notes:** Combo product ↓ daily pill burden **Interactions:** ↑ Effects w/ fluconazole, phenytoin, probenecid, trimethoprim, valproic acid, vinblastine, vincristine; ↑ hematologic toxicity w/ adriamycin, dapsone, ganciclovir, interferon-α; ↓ effects w/ rifampin, ribavirin, stavudine **NIPE:** Take w/o food; monitor for S/Sxs opportunistic infection; monitor for anemia

Zileuton (Zyflo) [Leukotriene Receptor Antagonist] Uses: *Chronic Rx of asthma* **Action:** Inhibitor of 5-lipoxygenase **Dose:** *Adults & Peds ≥ 12 y.* 600 mg PO qid **Caution:** [C, ?/–] **Contra:** Hepatic impair **Disp:** Tabs 600 mg **SE:** Hepatic damage, HA, GI upset, leukopenia **Interactions:** ↑ Effects OF propranolol, terfenadine, theophylline, warfarin **Labs:** ↓ WBCs; ↑ LFTs,; Monitor LFTs every month × 3, then q2–3 mo **NIPE:** Take w/o regard to food; take on a regular basis; not for acute asthma

Ziprasidone (Geodon) [Antipsychotic/Piperazine Derivative] **WARNING:** ↑ mortality in elderly w/ dementia-related psychoses Uses: *Schizophrenia, acute agitation* **Action:** Atypical antipsychotic **Dose:** 20 mg PO bid, may ↑ in 2-d intervals up to 80 mg bid; agitation 10–20 mg IM PRN up to 40 mg/d; separate 10 mg doses by 2 h & 20 mg doses by 4h (w/ food) **Caution:** [C, –] w/ ↓ Mg²⁺, ↓ K⁺ **Contra:** QT prolongation, recent MI, uncompensated heart failure, meds that prolong QT interval **Disp:** Caps 20, 40, 60, 80 mg; susp 10 mg/mL; Inj 20 mg/mL **SE:** Bradycardia; rash, somnolence, resp disorder, EPS, weight gain, orthostatic ↓ BP **Interactions:** ↑ Effects w/ ketoconazole; ↑ effects of antihypertensives; ↑ CNS depression w/ anxiolytics, sedatives, opioids, EtOH; TCAs, thioridazine, risk OF prolonged QT w/ cisapride, chlorpromazine, clarithromycin, diltiazem, erythromycin, levofloxacin, mefloquine, pentamidine, TCAs, thioridazine; ↓ effects w/ amphetamines, carbamazepine; ↓ effects OF levodopa **Labs:** ↑ Prolactin, cholesterol, triglycerides; monitor electrolytes **NIPE:** May take weeks before full effects, take w/ food, ↑ risk of tardive dyskinesia

Zoledronic Acid (Zometa) [Antihypercalcemic/Biphosphonate] Uses: *↑ Ca²⁺ of malignancy (HCM),* ↓ skeletal-related events in CAP, multiple myeloma, & metastatic bone lesions **Action:** Bisphosphonate; ↓ osteoclastic bone resorption **Dose:** *HCM:* 4 mg IV over at least 15 min; may re-treat in 7 d if adequate renal Fxn. *Bone lesions/myeloma:* 4 mg IV over at least 15 min, repeat q3–4wk PRN; prolonged w/ Cr ↑ **Caution:** [C, ?/–] Loop diuretics, aminoglycosides; ASA-sensitive asthmatics; avoid invasive dental procedures in cancer patients; renal dysfunction **Contra:** Bisphosphonate allergy; w/dental procedures **Disp:** Vial 4 mg **SE:** Adverse effects ↑ w/ renal dysfunction; fever, flu-like syndrome, GI upset, insomnia, anemia; electrolyte abnormalities, osteonecrosis of jaw **Interactions:** ↑ Risk OF hypocalcemia w/ diuretics; ↑ risk OF nephrotoxicity w/ aminoglycosides, thalidomide **Labs:** Follow Cr; effect prolonged w/Cr increase **NIPE:** ↑ Fluids to 2–3 L/d; Requires vigorous prehydration; do not exceed recommended doses/inf duration to ↓ dose-related renal dysfunction; avoid oral surgery; dental examination recommended prior to therapy; ↓ dose w/ renal dysfunction

Zolmitriptan (Zomig, Zomig XMT, Zomig Nasal) [Analgesic Migraine Agent/5-HT1 Receptor Agonist] Uses: *Acute Rx migraine* Action: Selective serotonin agonist; causes vasoconstriction Dose: Initial 2.5 mg PO, may repeat after 2 h, 10 mg max in 24 h; nasal 5 mg; HA returns, repeated after 2 h 10 mg max 24 h Caution: [C, ?/–] Contra: Ischemic heart Dz, Prinzmetal angina, uncontrolled HTN, accessory conduction pathway disorders, ergots, MAOIs Disp: Tabs 2.5, 5 mg; Rapid tabs (ZMT) 2.5, 5 mg; nasal 5.0 mg, SE: Dizziness, hot flashes, paresthesias, chest tightness, myalgia, diaphoresis Interactions: ↑ Effects w/ cimetidine, MAOIs, oral contraceptives, propranolol; ↑ risk of prolonged vasospasms w/ ergots; ↑ risk of serotonin syndrome w/ sibutramine, SSRIs NIPE: Admin to relieve migraines; not for prophylaxis

Zolpidem (Ambien, Ambien CR) [C-IV] [Sedative/Hypnotic] Uses: *Short-term Rx of insomnia* Action: Hypnotic agent Dose: 5–10 mg or 12.5 mg CR PO hs PRN; ↓ in elderly (use 6.25 mg CR), hepatic insuff Caution: [B, –] Contra: Breast-feeding Disp: Tabs 5, 10 mg; CR 6.25, 12.5 mg SE: HA, dizziness, drowsiness, nausea, myalgia Interactions: ↑ CNS depression w/ CNS depressants, sertraline, EtOH; ↑ effects of ketoconazole; ↓ effects OF rifampin NIPE: Take w/o food; ⊘ D/C abruptly if long-term use; may develop tolerance to drug; may be habit-forming; CR delivers a rapid then a longer lasting dose

Zonisamide (Zonegran) [Anticonvulsant/Sulfonamide] Uses: *Adjunct Rx complex partial Szs* Action: Anticonvulsant Dose: Initial 100 mg/d PO; may ↑ to 400 mg/d Caution: [C, –] Contra: Allergy to sulfonamides; oligohidrosis & hypothermia in peds Disp: Caps 25, 50, 100 mg SE: Dizziness, drowsiness, confusion, ataxia, memory impair, paresthesias, psychosis, nystagmus, diplopia, tremor; anemia, leukopenia; GI upset, nephrolithiasis, Stevens–Johnson syndrome; monitor for ↓ sweating & ↑ body temperature Interactions: ↑ tox w/ CYP3A4 inhibitor; ↓ Effects w/ carbamazepine, phenobarbital, phenytoin, valproic acid Labs: ↑ serum alkaline phosphatase, ALT, AST, creatinine, BUN, ↓ glucose, Na NIPE: ⊘ DC; swallow capsules whole

Zoster Vaccine, Live (Zostavax) [Vaccine] Uses: *Prevent varicella zoster in adults > 60 yrs* Action: Active immunization (live vaccine), to Herpes zoster Dose: *Adults.* 0.65 mL SQ Contra: Gelatin, neomycin anaphy-

laxis; untreated TB, immunocompromise **Caution:** [C,?/–] not for peds **Disp:** SDV **SE:** Inj site rxn, HA **Interactions:** ↑ Risk of extensive rash w/ corticosteroids **NIPE:** ⊘ pregnancy for at least 3 months > vaccination; once reconstituted use immediately

COMMONLY USED MEDICINAL HERBS

The following is a guide to some common herbal products. These may be sold separately or in combination with other products. According to the FDA: "manufacturers of dietary supplements can make claims about how their products affect the structure or function of the body, but they may not claim to prevent, treat, cure, mitigate, or diagnose a disease without prior FDA approval"*

Aloe Vera (*Aloe barbadensis*) **Uses:** Topically for burns, skin irritation, sunburn, wounds; internally used for constipation, amenorrhea, asthma, colds **Actions:** Multiple chemical components; aloinosides inhibit H_2O & electrolyte reabsorption & irritates colon, which ↑ peristalsis & propulsion; wound healing d/t ↓ production of thromboxane A2, inhibiting bradykinin & histamine **Available Forms:** Apply gel topically 3–5/d prn; capsules 100–200 mg po hs **Contra:** ⊘ Internally if pregnant, lactating, or in children < 12 years **Notes/SE:** Abdominal cramping, diarrhea, edema, hematuria, hypokalemia, muscle weakness, dermatitis **Interactions w/ internal use:** ↑ K^+ loss w/ BB, corticosteroids, diuretics, licorice; ↑ effects OF antiarrhythmics, corticosteroids, digoxin, diuretics, hyperglycemics, jimsonweed **Labs:** ↓ K^+, BS **NIPE:** Assess for dehydration, electrolyte imbalance, abdominal distress w/ internal use; stimulates uterine contracts & may cause spontaneous abortion

Arnica (*Arnica montana*) **Uses:** ↓ Swelling & inflammation from acne, blunt injury, bruises, rashes, sprains **Action:** Sesquiterpenoids have shown antibacterial, anti-inflammatory, & analgesic properties; **Available forms:** Topical cream, spray, oint, tinc; for poultice dilute tinc 3–10 × w/ water & apply PRN **Contra:** Poisonous, ⊘ take internally; ⊘ if pt allergic to arnica, chrysanthemums, marigold, sunflowers **Notes/SE:** Arrhythmias, abdominal pain, cardiac arrest, contact dermatitis, coma, death, hepatic failure, HTN, nervousness, restlessness **Interactions:** ↑ Risk OF bleeding w/ ASA, heparin, warfarin, angelica, anise, asafetida, bogbean, boldo, capsicum, celery, chamomile, clove, danshen, fenugreek, feverfew, garlic, ginger, ginkgo, ginseng, horse chestnut, horseradish, licorice, meadowsweet, onion, papain, passion flower, poplar bark, prickly ash, quassia wood, red clover, turmeric, wild carrot, wild lettuce, willow; ↓ effects of antihypertensives **Labs:** None **NIPE:** ⊘ Apply to broken skin, ⊘ use in PRG & lactation, serious liver & kidney damage w/ internal use, ingestion of flowers & root can cause death, prolonged topical use ↑ risk of allergic reaction

Astragalus (*Astragalus membranaceus*) **Uses:** Rx of resp infections, enhancement of immune system, & heart failure **Action:** Root saponins ↑ di-

286

uresis, ↓ BP; antiinflammatory action related to the stimulation of macrophages, ↑ antibody formation & ↑ T-lymphocyte proliferation **Available forms:** Caps/tabs 1–4 g tid, PO; liq ext 4–8 mL/d (1:2 ratio) ÷ doses; dry ext 250 mg (1:8 ratio) tid, PO **Notes/SE:** Immunosuppression w/ doses > 28 g **Interactions:** ↑ Effect OF acyclovir, anticoagulants, antihypertensives, antithrombotics, antiplts, interleukin-2, interferon; ↓ effect OF cyclophosphamide **Labs:** ↑ PT, INR **NIPE:** Use cautiously in immunosuppressed Pts or those w/ autoimmune Dz

Bilberry (*Vaccinium myrtillus*)

Uses: Prevent/treat visual problems such as cataracts, retinopathy, myopia, glaucoma, macular degeneration; treat vascular problems such as hemorrhoids, & varicose veins **Actions:** Contain anthocyanidins that: ↓ vascular permeability, inhibit platelet aggregation & thrombus formation, ↑ antioxidant effects on LDLs & liver, ↑ regeneration of rhodopsin in retina **Available Forms:** Products should have 25% anthocyanoside content; capsules, extracts, dried or fresh fruit, leaves; eye/vascular problems 240–480 mg po bid/tid; night vision 60–120 mg of extract po od **Contra:** ⊘ In pregnancy or lactation; caution in patients with diabetes and bleeding disorders **Notes/SE:** Constipation **Interactions:** ↑ Effects OF anticoagulants, antiplatelets, insulin, NSAIDs, oral hypoglycemics, ↓ effects OF iron **Labs:** ↑ PT; ↓ glucose, platelet aggregation **NIPE:** Large dose of leaves for long periods of time may be poisonous/fatal; take without regard to food

Black Cohosh (*Cimicifuga racemosa*)

Uses: Antitussive; smooth muscle relaxant; management of menopausal symptoms esp hot flashes, sleep disturbance & anxiety, premenstrual syndrome, & dysmenorrhea. Antiinflammatory, peripheral vasodilation, & sedative effects **Action:** Estrogenic activity w/ some studies showing ↓ in LH; vasodilation activity causing ↓ blood flow & hypotensive effects; antimicrobial activity **Available forms:** Dried root/rhizome caps 40–200 mg ONCE/D; fluid ext (1:1) 2–4 mL or 1 tsp once/d; tinc (1:5) 3–6 mL or 1–2 tsp once/d; powdered ext (4:1) 250–500 mg once/d; Remifemin Menopause (standardized ext brand name) 20 mg bid **Notes/SE:** Hypotension, bradycardia, N/V, anorexia, HA, miscarriage, nervous system & visual disturbances **Interactions:** ↑ Effects OF antihypertensives, estrogen HRT, oral contraceptives, hypnotics, sedatives; tinc may cause a reaction w/ disulfiram & metronidazole; ↑ antiproliferative effect w/ tamoxifen; ↓ effects OF ferrous fumarate, ferrous gluconate, ferrous sulfate **Labs:** May ↓ LH levels & plt counts **NIPE:** Tinc contains large % of EtOH, ⊘ use in PRG or lactation or give to children

Bogbean (*Menyanthes trifoliate*)

Uses: ↑ Appetite; treat GI distress; anti-inflammatory for arthritis **Action:** Several chemical constituents include alkaloids (choline, gentianin, gentianidine), flavonoids (hyperin, kaempferol, quercetin, rutin, trifolioside) that act as an anti-inflammatory, and acids (caffeic, chlorogenic, ferulic, folic, palmitic, salicylic, vanillic) that act as bile stimulants & other elements such as carotene, ceryl alcohol, coumarin, iridoid, scopeletin; two compounds produce considerable inhibition of prostaglandin synthesis **Available**

Forms: Extract (1:1 dilution) 1–2 ml po tid with fluid; dried leaf as tea 1–3 g po tid **Contra:** ⊘ if pregnant or lactating **Notes/SE:** N/V, bleeding **Interactions:** ↑ Risk OF bleeding w/ anticoagulants, antiplatelets, ANA, NSAIDs; ↑ effects OF stimulant laxatives; ↓ effects OF antacids, H2 antagonists, proton pump inhibitors, sucralfate **Labs:** None **NIPE:** May ↑ uterine contractions; extracts contain ETOH; monitor for S/Sys bleeding or ↑ bruising; ⊘ if h/o colitis, anemia

Borage (*Borage officinalis*) **Uses:** Oil used for eczema & dermatitis & as a GLA supplement; treat colds, coughs, & bronchitis; anti-inflammatory action used to treat arthritis **Action:** Oil contains GLA & its metabolites produce anti-inflammatory action; topical oil absorbed in skin ↑ fluid retention in stratum corneum; mucilage & malic acid components have expectorant & diuretic actions; contains alkaloids that are hepatotoxic **Available Forms:** Capsules with 10–25% GLA- 1.1–1.4 g GLA po od for joint inflammation; oil topical application bid for dermatitis & eczema; **Contra:** ⊘ In pregnancy, lactation, & pts with h/o liver disease or seizure disorder **Notes/SE:** ↑Constipation, flatulence, liver dysfunction, seizures **Interactions:** ↑ Risk OF bleeding w/ anticoagulants, antiplatelets; ↑ effects OF antihypertensives; ↓ effects OF anticonvulsants, phenothiazines, TCAs; ↓ effects OF herb w/ NSAIDs **Labs:** Monitor LFTs; may ↑ LFTs, PT & INR **NIPE:** Only use herb without UPA alkaloids

Buglewood (*Lycopus virginicus*) **Uses:** ↓ Hyperthyroid symptoms, analgesic, astringent **Action:** Inhibits gonadotropin, prolactin, TSH, & IgG antibody activity **Available Forms:** Teas, extracts, dried herb **Contra:** ⊘ Pregnancy or lactation, pts with hypothyroidism, pituitary or thyroid tumors, hypogonadism, & CHF **Notes/SE:** Thyroid gland enlargement **Interactions:** ↑ Effects OF insulin, oral hypoglycemics, ↑ thyroid suppressing effects w/ balm leaf & wild thyme plant; ↓ effect OF thyroid hormone **Labs:** ↓ FSH, LH, HCG, TSH; monitor BS **NIPE:** ⊘ substitute for antithyroid drugs; ⊘ if undergoing treatment or diagnostic procedures with radioisotopes; ⊘ stop abruptly

Butcher's Broom (*Ruscus aculeatus*) **Uses:** Rx of circulatory disorders such as PVD, varicose veins, & leg edema; hemorrhoids; diuretic; laxative; inflammation; arthritis **Action:** Vasoconstriction due to direct activation of the α-receptors of the smooth-muscle cells in vascular walls **Available forms:** Raw ext 7–11 mg once/d, PO; tea 1 tsp in 1 cup water; topical oint apply PRN **Notes/SE:** GI upset, N/V **Interactions:** ↑ Effects OF anticoagulants, MAOIs; ↓ effects OF antihypertensives **Labs:** None **NIPE:** Hypertensive crisis may occur if admin w/ MAOIs; ⊘ use in PRG & lactation

Capsicum (*Capsicum frutescens*) **Uses:** Topical use includes pain relief from arthritis, diabetic neuropathy, postherpetic neuralgia, postsurgical pain; internal uses include circulatory disorders, GI distress, HTN **Actions:** Stimulates skin pain receptors causing burning sensations; desensitization of pain receptors results in pain relief; ↓ lymphocyte production, antibody production, & platelet aggregation **Available Forms:** topical creams 0.025%–0.25% up to qid; capsules

400–500 mg po tid **Contra:** ⊘ on open sores, in pregnancy, children younger than 2 years; **Notes/SE:** GI irritation, sweating, bronchospasm, respiratory irritation, topical burning, stinging, erythema; **Interactions:** ↑ effects OF anticoagulants, antiplatelets, theophylline; ↑ risk of cough w/ ACEIs; ↑ risk of anticoagulant effects w/ feverfew, garlic, ginger, ginkgo, ginseng; ↑ risk of hypertension crisis w/ MAOIs; ↓ effects OF clonidine, methyldopa; **Labs:** none **NIPE:** pain relief may take several weeks; ⊘ apply heat on areas w/ topical capsicum cream; avoid contact w/ eyes or mucous membranes.

Cascara (*Rhamnus purshiana*) **Uses:** Laxative **Action:** Stimulates large intestine, ↑ bowel motility & propulsion **Available Forms:** Liquid extract 1–5 ml po od **Contra:** ⊘ Pregnancy, lactation, & IBD **Notes/SE:** N/V, abdominal cramps, urine discoloration **Interactions:** ↑ Effects OF antiarrhythmics, cardiac glycosides; ↑ K$^+$ loss w/ diuretics, corticosteroids, cardiac glycosides; ↓ effects w/ antacids, milk **Labs:** ↓ Serum K$^+$ **NIPE:** Short-term use; monitor electrolytes; caution w/ diuretics

Chamomile (*Matricaria recutita*) **Uses:** Anti-inflammatory, antipyretic, antimicrobial, antispasmodic, astringent, sedative **Action:** Ingredients include α-bisabolol oil, which ↓ inflammation, antispasmodic activity, ↑ healing times for burns & ulcers, & inhibits ulcer formation; apigenin contributes to the anti-inflammatory effect, antispasmodic & sedative effect; azulene inhibits histamine release; chamazulene reduces inflammation & has antioxidant & antimicrobial effects **Available forms:** Teas 3–5 g (1 tbsp) flower heads steeped in water tid–qid, also use as a gargle or compress; fluid ext 1:1 –45% EtOH 1–3 mL tid **Notes/SE:** Allergic reactions if Pt allergic to Compositae family (ragweed, sunflowers, asters), eg, angioedema, eczema, contact dermatitis & anaphylaxis **Interactions:** ↑ Effects OF CNS depressants, EtOH, anticoagulants, antiplts; ↑ risk of miscarriage; ↓ effects OF drugs metabolized by CY 450 3A4, eg, alprazolam, atorvastatin, diazepam, ketoconazole, verapamil **Labs:** Monitor anticoagulant levels **NIPE:** ⊘ in PRG, lactation, children < age 2 y, patients w/ asthma or hay fever

Chondroitin Sulfate **Uses:** Combine w/ glucosamine to Rx arthritis; use as an anticoagulant **Action:** Attracts fluid & nutrients into the joints; inhibits thrombi **Available forms:** 1200 mg once/d, PO, & usually given w/ glucosamine 1500 mg once/d, PO for normal weight adults; **Notes/SE:** Diarrhea, dyspepsia, HA, N/V, restlessness **Interactions:** ↑ Effects OF anticoagulants, aspirin, NSAIDs **Labs:** None **NIPE:** ⊘ in PRG & lactation

Comfrey (*Symphytum officinale*) **Uses:** Topical treatment of wounds, bruises, sprains, inflammation **Action:** Multiple chemical components, allantoin promotes cell division, rosmarinic acid has anti-inflammatory effects, tannin possesses astringent effects, mucilage is a demulcent with anti-inflammatory properties, pyrrolizidine alkaloids cause hepatotoxicity **Available Forms:** Topical application w/ 5–20% of herb applied on intact skin for up to 10 days **Contra:** ⊘ Internally due to hepatotoxicity, ⊘ in pregnancy or lactation **Notes/SE:** N/V, exfoliative dermatitis with topical use **Interactions:** ↑ Risk of hepatotoxicity w/ ingestion of borage, golden ragwort, hemp, petasties **Labs:** ↑ LFTs, total bilirubin, urine bilirubin **NIPE:** ⊘ Use for more than 6 wks in one yr; ⊘ use on broken skin

Coriander (*Coriandrum sativum*) **Uses:** ↑ Appetite, treat diarrhea, dyspepsia, flatulence **Action:** Stimulates gastric secretions, spasmolytic effects **Available Forms:** Tincture 10–30 gtts po od **Contra:** ⊘ In pregnancy or lactation **Notes/SE:** N/V, fatty liver tumors, allergic skin reactions **Interactions:** ↑ Effects OF oral hypoglycemics **Labs:** Monitor BS **NIPE:** ↑ Risk of photosensitivity—use sunscreen

Cranberry (*Vaccinium macrocarpon*) **Uses:** Prevention UTI; urinary deodorizer in urinary incontinence **Actions:** Interferes with bacterial adherence to epithelial cells of the bladder **Available Forms:** Capsules 300–500 mg po bid to qid; unsweetened juice 8–16 oz daily; tincture 3–5 mL **SE:** Diarrhea, irritation, nephrolithiasis if ↑ urinary calcium oxalate **Interactions:** ↑ Excretion OF alkaline drugs such as antidepressants & methotrexate will cause ↓ effectiveness OF drug, ↓ effectiveness OF Uva-ursi **Labs:** ↑ Urine pH **NIPE:** Not effective in treating UTI; tincture contains up to 45% etoh; only unsweetened form effective; regular use may ↓ frequency of bacteriuria with pyria

Dong Quai (*Angelica polymorpha, sinensis*) **Uses:** Dysmenorrhea, PMS, menorrhagia, chronic pelvic infection, irregular menstruation. Other reported uses include anemia, HTN, HA, rhinitis, neuralgia, & hepatitis **Action:** Root exts contain at least six coumarin derivatives that have anticoagulant, vasodilating, antispasmodic, & CNS-stimulating activity. Studies demonstrate weak estrogen-agonist actions of the ext **Available forms:** Caps 500 mg, 1–2 caps PO, tid; liq ext 1–2 gtt, tid; tea 1–2 g, tid **Notes/SE:** Diarrhea, bleeding, photosensitivity, fever **Interactions:** ↑ Effects OF anticoagulants, antiplts, estrogens, warfarin; ↑ anticoagulant activity w/ chamomile, dandelion, horse chestnut, red clover; ↑ risk OF disulfiram-like reaction w/ disulfiram, metronidazole; **Labs:** ↑ PT, PTT, INR **NIPE:** Photosensitivity—use sunscreen, ⊘ if breast-feeding or PRG; tincs & exts contain EtOH up to 60%; stop herb 14 d prior to dental or surgical procedures

Echinacea (*Echinacea purpurea*) **Uses:** Immune system stimulant; prevention/Rx of colds, flu; as supportive therapy for colds & chronic infections of the resp tract & lower urinary tract **Action:** Stimulates phagocytosis & cytokine production & ↓ resp cellular activity; topically exerts anesthetic, antimicrobial, & antiinflammatory effects **Available forms:** Caps w/ powdered herb equivalent to 300–500 mg, PO, tid; pressed juice 6–9 mL, PO, once/d; tinc 2–4 mL, PO, tid (1:5 dilution); tea 2 tsp (4 g) of powdered herb in 1 cup of boiling water **Notes/SE:** Fever, taste perversion, urticaria, angioedema; **Contra:** ⊘ in Pts w/ autoimmune Dz, collagen Dz, HIV, leukemia, MS, TB **Interactions:** ↑ Risk OF disulfiram-like reaction w/ disulfiram, metronidazole; ↑risk OF exacerbation of HIV or AIDS w/ echinacea & amprenavir, other protease inhibitors; ↓ effects OF azathioprine, basiliximab, corticosteroids, cyclosporine, daclizumab, econazole vaginal cream, muromonab-CD3, mycophenolate, prednisone, tacrolimus **Labs:** ↑ ALT, AST, lymphocytes, ESR **NIPE:** Large doses of herb interferes w/ sperm activity; ⊘ w/ breast-feeding or PRG; ⊘ continuously for longer than 8 wk w/o a 3-wk break in Rx

Ephedra/Ma Huang **Uses:** CNS stimulant, appetite suppressant, weight-loss herb, asthma, headaches, nasal congestion, arthralgia **Action:** Active ingredient of ext is ephedrine that stimulates CNS, ↑ HR, BP, & peripheral vasoconstriction; acts on β-receptors & α-receptors **Available forms:** Ext 1–3 mL, PO, tid; tea 1–5 g herb in 1 pt boiling water; caps max daily dose of 300 mg **Notes/SE:** Anxiety, confusion, dizziness, HA, insomnia, irritability, restlessness, nervousness, arrhythmias, HTN, palpitations, constipation, urinary retention, uterine contractions, dermatitis **Contra:** ⊘ Narrow-angle glaucoma, seizures, CAD, PRG, lactation **Interactions:** ↑ Sympathomimetic effects w/ BBs, guanethidine, yohimbe; ↑ cardiac rhythm disturbance w/ anesthetics, cardiac glycosides, halothane; ↑ psychotic effects w/ caffeine, EtOH; ↑ effects OF CNS stimulants, pseudoephedrine, theophylline ; ↑ risk OF HTN crisis w/ MAOIs, oxytocins, phenelzine, TCAs; ↓ effects OF oral hypoglycemics **Labs:** ↑ ALT, AST, total bilirubin, urine bilirubin, serum glucose **NIPE:** Tincs & exts contain EtOH; linked to several deaths; monitor for behavioral mood changes

Evening Primrose Oil (*Oenothera biennis*) **Uses:** PMS, diabetic neuropathy, ADHD, IBS, rheumatoid arthritis, mastalgia **Action:** Anti-inflammatory, antispasmodic, diuretic, sedative effects related to a high concentration of essential fatty acids especially GLA & CLA & their conversion into prostaglandins **Available Forms:** Capsules, gelcaps, liquid. Dose depends on GLA content. Diabetic Neuropathy 4000 mg–6000 mg po od, eczema 4000 mg po od, Mastalgia 3000 mg–4000 mg po divided doses, PMS 2000 mg–4000 mg po od, rheumatoid arthritis up to 5000 mg po od **Notes/SE:** Indigestion, N, soft stools, flatulence, HA, anorexia, rash **Contra:** ⊘ In pregnancy or lactation; ⊘ in persons with seizure disorders **Interactions:** ↑ Phenobarbital metabolism, ↓ Sz threshold, ↑ effects OF diuretics, sedatives **Labs:** None **NIPE:** May take up to 4 months for maximum effectiveness, take with food.

Feverfew (*Tanacetum parthenium*) **Uses:** Anti-inflammatory for arthritis, asthma, digestion problems, fever, migraines, menstrual complaints, threatened abortion **Action:** Active ingredient, parthenolide, inhibits serotonin release, prostaglandin synthesis, plt aggregation, & histamine release from mast cells; several ingredients inhibit activation of polymorphonucleear leukocytes & leukotriene synthesis **Available forms:** Freeze-dried leaf ext 25 mg once/d; caps 300 mg–400 mg tid PO; tinc 15–30 gtt once/d to 0.2–0.7 mg of parthenolide **Notes/SE:** Mouth ulcers, muscle stiffness, joint pain, GI upset, rash **Contra:** ⊘ in PRG & lactation or w/ ragweed allergy **Interactions:** ↑ Effects OF anticoagulants, antiplts, ↓ effects OF Fe absorption **Labs:** ↑ PT, INR, PTT **NIPE:** ⊘ D/C herb abruptly or may experience joint stiffness & pain, headaches, insomnia

Garlic (*Allium sativum*) **Uses:** Antithrombotic, antilipidemic, antitumor, antimicrobial, antiasthmatic, antiinflammatory **Action:** Inhibits gram(+) & gram(−) organisms, exerts cholesterol-lowering by preventing gastric lipase fat digestion & fecal excretion of sterols & bile acids & it inhibits free radicals **Available forms:** Teas, tabs, caps, ext, oil, dried powder, syrup, fresh bulb **Notes/SE:** Dizziness, diaphoresis, HA, N/V, hypothyroidism, contact dermatitis, allergic reactions, oral mucosa irritation, systemic garlic odor, ↓ Hgb production, lysis of RBCs **Interactions:** ↑ Effects OF anticoagulants, antiplts, insulin, oral hypoglycemics; ↓ effects w/ acidophilus **Labs:** ↓ Total cholesterol, LDL, triglycerides, plt aggregation, iodine uptake; ↑ PT, serum IgE **NIPE:** ⊘ in PRG, lactation, prior to surgery, GI disorders; report bleeding, bruising, petechiae, tarry stools, monitor CBC, PT

Gentiana (*Gentiana lutea*) **Uses:** ↑ Appetite, treat digestive disorders such as colitis, IBS, flatulence **Actions:** Chemical components stimulate digestive juices **Available Forms:** Liquid extract 2-4 g po od, tincture 1-3 g po od, dried root 2–4 g po od **Contra:** ⊘ Pregnancy, lactation, & hypertension; **Notes/SE:** N/V, HA **Interactions:** ↑ CNS sedation w/ barbiturates, benzodiazepines, ETOH if extract/tincture contains alcohol; ↓ absorption OF iron salts **Labs:** None **NIPE:** Caution—many herb preps contain up to 60% ETOH

Ginger (*Zingiber officinale*) **Uses:** Antiemetic ↓ N/V; antiinflammatory relieves pain & swelling of muscle injury, osteoarthritis & rheumatoid arthritis; antispasmodic action relieves colic, flatulence & indigestion; antiplt; antipyretic; antioxidant; antiinfective against gram(+) & gram(−) bacteria **Action:** Antiinflammatory effect inhibits prostaglandin, thromboxane, & leukotriene biosynthesis; antiemetic effects due to action on the GI tract; antiplt effect due to the inhibition of thromboxane formation; + inotropic effect on CV system **Available forms:** Dosage form & strength depends on Dz process *General use:* Dried ginger caps 1 g once/d, PO; fluid ext 0.7–2 mL once/d, PO, (2:1 ratio); tabs 500 mg bid–qid, PO; tinc 1.7–5 mL once/d, PO, (1:5 ratio) **Interactions:** ↑ Risk of bleeding w/ anticoagulants, antiplts; ↑ risk of disulfiram-like reaction w/ disulfiram, metronidazole **Labs:** ↑ PT **NIPE:** Store herb in cool, dry area; ⊘ in PRG, lactation; lack of standardization for herb dosing

Ginkgo Biloba **Uses:** Effective w/ circulatory disorders, cerebrovascular Dz, & dementia; used to improve alertness & attention span **Action:** Ext flavonoids release neurotransmitters & inhibit monoamine oxidase, which enhances cognitive function; vascular protective action results from relaxation of blood vessels, ↑ tissue perfusion, inhibition of plt aggregation; eradicates free radicals & ↓ polymorphonucleare neutrophils **Available forms:** Dosage depends on diagnosis *General uses:* Tabs & caps 40—80 mg tid, PO; tinc 0.5 mL tid, PO; ext 40–80 mg tid, PO **Notes/SE:** Anxiety, diarrhea, flatulence, HA, heart palpitations, N/V, restlessness **Interactions:** ↑ Effect OF MAOIs; ↑ risk of bleeding w/ anisindione, dalteparin, dicumerol, garlic, heparin, salicylates, warfarin; ↑ risk OF coma w/ trazodone; ↓ effect OF carbamazepine, gabapentin, insulin, oral hypoglycemics, phenobarbital, phenytoin; ↓ seizure threshold w/ bupropion, TCAs **Labs:** ↑ PT **NIPE:** ⊘ in PRG & lactation; tincs contain up to 60% EtOH; ⊘ 2 wk prior to surgery

Ginseng (*Panax quinquefolius*)
Uses: ↑ Physical endurance, concentration, appetite, sleep & stress resistance; ↓ fatigue; antioxidant; aids in glucose control **Action:** Dried root contains ginsenosides, which ↑ natural killer cell activity, & nuclear RNA synthesis, & motor activity **Available forms:** No standard dosage *General use:* Caps 200 mg–500 mg once/d, PO; tea 3 g steeped in boiling water tid PO, tinc 1–2 mg once/d, PO (1:1 dilution) **Notes/SE:** Anxiety, anorexia, chest pain, diarrhea, HTN, N/V, palpitations **Interactions:** ↑ Effects OF estrogen, hypoglycemics, CNS stimulants, caffeine, ephedra; ↑ risk OF bleeding w/ ibuprofen; ↑ risk OF HA, irritability & visual hallucinations w/ MAOIs; ↓ effects OF anisindione, dicumarol, furosemide, heparin, warfarin **Labs:** ↑ Digoxin level falsely; ↓ glucose, PT, INR **NIPE:** ⊘ Use continuously for > 3 mo; ⊘ during PRG or lactation; eval for ginseng abuse syndrome w/ symptoms of diarrhea, depression, edema, HTN, insomnia, rash & restlessness

Glucosamine Sulfate (chitosamine)
Uses: Used w/ chondroitin for the Rx of arthritis **Action:** Stimulate the production of cartilage components **Available forms:** Caps/tabs 1500 mg once/d, PO & chondroitin sulfate 1200 mg once/d, PO for adults of normal weight **Notes/SE:** Abdominal pain, anorexia, constipation or diarrhea, drowsiness, HA, heartburn, N/V, rash **Interactions:** ↑ Effects OF hypoglycemics; **Labs:** Monitor serum glucose levels in diabetics **NIPE:** Take w/ food to reduce GI effects; no uniform standardization of herb

Green Tea (*Camellia sinensis*)
Uses: Antioxidant, antibacterial, diuretic; prevention of CA, hyperlipidemia, atherosclerosis, dental caries **Actions:** Chemical components include anti-inflammatory, anti-CA polyphenols epigallocatechin & epigallocatechin-3-gallate, which inhibit tumor growth; fluoride & tannins demonstrate antimicrobial action against oral bacteria; antioxidant activity delays lipid peroxidation; antimicrobial action due to inhibition of growth of various bacteria, including *Staphylococcus aureus* **Available Forms:** Recommend 300–400 mg polyphenols po od (3 cups tea = 240–320 mg polyphenols) **Contra:** Caution—↑ intake may cause tannin-induced asthma **Notes/SE:** Tachycardia, insomnia, anxiety, n/v, ↑ BP, **Interactions:** ↑ Effects OF doxorubicin, ephedrine, stimulant drugs, theophylline; ↑ risk OF hypertensive crisis w/ MAOIs; ↑ bleeding risk w/anticoagulants, antiplatelets; ↓ effects w/ antacids, dairy products **Labs:** ↑ PT, PTT **NIPE:** Contains caffeine—caution in pregnancy, infants and small children, & pts w CAD, hyperthyroidism, & anxiety disorders; GI distress d/t tannins ↓ w the addition of milk; ↑ tannin content w ↑ brewing times

Guarana (*Paullinia cupana*)
Uses: Appetite suppressant, CNS stimulant, ↑ sexual performance, ↓ fatigue **Actions:** ↑ Caffeine content stimulates cardiac, CNS, & smooth muscle; ↑ diuresis; ↓ platelet aggregation **Available Forms:** Daily divided doses w/ a maximum of 3 g po daily **Contra:** Avoid in pregnancy &

lactation, CAD, hyperthyroidism, anxiety disorders d/t high caffeine content **Notes/SE:** Insomnia, tachycardia, anxiety, N/V, HA, HTN, seizures **Interactions:** ↑ Effects OF anticoagulants, antiplatelets, beta blockers, bronchodilators; ↑ risk of hypertensive crisis w/ MAOIs; ↑ effects w/ cimetidine, ciprofloxacin, ephedrine, hormonal contraceptives, theophylline, cola, coffee; ↓ effects OF adenosine, antihypertensives, benzodiazepines, iron, ↓ effects w/ smoking **Labs:** ↑ PT, PTT **NIPE:** Tinctures contain ETOH; may exacerbate GI disorders & HTN

Hawthorn (*Crataegus laevigata*)

Uses: Rx of HTN, arrhythmias, heart failure, stable angina pectoris, insomnia **Action:** ↑ myocardial contraction by ↓ oxygen consumption, ↓ peripheral resistance, dilating coronary blood vessels, ACE inhibition **Available forms:** Tinc 1–2 mL (1:5 ratio) tid, PO; liq ext 0.5–1 mL, (1:1 ration) tid, PO **Notes/SE:** Arrhythmias, fatigue, hypotension, N/V, sedation **Interactions:** ↑ Effects OF antihypertensives, cardiac glycosides, CNS depressants, & herbs such as adonis, lily of the valley, squill ↓; effects OF Fe **Labs:** False ↑ of digoxin **NIPE:** ⊘ in PRG & lactation; many tincs contain EtOH

Horsetail (*Equisetum arvense*)

Uses: ↑ Strength of bones, hair, nails, & teeth; diuretic, treat dyspepsia, gout; topically used to treat wounds **Actions:** Multiple chemical components; flavonoids ↑ diuretic activity; contains silica which strengthens bones, hair, nails, & hair **Available Forms:** Extract 20–40 gtts in H$_2$O po tid–qid; topically 10 g herb/L H$_2$O as compress prn **Contra:** ⊘ In pregnancy, lactation, w/ children, CAD; contains nicotine & large amts may cause nicotine toxicity **Notes/SE:** Nicotine toxicity (N/V, weakness, fever, dizziness, abnormal heart rate, wt. loss) **Interactions:** ↑ Effects OF digoxin, diuretics, lithium, adonis, lily of the valley; ↑ CNS stimulation w/ CNS stimulants, theophylline, coffee, tea, cola, nicotine; ↑ K$^+$ depletion w/ corticosteroids, diuretics, stimulant laxatives, licorice; ↑ risk of thiamine deficiency w/ ETOH use **Labs:** Monitor digoxin, electrolyte, thiamine levels **NIPE:** Tincture contains ETOH, which may cause disulfiram like reaction if taken with benzodiazepines or metronidazole; short-term use only; active components of herb absorbed thru skin

Kava Kava (*Piper methysticum*)

Uses: ↓ Anxiety, stress, & restlessness; sedative effect **Action:** Appears to act directly on the limbic system **Available forms:** Standardized ext (70% kavalactones) 100 mg bid–tid, PO **Notes/SE:** ↑ Reflexes, HA, dizziness, visual changes, hematuria, SOB **Interactions:** ↑ Effects OF antiplts, benzodiazepines, CNS depressants, MAOIs, phenobarbital; ↑ absorption when taken w/ food; ↑ in parkinsonian symptoms w/ kava & antiparkinsonian drugs **Labs:** ↑ ALT, AST, urinary RBCs; ↓ albumin, total protein, bilirubin, urea, plts, lymphocytes **NIPE:** ⊘ Take for > 3 mo; ⊘ during PRG & lactation

Licorice (*Glycyrrhiza glabra*)

Uses: Expectorant, shampoo, GI complaints **Action:** ↑ Mucous secretions, ↓ peptic activity, ↓ scalp sebum secretion **Available forms:** Liq ext, bulk dried root, tinc; 15 g once/d PO of licorice root; intake > 50 g once/d may cause toxicity **Notes/SE:** HTN, arrhythmias, edema, hypokalemia, HA, lethargy, rhabdomyolysis **Interactions:** ↑ Drug effects OF diuretics, corticosteroids, may prolong QT interval w/ loratadine, procainamide, quinidine, terfenadine; **Labs:** None **NIPE:** Monitor for electrolyte & ECG changes, HTN, mineralocorticoid-like effects; toxicity more likely w/ prolonged intake of small doses than one large dose

Melatonin (MEL) Uses: Insomnia, jet lag, antioxidant, immunostimulant
Action: Hormone produce by the pineal gland in response to darkness; declines w/ age **Available forms:** ER caps 1–3 mg once/d 2 h before hs, PO **Notes/SE:** HA, confusion, sedation, HTN, tachycardia, hyperglycemia **Interactions:** ↑ anxiolytic effects OF benzodiazepines; ↑ risk OF insomnia w/ cerebral stimulants, methamphetamine, succinylcholine **Labs:** None **NIPE:** ⊘ during PRG & lactation

Milk Thistle (Silybum marianum) Uses: Rx of hepatotoxicity, dyspepsia, liver protectorant **Action:** stimulates protein synthesis, which leads to liver cell regeneration **Available forms:** Tinc 70–120 mg (70% silymarin) tid, PO **Notes/SE:** Diarrhea, menstrual stimulation, N/V **Interactions:** ↑ Effects OF drugs metabolized by the cytochrome P-450, CYP3A4, CYP2C9 enzymes **Labs:** ↑ PT; ↓ LFTs, serum glucose **NIPE:** ⊘ in PRG & lactation; ⊘ in Pts allergic to ragweed, chrysanthemums, marigolds, daisies

Nettle: (Urtica dioica) Uses: Allergic rhinitis, asthma, cough, TB, BPH,
bladder nephritis, diuretic, antispasmodic, expectorant, astringent, and topically for oily skin, dandruff, & hair stimulant **Actions:** Multiple chemical components have different actions; scopoletin has anti-inflammatory action, root extract ↓ BPH; lectins display immunostimulant action **Available Forms:** Capsules 150–300 mg po od; liquid extract 2–8 mL po tid **Contra:** ⊘ If pregnant or lactating or in children ↓ 2 y.o. **Notes/SE:** N/V, edema, abdominal distress, diarrhea, oliguria, edema, local skin irritation **Interactions:** ↑ Effects OF diclofenac, diuretics, barbiturates, antipsychotics, opiates, ETOH; ↓ effects OF anticoagulants **Labs:** Monitor electrolytes **NIPE:** Skin contact w/ plant will result in stinging & burning; ↑ intake of foods high in K⁺

Rue: (Ruta graveolens) Uses: Sedative, spasmolytic for muscle cramps,
GI & menstrual disorders, promote lactation, promote abortion via uterine stimulation, anti-inflammatory effect for sports injuries, bruising, arthritis, joint pain **Action:** Contains essential oils, flavonoids, & alkaloids; shown mutagenic & cytotoxic action on cells; produced CV effects due to + chronotropic & inotropic effects on atria; vasodilatory effects reduce BP; shown strengthening effect on capillaries; alkaloids produce antispasmodic & abortifacient activity **Available Forms:** Capsules, extracts, teas, topical creams, topical oils; topical oil for earache; topical creams to affected areas prn; teas use 1 tsp/1/4 L H₂0; extract ¼–1 tsp po tid with food; capsules 1 po tid with food **Notes/SE:** Dizziness, tremors, hypotension, bradycardia, allergic skin reactions, spontaneous abortion **Contra:** ⊘ during pregnancy or lactation or give to children; caution in pts with CHF, arrhythmias, or receiving antihypertensive medication **Interactions:** ↑ Inotropic effects OF cardiac glycosides; ↑ effects OF antihypertensives & warfarin; ↓ effects OF fertility drugs

Labs: ↑ BUN, Crea, LFT **NIPE:** Large doses can be toxic or fatal; research does not establish a safe dose; tinctures & extracts contain ETOH; no data with use in children; ⊘ if h/o ETOH abuse or liver disease

Saw Palmetto (*Serenoa repens*) **Uses:** Rx of benign prostatic hypertrophy (BPH) stages 1 & 2 (inhibits testosterone-5-α-reductase), ↑ sperm production, ↑ breast size (estrogenic), ↑ sexual vigor, mild diuretic, treat chronic cystitis **Action:** Theorized that sitosterols inhibit conversion of testosterone to dihydrotestosterone (DHT), which reduces the prostate gland, also competes w/ DHT on receptor sites resulting in antiestrogenic effects **Available forms:** Caps/tabs 160 mg bid, PO; tinc 20–30 gtt qid (1:2 ration); fluid ext, standardized 160 mg bid PO or 320 mg once/d PO **Notes/SE:** Abdominal pain, back pain, diarrhea, dysuria, HA, HTN, N/V, impotence **Contra:** ⊘ PRG, lactation **Interactions:** ↑ Effects of adrenergics, anticoagulants, antiplts, hormones, Fe **Labs:** May affect semen analysis, may cause false – PSA **NIPE:** Take w/ meals to ↓ GI upset, do baseline PSA prior to taking herb, no standardization of herb content

Spirulina (*Spirulina spp*) **Uses:** Rx of obesity & as a nutritional supplement **Action:** Contains 65% protein, all amino acids, carotenoids, B-complex vitamins, essential fatty acids & Fe; has been shown to inhibit replicating viral cells **Available forms:** Caps/tabs or powder admin 3–5 g ac, PO **Notes/SE:** Anorexia, N/V **Interactions:** ↑ Effects OF anticoagulants; ↓ effects OF thyroid hormones due to high iodine content; ↓ absorption OF vitamin B_{12} **Labs:** ↑ Serum Ca, serum alkaline phosphatase; monitor PT, INR **NIPE:** May contain ↑ levels of Hg & radioactive ion content

Stevia (*Stevia rebaudiana*) **Uses:** Natural sweetener, hypoglycemic and hypotensive properties **Actions:** Multiple chemical components; sweetness d/t glycoside stevioside; hypotensive effect may be d/t diuretic action or vasodilation action **Available Forms:** Liquid extract, powder, capsules **Notes/SE:** HA, dizziness, bloating **Interactions:** ↑ Hypotensive effects w/antihypertensives esp CCB, diuretics **Labs:** Monitor BS **NIPE:** Monitor BP; does not encourage dental caries

St. John's Wort (*Hypericum perforatum*) **Uses:** Depression, anxiety, antiinflammatory, antiviral **Action:** MAOI in vitro, not in vivo; bacteriostatic & bactericidal, ↑ capillary blood flow, uterotonic activity in animals **Available forms:** Teas, tabs, caps, tinc, oil ext for topical use **Notes/SE:** Photosensitivity (use sunscreen) rash, dizziness, dry mouth, GI distress **Interactions:** Enhance MAOI activity, EtOH, narcotics, MAOIs, sympathomimetics **Labs:** ↑ GH; ↓ digoxin, serum iron, serum prolactin, theophylline; **NIPE:** ⊘ in PRG, breast-feeding, or in children, ⊘ w/ SSRIs, MAOIs, EtOH, ⊘ sun exposure

Tea Tree (*Melaleuca alternifolia*) **Uses:** Rx of superficial wounds (bacterial, viral, & fungal), insect bites, minor burns, cold sores, acne **Action:** Broad-spectrum antibiotic activity against *E. coli, S. aureus, C. albicans* **Available forms:** Topical creams, lotions, oint, oil apply topically PRN **Notes/SE:** Ataxia, contact dermatitis, diarrhea, drowsiness, GI mucosal irritation **Interactions:** ↓ Effects OF drugs that affect histamine release **Labs:** ↑ Neutrophil count **NIPE:** Caution Pt to use externally only; ⊘ apply to broken skin

Unsafe Herbs with Known Toxicity

Agent	Toxicities
Aconite	Salivation, N/V, blurred vision, cardiac arrhythmias
Aristolochic acid	Nephrotox
Calamus	Possible carcinogenicity
Chaparral	Hepatotox, possible carcinogenicity, nephrotox
"Chinese herbal mixtures"	May contain MaHuang or other dangerous herbs
Coltsfoot	Hepatotox, possibly carcinogenic
Comfrey	Hepatotox, carcinogenic
Ephedra/MaHuang	Adverse cardiac events, stroke, Sz
Juniper	High allergy potential, D, Sz, nephrotox
Kava kava	Hepatotox
Licorice	Chronic daily amounts (> 30 g/mo) can result in ↓ K⁺, Na/fluid retention w/HTN, myoglobinuria, hyporeflexia
Life root	Hepatotox, liver cancer
MaHuang/Ephedra	Adverse cardiac events, stroke, Sz
Pokeweed	GI cramping, N/D/V, labored breathing, ↓ BP, Sz
Sassafras	V, stupor, hallucinations, dermatitis, abortion, hypothermia, liver cancer
Usnic acid	Hepatotox
Yohimbine	Hypotension, abdominal distress, CNS stimulation (mania/& psychosis in predisposed individuals)

Valerian (*Valeriana officinalis*) **Uses:** Antianxiety, antispasmodic, dysmenorrheal, restlessness, sedative **Action:** Inhibits uptake & stimulates release of GABA, which ↑ GABA concentration extracellularly & causes sedation **Available forms:** Ext 400–900 mg PO 30 min < HS, tea 2–3 g (1 tsp of crude herb) qid, PRN, tinc 3–5 mL (½–1 tsp) (1:5 ratio) PO qid, PRN **Notes/SE:** GI upset, HA, insomnia, N/V, palpitations, restlessness, vision changes **Interactions:** ↑ Effects OF barbiturates, benzodiazepines, opiates, EtOH, catnip, hops, kava, passion flower, skullcap; ↓ effects OF MAOIs, phenytoin, warfarin **Labs:** ↑ ALT, AST, total bilirubin, urine bilirubin **NIPE:** Periodic check of LFTs, unknown effects in PRG & lactation, full effect may take 2–4 wk, taper herb to avoid withdrawal symptoms after long-term use

Yohimbine (*Pausinystalia yohimbe*) **Uses:** Rx for impotence, aphrodisiac **Action:** Peripherally affects autonomic nervous system by ↓ adrenergic activity & ↑ cholinergic activity; ↑ blood flow **Available forms:** Tabs 5.4 mg tid, PO; doses at 20–30 mg/d may ↑ BP & heart rate **Notes/SE:** Anxiety, dizziness, dysuria, genital pain, HTN, tachycardia, tremors **Interactions:** ↑ Effects OF CNS stimulants, MAOIs, SSRIs, caffeine, ETOH; ↑ risk OF toxicity w/ α-adrenergic blockers, phenothiazines; ↑ yohimbe toxicity w/ sympathomimetics; ↑ BP w/ foods containing tyramine **Labs:** ↑ BUN, creatinine **NIPE:** ⊘ w/ caffeine-containing foods w/ herb, may exacerbate mania in patients w/ psychiatric disorders

Tables

TABLE 1
Quick Guide to Dosing of Acetaminophen Based on the Tylenol Product Line

	Suspension[a] Drops and Original Drops 80 mg/0.8 mL Dropperful	Chewable[a] Tablets 80-mg tabs	Suspension[a] Liquid and Original Elixir 160 mg/5 mL	Junior[a] Strength 160-mg Caplets/Chewables	Regular[b] Strength 325-mg Caplets/Tablets	Extra Strength[b] 500-mg Caplets/Gelcaps
Birth–3 mo/ 6–11 lb/ 2.5–5.4 kg	$\frac{1}{2}$ dppr[c] (0.4 mL)					
4–11 mo/ 12–17 lb/ 5.5–7.9 kg	1 dppr[c] (0.8 mL)		$\frac{1}{2}$ tsp			
12–23 mo/ 18–23 lb/ 8.0–10.9 kg	$1\frac{1}{2}$ dppr[c] (1.2 mL)		$\frac{3}{4}$ tsp			
2–3 y/24–35 lb/ 11.0–15.9 kg	2 dppr[c] (1.6 mL)	2 tab	1 tsp			
4–5 y/36–47 lb/ 16.0–21.9 kg		3 tab	$1\frac{1}{2}$ tsp			

6–8 y/48–59 lb/ 22.0–26.9 kg	4 tab	2 tsp	2 cap/tab
9–10 y/60–71 lb/ 27.0–31.9 kg	5 tab	$2\frac{1}{2}$ tsp	$2\frac{1}{2}$ cap/ tab
11 y/72–95 lb/ 32.0–43.9 kg	6 tab	4 tsp	3 cap/tab
Adults & children ≥ 12 y ≥ 96 lb ≥ 44.0 kg		4 cap/tab	1 or 2 caps/ tabs	2 caps/ gel

aDoses should be administered 4 or 5 times daily. Do not exceed 5 doses in 24 h.

bNo more than 8 dosage units in any 24-h period. Not to be taken for pain for more than 10 days or for fever for more than 3 days unless directed by a physician.

cDropperful.

301

TABLE 2
Common Drug Levels[a]

Drug	When to Sample	Therapeutic Levels	Usual Half-Life	Potentially Toxic Levels
Antibiotics				
Gentamicin, Tobramycin	*Peak:* 30 min after 30-min infusion (peak level not necessary if extended-interval dosing: 6 mg/kg/dose) *Trough:* <0.5 h before next dose	*Peak:* 5–8 mcg/mL *Trough:* <2 mcg/mL <1.0 mcg/mL for extended intervals (6 mg/kg/dose) (peak levels not needed with extended-interval dosing)	2 h	Peak: >12 mcg/mL
Amikacin Vancomycin	Same as above *Peak:* 1 h after 1-h infusion *Trough:* <0.5 h before next dose	*Peak:* 20–30 mcg/mL *Peak:* 30–40 mcg/mL	2 h 6–8 h	Peak: >35 mcg/mL Peak: >50 mcg/mL Trough: >15 mcg/mL

302

Anticonvulsants

Carbamazepine	*Trough:* just before next oral dose	8–12 mcg/mL (monotherapy) 4–8 mcg/mL (polytherapy)	15–20 h	Trough: >12 mcg/mL
Ethosuximide	*Trough:* just before next oral dose	40–100 mcg/mL	30–60 h	Trough: >100 mcg/mL
Phenobarbital	*Trough:* just before next dose	15–40 mcg/mL	40–120 h	Trough: >40 mcg/mL
Phenytoin	May use free phenytoin to monitor[b] *Trough:* just before next dose	10–20 mcg/mL	Concentration-dependent	>20 mcg/mL
Primidone	*Trough:* just before next dose (primidone is metabolized to phenobarb; order levels separately)	5–12 mcg/mL	10–12 h	>12 mcg/mL
Valproic acid	*Trough:* just before next dose	50–100 mcg/mL	5–20 h	>100 mcg/mL

303

TABLE 2
(Continued)

Drug	When to Sample	Therapeutic Levels	Usual Half-Life	Potentially Toxic Levels
Bronchodilators				
Caffeine	*Trough:* just before next dose	Adults 5–15 mcg/mL Neonates 6–11 mcg/mL	Adults 3–4 h Neonates 30–140 h	20 mcg/mL
Theophylline (IV)	IV: 12–24 h after infusion started	5–15 mcg/mL	Nonsmoking adults 8 h Children and smoking adults 4 h	>20 mcg/mL
Theophylline (PO)	*Peak levels:* not recommended *Trough level:* just before next dose	5–15 mcg/mL		

Amiodarone	Trough: just before next dose	1–2.5 mcg/mL	30–100 days	>2.5 mcg/mL
Digoxin	Trough: just before next dose (levels drawn earlier than 6 h after a dose willbe artificiallyelevated)	0.8–2.0 ng/mL	36 h	>2 ng/mL
Disopyramide	Trough: just before next dose	2–5 mcg/mL	4–10 h	>5 mcg/mL
Flecainide	Trough: just before next dose	0.2–1 mcg/mL	11–14 h	>1 mcg/mL
Lidocaine	Steady-state levels are usually achieved after 6–12 h	1.2–5 mcg/mL	1.5 h	>6 mcg/mL
Procainamide	Trough: just before next oral dose	4–10 mcg/mL NAPA + procaine: 5–30 mcg/mL	Procaine: 3–5 h NAPA: 6–10 h	>10 mcg/mL NAPA + procaine: >30 mcg/mL 0.5 mcg/mL
Quinidine	Trough: just before next oral dose	2–5 mcg/mL	6 h	
Other Agents				
Amitriplyline plus nortriptyline	Trough: just before next dose	120–250 ng/mL		
Nortriptyline	Trough: just before next dose	50–140 ng/mL		
Lithium	Trough: just before next dose	0.5–1.5 mEq/mL	18–20 h	>1.5 mEq/mL

TABLE 2
(Continued)

Drug	When to Sample	Therapeutic Levels	Usual Half-Life	Potentially Toxic Levels
Imipramine plus desipramine	*Trough:* just before next dose	150–300 ng/mL		
Desipramine	*Trough:* just before next dose	50–300 ng/mL		
Methotrexate	By protocol	<0.5 mcmol/L after 48 h		
Cyclosporine	*Trough:* just before next dose	Highly variable *Renal:* 150–300 ng/mL (RIA) *Hepatic:* 150–300 ng/mL	Highly variable	
Doxepin	*Trough:* just before next dose	100–300 ng/mL		
Trazodone	*Trough:* just before next dose	900–2100 ng/mL		

^aResults of therapeutic drug monitoring *must* be interpreted in light of the complete clinical situation. For information on dosing or interpretation of drug levels contact the pharmacist or an order for a pharmacokinetic consult may be written in the patient's chart. Modified and reproduced with permission from the *Pharmacy and Therapeutics Committee Formulary,* 41st ed., Thomas Jefferson University Hospital, Philadelphia, PA.

^bMore reliable in cases of uremia and hypoalbuminemia.

TABLE 3
Local Anesthetic Comparison Chart for Commonly Used Injectable Agents

Agent	Proprietary Names	Onset	Duration	Maximum Dose	
				mg/kg	Volume in 70-kg Adult[a]
Bupivacaine	Marcaine	7–30 min	5–7 h	3	70 mL of 0.25% solution
Lidocaine	Xylocaine, Anestacon	5–30 min	2 h	4	28 mL of 1% solution
Lidocaine with epinephrine (1:200,000)		5–30 min	2–3 h	7	50 mL of 1% solution
Mepivacaine	Carbocaine	5–30 min	2–3 h	7	50 mL of 1% solution
Procaine	Novocaine	Rapid	30 min–1 h	10–15	70–105 mL of 1% solution

[a]To calculate the maximum dose if not a 70-kg adult, use the fact that a 1% solution has 10 mg of drug per milliliter.

307

TABLE 4
Comparison of Systemic Steroids

Drug	Relative Equivalent Dose (mg)	Mineralo-corticoid Activity	Duration (h)	Route
Betamethasone	0.75	0	36–72	PO, IM
Cortisone (Cortone)	25	2	8–12	PO, IM
Dexamethasone (Decadron)	0.75	0	36–72	PO, IV
Hydrocortisone (Solu-Cortef, Hydrocortone)	20	2	8–12	PO, IM, IV
Methylprednisolone acetate (Depo-Medrol)	4	0	36–72	PO, IM, IV
Methylprednisolone succinate (Solu-Medrol)	4	0	8–12	PO, IM, IV
Prednisone (Deltasone)	5	1	12–36	PO
Prednisolone (Delta-Cortef)	5	1	12–36	PO, IM, IV

TABLE 5
Topical Steroid Preparations

Agent	Common Trade Names	Potency	Apply
Alclometasone dipropionate	Aclovate, cream, oint 0.05%	Low	bid/tid
Amcinonide	Cyclocort, cream, lotion, oint 0.1%	High	bid/tid
Betamethasone			
Betamethasone valerate	Valisone cream, lotion 0.01%	Low	qd/bid
Betamethasone valerate	Valisone cream 0.01, 0.1%, oint, lotion 0.1%	Intermediate	qd/bid
Betamethasone dipropionate	Diprosone cream 0.05%	High	qd/bid
Betamethasone dipropionate	Diprosone aerosol 0.1%		
Betamethasone dipropionate, augmented	Diprolene oint, gel 0.05%	High	qd/bid
Clobetasol propionate	Temovate cream, gel, oint, scalp, soln 0.05%	Ultrahigh	bid (2 wk max)
Clocortolone pivalate	Cloderm cream 0.1%	Intermediate	qd–qid
Desonide	DesOwen, cream, oint, lotion 0.05%	Low	bid–qid
Desoximetasone			
Desoximetasone 0.05%	Topicort LP cream, gel 0.05%	Intermediate	
Desoximetasone 0.25%	Topicort cream, oint	High	
Dexamethasone base	Aeroseb-Dex aerosol 0.01%	Low	bid–qid
	Decadron cream 0.1%		
Diflorasone diacetate	Psorcon cream, oint 0.05%	Ultrahigh	bid/tid
Fluocinolone			
Fluocinolone acetonide 0.01%	Synalar cream, soln 0.01%	Low	bid/tid
Fluocinolone acetonide 0.025%	Synalar oint, cream 0.025%	Intermediate	bid/tid

(continued)

TABLE 5
(Continued)

Agent	Common Trade Names	Potency	Apply
Fluocinolone acetonide 0.2%	Synalar-HP cream 0.2%	High	bid/tid
Fluocinonide 0.05%	Lidex, anhydrous cream, gel, soln 0.05%	High	bid/tid oint
	Lidex-E aqueous cream 0.05%		
Flurandrenolide	Cordran cream, oint 0.025%	Intermediate	bid/tid
	cream, lotion, oint 0.05%	Intermediate	bid/tid
	tape, 4 mcg/cm²	Intermediate	
Fluticasone propionate	Cutivate cream 0.05%, oint 0.005%	Intermediate	bid
Halobetasol	Ultravate cream, oint 0.05%	Very high	bid
Halcinonide	Halog cream 0.025%, emollient base 0.1% cream, oint, sol 0.1%	High	qd/tid
Hydrocortisone			
Hydrocortisone	Cortizone, Caldecort, Hycort, Hytone, etc. aerosol 1%, cream 0.5, 1, 2.5%, gel 0.5%, oint 0.5, 1, 2.5%, lotion 0.5, 1, 2.5%, paste 0.5%, soln 1%	Low	tid/qid
Hydrocortisone acetate	Corticaine cream, oint 0.5, 1%	Low	tid/qid
Hydrocortisone butyrate	Locoid oint, soln 0.1%	Intermediate	bid/tid
Hydrocortisone valerate	Westcort cream, oint 0.2%	Intermediate	bid/tid

Mometasone furoate	Elocon 0.1% cream, oint, lotion	Intermediate	qd
Prednicarbate	Dermatop 0.1% cream	Intermediate	bid
Triamcinolone			
Triamcinolone acetonide 0.025%	Aristocort, Kenalog cream, oint, lotion 0.025%	Low	tid/qid
Triamcinolone acetonide 0.1%	Aristocort, Kenalog cream, oint, lotion 0.1%	Intermediate	tid/qid
	Aerosol 0.2-mg/2-sec spray		
Triamcinolone acetonide 0.5%	Aristocort, Kenalog cream, oint 0.5%	High	tid/qid

TABLE 6
Comparison of Insulins

Type of Insulin	Onset (h)	Peak (h)	Duration (h)
Ultra Rapid			
Apidra (glulisine)	Immediate	0.5–1.5	3–5
Humalog (lispro)	Immediate	0.5–1.5	3–5
NovoLog (insulin aspart)	Immediate	0.5–1.5	3–5
Rapid			
Regular Iletin II	0.25–0.5	2–4	5–7
Humulin R	0.5	2–4	6–8
Novolin R	0.5	2.5–5	5–8
Velosulin	0.5	2–5	6–8
Intermediate			
NPH Iletin II	1–2	6–12	18–24
Lente Iletin II	1–2	6–12	18–24
Humulin N	1–2	6–12	14–24
Novulin L	2.5–5	7–15	18–24
Novulin 70/30	0.5	7–12	24
Prolonged			
Ultralente	4–6	14–24	28–36
Humulin U	4–6	8–20	24–28
Lantus (insulin glargine)	4–6	No peak	24
Combination Insulins			
Humalog Mix (lispro protamine/ lispro)	0.25–0.5	1–4	24

TABLE 7
Commonly Used Oral Contraceptives[a]

Monophasics

Drug (Manufacturer)	Estrogen (mcg)	Progestin (mg)
Alesse 21, 28 (Wyeth)	Ethinyl estradiol (20)	Levonorgestrel (0.1)
Apri 28 (Barr)	Ethinyl estradiol (30)	Desogestrel (0.15)
Aviane 28 (Barr)	Ethinyl estradiol (20)	Levonorgestrel (0.1)
Brevicon 28 (Watson)	Ethinyl estradiol (35)	Norethindrone (0.5)
Cryselle 28 (Barr)	Ethinyl estradiol (30)	Norgestrel (0.3)
Demulen 1/35 21, 28 (Pfizer)	Ethinyl estradiol (35)	Ethynodiol diacetate (1)
Demulen 1/50 21, 28 (Pfizer)	Ethinyl estradiol (50)	Ethynodiol diacetate (1)
Desogen 28 (Organon)	Ethinyl estradiol (30)	Desogestrel (0.15)
Estrostep 28 (Warner-Chilcott)[b]	Ethinyl estradiol (20, 30, 35)	Norethindrone acetate (1)
Junel Fe 1/20, 21, 28 (Barr)	Ethinyl estradiol (20)	Norethindrone acetate (1)
Junel Fe 1.5/30 21, 28 (Barr)	Ethinyl estradiol (30)	Norethindrone acetate (1.5)
Kariva 28 (Barr)	Ethinyl estradiol (20, 0, 10)	Desogestrel (0.15)
Lessina 28 (Barr)	Ethinyl estradiol (20)	Levonorgestrel (0.1)
Levlen 28 (Berlex)	Ethinyl estradiol (30)	Levonorgestrel (0.15)
Levlite 28 (Berlex)	Ethinyl estradiol (20)	Levonorgestrel (0.1)
Levora 28 (Watson)	Ethinyl estradiol (30)	Levonorgestrel (0.15)
Loestrin Fe 1.5/30 21, 28 (Warner-Chilcott)	Ethinyl estradiol (30)	Norethindrone acetate (1.5)
Loestrin Fe 1/20 21, 28 (Warner-Chilcott)	Ethinyl estradiol (20)	Norethindrone acetate (1)
Lo/Ovral 21, 28 (Wyeth)	Ethinyl estradiol (30)	Norgestrel (0.3)
Low-Ogestrel 28 (Watson)	Ethinyl estradiol (30)	Norgestrel (0.3)
Microgestin Fe 1/20 21, 28 (Watson)	Ethinyl estradiol (20)	Norethindrone acetate (1)
Microgestin Fe 1.5/30 21, 28 (Watson)	Ethinyl estradiol (30)	Norethindrone acetate (1.5)

TABLE 7
(Continued)

Drug (Manufacturer)	Estrogen (mcg)	Progestin (mg)
Mircette 28 (Organon)	Ethinyl estradiol [20, 0, 10]	Desogestrel (0.15)
Modicon 28 (Ortho-McNeil)	Ethinyl estradiol [35]	Norethindrone (0.5)
MonoNessa 28 (Watson)	Ethinyl estradiol [35]	Norgestimate (0.25)
Necon 1/50 28 (Watson)	Mestranol [50]	Norethindrone (1)
Necon 0.5/35, 28 (Watson)	Ethinyl estradiol [35]	Norethindrone (0.5)
Necon 1/35 28 (Watson)	Ethinyl estradiol [35]	Norethindrone (1)
Nordette 21, 28 (King)	Ethinyl estradiol [30]	Levonorgestrel (0.15)
Nortrel 0.5/35 28 (Barr)	Ethinyl estradiol [35]	Norethindrone (0.5)
Nortrel 1/35 21, 28 (Barr)	Ethinyl estradiol [35]	Norethindrone (1)
Norinyl 1/35 28 (Watson)	Ethinyl estradiol [35]	Norethindrone (1)
Norinyl 1/50 28 (Watson)	Mestranol [50]	Norethindrone (1)
Ogestrel 28 (Watson)	Ethinyl estradiol [50]	Norgestrel (0.5)
Ortho-Cept 28 (Ortho-McNeil)	Ethinyl estradiol [30]	Desogestrel (0.15)
Ortho-Cyclen 28 (Ortho-McNeil)	Ethinyl estradiol [35]	Norgestimate (0.25)
Ortho-Novum 1/35 28 (Ortho-McNeil)	Ethinyl estradiol [35]	Norethindrone (1)
Ortho-Novum 1/50 28 (Ortho-McNeil)	Mestranol [50]	Norethindrone (1)
Ovcon 35 21, 28 (Warner-Chilcott)	Ethinyl estradiol [35]	Norethindrone (0.4)
Ovcon 50 28 (Warner-Chilcott)	Ethinyl estradiol [50]	Norethindrone (1)
Ovral 21, 28 (Wyeth-Ayerst)	Ethinyl estradiol [50]	Norgestrel (0.5)
Portia 28 (Barr)	Ethinyl estradiol [30]	Levonorgestrel (0.15)
Sprintec 28 (Barr)	Ethinyl estradiol [35]	Norgestimate (0.25)
Yasmin 28 (Berlex)	Ethinyl estradiol [30]	Drospirenone (3)
Zovia 1/50E 28 (Watson)	Ethinyl estradiol [50]	Ethynodiol diacetate (1)
Zovia 1/35F 28 (Watson)	Ethinyl estradiol [35]	Ethynodiol diacetate (1)

Multiphasics

Drug	Estrogen (mcg)	Progestin (mg)
Cyclessa 28 (Organon)	Ethinyl estradiol (25)	Desogestrel (0.1, 0.125, 0.15)
Enpresse 28 (Barr)	Ethinyl estradiol (30, 40, 30)	Levonorgestrel (0.05, 0.075, 0.125)
Necon 10/11 21, 28 (Watson)	Ethinyl estradiol (35)	Norethindrone (0.5, 1)
Necon 7/7/7 (Watson)	Ethinyl estradiol (35)	Norethindrone (0.5, 0.75, 1)
Nortrel 7/7/7 28 (Barr)	Ethinyl estradiol (35)	Norethindrone (0.5, 0.75, 1)
Ortho Tri-Cyclen 21, 28 (Ortho-McNeil)[b]	Ethinyl estradiol (25)	Norgestimate (0.18, 0.215, 0.25)
Ortho Tri-Cyclen lo 21, 28 (Ortho-McNeil)	Ethinyl estradiol (35, 35, 35)	Norgestimate (0.18, 0.215, 0.25)
Ortho-Novum 10/11 21 (Ortho-McNeil)	Ethinyl estradiol (35, 35, 35)	Norethindrone (0.5, 1.0)
Ortho-Novum 7/7/7 21 (Ortho-McNeil)	Ethinyl estradiol (35, 35, 35)	Norethindrone (0.5, 0.75, 1.0)
Tri-Levlen 28 (Berlex)	Ethinyl estradiol (30, 40, 30)	Levonorgestrel (0.05, 0.075, 0.125)
Tri-Nessa 28 (Watson)	Ethinyl estradiol (35)	Norgestimate (0.18, 0.215, 0.25)
Tri-Norinyl 21, 28 (Watson)	Ethinyl estradiol (35, 35, 35)	Norethindrone (0.5, 1.0, 0.5)
Triphasil 21, 28 (Wyeth)	Ethinyl estradiol (30, 40, 30)	Levonorgestrel (0.05, 0.075, 0.125)
Tri-Sprintec (Barr)	Ethinyl estradiol (35)	Norgestimate (0.18, 0.215, 0.25)
Trivora-28 (Watson)	Ethinyl estradiol (30, 40, 30)	Levonorgestrel (0.05, 0.075, 0.125)
Velivet (Barr)	Ethinyl estradiol (25)	Desogestrel (0.1, 0.125, 0.15)

TABLE 7
(Continued)

Progestin Only

Drug	Estrogen (mcg)	Progestin (mg)
Camila (Barr)	None	Norethindrone (0.35)
Errin (Barr)	None	Norethindrone (0.35)
Jolivette (Watson)	None	Norethindrone (0.35)
Micronor (Ortho-McNeil)	None	Norethindrone (0.35)
Nor-QD (Watson)	None	Norethindrone (0.35)
Nora-BE 28 (Ortho-McNeil)	None	Norethindrone (0.35)
Ovrette (Wyeth-Ayerst)	None	Norgestrel (0.075)

Extended-Cycle Combination

Drug		
Seasonale (Duramed)	Ethinyl estradiol (30)	Levonorgestrel (0.15)

Based in part on data published in the *Medical Letter* Volume 2 (Issue 24) August 2004.

[a]The designations 21 and 28 refer to number of days in regimen available.

[b]Also approved for acne.

TABLE 8
Some Common Oral Potassium Supplements

Brand Name	Salt	Form	mEq Potassium/ Dosing Unit
Glu-K	Gluconate	Tablet	2 mEq/tablet
Kaochlor 10%	KCl	Liquid	20 mEq/15 mL
Kaochlor S-F 10% (sugar-free)	KCl	Liquid	20 mEq/15 mL
Kaochlor Eff	Bicarbonate/ KCl/citrate	Effervescent tablet	20 mEq/tablet
Kaon elixir	Gluconate	Liquid	20 mEq/15 mL
Kaon	Gluconate	Tablet	5 mEq/tablet
Kaon-Cl	KCl	Tablet, SR	6.67 mEq/tablet
Kaon-Cl 20%	KCl	Liquid	40 mEq/15 mL
KayCiel	KCl	Liquid	20 mEq/15 mL
K-Lor	KCl	Powder	15 or 20 mEq/packet
Klorvess	Bicarbonate/ KCl	Liquid	20 mEq/15 mL
Klotrix	KCl	Tablet, SR	10 mEq/tablet
K-Lyte	Bicarbonate/ citrate	Effervescent tablet	25 mEq/tablet
K-Tab	KCl	Tablet, SR	10 mEq/tablet
Micro-K	KCl	Capsule, SR	8 mEq/capsule
Slow-K	KCl	Tablet, SR	8 mEq/tablet
Tri-K	Acetate/bicar- bonate and citrate	Liquid	45 mEq/15 mL
Twin-K	Citrate/gluconate	Liquid	20 mEq/5 mL

SR = sustained release.

TABLE 9
Tetanus Prophylaxis

History of Absorbed Tetanus Toxoid Immunization	Clean, Minor Wounds		All Other Wounds[a]	
	Td[b]	TIG[c]	Td[d]	TIG[c]
Unknown or <3 doses	Yes	No	Yes	Yes
=3 doses	No[e]	No	No[f]	No

[a]Such as, but not limited to, wounds contaminated with dirt, feces, soil, saliva, etc; puncture wounds; avulsions and wounds resulting from missiles, crushing, burns, and frostbite.

[b]Td = tetanus-diphtheria toxoid (adult type), 0.5 mL IM.
  • For children <7 y, DPT (DT, if pertussis vaccine is contraindicated) is preferred to tetanus toxoid alone.
  • For persons >7 y, Td is preferred to tetanus toxoid alone.
  • DT = diphtheria-tetanus toxoid (pediatric), used for those who cannot receive pertussis.

[c]TIG = tetanus immune globulin, 250 U IM.

[d]If only 3 doses of fluid toxoid have been received, then a fourth dose of toxoid, preferably an absorbed toxoid, should be given.

[e]Yes, if >10 y since last dose.

[f]Yes, if >5 y since last dose.

Source: Based on guidelines from the Centers for Disease Control and Prevention and reported in *MMWR.*

TABLE 10
Oral Anticoagulant Standards of Practice

Thromboembolic Disorder	INR	Duration
Deep Venous Thrombosis & Pulmonary Embolism		
Treatment single episode		
Transient risk factor	2–3	3 mo
Idiopathic	2–3	6–12 mo
Recurrent systemic embolism	2–3	Indefinite
Prevention of Systemic Embolism		
Atrial fibrillation (AF)[a]	2–3	Indefinite
AF: cardioversion	2–3	3 wk prior; 4 wk post sinus rhythm
Valvular heart disease	2–3	Indefinite
Cardiomyopathy	2–3	Indefinite
Acute Myocardial Infarction		
High risk patients[c]	2–3 + low dose aspirin	3 mo
Prosthetic Valves		
Tissue heart valves	2–3	3 mo
Bileaflet mechanical valves in aortic position	2–3	2–3 mo Indefinite
Other mechanical prosthetic valves[b]	2.5–3.5	Indefinite

[a]With high-risk factors or multiple moderate risk factors.

[b]May add aspirin 81 mg to warfarin in patients with caged ball or caged disk valves or with additional risk factors.

[c]Large anterior MI, significant heart failure, intracardiac thrombus, and/or history of thromboembolic event.

[d]INR = international normalized ratio.

Source: Based on data published in *Chest* 2004 Sep; 126 (Suppl): 163S–696S.

TABLE 11
Serotonin 5-HT₁ Receptor Agonists

Drug	Initial Dose	Repeat Dose	Max. Dose/24h	Supplied
Almotriptan (Axert)	6.25 or 12.5 mg PO	× 1 in 2 h	25 mg	Tabs 6.25, 12.5 mg
Frovatriptan (Frova)	2.5 mg PO	in 2 h	7.5 mg	Tabs 2.5 mg
Naratriptan (Amerge)	1 or 2.5 mg PO[a]	in 4 h	5 mg	Tabs 1, 2.5 mg
Rizatriptan (Maxalt)	5 or 10 mg PO[b]	in 2 h	30 mg	Tabs 5, 10 mg; Disintegrating tabs 5, 10 mg
Sumatriptan (Imitrex)	25, 50, or 100 mg PO	in 2 h	200 mg	Tabs 25, 50 mg
	5–20 mg intranasally	in 2 h	40 mg	Nasal spray 5, 20 mg
	6 mg SQ	in 1 h	12 mg	Inj 12 mg/mL
Zolmitriptan (Zomig)	2.5 or 5 mg PO	in 2 h	10 mg	Tabs 2.5, 5 mg

Precautions/contraindications: [C, M]: ischemic heart disease, coronary artery vasospasm, Prinzmetal's angina, uncontrolled HTN, hemiplegic or basilar migraine, ergots, use of another serotonin agonist within 24 h, use with MAOI. Side effects: dizziness, somnolence, paresthesias, nausea, flushing, dry mouth, coronary vasospasm, chest tightness, HTN, GI upset.

[a]Reduce dose in mild renal and hepatic insufficiency (2.5 mg/d MAX); contraindicated with severe renal (CrCl <15 mL/min) or hepatic impairment.

[b]Initiate therapy at 5 mg PO (15 mg/d max) in patients receiving propranolol.

320

TABLE 12
Antiarrhythmics: Vaughn Williams Classification

Class I: Sodium Channel Blockade

A. **Class Ia:** Lengthens duration of action potential ($\uparrow$ the refractory period in atrial and ventricular muscle, in SA and AV conduction systems, and Purkinje fibers)
　1. Amiodarone (also class II, III, IV)
　2. Disopyramide (Norpace)
　3. Imipramine (MAO inhibitor)
　4. Procainamide (Pronestyl)
　5. Quinidine

B. **Class Ib:** No effect on action potential
　1. Lidocaine (Xylocaine)
　2. Mexiletine (Mexitil)
　3. Phenytoin (Dilantin)
　4. Tocainide (Tonocard)

C. **Class Ic:** Greater sodium current depression (blocks the fast inward Na^+ current in heart muscle and Purkinje fibers, and slows the rate of $\uparrow$ of phase 0 of the action potential)
　1. Flecainide (Tambocor)
　2. Propafenone

Class II: Beta blocker

D. Amiodarone (also class Ia, III, IV)
E. Esmolol (Brevibloc)
F. Sotalol (also class III)

Class III: Prolong refractory period via action potential

G. Amiodarone (also class Ia, II, IV)
H. Sotalol

Class IV: Calcium channel blocker

I. Amiodarone (also class Ia, II, III)
J. Diltiazem (Cardizem)
K. Verapamil (Calan)

TABLE 13
Cytochrome P-450 Isoenzymes and the Drugs They Metabolize,
Inhibit, and Induce^a

CYP1A2

Substrates:	Acetaminophen, caffeine, clozapine, imipramine, theophylline, propranolol
Inhibitors:	Most fluoroquinolone antibiotics, fluvoxamine, cimetidine
Inducer:	Tobacco smoking, charcoal-broiled foods, cruciferous vegetables, omeprazole

---

CYP2C9

Substrates:	Most NSAIDs (including COX-2), warfarin, phenytoin
Inhibitors:	Fluconazole
Inducer:	Barbiturates, rifampin

CYP2C19

Substrates:	Diazepam, lansoprazole, omeprazole, phenytoin, pantoprazole
Inhibitors:	Omeprazole, isoniazid, ketoconazole
Inducer:	Barbiturates, rifampin

CYP206

Substrates:	Most β-blockers, codeine, clomipramine, clozapine, codeine, encainide, flecainide, fluoxetine, haloperidol, hydrocodone, 4-methoxy-amphetamine, metoprolol, mexiletine, oxycodone, paroxetine, propafenone, propoxyphene, risperidone, selegiline (deprenyl), thioridazine, most tricyclic antidepressants, timolol
Inhibitors:	Fluoxetine, haloperidol, paroxetine, quinidine
Inducer:	Unknown

CYP3A

Substrates:	**Anticholinergics:** Darifenacin, oxybutynin, solifenacin, tolterodine
	Benzodiazepines: Alprazolam, midazolam, triazolam
	Ca channel blockers: Diltiazem, felodipine, nimodipine, nifedipine, nisoldipine, verapamil

(continued)

TABLE 13 (continued)
Cytochrome P-450 Isoenzymes and the Drugs They Metabolize, Inhibit, and Induce[a]

	Chemotherapy: Cyclophosphamide, erlotinib, ifosfamide, paclitaxel, tamoxifen, vinblastine, vincristine
	HIV protease inhibitors: Amprenavir, atazanavir, indinavir, nelfinavir, ritonavir, saquinavir
	HMG-CoA reductase inhibitors: Atorvastatin, lovastatin, simvastatin
	Immunosuppressive agents: Cyclosporine, tacrolimus
	Macrolide-type antibiotics: Clarithromycin, erythromycin, telithromycin, troleandomycin
	Opioids: Alfentanil, cocaine, fentanyl, sufentanil
	Steroids: Budesonide, cortisol, 17-β-estradiol, progesterone
	Others: Acetaminophen, amiodarone, carbamazepine, delavirdine, efavirenz, nevirapine, quinidine, repaglinide, sildenafil, tadalafil, trazodone, vardenafil
Inhibitors:	Amiodarone, amprenavir, atazanavir, ciprofloxacin, cisapride, clarithromycin, diltiazem, erythromycin, fluconazole, fluvoxamine, grapefruit juice (in high ingestion), indinavir, itraconazole, ketoconazole, nefazodone, nelfinavir, norfloxacin, ritonavir, telithromycin, troleandomycin, verapamil, voriconazole
Inducer:	Carbamazepine, efavirenz, glucocorticoids, macrolide antibiotics, nevirapine, phenytoin, phenobarbital, rifabutin, rifapentine, rifampin, St. John's wort

[a]Increased or decreased (primarily hepatic cytochrome P-450) metabolism of medications may influence the effectiveness of drugs or result in significant drug-drug interactions. Understanding the common cytochrome P-450 isoforms (eg, CYP2C9, CYP2D9, CYP2C19, CYP3A4) and common drugs that are metabolized by (aka "substrates"), inhibit, or induce activity of the isoform helps minimize significant drug interactions. CYP3A is involved in the metabolism of >50% of drugs metabolized by the liver.

Based on data from Katzung B (ed): *Basic and Clinical Pharmacology,* 9th ed. McGraw-Hill, New York, 2004; *The Medical Letter,* Volume 47, July 4, 2004; http://www.fda.gov/cder/drug/drugreactions (accessed September 16, 2005).

TABLE 14
Serotonin syndrome as a result of combined use of selective serotonin reuptake inhibitors (SSRI) and triptans

Serotonin syndrome is a life-threatening condition that can develop when SSRIs and 5-hydroxytryptamine receptor agonists (triptans) are used together. Serotonin syndrome may be more likely to occur when starting or increasing the dose of an SSRI or a triptan.

Signs and symptoms of serotonin syndrome include the following:

restlessness	fast heartbeat
diarrhea	vomiting
hallucinations	increased body temperature
coma	fast changes in blood pressure
loss of coordination	overactive reflexes
nausea	

TABLE 15
Composition of selected multivitamins and multivitamins with mineral and trace element supplements

| | Vitamins | | | | | | | | | | | | |
| | Fat Soluble | | | | Water Soluble | | | | | | | | |
	A	D	E	K	C	B_1	B_2	B_3	B_6	Folate	B_{12}	Biotin	B_5
Centrum	70	100	100	31	100	100	100	100	100	100	100	10	100
Centrum Performance	70	100	200	31	200	300	300	200	300	100	300	13	100
Centrum Silver	70	100	150	13	100	100	100	100	150	100	417	10	100
NatureMade Multi	60	100	167	31	200	100	100	100	100	100	100	10	100
NatureMade Multi Complete	60	100	100	NA	100	100	100	100	100	100	100	NA	100
NatureMade Multi Daily													
NatureMade Multi Max	60	100	500	50	500	3333	2941	250	2500	100	833	17	500
NatureMade Multi 50+	100	100	200	13	200	200	200	100	200	100	417	10	100
One-A-Day 50 Plus	50	100	110	25	200	300	200	100	300	100	417	10	150
One-A-Day Essential	100	100	100	NA	100	100	100	100	100	100	100	NA	100

TABLE 15
Composition of selected multivitamins and multivitamins with mineral and trace element supplements (continued)

| | Vitamins | | | | | | | | | | | | |
| | Fat Soluble | | | | Water Soluble | | | | | | | | |
	A	D	E	K	C	B$_1$	B$_2$	B$_3$	B$_6$	Folate	B$_{12}$	Biotin	B$_5$
One-A-Day Maximum	50	100	100	31	100	100	100	100	100	100	100	10	100
Therapeutic Vitamin	100	100	100	NA	150	200	200	100	150	100	150	10	100
Theragran-M Advanced Formula High Potency	100	100	200	35	150	200	200	100	300	100	200	10	100
Theragran-M Premier High Potency	70	100	200	31	200	267	235	125	200	100	150	10	100
Theragran-M Premier 50 Plus High Potency	70	100	200	13	125	200	176	125	300	100	500	12	150

	Minerals								Trace Elements				Other
	Ca	P	Mg	Fe	Zn	I	Se	K	Mn	Cu	Cr	Mo	
Therapeutic Vitamin + Minerals Enhanced	100	100	200	NA	150	200	200	100	300	100	200	10	100
Unicap M	100	100	50	100	100	100	100	100	100	100	100	NA	100
Unicap Senior	100	50	10	100	100	80	82	80	110	100	50	NA	100
Unicap T	100	100	100	NA	833	667	588	500	300	100	300	NA	250
Centrum	16	11	25	100	100	100	29	2	100	100	100	100	
Centrum Performance	10	5	10	100	100	100	100	2	200	100	100	100	Lycopene
Centrum Silver	20	5	25	NA	100	100	29	2	100	100	125	100	
NatureMade Multi Complete	10	8	25	50	100	100	35	1	100	100	100	33	Ginseng Ginkgo
NatureMade Multi Daily	45	NA	NA	100	100	NA	NA	NA	NA	NA	NA	NA	Lycopene
NatureMade Multi Max	10	4	6	50	100	100	100	1	100	100	100	NA	Lutein

TABLE 15
Composition of selected multivitamins and multivitamins with mineral and trace element supplements (continued)

	Minerals						Trace Elements						
	Ca	P	Mg	Fe	Zn	I	Se	K	Mn	Cu	Cr	Mo	Other
NatureMade Multi 50+	20	5	25		100	100	71	2	100	100	100	33	
One-A-Day 50 Plus	12	NA	25	NA	150	100	150	1	200	100	150	120	Lutein
One-A-Day Essential	NA	NA	NA	NA	NA	NA	NA	NA	NA	NA	NA	NA	
One-A-Day Maximum	16	11	25	100	100	100	29	2	175	100	54	213	
Therapeutic 7 Vitamin	NA	NA	NA	NA	NA	NA	NA	NA	NA	NA	NA		
Theragran-M Advanced Formula High Potency	4	3	26	50	100	100	100	1	100	100	42	100	
Theragran-M Premier High Potency	17	11	25	100	100	100	286	2	100	175	100	107	Lutein
Theragran-M Premier 50 Plus High Potency	20	5	25	0	113	100	286	2	175	100	125	100	Lutein

Therapeutic Vitamin + Minerals Enhanced	4	3	25		100	100	<1	100	100	42	100
Unicap M	6	5	NA	100	100	100	NA	50	100	NA	NA
Unicap Senior	10	8	8	56	100	100	NA	50	100	NA	NA
Unicap T	NA	NA	NA	100	100	14	<1	50	100	NA	NA

Common multivitamins available without a prescription are listed. Most chain stores have generic versions of many of the multivitamin supplements listed above; thus, specific generic brands are not listed.[1] Many specialty vitamin combinations are available, but not included in this list. (Examples are B vitamins plus C, supplements for a specific condition or organ, pediatric and infant formulations, and prenatal vitamins.)

Values are listed as percentages of the Daily Value based on Recommended Dietary Allowances of vitamins and minerals based on Dietary Reference Intakes (Food and Nutrition Board, Institute of Medicine, National Academy of Science).

[1] Common generic brands (when other than the store name itself) are: Osco Drug CentraVite (Albertson's); Spectravite (CVS); Kirkland Signature Daily Multivitamin (Costco); Whole Source, PharmAssure (Rite Aid); CentraVite (Safeway); Member's Mark (Sam's Club); Vitasmart (Kmart); Century (Target); A thru Z Select, Super Aytinal, Ultra Choice (Walgreens) Equate Complete or Spring Valley Sentury-Vite (Wal-Mart).

Vitamins: B1 = Thiamine; B2 = Riboflavin; B3 = Niacin; B5 = Pantothenic Acid; B6 = Pyridoxine; B12 = Cyanocobalamin. **Elements:** Ca = calcium; Cr = chromium; Cu = copper; Fe = iron; Fl = fluoride; I = iodine; K = potassium; Mg = magnesium; Mn = manganese; Mo = Molybdenum; P = phosphorus; Se = selenium; Zn = zinc; NA = not applicable or not available.

Index

NOTE: Page numbers followed by t indicate tables.

331

CONTENTS

iii

1 2 3 4 5 6 7 8 9 0   TRA/TRA   0 9 8 7

ISBN: 13: 978-0-07-149246-1
     10: 0-07-149246-1
ISSN: 1550-2554

Notice

Medicine is an ever-changing science. As new research and clinical experience broaden our knowledge, changes in treatment and drug therapy are required. The authors and the publisher of this work have checked with sources believed to be reliable in their efforts to provide information that is complete and generally in accord with the standards accepted at the time of publication. However, in view of the possibility of human error or changes in medical sciences, neither the authors nor the publisher nor any other party who has been involved in the preparation or publication of this work warrants that the information contained herein is in every respect accurate or complete, and they disclaim all responsibility for any errors or omissions or for the results obtained from use of the information contained in this work. Readers are encouraged to confirm the information contained herein with other sources. For example and in particular, readers are advised to check the product information sheet included in the package of each drug they plan to administer to be certain that the information contained in this work is accurate and that changes have not been made in the recommended dose or in the contraindications for administration. This recommendation is of particular importance in connection with new or infrequently used drugs.

The book was set in Times Roman by Pine Tree Composition, Inc.
The editors were Quincy McDonald and Karen Davis.
The senior production supervisor was Sherri Souffrance.
Project management was provided by Pine Tree Composition, Inc.
The text designer was Marsha Cohen/Parallelogram Graphics.
The indexer was Katherine Pitcoff.
Transcontinental Gagne was printer and binder.

This book is printed on acid-free paper.

NURS
DRUG
2008

EDITOR
Judith A. Barberio, PhD, APN,C, ANP, FNP, GNP

CONSULTING EDITOR
Leonard G. Gomella, MD, FACS

ASSOCIATE EDITORS
Steven A. Haist, MD, MS, FACP
Aimee Gelhot Adams, PharmD
Kelly M. Smith, PharmD

MEDICAL PUBLISHING DIVISION
New York   Chicago   San Francisco   Lisbon
London   Madrid   Mexico City   Milan   New Delhi
San Juan   Seoul   Singapore   Sydney   Toronto